W9-CLU-021

PLURAL+PLUS

COMPANION WEBSITE

Purchase of *Anatomy & Physiology for Speech, Language, and Hearing, Sixth Edition* comes with access to supplementary student and instructor materials on a PluralPlus companion website.

The companion website is located at:
https://www.pluralpublishing.com/publication/apslh6e

STUDENTS:

To access the **student** materials, you must register on the companion website and log in using the access code below.*

Access Code: APSLH6E-NRF76W

INSTRUCTORS:

To access the **instructor** materials, you must contact Plural Publishing, Inc. to be verified as an instructor and receive your access code.

Email: information@pluralpublishing.com
Tel: 866-758-7251 (toll free) or 858-492-1555

 ANAQUEST LESSON ▶

Look for this icon throughout the text indicating there is a related lesson in the ANAQUEST study software on the companion website.

Note for students: If you have purchased this textbook used or have rented it, your access code will not work if it was already redeemed by the original buyer of the book. Plural Publishing does not offer replacement access codes for used or rented textbooks.

Anatomy & Physiology

for Speech, Language, and Hearing

SIXTH EDITION

Anatomy & Physiology

for Speech, Language, and Hearing

SIXTH EDITION

J. Anthony Seikel, PhD
David G. Drumright, BS
Daniel J. Hudock, PhD, CCC-SLP

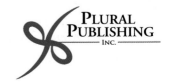

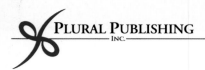

5521 Ruffin Road
San Diego, CA 92123

e-mail: information@pluralpublishing.com
Website: https://www.pluralpublishing.com

Copyright © 2021 by Plural Publishing, Inc.

Typeset in 12/14 Adobe Garamond Pro by Flanagan's Publishing Services, Inc.
Printed in China by Regent Publishing Services Ltd.
25 24 23 22   5 6 7 8

All rights, including that of translation, reserved. No part of this publication may be reproduced, stored in a retrieval system, or transmitted in any form or by any means, electronic, mechanical, recording, or otherwise, including photocopying, recording, taping, Web distribution, or information storage and retrieval systems without the prior written consent of the publisher.

Photography by Sarah Moore, Susan Duncan, Eric Gordon, and Brian Smith.

For permission to use material from this text, contact us by
Telephone: (866) 758-7251
Fax: (888) 758-7255
e-mail: permissions@pluralpublishing.com

Every attempt has been made to contact the copyright holders for material originally printed in another source. If any have been inadvertently overlooked, the publisher will gladly make the necessary arrangements at the first opportunity.

Library of Congress Cataloging-in-Publication Data:

Names: Seikel, John A., author. | Drumright, David G., author. | Hudock, Daniel J., author.
Title: Anatomy & physiology for speech, language, and hearing / J. Anthony Seikel, David G. Drumright, Daniel J. Hudock.
Other titles: Anatomy and physiology for speech, language, and hearing
Description: Sixth edition. | San Diego, CA : Plural Publishing, [2020] | Includes bibliographical references and index.
Identifiers: LCCN 2019029690 | ISBN 9781635502794 (hardcover) | ISBN 1635502799 (hardcover) | ISBN 9781635503005 (ebook)
Subjects: MESH: Speech—physiology | Language | Hearing—physiology | Nervous System—anatomy & histology | Respiratory System—anatomy & histology | Respiratory Physiological Phenomena
Classification: LCC QP306 | NLM WV 501 | DDC 612.7/8—dc23
LC record available at https://lccn.loc.gov/2019029690

Contents

Chapter 7 Physiology of Articulation and Resonation 417

Chapter 8 Physiology of Mastication and Deglutition 455

Chapter 9   Anatomy of Hearing   515

Chapter 12   Neurophysiology   745

Appendix A   Anatomical Terms   807

Appendix B   Useful Combining Forms   809

Preface

Anatomy & Physiology for Speech, Language, and Hearing, Sixth Edition, provides a sequential tour of the anatomy and physiology associated with speech, language, and hearing. We aspire to keep the content alive for students of today by providing not only basic anatomy and physiology, but also by forging the relationship between the structures and functions and the dysfunction that occurs when the systems fail. We know that students in audiology and speech-language pathology have their future clients in mind as they read this content, and we hope that by integrating information about pathology we can bring anatomy to life and to relevancy for you.

We have designed this text and the support materials to serve the upper division undergraduate or graduate student in the fields of speech-language pathology and audiology, and hope that it can serve you as a reference for your professional life as well. We aspire for it to be a learning tool and resource for both the developing and the accomplished clinician. We, the authors of this text, are first and foremost teachers ourselves. We are committed to the students within our professions and to the instructors who have made it their life work to teach them. Learning is a lifelong process, and our goal is to give instructors the tools to start students on that lifelong professional path and to inspire learning throughout your life. We know that learning is not a spectator sport because we continue to engage ourselves as learners. Our goal is to make the text and its ancillary materials as useful to 21st-century students as possible. This new edition not only provides students with great interactive study tools in the revised and renamed ANAQUEST study software, but also makes available a wealth of student and instructor resources to facilitate learning. We want you to be the best clinician and scientist you can be and sincerely hope that these materials move you along the path of your chosen career.

Organization

The text is organized around the five "classic" systems of speech and hearing: the respiratory, phonatory, articulatory/resonatory, nervous, and auditory systems. The respiratory system (involving the lungs) provides the "energy source" for speech, whereas the phonatory system (involving the larynx) provides voicing. The articulatory/resonatory system modifies the acoustic source provided by voicing (or other gestures) to produce the sounds we acknowledge as speech. The articulatory system is responsible for the mastication (chewing) and deglutition (swallowing) function, an increasingly important area within the field of speech-language pathology. The nervous system lets us control musculature, receive information, and make sense of the information. Finally, the auditory mechanism processes speech and nonspeech acoustic signals received by the listener who is trying to make sense of her or his world.

There are few areas of study where the potential for overwhelming detail is greater than in the disciplines of anatomy and physiology. Our desire with this text and the accompanying software lessons is to provide a stable foundation upon which detail may be learned. In the text, we provide you with an introductory section that sets the stage for the detail to follow, and we bring you back to a more global picture with summaries. We have also provided derivations of words to help you remember technical terms.

New to the Sixth Edition

This new edition of *Anatomy & Physiology for Speech, Language, and Hearing, Sixth Edition* includes many exciting enhancements:

- Revised and updated physiology of swallowing includes discussion of orofacial-myofunctional disorders and other swallowing dysfunction arising from physical etiologies.
- An introduction to the effects of pathology on communication is included within each of the physical systems of communication.
- Many new photographs of specimens have been added, with a focus on a clear and accurate understanding of the classical framework of the speech, language, and hearing systems.
- *Clinical Notes* boxes link anatomy and physiology with disorders seen by speech-language pathologists and audiologists to provide real-world applications for students.
- The ANAQUEST study software is Internet-based and accessible on the PluralPlus companion website that comes with the text. ANAQUEST provides on-the-go learning, with animation lessons, simulations, and updates to content. The software now includes a set of video lab experiences narrated by new contributor Katrina Rhett, an anatomist and lecturer in the Department of Biological Sciences at Idaho State University. We have added three-dimensional views with animations that explore the important processes of hearing, phonation, respiration, swallowing, and more.

See the beginning of the textbook for instructions on how to access the PluralPlus companion website.

The PluralPlus companion website is divided into two areas: one housing materials for the instructor and the other just for students.

For the Instructor

The PluralPlus companion website contains a variety of tools to help instructors successfully prepare lectures and teach within this subject area. This comprehensive package provides something for all instructors, from those teaching anatomy and physiology for the first time to seasoned instructors who want something new. The following materials have been made available just for instructors:

- An *Instructor's Manual* containing materials and suggested activities for the lecture and lab guides to facilitate learning outside of the classroom.
- A *test bank* with approximately 1,000 questions and answers, for use in instructor-created quizzes and tests.
- *PowerPoint lecture slides* for each chapter to use as in-class lecture material and as handouts for students.
- A version of the ANAQUEST study software created for upload to a Learning Management System (LMS).

For the Student

ANAQUEST study software comes with purchase of the textbook and can be accessed on the PluralPlus companion website. ANAQUEST software is your true partner in learning. The available labs give you the opportunity to examine structures and functions of the speech mechanism in an interactive digital environment. The ANAQUEST software is keyed to the text, reinforcing identification of the structures presented during lecture, but more importantly illustrating the function of those structures. An icon in the margin of the text indicates that you'll find related lessons and video labs in ANAQUEST, where you can examine speech physiology through the interactive manipulation of the structures under study, and learn the relationship of the body parts and how they function together. See the beginning of the textbook for the website URL and your access code.

J. Anthony Seikel
David G. Drumright
Daniel J. Hudock

About the Authors

J. Anthony (Tony) Seikel, PhD, is emeritus faculty at Idaho State University, where he taught graduate and undergraduate coursework in neuroanatomy and neuropathology over the course of his career in Communication Sciences and Disorders. He is coauthor of numerous chapters, books, and research publications in the fields of speech-language pathology and audiology. His current research is examining the relationship between orofacial myofunctional disorders and oropharyngeal dysphagia. Dr. Seikel is also coauthor of *Neuroanatomy & Neurophysiology for Speech and Hearing Sciences,* also published by Plural Publishing in 2018.

David G. Drumright, BS, grew up in Oklahoma and Kansas, taught electronics at DeVry for several years, then spent 20 years as a technician in acoustics and speech research. He developed many programs and devices for analysis and instruction in acoustics and speech/hearing. He has been semiretired since 2002, working on graphics and programming for courseware. He is also coauthor of *Neuroanatomy & Neurophysiology for Speech and Hearing Sciences,* published by Plural Publishing in 2018.

Daniel J. Hudock, PhD, CCC-SLP, is an Associate Professor of Communication Sciences and Disorders at Idaho State University who has taught courses on Anatomy & Physiology of the Speech and Hearing Mechanisms and Speech & Hearing Science for over a decade. He has published more than 30 articles and has given over 100 presentations. In his TEDx Talk (https://bit .ly/2oAYeKC) entitled "Please Let Me Finish My Sentence," he presents about his experience living with a stutter. Dr. Hudock is also the founding director of the Northwest Center for Fluency Disorders that offers an intensive interprofessional stuttering clinic with speech language pathologists collaborating with counselors and clinical psychologists through an Acceptance and Commitment Therapy (ACT) informed framework in the treatment of adolescent and adult stuttering, which is his main area of research.

About the Contributor

Katrina Rhett, MS, is an Assistant Lecturer in the Department of Biological Sciences at Idaho State University where she administers dissection-based and prosection-based human gross anatomy courses. She teaches undergraduate anatomy and physiology lab, graduate anatomy lab for the physical and occupational therapy programs, and advanced medical workshops. Prior to joining the faculty at Idaho State University, she taught undergraduate and medical human gross anatomy courses and conducted research in cardiovascular and muscular research labs at the University of Minnesota.

Acknowledgments

We are deeply indebted to our friends at Plural Publishing who have worked so hard to make this new edition happen. Frankly, we feel that we have returned home after a long time away, because this text began as a "twinkle in the eye" of Dr. Sadanand Singh, then owner of Singular Publishing. We were affiliated with another publisher for many years after, but are excited and relieved to have returned to our home in Plural Publishing, and to the capable and compassionate hands of Angie Singh and Valerie Johns. Angie and Val have had the vision to see this text through to its sixth edition, and we are forever grateful for their support and determination.

We would like to acknowledge the effort that reviewers put into their examination of our material and hope we have done justice to their work. Reviewers are the unsung heroes of textbook preparation. They put in long and often tedious hours, examining our work with an unflinching eye. The deadlines that they faced in reviewing the material for this sixth edition were daunting, and yet they persevered. We are very deeply indebted to them for their careful review and willingness to call our attention to areas that need refinement and improvement. We also are grateful for their keen insight and discernment, and hope that we have in some measure answered their suggestions. This textbook is written, quite literally, on their shoulders.

We also wish to acknowledge all those who have, over the course of the past few years, given us corrections and suggestions for improving the text. Patrick Walden, Mayrose McInerney, Nelson Roy, and Shawn Nissen have provided inspiration to us through their love of teaching. It has been inspiring to be once again in communication with Tanis Tranka and Lyn Russell. There are many other instructors and students with whom we have had the fortune to work and who have provided valuable feedback on the text, and we appreciate every one of you.

To you, our students, please realize that your future clients support your present intention and also will serve as your inspiration as you move through life. As speech-language pathologists and audiologists, we must acknowledge the tremendous debt we owe to the great researchers and teachers who have formed the profession, our colleagues with whom we consult and work, and, always, our clients, who have taught us more than any textbook could.

As authors, we must also acknowledge the source of our inspiration. We have been actively involved in teaching students in speech-language pathology and audiology for some time, and not a semester goes by that we don't realize how very dedicated our students are. There is something special about our field that attracts not just the brightest, but the most compassionate. You, students, keep us as teachers alive and vital. Thank you.

Introduction to the Learner

We continue to be impressed with the complexity and beauty of the systems of human communication. Humans use an extremely complex system for communication, requiring extraordinary coordination and control of an intensely interconnected sensorimotor system. It is our heartfelt desire that the study of the physical system will lead you to an appreciation of the importance of your future work as a speech-language pathologist or audiologist.

We also know that the intensity of your study will work to the benefit of your future clients and that the knowledge you gain through your effort will be applied throughout your career. We appreciate the fact that the study of anatomy is challenging, but we also recognize that the effort you put forth now will provide you with the background for work with the medical community.

A deep understanding of the structure and function of the human body is critical to the individual who is charged with the diagnosis and treatment of speech, language, and hearing disorders. As beginning clinicians, you are already aware of the awesome responsibility you bear in clinical management. It is our firm belief that knowledge of the human body and how it works will provide you with the background you need to make informed and wise decisions. We welcome you on your journey into the world of anatomy.

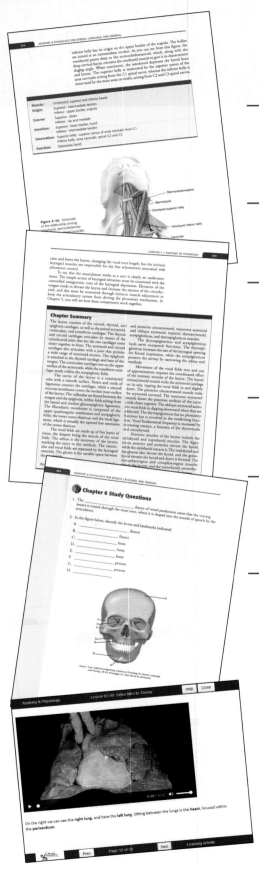

- **"To Summarize" sections** provide a succinct listing of the major topics covered in a chapter or chapter section. These summaries provide a helpful recap of the general areas where you should focus your time while reviewing for examinations.

- **Muscle Tables** describe the origin, course, insertion, innervation, and function of key muscles and muscle groups. Use these tables to stay organized and keep track of the numerous muscles studied in each chapter.

- **Chapter Summaries** provide precise reviews of content. The summary is offset from the running text to make it easily identifiable for quick review.

- **Study Questions and Answers** can be completed after reading a chapter to help you identify areas you may need to reread or focus on while studying. Complete the questions again as you review for a midterm or final examination to help keep the content fresh in your memory.

- A **Bibliography** with a comprehensive list of references at the end of each chapter offers great sources to start your research for a paper or class project.

- **Appendices** include an alphabetical listing of anatomical terms, useful combining forms, and listings of sensors and cranial nerves. You will also find a complete **Glossary** of all key terms found throughout the text.

- The **ANAQUEST** software labs and videos are self-paced, with frequent quizzes to help you examine the effectiveness of your study habits. If you spend two or three half-hour sessions per week with the ANAQUEST software, you will get the greatest benefit from your classes and readings. The software will also prove a great refresher in preparing for quizzes and examinations.

The authors wish to dedicate this text to the many clients we have known over our years of practice who have inspired us with their courage and wisdom. We also wish to dedicate this text to the students and faculty in speech and hearing who do the work of helping people with communication and swallowing difficulties. We have been blessed with our associations with you for many decades, and we know that audiologists and speech-language pathologists are compassionate and generous people who dedicate their lives to improving the well-being of others in what we, the authors, consider the most important aspect of life: communication. We thank you, the faculty and students of our fields, for your dedication.

—*JAS, DGD, and DJH*

I also dedicate the text to my four research mentors. Robert McCroskey, my first research mentor, would exclaim "data!" when he saw a printout, gleeful that he could pry some more meaning from observations. John Brandt gave me an "Occam's razor" with which to discern signal from noise, figure from ground. John Ferraro gave me a love of electrophysiological processes (as well as loan of his electrophysiological lab facility!) that has inspired my love of the hearing mechanism throughout my career. Kim Wilcox blessed me with passion for research and a sense of humor that has sustained me throughout my career. To all of these giants, I say "thank you" for the gift.

— *Tony Seikel*

I also dedicate the accompanying software to Professor Merle Phillips, who taught me something about audiology and a lot about life.

—*David Drumright*

I wish to dedicate my contributions to the text to the first author, "Tony," who has been a beloved colleague, mentor, and dear friend over the past several years. Tony's passion for the field, colleagues, teaching, and students knows no bounds as he has tirelessly and compassionately given of himself for the betterment of others. I would also like to dedicate my contributions to this book to the many speech-language pathologists, teachers, professors, students, friends, and family that have supported him along the way. There are no words that can fully express my gratitude and appreciation for the kindness and support shown to me. Thank you.

—*Dan Hudock*

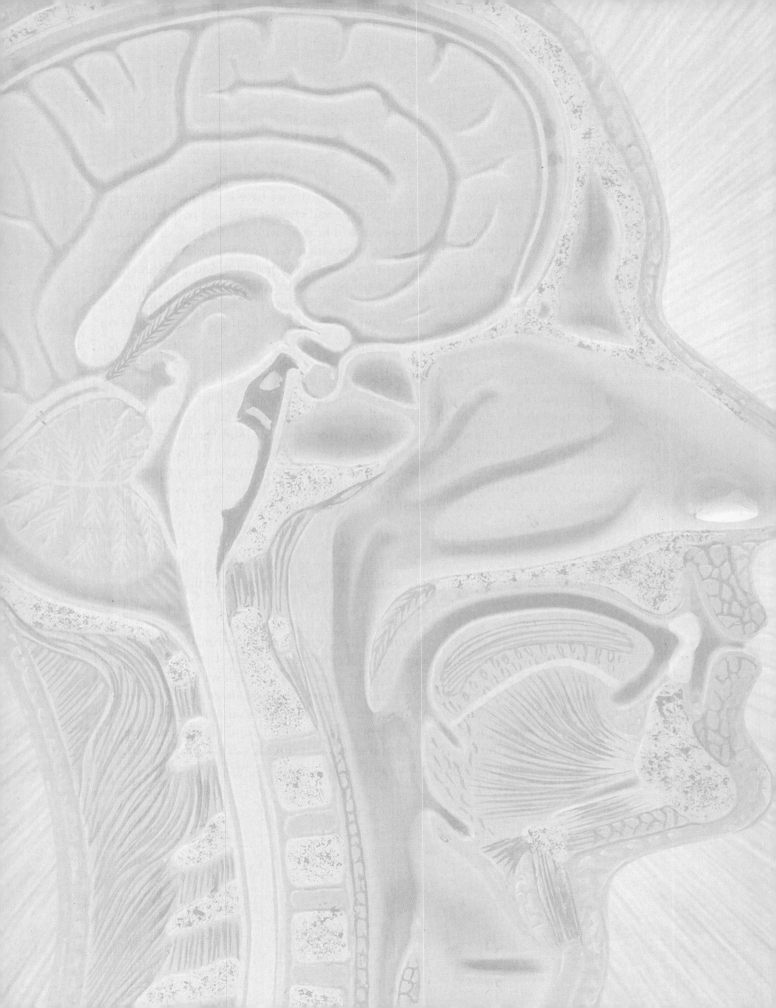

Basic Elements of Anatomy

You are entering into study of the human body that has a long and rich tradition. We are fortunate to have myriad instruments and techniques at our avail for this study, but it has not always been so. You will likely struggle with arcane terminology that seems confusing and strange, and yet if you look closely, you will see what the early anatomists first saw. The amygdala of the brain is a small almond-shaped structure, and *amygdala* means almond. *Lentiform* literally means lens-shaped, and the lentiform nucleus is just that. The fact that the terminology remains in our lexicon indicates the accuracy with which our academic ancestors studied their field, despite extraordinarily limited resources.

This chapter provides you with some basic elements to prepare you for your study of the anatomy and physiology of speech, language, and hearing. We provide a broad picture of the field of anatomy and then introduce you to the basic tissues that make up the human body. Tissues combine to form structures, and those structures combine to form systems. This chapter sets the stage for your understanding of the new and foreign anatomical terminologies.

Anatomy and Physiology

Anatomy refers to the study of the *structure* of an organism. **Physiology** is the study of the *function* of the living organism and its parts, as well as the chemical processes involved. **Applied anatomy** (also known as **clinical anatomy**) involves the application of anatomical study for the diagnosis and treatment of disease and surgical procedures. **Descriptive anatomy** (also known as **systemic anatomy**) is description of individual parts of the body without reference to disease conditions, viewing the body as a composite of systems that function together.

Gross anatomy studies structures that are visible without a microscope, while **microscopic anatomy** examines structures not visible to the unaided eye. **Surface anatomy** (also known as **superficial anatomy**) studies the form and structure of the surface of the body, especially with reference to the organs beneath the surface (Agur & Dalley, 2012; Gilroy, MacPherson, & Ross, 2012; Rohen, Lutjen-Drecoll, & Yokochi, 2010; Standring, 2008).

ANAQUEST LESSON

anatomy: Gr., anatome, **dissection**

dissection: L., dissecare, the process of cutting up

physiology: Gr., physis, nature; and logos, study; function of an organism

applied anatomy or **clinical anatomy:** application of anatomical study for the diagnosis and treatment of disease, particularly as it relates to surgical procedures

descriptive anatomy or **systemic anatomy:** anatomical specialty involving the description of individual parts of the body without reference to disease conditions

gross anatomy: study of the body and its parts as visible without the aid of microscopy

microscopic anatomy: study of the structure of the body by means of microscopy

surface anatomy or **superficial anatomy:** study of the body and its surface markings as related to underlying structures

developmental anatomy: study of anatomy with reference to growth and development from conception to adulthood

pathological anatomy: study of parts of the body with respect to the pathological entity

comparative anatomy: study of homologous structures of different animals

electrophysiological techniques: those techniques that measure the electrical activity of single cells or groups of cells, including muscle and nervous system tissues

cytology: Gr., kytos, cell; logos, study

histology: Gr., histos, web, tissue; logos, study

osteology: Gr., osteon, bone; logos, study

myology: Gr., mys, muscle; logos, study

arthrology: Gr., arthron, joint; logos, study

angiology: Gr., angio, blood vessels; logos, study

neurology: Gr., neuron, sinew, nerve; logos, study

Developmental anatomy deals with the development of the organism from conception (Moore, Persaud, & Torchia, 2013).

When your study examines disease conditions or structural abnormalities, you have entered the domain of **pathological anatomy**. When we make comparisons across species boundaries, we are engaged in **comparative anatomy**.

Examination of physiological processes may entail the use of a range of methods, from simply measuring forces exerted by muscles, to highly refined **electrophysiological techniques** that measure electrical activity of single cells or groups of cells, including muscle and nervous system tissues. For example, audiologists are particularly interested in procedures that measure the electrical activity of the brain caused by auditory stimuli (**evoked auditory potentials**). We rely heavily on descriptive anatomy to guide our understanding of the physical mechanisms of speech and to aid our discussion of its physiology (e.g., Duffy, 2012). Study of pathological anatomy occurs naturally as you enter your clinical process, because many of the acquired conditions speech-language pathologists or audiologists work with arise from pathological changes in structure.

We will need to call on knowledge from related fields to support your study of anatomy and physiology. **Cytology** is the discipline that examines structure and function of cells; **histology** is the microscopic study of cells and tissues. **Osteology** studies structure and function of bones, while **myology** examines muscle form and function. **Arthrology** studies the joints uniting bones, and **angiology** is the study of blood vessels and the lymphatic system. **Neurology** is the study of diseases of the nervous system.

Teratogens

A **teratogen** or teratogenic agent is anything causing teratogenesis, the development of a severely malformed fetus. For an agent to be teratogenic, its effect must occur during prenatal development.

Because the development of the fetus involves the proliferation and differentiation of tissues, the timing of the teratogen is particularly critical. The heart undergoes its most critical period of development from the third embryonic week to the eighth, while the critical period for the palate begins around the fifth week and ends around the 12th week. The critical period for neural development stretches from the third embryonic week until birth. These critical periods for development mark the points at which the developing human is most susceptible to insult. An agent destined to have an effect on the development of an organ or system will have its greatest impact during that critical period.

Many teratogens have been identified, including organic mercury (which causes cerebral palsy, mental retardation, blindness, cerebral atrophy, and seizures), heroin and morphine (causing neonatal convulsions, tremors, and death), alcohol (fetal alcohol syndrome, mental retardation, microcephaly, joint anomalies, and maxillary anomalies), and tobacco (growth retardation), to name just a few.

✅ *To summarize:*

- **Anatomy** is the study of the structure of an organism; **physiology** is the study of function.

- **Descriptive anatomy** relates the individual parts of the body to functional systems.

- **Pathological anatomy** refers to changes in structure as they relate to disease.

- **Gross** and **microscopic anatomy** refer to levels of visibility of structures under study.

- **Developmental anatomy** examines growth and development of an organism.

- **Cytology** and **histology** study cells and tissues, respectively. **Myology** examines muscle form and function.

- **Arthrology** refers to the study of the joint system for bones, while **osteology** is the study of form and function of bones.

- **Neurology** refers to the study of diseases of the nervous system.

Terminology of Anatomy

Terminology allows us to communicate relevant information concerning the location and orientation of various body parts and organs, so clarity of terminology is of the utmost importance in the study of anatomy. Terminology also links us to the historic roots of this field of study. To the budding scholar of Latin or Greek, learning the terms of anatomy is an exciting reminder of our linguistic history. To the rest of us, the terms we are about to discuss may be less easily digested but are nonetheless important.

As you prepare for your study of anatomy, please realize that this body of knowledge is extremely hierarchical. *What you learn today will be the basis for what you learn tomorrow.* Not only are the terms the bedrock for understanding anatomical structures, but also mastery of their usage will let you gain the maximum benefit from new material presented.

Terms of Orientation

In the **anatomical position**, the body is erect, and the palms, arms, and hands face forward, as shown in Figure 1–1A. Terms of direction assume this position. The body and brain (and many other structures) are seen to have axes (plural of axis) or midlines from which other structures arise. The **axial skeleton** is the head and trunk, with the spinal column being the axis, while the **appendicular skeleton** includes the upper and lower limbs. The **neuraxis**, or the axis of the brain, is slightly less straightforward due to morphological changes of the brain during development. The embryonic nervous system is essentially tubular, but as the cerebral cortex develops, a

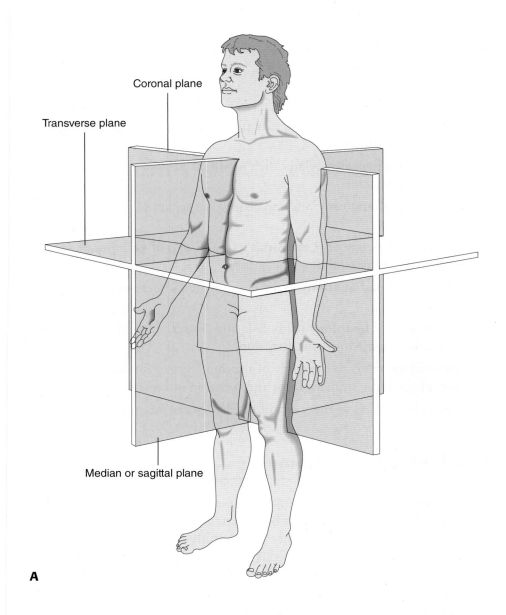

Coronal plane

Transverse plane

Median or sagittal plane

A

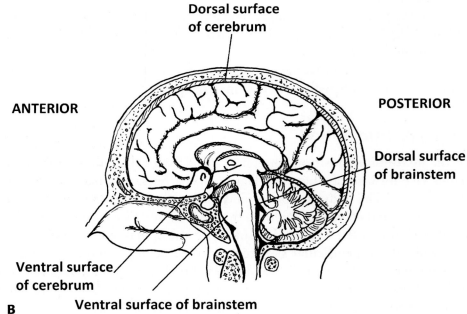

Dorsal surface of cerebrum

ANTERIOR

POSTERIOR

Dorsal surface of brainstem

Ventral surface of cerebrum

Ventral surface of brainstem

B

Figure 1–1. A. Terms and planes of orientation. *Source:* From Seikel/Drumright/ King. *Anatomy & Physiology for Speech, Language, and Hearing, 5th Ed.* ©Cengage, Inc. Reproduced by permission. **B.** The neuraxis of the brain. *Source:* From *Neuroanatomy & Neurophysiology for Speech, Language and Hearing* by Seikel, J. A., Konstantopoulos, K. & Drumright, D. G. Copyright © 2020 Plural Publishing, Inc. *continues*

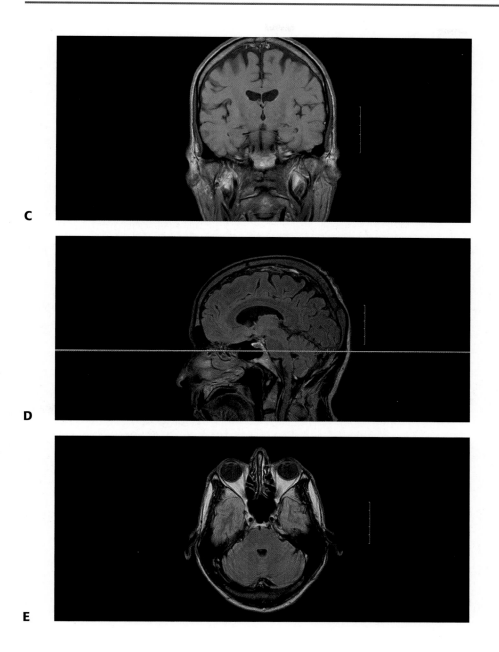

C

D

E

Figure 1–1. *continued*
C. Coronal section through the brain and skull using magnetic resonance imaging (MRI). **D.** Sagittal or median section through the brain and skull using MRI. **E.** Transverse section through the brain and skull using MRI. *Source:* From Seikel/Drumright/ King. *Anatomy & Physiology for Speech, Language, and Hearing, 5th Ed.* ©Cengage, Inc. Reproduced by permission. *continues*

flexure occurs and the telencephalon (the region that will become the cerebrum) folds forward. As a result, the neuraxis assumes a T-formation (Moore et al., 2013). The spinal cord and brain stem have dorsal (back) and ventral (front) surfaces corresponding to those of the surface of the body. Because the cerebrum folds forward, the dorsal surface is also the superior surface, and the ventral surface is the inferior surface. Most anatomists avoid this confusing state by referring to the ventral and dorsal surfaces of the embryonic brain as inferior and superior surfaces, respectively (Figure 1–1G).

Some terms are related to the physical orientation of the body (such as *vertical* or *horizontal*). Other terms (such as *frontal*, *coronal*, and *longitudinal*) refer to planes or axes of the body and are therefore insensitive to the position of the body.

Those of you who play cards may remember "ante up," meaning "put your money up front!" You may remember the term antebellum, meaning "before the war."

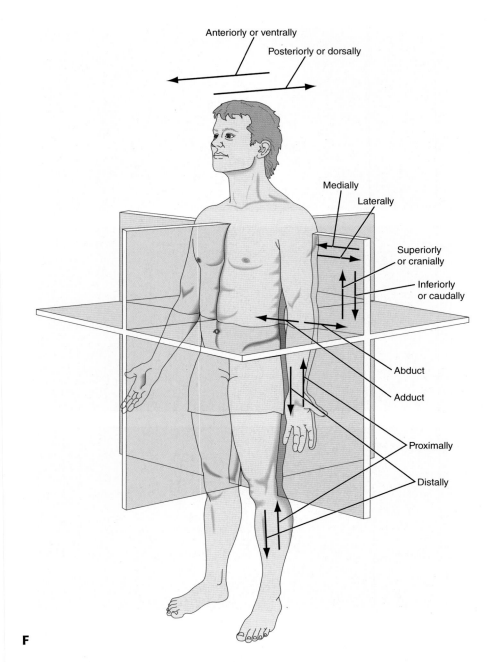

Figure 1–1. *continued* **F.** Terms of movement. *Source: From Seikel/Drumright/ King. Anatomy & Physiology for Speech, Language, and Hearing, 5th Ed.* ©Cengage, Inc. Reproduced by permission. *continues*

F

frontal section or **frontal view:** divides body into front and back halves

midsagittal section: an anatomical section that divides the body into left and right halves in the median plane

sagittal section: divides the body or body part into right and left halves

You may think of the following planes as referring to sections of a standing body, but they are actually defined relative to imaginary axes of the body. If you were to divide the body into front and back sections, you would have produced a **frontal section** or **frontal view**. If you cut the body into left and right halves, this would be along the median plane and it would produce **midsagittal sections**. A **sagittal section** is any cut that is parallel to the median plane and divides the body into left and right portions: The cut is in the sagittal plane. The **transverse plane** divides the body into upper and lower portions (this plane is often referred to by radiologists as *transaxial* or *axial*, and the radiological orientation always assumes you are looking from the feet toward the head). Figure 1–1A illustrates these sections. Armed with

cells to the damaged site for protective purposes. This protective function can go awry, as seen in anaphylactic shock, which is a runaway hypersensitive inflammatory reaction.

Muscular Tissue

Muscle is specialized contractile tissue that has muscle fibers capable of being stimulated to contract. Muscle is generally classified as being striated, smooth, or cardiac (Figure 1–2). **Striated** muscle, which has a striped appearance on microscopic examination, is more commonly known as **skeletal muscle** because it is used to move skeletal structures. It is also known as **voluntary** or **somatic muscle**, because it can be moved in response to conscious, voluntary processes. In contrast, **smooth muscle**, which includes the visceral muscular tissue of the digestive tract and blood vessels, is generally sheet-like, with spindle-shaped cells. **Cardiac muscle** is composed of cells that interconnect in a net-like fashion. Smooth and cardiac muscle are generally outside of voluntary control, relegated to the **autonomic** or involuntary nervous system.

striated: L., stria, striped; streaked

smooth muscle: muscle that is found in the **viscera**, including digestive tract and blood vessels

viscera: L., body organs

cardiac muscle: muscle of the heart, composed of cells that interconnect in a net-like fashion

autonomic: Gr., autos, self; nomos, law; self-regulating

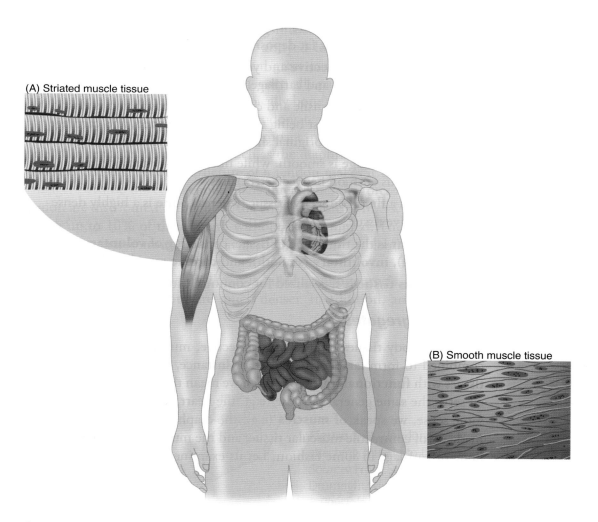

(A) Striated muscle tissue

(B) Smooth muscle tissue

Figure 1–2. Striated and smooth muscle. *Source:* From Seikel/Drumright/King. *Anatomy & Physiology for Speech, Language, and Hearing, 5th Ed.* ©Cengage, Inc. Reproduced by permission.

Osteoporosis

Osteoporosis is a condition wherein bone becomes increasingly porous due to loss of calcium. The reduction in calcium may be the result of aging or may arise from vitamin D deficiency, as in osteomalacia. Loss of calcium may also arise from disuse, as found in individuals confined to bed during illness. Individuals with osteoporosis are particularly susceptible to bone fractures from normal application of force. The elderly individual who has fallen and broken a hip may actually have broken the hip prior to the fall. An individual with osteoporosis may break ribs while coughing. Osteoporosis may be localized, as seen in the bones of the skull in Paget's disease (osteitis deformans).

retains the longitudinal orientation of the connective tissue fibers, whereas a fascia is made up of matted fibers.

The dense packing of longitudinal fibers makes tendons quite strong. A tendon can withstand pulling of more than 8,000 times the stretching force that a muscle the same diameter can. In fact, the tendon for a given muscle is able to withstand at least twice the pulling force of the muscle itself. That is, a sudden pull on a muscle will damage the muscle itself or the musculotendinous junction well before the tendon itself is actually damaged.

Bones

Bones and cartilage have an interesting relationship. Developing bone typically has a portion that is cartilage, and all bone begins as a cartilaginous mass. Many points of **articulation** (or joining) between bones are composed of cartilage, because cartilaginous surfaces are smoother and glide across each other more freely than surfaces of bone. Likewise, cartilage replaces bone where elasticity is beneficial. We see this in the cartilaginous portion of the rib cage, in the cartilage of the larynx, and in the nasal cartilages. As cartilage becomes impregnated with inorganic salts, it begins to harden, ultimately becoming bone.

articulation: the point of union between two structures

Bones provide rigid skeletal support and protect organs and soft tissues. Thirty percent of a bone is collagen, providing great tensile strength. The rigidity and compressive strength of bone tissue comes from the even greater proportion of calcium deposited within it. Indeed, bones in older individuals become more susceptible to compression as a result of loss of calcium through the aging process.

Bones are broadly characterized by length (long or short) or shape (flat), or generally as having irregular morphology. The **periosteum** (fibrous membrane covering of a bone) extends along its entire surface except regions with cartilage. This outer periosteum layer is most tightly bound to the bone at the tendinous junctures. Although the outer periosteum layer is tough and fibrous, the inner layer of periosteum contains fibroblasts that facilitate bone repair.

Blood cell production occurs within the cavities of the spongy bone trabeculae (trabeculae are supporting "beams" of a structure). As you can see from Figure 1–4, the cavities within the spongy bone are protected by the

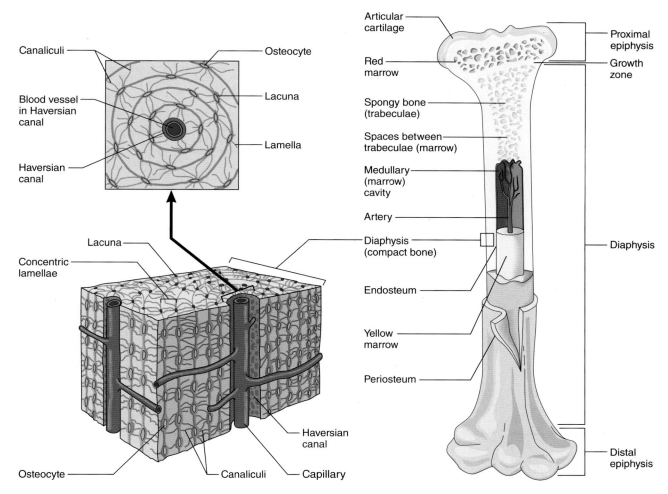

Figure 1–4. Microscopic structure of bone, revealing periosteum, haversian canals, and spongy bone trabeculae. *Source:* From Seikel/Drumright/King. *Anatomy & Physiology for Speech, Language, and Hearing, 5th Ed.* ©Cengage, Inc. Reproduced by permission.

compact bone. Notice the periosteum bound to the compact bone, and the blood supply to the entire bony structure.

Bone growth and development stand as a classic example of "use it or lose it." The density of a bone and its conformation are directly related to the amount of force placed on the bone. Using muscles causes bone to strengthen and become denser in regions stressed by that activity. Males tend to have greater muscle mass than females, and the bones of males often have more readily identifiable landmarks.

Joints

The union of bones with other bones, or cartilage with other cartilage, is achieved by means of **joints** (Figure 1–5). Joints take a variety of forms. Generally, joints are classified based on the degree of movement they permit: high mobility (**diarthrodial** joints), limited mobility (**amphiarthrodial**), or no mobility (**synarthrodial**) (Table 1–2). The joints are also classified based

diarthrodial: the class of joints of the skeletal system that permits maximum mobility

amphiarthrodial: the class of joints of the skeletal system that permit limited movement

synarthrodial: the class of joints of the skeletal system that permit no movement

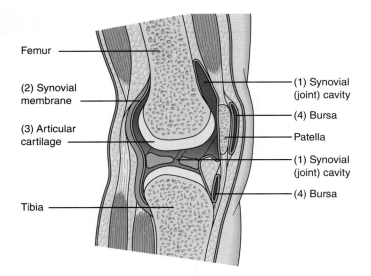

Femur

(2) Synovial membrane

(3) Articular cartilage

Tibia

(1) Synovial (joint) cavity

(4) Bursa

Patella

(1) Synovial (joint) cavity

(4) Bursa

SIMPLE SYNOVIAL JOINT

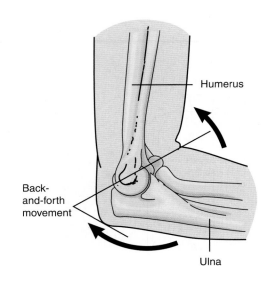

Humerus

Back-and-forth movement

Ulna

HINGE JOINT

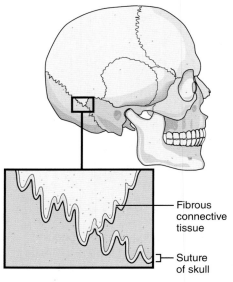

Fibrous connective tissue

Suture of skull

SUTURE

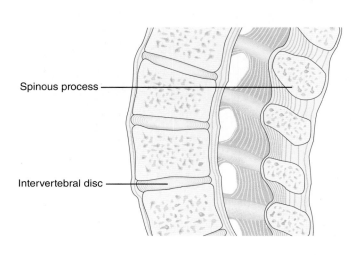

Spinous process

Intervertebral disc

SYMPHYSIS

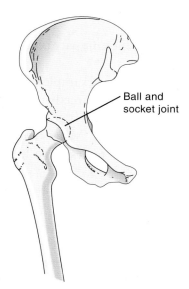

Ball and socket joint

ELLIPSOID JOINT

Figure 1–5. Different types of joints. *Source:* From Seikel/Drumright/King. *Anatomy & Physiology for Speech, Language, and Hearing, 5th Ed.* ©Cengage, Inc. Reproduced by permission.

Table 1–2

Types of Joints

  I. **Fibrous joints** (Immobile)
    A. Syndesmosis: Banded by ligament
    B. Suture: Skull bone union
    C. Gomphosis: Tooth in alveolus

  II. **Cartilaginous joints** (Limited movement)
    A. Synchondrosis: Cartilage that ossifies through aging
    B. Symphysis: Bone connected by fibrocartilage

  III. **Synovial joints** (Highly mobile)
    A. Plane (gliding joint; arthrodial): Shallow or flat surfaces
    B. Spheroid (cotyloid): Ball and socket variant allowing wide range of movement
    C. Condylar: Shallow ball-and-socket joint
    D. Ellipsoid: Football-shaped ball-and-socket joint
    E. Trochoid (pivot): head rotates or pivots in fossa
    F. Sellar (saddle): convex and concave joint with a long axis
    G. Ginglymus (hinge) One member rotates, allowing only flexion and extension

on the primary component involved in the union between bones. Synarthrodial joints are anatomically classified as **fibrous joints**, amphiarthrodial joints are **cartilaginous joints**, and diarthrodial joints are **synovial joints**, or joints containing synovial fluid within a joint space.

Fibrous Joints. There are two major types of fibrous or synarthrodial joints: syndesmoses and sutures. **Syndesmosis** joints are bound by fibrous ligaments but have little movement. **Sutures** are joints between bones of the skull that are not intended to move at all. The mating surfaces of the bones form a rough and jagged line that enhances the strength of the joint. Sutures take several forms (Figure 1–6). A **gomphosis** (peg) suture (Figure 1–6A) is one in which a peg fits into a hole. A socket (alveolus) and tooth is one such joint. A dentate (or serrate) suture (Figure 1–6B) gains its strength from the jagged (i.e., serrated) edge that mates the two bones together. This is the type of suture found, for instance, between the two parietal bones. A squamous suture (Figure 1–6C) is one in which the two mating bones actually overlap in a "keying" formation, much like current-day joining of wood sheets. A final joint, the plane joint (Figure 1–6D), is simply the direct union of two edges of bone.

Cartilaginous Joints. As the name implies, cartilaginous joints (also called amphiarthrodial joints) are those in which cartilage provides the union

fibrous joints: joints that are connected by fibrous tissue

cartilaginous joints: joints in which cartilage serves to connect two bones

synovial joints: a type of diarthrodial joint that has encapsulated fluid as a cushion

syndesmosis: Gr., syndesmos, ligament; osis, condition

sutures: L., sutura, seam; immobile joints between plates of bone

gomphosis: Gr., bolting together

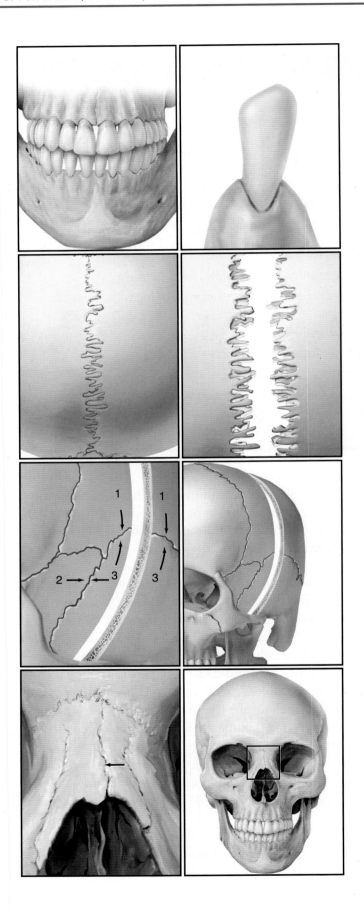

Figure 1–6. Sutures are immobile joints between plates of bone. **A.** Gomphosis or peg suture, in which a structure such as a tooth is embedded in an alveolus or hole. **B.** Dentate (serrated) suture, so called because of the jagged edge. **C.** Squamous suture, in which the two plates of bone are "keyed" by means of interlocked, overlapping phalanges. **D.** Plane suture, which involves a simple edge-to-edge union between two bones. *Source:* From Seikel/Drumright/King. *Anatomy & Physiology for Speech, Language, and Hearing, 5th Ed.* ©Cengage, Inc. Reproduced by permission.

(A) Gomphosis or peg suture

(B) Dentate (serrated) suture

(C) Squamous suture (*arrows*)

(D) Plane suture (*arrow*)

between two bones. Considering that bone arises from cartilage during development, it makes sense that in some cases cartilage would persist. In **synchondrosis**, the cartilaginous union is maintained, as in the junction of the manubrium sterni and the corpus sterni, although the junction ossifies as the individual ages. The second type of cartilaginous joint is a **symphysis**, such as that found between the pubic bones (pubic symphysis) or between the disks of the vertebral column.

Synovial Joints. The distinguishing feature of synovial or diarthrodial joints is that they all include some form of joint cavity within which is found **synovial fluid**, a lubricating substance, and around which is an articular capsule. The **articular capsule** is made up of an outer fibrous membrane of collagenous tissue and ligament to which the bone and an inner synovial membrane lining bind. Hyaline cartilage covers the surface of each bone of the joint, providing a smooth, strong mating surface.

Synovial joints are either simple or composite, depending on whether two bone surfaces are being joined or more than two, respectively. **Plane synovial joints** (gliding joints; arthrodial) are those in which the mating surfaces of the bone are more or less flat. Bones joined in this manner are permitted some gliding movement. **Spheroid** (or **cotyloid**) joints are **reciprocal** in nature (as are all but plane joints), in that one member of the union has a convex portion that mates with a concave portion of the other member. The spheroid joint is a ball-and-socket joint, in which a convex ball or head fits into a cup or **cotylica**. This joint permits a wide range of movement, including rotation.

Condylar joints are more shallow versions of the ball-and-socket joint, and their movement is more limited. **Ellipsoid joints** capitalize on an elliptical (football-shaped) member. These joints permit a wide range of movements, but not rotation. A **trochoid joint** (**pivot joint**), in contrast, is designed for rotation, and little else. It consists of a bony process protruding into a fossa. A **sellar** (or **saddle) joint** (is perhaps the most descriptive of the joint names. One member of the saddle joint is convex, like a saddle, while

synchondrosis: Gr., syn, together; chondros, cartilage; osis, condition

symphysis: Gr., growing together

articular capsule: the fibrous connective tissue covering of a synovial joint

plane synovial joints: joints with mating surfaces that are predominantly flat

cotyloid: Gr., kotyloeides, cup-shaped

condylar joint: a shallow ball-and-socket joint with limited mobility

trochoid joint (pivot joint): a joint consisting of a process and fossa, permitting only rotation

Sellar (or saddle) joint : a ball-and-socket joint in which the concave member rests on an elongated convex member

Craniosynostosis

As the infant develops, the sutures of the skull become ossified, a process called **synostosis**. Complete synostosis normally occurs well into childhood, but in some instances, synostosis may occur prenatally, called **craniosynostosis**. Continued normal growth of the brain, especially during the first postnatal year, places pressure on the skull. The effects of premature craniosynostosis on skull development are quite profound. With **sagittal craniosynostosis**, the child's head becomes peaked along the suture and elongated in back. In Apert syndrome, a genetic condition, the affected child's stereotypic peaked head is the result of premature closure of the coronal suture, resulting in pronounced bulging along that articulation.

synostosis: ossification of sutures

craniosynostosis: premature closure of cranial sutures

sagittal craniosynostosis: premature closure of sagittal suture

ginglymus (or hinge) joint: a joint that acts like a hinge, permitting only flexion and extension

sellar: L., sella; Turkish saddle

epimysium: Gr., epi, upon, over; mys, muscle

the other concave member sits on the saddle. A **ginglymus** (or **hinge**) **joint** acts like the hinge of a cabinet door: One member rotates on that joint with a limited range, permitting only flexion and extension.

✓ To summarize:

- Tissues combine to form larger structures.
- **Fascia** is a sheet-like membrane surrounding organs.
- **Ligaments** bind organs together or hold bones to bones or cartilage.
- **Tendons** attach muscle to bone or to cartilage; if a tendon is flat, it is referred to as an **aponeurosis**.
- Bones and cartilage provide the structure for the body, articulating by means of joints.
- **Diarthrodial** (synovial) **joints** are highly mobile, **amphiarthrodial** (cartilaginous) **joints** permit limited mobility, and **synarthrodial** (fibrous) **joints** are immobile.
- **Fibrous joints** bind immobile bodies together, **cartilaginous joints** are those in which cartilage serves the primary joining function, and **synovial joints** are those in which lubricating synovial fluid is contained within an articular capsule.
- Among synovial joints are **plane** (gliding) joints, **spheroid**, **condylar**, **trochoid**, **sellar**, and **ellipsoid** joints (all variants of ball-and-socket joints), as well as ginglymus joints.

Muscles

The combination of muscle fibers into a cohesive unit is both functionally and anatomically defined. Anatomically, muscles are bound groups of muscle fibers with functional unity. A fascia of connective tissue termed the **epimysium** surrounds the muscles, and the muscles are endowed with a tendon to permit attachment to skeletal structure. Muscles have a nerve supply to provide stimulation of the contracting bundle of tissue; muscles also have a vascular supply to meet their nutrient needs, as will be discussed in Chapter 12. Muscle morphology varies widely, depending on function. Fibers of wide, flat muscles tend to radiate from a broad point of origination to a more focused insertion. More cylindrical muscles have unitary points of attachment on either end. In all cases, the orientation of the muscle fibers defines the region on which force will be applied, because muscle fiber can only actively shorten. Muscle bundles can contract to approximately half their length.

A muscle can contract to approximately one-third its original length, and thus long muscles can contract more than short muscles. The diameter of a muscle is directly related to its strength, because the diameter represents the number of muscle fibers allocated to perform the task.

The work performed by the body is widely varied between extremes of muscular effort (very little to great amounts) and extremes of muscle rate of contraction (very rapid to slow and sustained). Although muscle morphology accounts for much of the variation in function, the physical relationship between muscle and bone provides a great deal of flexibility in muscle use.

Muscles can exert force only by shortening the distance between two points and can contract only in a straight line (with the exception of sphincteric muscles). By convention, the point of attachment of the least mobile element is termed the **origin**, and the point of attachment that moves as a result of muscle contraction is termed the **insertion**. When referring to limbs, the insertion point is more distant from the body. Muscles that move a structure are referred to as **agonists** (**prime movers**), whereas those that oppose a given movement are called **antagonists**. Thus, an agonist for one movement may become an antagonist for the opposite movement. Muscles that stabilize structures are termed **fixators**, while those that aid in movement are termed **synergists**. For example, in the middle ear, when the stapedius muscle contracts, it pulls the stapes posteriorly, so that it inhibits movement of the footplate in the oval window. When the tensor tympani of the middle ear contracts, it pulls the malleus anteromedially, reducing the movement of the malleus and, subsequently, the movement of the tympanic membrane in response to sound. In this sense, these two muscles are antagonistic to each other (the stapedius works to oppose the action of the tensor tympani). In another sense, these two muscles work together, because co-contraction causes the ossicular chain to stiffen or become relatively less mobile, reducing sound conduction to the inner ear. Thus, acting together, these muscles work synergistically to stabilize the ossicular chain, reducing the impact of loud noise.

Another, more direct example of the fixative function is the interaction of the genioglossus and intrinsic muscles of the tongue. The *genioglossus* is a large muscle of the tongue that moves the tongue into its gross position, but the intrinsic muscles of the tongue do the job of making fine movements. In this sense, the genioglossus is responsible for stabilizing the tongue so that the fine gestures associated with articulation can be accomplished.

Muscle action that does not result in movement of a structure is termed **isometric**. Agonists and antagonists often co-contract, providing a **fixator** function that stabilizes a structure. This is a critically important component of motor control. We need to make another very important point here, specifically related to speech and hearing. As we mentioned earlier, humans have done a marvelous job of getting double duty from systems. For instance, the larynx is responsible for protecting the airway from foreign matter, but we use it for voice production. When we discuss origins and insertions of muscles, we define those as the *functional* origins and insertions. We will differ from classical anatomical texts in some cases, because *our* speech-based piggybacked function differs from the *stated* classic or primary functions for a few of the muscles. For instance, contraction of the pectoralis major adducts the humerus and with it the shoulder, so for its primary (classical) function the origin is at the sternum and the insertion is the greater tubercle of the humerus. The pectoralis major is also a muscle of respiration, in which case its job is to expand the rib cage. When we use pectoralis to help us expand the chest cavity and inhale, the origin is the humerus, while the insertion is the sternum (the humerus is holding still and the sternum is moving).

agonist: muscle contracted for purpose of a specific motor act (in contrast to the antagonist)

prime mover: agonist; the muscle responsible for the primary or desired movement

antagonist: a muscle that opposes the contraction of another muscle (the agonist)

fixators: muscles that stabilize structures through contraction

synergist: muscle that assists the agonist accomplishing a movement

isometric: muscle action that does not result in movement

We will remind you of this again later but *recognize that we are using the functional definition of origin and insertion as related to speech function.* As you can see in Figure 1–7, the points of muscle attachment have a great deal to do with how much force can be exerted by muscle contraction to achieve work. A muscle attached closer to a joint moves the bone farther and faster than the one attached farther from the joint. In contrast, the muscle farther from the joint is able to exert more force through its range, because of the leverage advantage. The more distally placed muscle has an advantage for lifting, while the muscle closer to the joint provides greater range to the bone to which it is attached.

Muscles are **innervated** or supplied by a single nerve. **Innervation** refers to the process of stimulating a muscle or gland, or receiving output from a

innervation: stimulation of a muscle, gland, or structure by means of a nerve

Neuromuscular Diseases

A host of neuromuscular conditions prey on the muscular system and the nerve components that supply it. Amyotrophic lateral sclerosis is a condition in which the motor neuron is destroyed, resulting in loss of muscle function. Myelin destruction occurs in multiple sclerosis, with manifestation of the disease varying by site of lesion. Myasthenia gravis is a condition in which the nerve–muscle junction is compromised as a result of an immune system response. The result is weakness and loss of muscle range due to inability of the nerve and muscle to communicate, as will be discussed in Chapter 12.

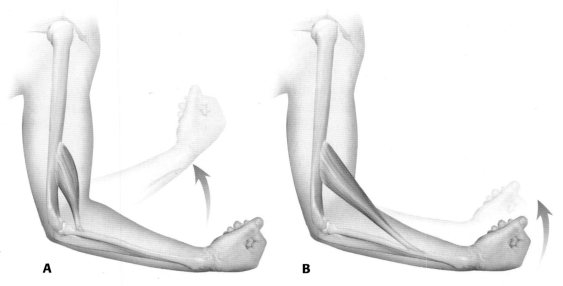

A   **B**

Figure 1–7. Mechanical advantage derived from point of insertion. **A.** The muscle inserts closer to the point of rotation and the movable point undergoes a greater excursion on contraction of the muscle. **B.** The muscle is attached a greater distance from the point of rotation so that the bone moves a smaller distance, but the muscle is capable of exerting greater force in the direction of movement. *Source:* From Seikel/Drumright/King. *Anatomy & Physiology for Speech, Language, and Hearing, 5th Ed.* ©Cengage, Inc. Reproduced by permission.

body sensor. Innervation can be sensory (generally termed **afferent**) or excitatory (**efferent**) in nature. A **motor unit** consists of one efferent nerve fiber and the muscle fibers to which it attaches. Every muscle fiber is innervated. In addition, muscles have sensory components providing information to the central nervous system concerning the state of the muscle.

afferent: L., ad, to; ferre, carry

efferent: L., ex, from; ferre, carry

 To summarize:

- **Muscle** is contractile tissue, with muscle bundles capable of contracting to about half their length.
- The point of attachment with the least movement is termed the **origin**, while the **insertion** is the point of attachment of relative mobility.
- Muscles that move a structure are **agonists** and those that oppose movement are called **antagonists**.
- Muscles that stabilize structures are termed **fixators**, while **synergists** are muscles that aid primary movement.
- Muscles are innervated by a single nerve.
- A **motor unit** is the efferent nerve fiber and muscle fibers it innervates.

Body Systems

In the same way that tissues combine to form organs, organs combine to form functional systems. **Systems** of the body are groups of organs with functional unity. That is, the combination of organs performs a basic function, and failure or deficiency of an organ will result in a change in the function of the system. Because systems are functionally defined, organs can belong to more than one system. Similarly, we can define the physical communication systems of the human organism through combinations of organs.

The basic systems of the body are fairly straightforward. The **muscular system** includes the smooth, striated, and cardiac muscles of the body. The **skeletal system** includes the bones and cartilages that form the structure of the body. The **respiratory system** includes the passageways and tissues involved in gas exchange with the environment, including the oral, nasal, and pharyngeal cavities; the trachea and bronchial passageway; and lungs. The **digestive system** also includes the oral cavity and pharynx, in addition to the esophagus, liver, intestines, and associated glands. The **reproductive system** includes the organs involved with reproduction (ovaries and testes), and the **urinary system** includes the kidneys, ureters, bladder, and urethra. The **endocrine system** involves production and dissemination of hormones, so it includes glands, such as the thyroid gland, testes, and ovaries. The **nervous system** includes the nerve tissues and structures of the central and peripheral nervous systems that are responsible for muscle control and sensory function.

system: a functionally defined group of organs

muscular system: the anatomical system that includes smooth, striated, and cardiac muscle

skeletal system: the anatomical system that includes the bones and cartilages that make up the body

respiratory system: the physical system involved in respiration, including the lungs, bronchial passageway, trachea, larynx, pharynx, oral cavity, and nasal cavity

reproductive system: the system of the body involved in reproduction

urinary system: the body system including kidneys, ureters, bladder, and urethra

endocrine system: the system involved in production and dissemination of hormones

nervous system: the system of nervous tissue, comprising the central and peripheral nervous systems

information between the environment and the brain, for communicating among the components of the nervous system, and for activating glands and muscles. The processes of receiving or sensing information are termed *sensory* or *afferent* processes, and the processes of activating muscles and glands are called *motor* or *efferent* processes. We refer to sensory pathways as afferent pathways, and motor pathways as efferent pathways. Both these broad neurophysiological processes are the product of interactions among neurons, so let us look at some of the basic parts so they make sense in the following chapters.

A neuron is made up of three basic components: the dendrite, soma, and axon (Figure 1–10). The dendrite or dendritic tree is the input side of a neuron. Information, such as touch sensation, is received by the dendrite. The soma is the cell body of the neuron, and it houses many organelles or components that are essential for the function and maintenance of the neuron. The axon is the point at which information leaves the neuron.

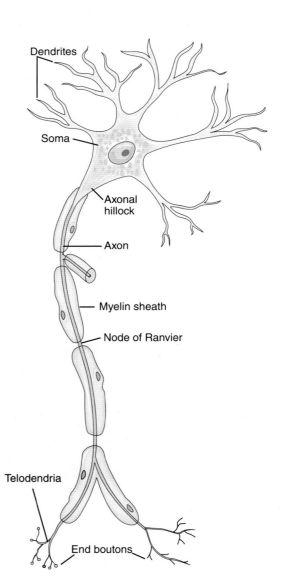

Figure 1–10. Schematic of basic elements of a neuron. *Source:* From Seikel/Drumright/King. *Anatomy & Physiology for Speech, Language, and Hearing, 5th Ed.* ©Cengage, Inc. Reproduced by permission.

If the information at the dendrite is sufficiently robust or "loud" enough to cause the neuron to be excited, an impulse travels from the dendrite, through the soma, and to the axon. At the axon, an action potential is generated that causes a wave of depolarization down the axon to its end. Depolarization is the process whereby the membranous surface of the axon opens to allow passage of ions that, in turn, communicate information toward the end of the axon, an area known as the *end bouton* (or "end button"). End boutons have small sacs or vesicles filled with neurotransmitter (Figure 1–11), and the wave of depolarization passing through the axon

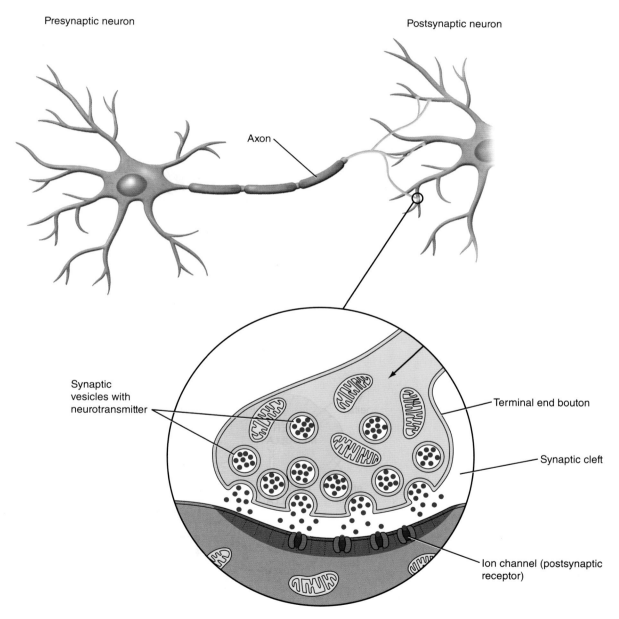

Figure 1–11. Presynaptic and postsynaptic nerves. Note expanded view of synapse between the two neurons. *Source:* From Seikel/Drumright/King. *Anatomy & Physiology for Speech, Language, and Hearing, 5th Ed.* ©Cengage, Inc. Reproduced by permission.

brain stem: the subcortical region including the medulla, pons, and midbrain

breathing. The reflexes mediated by cranial nerves tend to be more complex than spinal reflexes, so the stakes are much higher when we have damage to the **brain stem** area from which cranial nerves arise. This damage usually comes in the form of a stroke (cerebrovascular accident), and those of you choosing to be speech-language pathologists will be very much involved in rehabilitation of a person with this kind of a problem.

What follows is a brief discussion of cranial nerves so that you are familiar with them as you delve into anatomy and physiology. Please realize that some cranial nerves have multiple functions: Some are only sensory, some are only motor, and some are mixed sensory and motor. Some serve not only skeletal muscle but also smooth muscle, and some of the sensations mediated by cranial nerves do not even reach consciousness. We will cover the cranial nerves in more depth in Chapters 11 and 12 on neuroanatomy and neurophysiology, respectively. We use the convention here of giving number and name of the cranial nerve, and we always use the Roman numerals (Figure 1–14). We have found that if we always refer to the cranial nerve by name and number, we will always have those two mentally linked. Pay particular attention to cranial nerves I olfactory, V trigeminal, VII facial, VIII vestibulocochlear, IX glossopharyngeal, X vagus, XI accessory, and XII hypoglossal. These are all important to speech and hearing functions.

I. Olfactory nerve: This afferent cranial nerve mediates the sense of smell through sensors within the mucous membrane of the nasal cavity. It is only a sensory nerve. This is an important cranial nerve related to eating and swallowing, and damage to it can affect our taste perception.

II. Optic nerve: This afferent cranial nerve mediates the special sense of vision.

III. Oculomotor nerve: This efferent cranial nerve mediates most of the movement of the eyeball. It also is responsible for accommodation to light.

IV. Trochlear nerve: This efferent cranial nerve is responsible for moving the eyeball down.

V. Trigeminal nerve: This is an important mixed cranial nerve that mediates the sense of touch for the face (sensory) and controls many of the muscles of chewing (mastication). It is divided into three branches: the V trigeminal ophthalmic branch, V trigeminal maxillary branch, and V trigeminal mandibular branch. The ophthalmic branch mediates the sense of touch for the upper face, including forehead, front of scalp, upper eyelid, and iris. The maxillary branch sends information about sensation from the lower eyelid, nose, palate, upper teeth, and upper jaw (maxilla) regions. The maxillary branch has a double function: The sensory component mediates sensory information for the lower teeth and jaw (mandible), cheeks, and touch sense for the anterior two-thirds of the tongue; the motor component

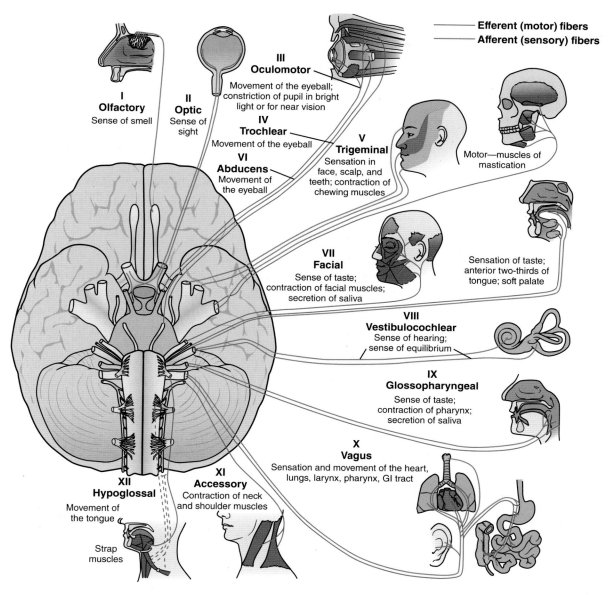

Figure 1–14. Brain stem and cranial nerves serving the head and neck. *Source:* From Seikel/Drumright/King. *Anatomy & Physiology for Speech, Language, and Hearing, 5th Ed.* ©Cengage, Inc. Reproduced by permission.

controls contraction of the muscles of mastication, one muscle of the soft palate, and one of the tiny muscles in the middle ear.

VI. Abducens: This motor nerve is responsible for abduction of the eyeball.

VII. Facial nerve: This mixed nerve provides motor activation of the muscles of the face and the lacrimal (tearing), and sublingual and submandibular (salivary) glands. The sensory component includes body sense of the ear canal and skin of the outer ear, as well as taste for the anterior two-thirds of the tongue.

VIII. Vestibulocochlear nerve: This sensory nerve is often called the auditory nerve because it mediates the sense of sound from the cochlea to the brain stem. It also transmits information from the vestibular mechanism of the inner ear, which is critical for balance and movement.

IX. Glossopharyngeal nerve: This is a mixed motor/sensory nerve, responsible for many important functions. The sensory component mediates sense of taste for the posterior third of the tongue and upper airway region (upper pharynx), as well as body sense for the ear (in conjunction with the VII facial nerve). It also mediates the sensation associated with initiating the swallow, gag, and vomit reflexes. The motor component is responsible for helping to constrict the upper airway (pharynx) for swallowing, as well as for elevation of the pharynx.

X. Vagus nerve: This mixed nerve has various functions, but we mention just a few here. There are two main branches of concern for us right now. The X vagus recurrent laryngeal nerve (RLN) controls nearly all the musculature of the larynx, so it is responsible for protection of the airway. The X vagus superior laryngeal nerve controls the muscles associated with pitch changing in voice. The sensory components of the X vagus provide body sensation for the pharynx, larynx, trachea, esophagus, thorax, and abdomen. There are even taste sensors in the entry to the larynx that are innervated by the X vagus.

XI. Accessory nerve: This efferent nerve joins with the X vagus to serve the intrinsic muscles of the larynx, as well as innervates two muscles associated with respiration.

XII. Hypoglossal nerve: This efferent nerve is responsible for controlling all the muscles of the tongue. As you can probably guess, it's highly important for articulation.

Cerebral Cortex

The cerebral cortex is by far the most complex structure of the nervous system. It is responsible for all conscious thought and voluntary action. It is the seat of cognitive function and is responsible for making sense of the world we live in. It is composed of two hemispheres (left and right), with five lobes in each hemisphere (Figure 1–15). Because of the construction of the pathways to and from the cortex, the left hemisphere governs motor activity on the right side of the body, while the right hemisphere governs the left. Likewise, sensations from the right body are sent to the left hemisphere (fortunately, there is a structure—the corpus callosum—that guarantees the right side knows what the left side knows).

Frontal Lobe. The frontal lobe is responsible for cognition, which is how we make sense of the world. It is also responsible for initiation of all voluntary motor activity, through activation of the motor strip (precentral gyrus). Immediately anterior to the motor strip is the premotor region, responsible

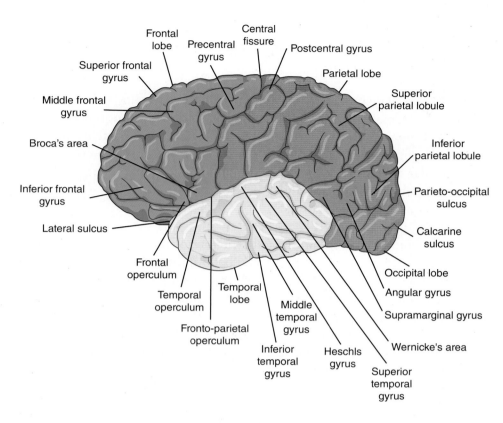

Figure 1–15. Landmarks of the left cerebral hemisphere. *Source:* From Seikel/Drumright/King. *Anatomy & Physiology for Speech, Language, and Hearing, 5th Ed.* ©Cengage, Inc. Reproduced by permission.

for motor planning. A very important cortical structure within the dominant hemisphere for speech and language is the area known as **Broca's area**, which is responsible for the expression of language (i.e., spoken language).

Parietal Lobe. The parietal lobe is responsible for processing body (somatic) sense. Body sense includes the sense of touch, vibration, pressure, pain, and temperature sense, but not the special senses of hearing, smell, vision, and speech. Information arriving in the parietal lobe is used by the frontal lobe to plan the motor act as well as to identify the environment in which cognition functions (e.g., if you have a significant pain, you'll direct your cognitive functions to figuring out how to stop it). The parietal lobe is also an area of integration with other areas, particularly with vision. Damage to the parietal lobe can result in dressing apraxia, a problem in which a person cannot organize their motor plan to put on clothes.

Occipital Lobe. The occipital lobe has the responsibility for receiving and processing visual information. It projects its output to many different areas, including the parietal and temporal lobes.

Temporal Lobe. The temporal lobe is a very important lobe for those of us in speech and hearing. This lobe receives the auditory input that arises from the cochlea. The left temporal lobe also houses the very important language zone, Wernicke's area. Wernicke's area is responsible for auditory comprehension, particularly of language, and damage to this area can result in a severe form of language comprehension deficit, fluent (Wernicke's) aphasia. The temporal lobe also houses the hippocampus, which is responsible for mediating short-term memory.

Insular Lobe. The insular lobe is hidden from view, residing beneath Broca's area of the frontal lobe. The left insular lobe is critically important for planning and organization of speech output. Damage to the left insular lobe results in apraxia of speech, which is a difficulty planning the speech act. The insular cortex has many other functions as well, including mediating the sense of taste (gustation) and a sense of self.

Cerebellum

The cerebellum is the second largest structure of the nervous system. It is situated beneath the cerebral cortex and behind the brain stem. It is responsible for integrating all body sense with the motor plan so that what we do (motor act) is planned appropriately for the context of our body condition. That is, picking up a glass from the floor while standing is a completely different task from picking up the same glass while lying on the floor, so the motor plan needs to take all body conditions into consideration. The cerebellum is the great coordinator for motor activity.

Brain Stem

The brain stem is divided into three regions: the medulla oblongata (medulla), pons, and midbrain. The medulla houses many cranial nerve nuclei and other nuclei that are critical for life function. The pons is a major communication bridge (*pons* is Latin for bridge) among the spinal cord, vestibular mechanism, brain stem, cerebral cortex, and cerebellum. The midbrain has cranial nerve nuclei and is also the recipient of the motor pathway as the fibers exit the cortex to enter the brain stem.

Subcortical Structures

Beneath the cortex are a group of nuclei that are very important for sensory and motor function. The basal ganglia are responsible for repetitive movement, muscle tone control, and control of background movement (e.g., arm swing when walking). The thalamus is the last way station for sensory information that goes to the cortex. The subthalamus works with the basal ganglia for motor control.

✓ *To summarize:*

- Organs combine to form **functional systems**, including the system concerned with muscles (**muscular system**), the framework of the body (**skeletal system**), breathing (**respiratory system**), digestion (**digestive system**), and reproduction (**reproductive system**), as well as the **urinary** and **endocrine systems**, and the **nervous system**.
- Within the discipline of speech pathology, we have functionally defined four systems.

- The **respiratory system** is concerned with respiration, the **phonatory system** is made up of the components of the respiratory and digestive systems associated with production of voiced sounds (the larynx), the **articulatory/resonatory system** (including the structures of the face, mouth, and nose), and the **nervous system** (related to central nervous system's control of speech process).

- The nervous system is broken into the peripheral nervous system (PNS) and central nervous system (CNS). The basic unit of the nervous system is the neuron, which is responsible for communication within the nervous system. Glial cells support neuron function and are responsible for development of myelin, which greatly reduces conduction time in the nervous system.

- The PNS is made up of cranial and spinal nerves, with cranial nerves being the most critical part of the PNS for speech and hearing.

- Cranial nerves are identified with Roman numerals. I olfactory is responsible for the sense of smell. II optic mediates vision. III oculomotor, IV trochlear, and VI abducens serve eye movement. V trigeminal innervates muscles of mastication, some muscles of the soft palate, and a muscle of the middle ear. VII facial nerve innervates muscles of facial expression, as well as the sense of taste for a portion of the tongue. VIII vestibulocochlear nerve is responsible for hearing and balance, and IX glossopharyngeal is involved in both sensory and motor function related to swallowing. X vagus innervates a number of motor systems, including laryngeal musculature. XI accessory functions largely as a support system for IX and X. XII hypoglossal nerve innervates the tongue muscles.

- The CNS is made up of larger neural structures, including the cerebral cortex, brain stem, cerebellum, spinal cord, and other subcortical structures.

- The cerebral cortex is responsible for conscious and voluntary function, while the cerebellum coordinates sensory and motor plans. The brain stem mediates many life functions, as well as serves as the origination for cranial nerves. The thalamus is the last way station for sensation from the body, while the basal ganglia control muscle tone and some stereotyped movements.

Chapter Summary

Anatomy and physiology are the study of structure and function of an organism, respectively. Subspecializations of anatomy interact to provide the detail required for understanding the anatomy and physiology of speech. Descriptive anatomy relates the individual parts of the body to functional systems, and pathological anatomy relates to changes in structure from disease. Disciplines such as cytology and histology study cells and tissues, respectively; and myology examines muscle form and function. Arthrology refers to the study of the joint system for bones, while osteology is the study of the form and function of bones. Neurology relates to the study of diseases of the nervous system.

The axial skeleton supports the trunk and head, and the appendicular skeleton supports the extremities. Anatomical terminology relates position and orientation of the body and its parts. A frontal plane involves a cut that produces front and back halves of a body, a sagittal plane is produced by a cut dividing the body into left and right halves, and a transverse plane is produced by dividing the body into upper and lower halves. Anterior and posterior refer to the front and back of a body, respectively, as do ventral and dorsal for the human. Peripheral refers to a direction toward the surface or superficial region, while deep refers to direction away from the surface. Distal and proximal refer to away from and toward the root of a free extremity, respectively. Superior and inferior refer to upper and lower regions, respectively. Lateral and medial refer to the side and midline, respectively. Flexion refers to bending ventral surfaces toward each other at a joint, and extension is moving those surfaces farther apart. Plantar and palmar refer to ventral surfaces of the feet and hands, respectively.

The four basic tissues of the human body are epithelial, connective, muscular, and nervous. Epithelial tissue provides the surface covering of the body and linings of cavities and passageways. Connective tissue provides the variety of tissue linking structures together—those comprising ligaments, tendons, cartilage, bone, and blood. Muscular tissue is contractile in nature, composed of striated, smooth, and cardiac. Nervous tissue is specialized for communication.

Tissues combine to form structures and organs. Fascia surrounds organs, ligaments bind bones or cartilage, tendons attach muscle to bone or to cartilage, and bones and cartilage provide the structure for the body. Joints between skeletal components may be diarthrodial (synovial; highly mobile), amphiarthrodial (cartilaginous; slightly mobile), or synarthrodial (fibrous; immobile). Fibrous joints bind immobile bodies together, cartilaginous joints are those in which cartilage serves the primary joining function, and synovial joints are those in which lubricating synovial fluid is contained within an articular capsule.

Muscle bundles are capable of contracting to about half their length. The origin is the point of attachment with the least movement, and the insertion is the relatively mobile point of attachment. Agonists are muscles that move a structure, antagonists oppose movement, and fixators stabilize a structure. Synergists are muscles that assist in the primary movement. Muscles are innervated by a single nerve, and innervation can be afferent or efferent. A motor unit is the efferent nerve fiber and muscle fibers it innervates.

Systems of the body include the muscular, skeletal, respiratory, digestive, reproductive, urinary, endocrine, and nervous systems. Systems of speech production include the respiratory, phonatory, articulatory/resonatory, and nervous systems. The peripheral nervous system (PNS) and central nervous system (CNS) are made up of neurons, which transmit information, and glial cells, which support neuron function. The PNS is made up of cranial and spinal nerves. The CNS is made up of larger structures, including the cerebral cortex, brain stem, cerebellum, spinal cord, and others. The cerebral cortex is responsible for conscious and voluntary function, while the cerebellum coordinates sensory and motor plans. The brain stem mediates many life functions, as well as serves as the origination for cranial nerves. The thalamus is the last way station for sensation from the body, while the basal ganglia control muscle tone and some stereotyped movements.

Chapter 1 Study Questions

1. _____ is the study of the structure of an organism.

2. _____ is the study of the function of a living organism and its parts.

3. _____ anatomy is anatomical study for diagnosis and treatment of disease.

4. _____ anatomy is involved in the description of individual parts of the body without reference to disease conditions, viewing the body as a composite of systems that function together.

5. _____ is the study of structure and function of cells.

6. _____ is the study of structure and function of bones.

7. _____ is the study of form and function of muscle.

8. _____ is the study of diseases of the nervous system.

9. _____ is the type of tissue that makes up the skin and mucous membrane.

10. _____ is a particularly important connective tissue because it is both strong and elastic.

11. _____ is a contractile tissue.

12. _____ bind organs together or hold bones to bone or cartilage.

13. _____ is a sheet-like membrane surrounding organs.

14. _____ attach muscle to bone or to cartilage.

15. The relatively immobile point of attachment of a muscle is termed the _____.

16. The relatively mobile point of attachment of a muscle is termed the _____.

17. Identify the systems defined below:

    A. _____ This system includes smooth, striated, and cardiac muscle of the body.

    B. _____ This system includes the bones and cartilages that form the structure of the body.

    C. _____ This system includes the passageways and tissues involved in gas exchange with the environment, including the oral, nasal, and pharyngeal cavities, the trachea and bronchial passageway, and lungs.

    D. _____ This system includes the esophagus, liver, intestines, and associated glands.

    E. _____ This system includes the nerve tissue and structures of the central and peripheral nervous system.

18. Identify the systems of speech defined below:

   A. _____ This system provides the energy source for speech production.

   B. _____ This system is involved in production of voiced sound and uses components of the respiratory system (the laryngeal structures).

   C. _____ This system is the combination of structures used to alter the characteristics of the sounds of speech, including parts of the anatomically defined digestive and respiratory systems (e.g., tongue, lips, teeth, soft palate).

   D. _____ This system includes the nasal cavity and soft palate and portions of the anatomically defined respiratory and digestive systems.

19. Terms of orientation: On the following figure, identify the descriptive terms indicated.

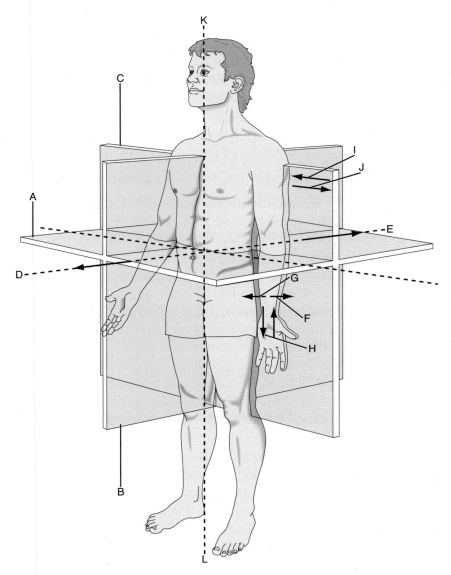

Source: From Seikel/Drumright/King. *Anatomy & Physiology for Speech, Language, and Hearing, 5th Ed.* ©Cengage, Inc. Reproduced by permission.

A. _____ plane

B. _____ plane

C. _____ plane

D. _____ aspect

E. _____ aspect

F. _____ (movement away from midline)

G. _____ (movement toward midline)

H. _____ (located away from root of free extremity)

I. _____ (located near root of free extremity)

J. _____ (related to the side)

K. _____ (above)

L. _____ (below)

20. The _____ system refers to that group of nervous system components that include the cerebrum, cerebellum, brain stem, and spinal cord.

21. The _____ system includes cranial and spinal nerves.

22. The _____ is responsible for coordinating the motor act by integrating motor and sensory information.

23. The _____ contains the medulla oblongata, pons, and midbrain.

24. The _____ (number and name) nerve mediates the sense of smell.

25. The _____ (number and name) nerve mediates the sense of taste for the anterior two-thirds of the tongue.

26. The _____ (number and name) nerve is responsible for activation of muscles of the face.

27. The _____ (number and name) nerve is responsible for movement of the muscles of mastication.

28. The _____ (number and name) nerve mediates the sense of taste for the posterior third of the tongue.

29. The _____ (number and name) nerve innervates all the tongue muscles.

30. As our field has developed, the professionals working with speech and language became known as "speech-language pathologists." Reflecting on the terminology you have just reviewed, to what does the term "pathologist" refer?

❓ Chapter 1 Study Question Answers

1. **ANATOMY** is the study of the structure of an organism.

2. **PHYSIOLOGY** is the study of the function of a living organism and its parts.

3. **CLINICAL OR APPLIED** anatomy is anatomical study for diagnosis and treatment of disease.

4. **SYSTEMIC ANATOMY** is involved in the description of individual parts of the body without reference to disease conditions, viewing the body as a composite of systems that function together.

5. **CYTOLOGY** is the study of structure and function of cells.

6. **OSTEOLOGY** is the study of structure and function of bones.

7. **MYOLOGY** is the study of form and function of muscle.

8. **NEUROLOGY** is the study of the nervous system.

9. **EPITHELIAL** is the type of tissue that makes up the skin and mucous membrane.

10. **CARTILAGE** is a particularly important connective tissue because it is both strong and elastic.

11. **MUSCLE** is a contractile tissue.

12. **LIGAMENTS** bind organs together or hold bones to bone or cartilage.

13. **FASCIA** is a sheet-like membrane surrounding organs.

14. **TENDONS** attach muscle to bone or to cartilage.

15. The relatively immobile point of attachment of a muscle is termed the **ORIGIN**.

16. The relatively mobile point of attachment of a muscle is termed the **INSERTION**.

17. The defined systems are as follows:

    A. **MUSCULAR SYSTEM** includes smooth, striated, and cardiac muscle of the body.

    B. **SKELETAL SYSTEM** includes the bones and cartilages that form the structure of the body.

    C. **RESPIRATORY SYSTEM** includes the passageways and tissues involved in gas exchange with the environment, including the oral, nasal, and pharyngeal cavities, the trachea and bronchial passageway, and lungs.

    D. **DIGESTIVE SYSTEM** includes the esophagus, liver, intestines, and associated glands.

    E. **NERVOUS SYSTEM** includes the nerve tissue and structures of the central and peripheral nervous system.

18. The defined systems of speech are as follows:

    A. **RESPIRATORY SYSTEM** This system provides the energy source for speech production.

    B. **PHONATORY SYSTEM** is involved in production of voiced sound and uses components of the respiratory system (the laryngeal structures).

C. **ARTICULATORY SYSTEM** is the combination of structures used to alter the characteristics of the sounds of speech, including parts of the anatomically defined digestive and respiratory systems (e.g., tongue, lips, teeth, soft palate).

D. **RESONATORY SYSTEM** includes the nasal cavity and soft palate and portions of the anatomically defined respiratory and digestive systems.

19. The descriptive terms of orientation are as follows:

A. **TRANSVERSE** plane

B. **SAGITTAL OR MEDIAN** plane

C. **CORONAL OR FRONTAL** plane

D. **ANTERIOR OR VENTRAL** aspect

E. **POSTERIOR OR DORSAL** aspect

F. **ABDUCT** (movement away from midline)

G. **ADDUCT** (movement toward midline)

H. **DISTAL** (located away from root of free extremity)

I. **PROXIMAL** (located near root of free extremity)

J. **LATERAL** (related to the side)

K. **SUPERIOR** (above)

L. **INFERIOR** (below)

20. The **CENTRAL NERVOUS** system refers to that group of nervous system components that include the cerebrum, cerebellum, brain stem, and spinal cord.

21. The **PERIPHERAL NERVOUS** system includes cranial and spinal nerves.

22. The **CEREBELLUM** is responsible for coordinating the motor act by integrating motor and sensory information.

23. The **BRAIN STEM** contains the medulla oblongata, midbrain, and pons.

24. The **I OLFACTORY** nerve mediates the sense of smell.

25. The **VII FACIAL** nerve mediates the sense of taste for the anterior two-thirds of the tongue.

26. The **VII FACIAL** nerve is responsible for activation of muscles of the face.

27. The **V TRIGEMINAL** nerve is responsible for movement of the muscles of mastication.

28. The **IX GLOSSOPHARYNGEAL** nerve mediates the sense of taste for the posterior third of the tongue.

29. The **XII HYPOGLOSSAL** nerve innervates all the tongue muscles.

30. Pathology is the study of diseased tissue. By extension, a speech-language pathologist is one who studies the pathology of our field, communication disorders.

Bibliography

Agur, A., & Dalley, A. (2012). *Grant's atlas of anatomy* (13th ed.). New York, NY: Lippincott Williams & Wilkins.

Duffy, J. R. (2012). *Motor speech disorders* (3rd ed.). St. Louis, MO: Mosby.

Gilroy, A. M., MacPherson, B. R., & Ross, L. M. (2012). *Atlas of anatomy* (2nd ed.). New York, NY: Thieme.

Moore, K. L., Persaud, T. V. N., & Torchia, M. G. (2013). *The developing human: Clinically oriented embryology* (9th ed.). Philadelphia, PA: W. B. Saunders.

Rohen, J. W., Lutjen-Drecoll, E., & Yokochi, C. (2010). *Color atlas of anatomy: A photographic study of the human body*. New York, NY: Lippincott Williams & Wilkins.

Seikel, J. A., Konstantopoulos, K., & Drumright, D. G. (2020). *Neuroanatomy and neurophysiology for speech and hearing sciences*. San Diego, CA: Plural Publishing.

Standring, S. (2008). *Gray's anatomy* (40th ed.). London, UK: Churchill Livingstone Elsevier.

Anatomy of Respiration

Breathe! You are alive!
—Thich Nhat Hanh, Zen Master

We *must* breathe with great regularity to maintain body systems that are dependent on efficient oxygen exchange. Respiration is simultaneously a very robust and a very delicate system. Our respiratory rate and depth of breathing are governed by a number of involuntary sensory systems, and we take these involuntary processes for granted as they meet our everyday needs. Yet, changes in respiratory tissues arising from environmental or disease-related issues can quickly destabilize this system, leaving us in peril for our lives. Most of the degenerative neurological diseases with which we work in speech-language pathology ultimately end with respiratory failure. Even when these automatic life processes are functioning well, we, as humans, regularly tax them by hijacking the respiratory system to provide the energy source for oral communication. We exercise a great deal of external control over the respiratory mechanism while still working within the bounds of the biological requirements for life (Des Jardins & Burton, 2017; Ganong, 2003). In this chapter, we discuss respiration as it is needed to sustain life, and then we discuss respiration for speech.

Respiration is defined as the exchange of gas between an organism and its environment. We bring oxygen to the cells of the body to sustain life by breathing in, the process of **inspiration**, and eliminate waste products by breathing out, or **expiration**.

Gas exchange happens within the minuscule air sacs known as the **alveoli**. Bringing air into the lungs is an active, muscular process. It capitalizes on the fact that all forces in nature seek balance and equilibrium. The basic mechanism for inspiration may be likened to that of a hypodermic needle. When the plunger on the hypodermic needle in Figure 2–1 is pulled down, whatever is near the opening enters the tube and is drawn into the awaiting chamber. If you envision the respiratory system as a syringe, with your mouth or nose as the tip, you can realize that pulling on the plunger (your diaphragm) causes air to enter the chamber (your lungs). If you hold your finger over the opening as you pull back the plunger, you can feel the suction on your finger. This suction is the product of *lowering* the relative air pressure within the chamber, producing an imbalance in relation to atmospheric pressure. Let us examine the physical principles involved a little more deeply.

Air pressure is the force exerted on the walls of a chamber by molecules of air. Because of the molecular charge, air molecules tend to keep their

inspiration: Gr. spiro, breath

alveoli: L., small hollows or cavities in a structure

ANAQUEST LESSON ▶

air pressure: the force exerted on a surface by air molecules

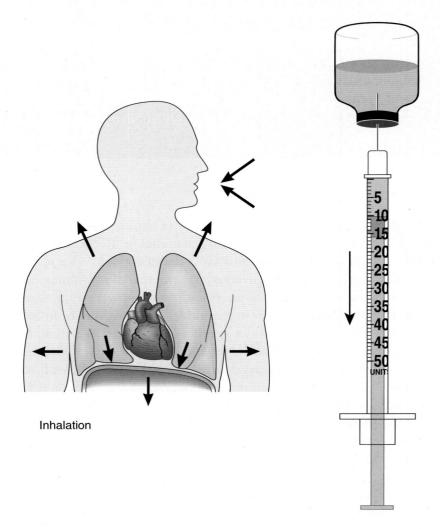

Inhalation

Figure 2–1. Comparison of the action of the diaphragm with that of a plunger on a syringe. As the diaphragm pulls down, air enters the lungs, just as it enters the chamber of the syringe when the plunger is pulled down. *Source:* From Seikel/Drumright/King. *Anatomy & Physiology for Speech, Language, and Hearing, 5th Ed.* ©Cengage, Inc. Reproduced by permission.

distance from other air molecules. If the chamber is opened to the atmosphere, the pressure exerted on the inner walls of the chamber will be the same as that exerted on the outer walls.

The action starts when you close the chamber and change the volume. Making the chamber smaller does not change the forces that keep molecules apart, but rather lets those forces manifest on the walls of the chamber. Although the forces have not changed, the area on which they exert themselves has (you made it smaller, remember?), and that results in an increase in pressure. That is, **pressure** is *Force* exerted on *Area*, or P = F/A. You have just increased pressure by decreasing area.

Boyle's law states that, given a gas of constant temperature, if you increase the volume of the chamber in which the gas is contained, the pressure will decrease. If you increase the size (volume) of the chamber of a syringe, the air pressure within that chamber will decrease. The opposite is also true: If you decrease the volume of the chamber, the pressure will increase. When volume increases, pressure decreases, and natural law says that air will flow to equalize that pressure. Thus, air flows into the chamber—in our case, the lungs.

Figure 2–2 shows the same effect graphically. The chamber has 11 molecules in it in both cases. On the left, the volume of the chamber has been reduced, so the 11 molecules are much closer together and the pressure has increased (known as **positive pressure**). Likewise, when you pull back the plunger so the molecules are farther apart than the forces dictate, the pressure decreases, and the pressure is now referred to as **negative pressure**. The beauty of this arrangement is that it provides all the principles we need to discuss respiratory physiology at the macro- or microscopic level. The forces that draw air into the lungs are also responsible for drawing carbon dioxide out.

positive pressure: air pressure that exceeds atmospheric pressure

negative pressure: air pressure that is less than atmospheric pressure

⊘ *To summarize:*

- **Pressure** is defined as force distributed over area, P = F/A.
- **Boyle's law** tells us that as the volume of a container increases, the air pressure within the container decreases.
- This relatively **negative pressure** will cause air to enter the container until the pressure is equalized.
- If volume is decreased, pressure increases and air flows out until the pressures inside and outside are equal.
- This principle forms the basis for movement of air into and out of the lungs.

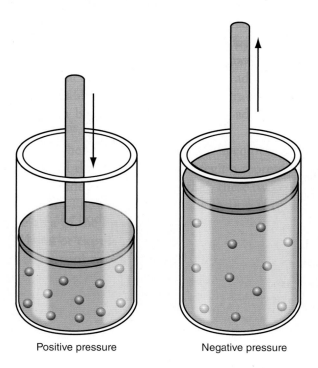

Positive pressure   Negative pressure

Figure 2–2. The piston on the left has been depressed, compressing the air in the chamber and increasing the air pressure. On the right, the piston has been retracted, increasing the space between the molecules and creating a relatively negative pressure. *Source:* From Seikel/Drumright/King. *Anatomy & Physiology for Speech, Language, and Hearing, 5th Ed.* ©Cengage, Inc. Reproduced by permission.

The Support Structure of Respiration

Overview

The respiratory system consists of a gas-exchanging mechanism supported and protected by a bony cage (Table 2–1). Gas exchange is carried out by the lungs, while the rib cage performs a protective function.

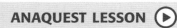

ANAQUEST LESSON

Let us take a guided tour of the respiratory system. To begin, pay attention to your own breathing. Try the following. While sitting up straight with your eyes closed, take 10 quiet breaths through your nose. First, concentrate your attention on your nose, feeling the air entering and leaving your nostrils. Then feel your abdominal region stretch out a little with each inspiration, and then become aware that your thorax (rib cage) is expanding a little with each inhalation. Now take a good, deep breath (still through your nose) and feel your whole chest rise and your shoulders straighten out a little.

Besides relaxing you, attending to your breathing has given you a sense of the parts of your body that are activated for inspiration and expiration. At first you directed your attention to your nostrils, the part of the respiratory passageway that warms and moistens the air going into the lungs. Then you noticed your abdomen protruding, which is a natural process associated with inspiration, because the diaphragm is pushing against the abdomen when it contracts to bring in air. Then you noticed that your thorax was expanding a

Table 2–1

Structures of Respiration
Bony thorax
Vertebrae and vertebral column
Ribs and their attachment to vertebral column
Pectoral girdle
Scapula and clavicle
Sternum
Pelvic girdle
Ischium
Pubic bone
Sacrum
Ilium
Visceral thorax
Respiratory passageway
Mouth and nose
Trachea and bronchi
Lungs
Mediastinum

little as you breathed in quietly, and then you noted that your thorax expanded markedly as you breathed in deeply. If you missed any of these things happening, take a minute and breathe a little more. This exercise sets the stage for understanding what is going on with the bones and muscles of respiration.

The lungs are housed within the thorax, an area bounded in the superior aspect by the first rib and clavicle, and in the inferior by the 12th rib (Figure 2–3). The lateral and anterior aspects are composed of the ribs and **sternum**. The entire thorax is suspended from the **vertebral column** (spinal column), a structure that doubles as the conduit for the **spinal cord**, which is the nervous system supply for the body and extremities.

Vertebral Column

The vertebral column is made up of a series of individual bones called vertebrae (singular: **vertebra**; plural: vertebrae). The vertebral column has five divisions: cervical, thoracic, lumbar, sacral, and coccygeal (Figure 2–4). The anatomical shorthand associated with the vertebral column and spinal nerves is as follows. The vertebrae are numbered sequentially from superior to inferior by section, so that the uppermost of the **cervical vertebrae** is C1, the second is C2, and so forth to C7. Likewise, the first **thoracic vertebra** is T1, and the last is T12. **Lumbar vertebrae** include L1 through L5, **sacral vertebrae** include S1 through S5, and the **coccygeal vertebrae** are considered a fused unit, known as the coccyx. The vertebrae are separated by intervertebral discs, which are made of fibrocartilage. Each disc consists of a gelatinous core that equalizes forces placed on the disc (the *nucleus pulposus*) and a fibrous ring known as the *annulus fibrosus*. The role of the disc is to keep the vertebrae separated, to cushion the forces exerted on the vertebrae, and

sternum: L., sternum, breastplate

vertebral column: the bony structure made of vertebrae

spinal cord: the nerve tracks and cell bodies within the spinal column

ANAQUEST LESSON

vertebra: bony segment of the vertebral (spinal) column

cervical vertebra: vertebra of the cervical spinal column

thoracic vertebra: vertebra of the thoracic spinal column

lumbar vertebra: vertebra of the lumbar spinal column

sacral vertebrae: vertebral components of the sacrum

coccygeal vertebrae: fused vestigial vertebral components of the coccyx

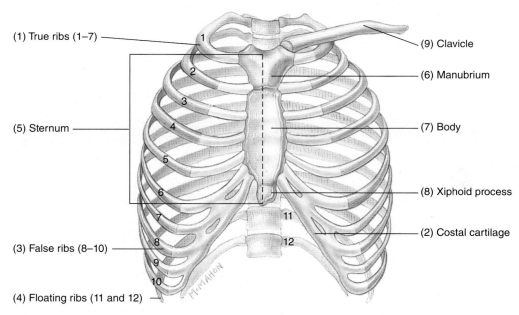

Figure 2–3. Anterior view of the thorax. *Source:* From Seikel/Drumright/King. *Anatomy & Physiology for Speech, Language, and Hearing, 5th Ed.* ©Cengage, Inc. Reproduced by permission.

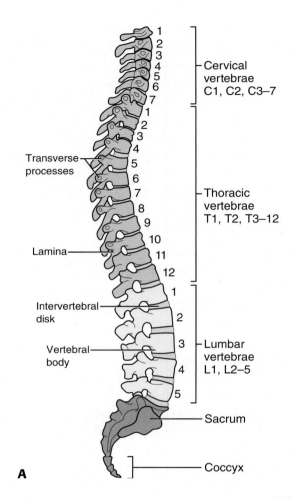

Figure 2–4. A. Components of the vertebral column. *Source:* From Seikel/Drumright/King. *Anatomy & Physiology for Speech, Language, and Hearing, 5th Ed.* ©Cengage, Inc. Reproduced by permission. *continues*

to allow free space for passage of the spinal nerves from the spinal cord to the periphery.

The vertebral column is composed of 33 segments of bone with a rich set of fossa and protuberances. Although vertebrae have roughly the same shape, their form and landmarks vary depending on the location and the area they serve, their attachments (such as ribs), and the size of the spinal

Palpation

Palpation, or the process of examining structures with the hands, can be a very useful tool for understanding anatomy. As a clinician, when you perform an oral peripheral examination, you need to be comfortable with the process of palpating because it is a means of gathering information about your client's physical condition that may help you in your diagnosis and in the remediation of speech problems. For instance, palpation of the temporomandibular joint (the joint forming the articulation of the mandible and the temporal bone) while your client moves the jaw provides you with insight into the integrity of the joint as well as the degree of muscular control your client is able to exert.

Throughout these chapters, we provide you with palpation activities that you can perform on yourself. Identifying the landmarks of the bones, joints, and muscles helps you understand the structures with which we deal in speech-language pathology.

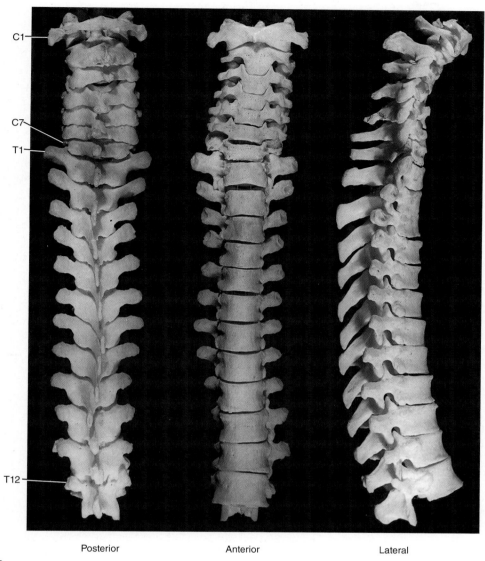

C1

C7

T1

T12

Posterior   Anterior   Lateral

B

Figure 2–4. *continued* **B.** Articulated cervical and thoracic vertebrae. *Source:* From Seikel/ Drumright/King. *Anatomy & Physiology for Speech, Language, and Hearing, 5th Ed.* ©Cengage, Inc. Reproduced by permission.

cord passing through them. The area serving the head requires more security for the vertebral artery and vein, so the cervical vertebrae have **foramina** (or openings) through which these arteries pass. In lower regions, there is a great deal more bone in the **corpus** or body of the vertebra, supporting the powerful muscles used for lifting.

foramina: L., openings (sing., *foramen*)

corpus: L., body

Cervical Vertebrae

Major landmarks of the vertebrae include a prominent **spinous process**, which can be felt by rubbing the spine of your friend's back, and **transverse processes** on both sides (Figure 2–5). The corpus of the vertebra makes

spinous process: posterior-most process of vertebra

transverse processes: lateral processes of vertebra

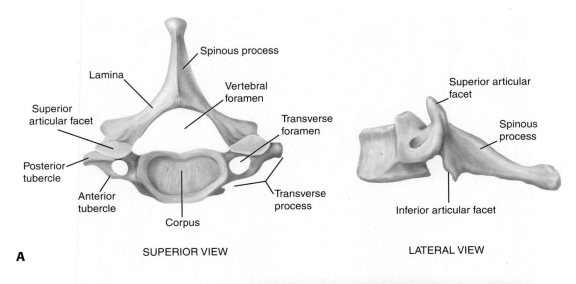

Figure 2–5. A. Superior and lateral views of cervical vertebra. **B.** Photograph of cervical vertebra. *Source:* From Seikel/Drumright/King. *Anatomy & Physiology for Speech, Language, and Hearing, 5th Ed.* ©Cengage, Inc. Reproduced by permission.

vertebral foramena: foramen of vertebral segment through which spinal cord passes

intervertebral foramena: foramena through which spinal nerves exit and/or enter the spinal cord

up the anterior portion, with a prominent hole or **vertebral foramen** just posterior to that. The tracts of the spinal cord pass through the vertebral foramen. The spinal nerves must somehow exit and enter the spinal cord; the **intervertebral foramina** on either side of the vertebra permit this. Vertebral segments ride one atop another to form the vertebral column. Superior and inferior articular facets provide the mating surfaces for two adjacent vertebrae, limiting movement in the anterior–posterior dimension, and thus protecting the spinal cord and allowing limited rotatory and rocking motion. We must be able to move freely, but not *too* freely, considering the importance of the spinal cord within that column.

The uppermost cervical vertebra, C1, is the **atlas**, so named after the mythical figure supporting the earth for its singular role in supporting the skull for rotation. C2 (the **axis**) articulates with the inferior surface of the atlas, allowing the skull to pivot (Figure 2–6). C1 and C2 differ markedly from C3 through C7. The posterior of C1 has a reduced prominence,

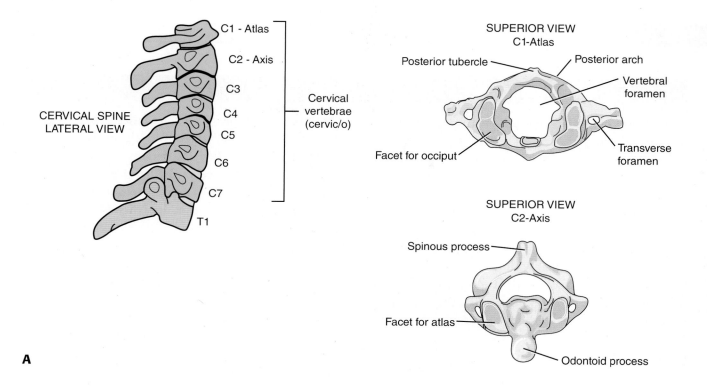

CERVICAL SPINE
LATERAL VIEW

C1 - Atlas
C2 - Axis
C3
C4
C5
C6
C7
T1

Cervical
vertebrae
(cervic/o)

SUPERIOR VIEW
C1-Atlas

Posterior tubercle
Posterior arch
Vertebral foramen
Facet for occiput
Transverse foramen

SUPERIOR VIEW
C2-Axis

Spinous process
Facet for atlas
Odontoid process

A

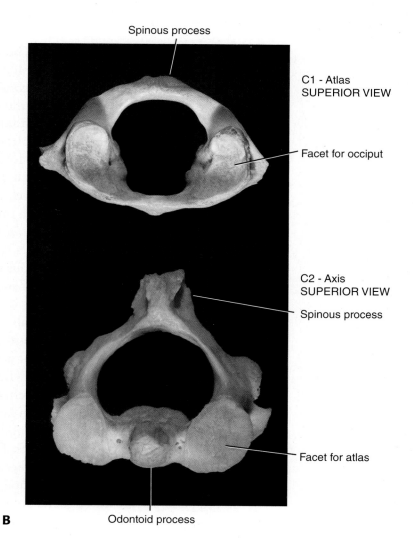

Spinous process

C1 - Atlas
SUPERIOR VIEW

Facet for occiput

C2 - Axis
SUPERIOR VIEW

Spinous process

Facet for atlas

Odontoid process

B

Figure 2–6. A. Cervical vertebrae. On the right are atlas (C1, upper) and axis (C2, lower). On the left are the articulated cervical vertebrae. **B.** Superior view of atlas and axis. *Source:* From Seikel/Drumright/King. *Anatomy & Physiology for Speech, Language, and Hearing, 5th Ed.* ©Cengage, Inc. Reproduced by permission.

Odontoid Malformations

Odontoid malformations are those in which the odontoid process of C2 fails to develop. In cases such as these, the atlas (C1) is free to rotate on the axis (C2), providing the potential for significant spinal cord and medulla oblongata injury during hyperrotation or hyperextension. Because the medulla oblongata is a vital component of the brain stem, these malformations can be life-threatening. The individual with undiagnosed odontoid malformation may complain of joint pain or stiffness in the neck, but otherwise may be asymptomatic. It is not until a radiograph of the neck region is performed for other purposes that the absent process is identified. Often the individual undergoes a minor trauma, such as a fall, that has a result that is greater than expected. In the literature on odontoid malformations are cases of wrestlers who suffer repeated syncope (significant reduction in blood pressure that results in light-headedness), transient limb weakness, and even seizure disorder. A more serious malformation is the **os odontoideum** malformation, in which the anterior tip of the vertebra is separated. In this condition, the tip typically continues to receive vascular supply and often grows into the foramen magnum. The result is that the tip places pressure on the spinal cord and lower brain stem, resulting in muscular weakness, pain, and reduction in motor coordination (ataxia), depending on the location of the injury. If the tip compresses an artery, there can be further complications due to reduction in vascular supply.

tubercle: L., tuberculum, little swelling

facet: Fr., facette, small face

odontoid: Gr. odont-, tooth; eido, form

dens: L., tooth

pedicle: L., pedalis, foot

here called the posterior **tubercle**. The superior articular **facet** is larger than those of C3 through C7, providing increased surface area for vertebra–skull articulation. Similarly, the C1 vertebral foramen is larger than those in the lower cervical vertebrae, reflecting the transition from spinal cord to brain stem that begins at that level. The **odontoid** (or **dens**) process of the axis (also known as the odontoid process) protrudes through the vertebral foramen of C1. The relationship between the odontoid process and vertebral foramen is protective, because unchecked lateral or rotatory movement could result in damage to the spinal cord at this level, which would be life-threatening. You might notice that the axis (C2) has a rudimentary spinous process, although the atlas does not. The articulation of C1 and C2 is shown in Figure 2–6.

As you can see in Figure 2–5, a typical cervical vertebra has a number of landmarks. The corpus and spinous process provide a clue to orientation: The corpus is in the anterior aspect, and the posterior spinous process slants downward.

Examination of Figure 2–5 also reveals lateral wings known as the transverse processes, which are directed in a posterolateral (*postero* = back; *lateral* = side) direction. The superior surface is marked by a superior articular facet, which rests atop the **pedicle**. The inferior surface contains an inferior articular facet. In the articulated vertebral column, these facets mate. The pair of transverse foramina shown in Figure 2–5 is found only in the cervical vertebrae and may even be absent in C7. Figure 2–7 shows that the vertebral artery and vein pass through this foramen. You can palpate the seventh cervical vertebra by bending your head forward so that your chin touches your chest. The first prominent spinous process you feel on your neck is C7. You can also palpate the large transverse processes of the atlas, inferior to the mastoid process of the temporal bone.

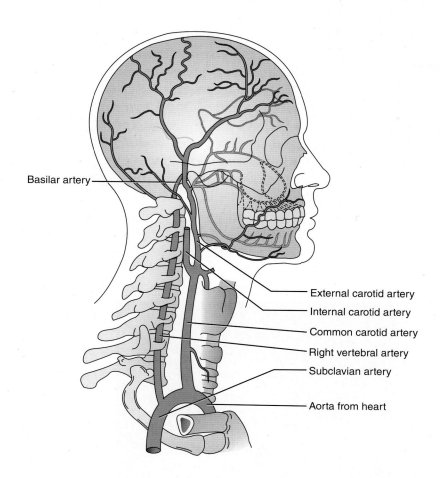

Basilar artery

External carotid artery

Internal carotid artery

Common carotid artery

Right vertebral artery

Subclavian artery

Aorta from heart

Figure 2–7. Course of vertebral artery through the transverse foramina of cervical vertebrae. *Source:* From Seikel/Drumright/King. *Anatomy & Physiology for Speech, Language, and Hearing, 5th Ed.* ©Cengage, Inc. Reproduced by permission.

Thoracic Vertebrae

The 12 thoracic vertebrae (T1 to T12) provide the basis for the respiratory framework, because they form the posterior point of attachment for the ribs of the bony thorax. As seen in Figure 2–8, the thoracic vertebrae have larger spinous and transverse processes than the cervical vertebrae. Between vertebrae is the intervertebral foramen, formed by the articulation of the inferior and superior vertebral notches of the vertebrae. Spinal nerves pass through these foramena, as they pass to and from the periphery. Note the superior and inferior costal facets: These are the points of attachment for the ribs, as seen in Figure 2–9.

The articulation of rib and thoracic vertebrae is complicated. Although it would have been simpler for us had the second rib been attached to the second vertebra, had the third rib been attached to the third vertebra, and so forth, only the first rib and the last three ribs (1, 10, 11, 12) have this nice one-to-one arrangement. Each of the remaining ribs (2 through 9) attaches to the transverse process and corpus of the same-numbered vertebra and also attaches to the body of the vertebra above it (e.g., rib 2 attaches to transverse process of T2 and body of T1 and T2). The utility of this articulation will become apparent when we discuss movement of the rib cage for respiration.

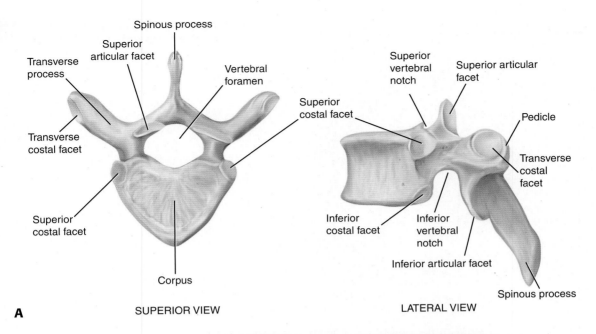

A   SUPERIOR VIEW   LATERAL VIEW

Superior view labels: Spinous process, Superior articular facet, Transverse process, Transverse costal facet, Vertebral foramen, Superior costal facet, Superior costal facet, Corpus

Lateral view labels: Superior vertebral notch, Superior articular facet, Pedicle, Transverse costal facet, Inferior costal facet, Inferior vertebral notch, Inferior articular facet, Spinous process

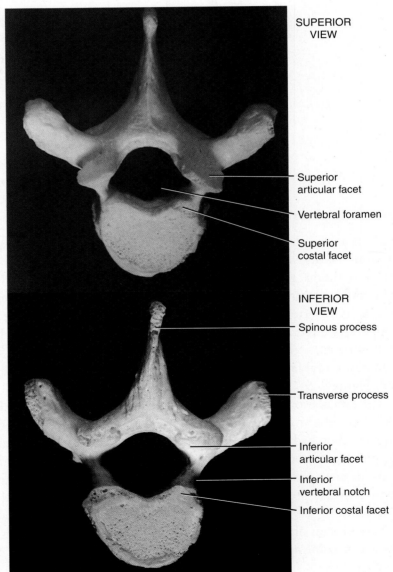

SUPERIOR VIEW

Superior articular facet

Vertebral foramen

Superior costal facet

INFERIOR VIEW

Spinous process

Transverse process

Inferior articular facet

Inferior vertebral notch

Inferior costal facet

Figure 2–8. A. Superior and lateral views of thoracic vertebrae. **B.** Superior (upper) and inferior (lower) view of thoracic vertebra. *Source:* From Seikel/Drumright/ King. *Anatomy & Physiology for Speech, Language, and Hearing, 5th Ed.* ©Cengage, Inc. Reproduced by permission.

B

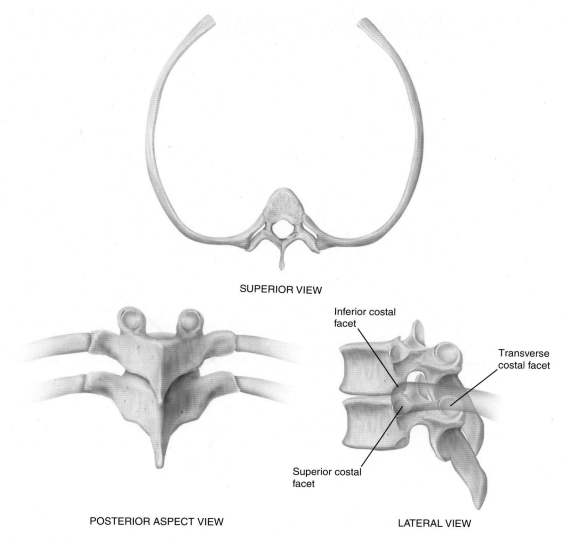

SUPERIOR VIEW

Inferior costal facet

Transverse costal facet

Superior costal facet

POSTERIOR ASPECT VIEW   LATERAL VIEW

Figure 2–9. Articulation of rib and vertebrae. *Source:* From Seikel/Drumright/King. *Anatomy & Physiology for Speech, Language, and Hearing, 5th Ed.* ©Cengage, Inc. Reproduced by permission.

Lumbar Vertebrae

The five lumbar vertebrae are quite large in comparison to those of the thoracic or cervical region, reflecting the stress placed on them during lifting and **ambulation** (walking). They provide direct or indirect attachment to a host of back and abdominal muscles, as well as to the posterior fibers of the diaphragm. The transverse and spinous processes are relatively smaller, and the corpus is much larger than in the thoracic and cervical vertebrae.

Sacrum and Coccyx

The five sacral vertebrae are actually a fused mass known as the **sacrum**. The sacrum and its ossified intervertebral discs retain vestiges of the vertebrae from which they are formed, with remnants of spinous and transverse

ANAQUEST LESSON

sacrum: L., sacralis, sacred

Herniation of Intervertebral Discs

The vertebral column is made up of individual vertebrae that are separated by intervertebral discs. These discs are an elegant solution to the problem of how to allow the vertebral column to move while still protecting the integrity of the column and its precious cargo, the spinal cord. Each intervertebral disc is made up of a ring of fibrocartilage surrounding a gelatinous core. The spinal cord takes a tremendous beating in day-to-day life. Every time you lift something, push on an object, or throw a baseball, you are putting compressive force on the vertebral column as muscles attached to the thorax and or vertebral column contract forcefully. Discs are exquisite in design, as the fibrocartilage rings flex with each movement. The gelatinous core evenly distributes forces placed on the ring throughout the disc. As an example, blow up a balloon and push your finger into it. The compression of your finger causes the entire balloon to change shape and expand because the forces are distributed evenly throughout the balloon.

The problem with this design is age. Nothing lasts forever, and the intervertebral disc is no exception. The fibrocartilage weakens and bulges under the pressure. Sometimes the disc ruptures and allows the core (the **nucleus pulposus**) to leak out. When the disc collapses, it allows the vertebrae to come closer, and the disc tends to bulge in the process. Both of these processes can compress the spinal nerve roots that emerge through the intervertebral foramina. The result can be pain and muscular weakness of the areas and muscles served by the nerve.

coccyx: Gr., kokkus, cuckoo (shaped like a cuckoo's beak)

processes. The sacral foramina perform the function of the intervertebral foramina, providing a passage for the sacral nerves (Figure 2–10).

The **coccyx** is composed of the fused coccygeal vertebrae. It is so named because of its beaklike appearance, and it articulates with the inferior sacrum by means of a small disc.

✅ To summarize:

- The **vertebral column** is composed of vertebral segments that combine to form a strong but flexible column.
- **Vertebrae** are identified based on their level: C1 to C7 (**cervical**), T1 to T12 (**thoracic**), L1 to L5 (**lumbar**), S1 to S5 (**sacral**).
- The fused **coccygeal vertebrae** are referred to as the **coccyx**.
- This spinal column provides the points of attachment for numerous muscles by means of the **spinous** and **transverse processes**.
- It also houses the **spinal cord**, with **spinal nerves** emerging and entering the spinal cord through spaces between the vertebrae.
- The ribs of the rib cage articulate with the spinal column in a fashion that permits the rib cage some limited movement for respiration.

Pelvic and Pectoral Girdles

The vertebral column is central to the body, and if we are to interact physically with our environment, we must use our appendages attached to this column.

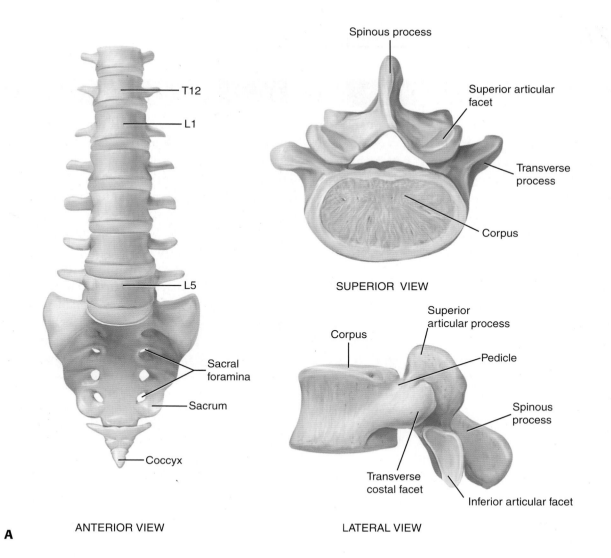

ANTERIOR VIEW

SUPERIOR VIEW

LATERAL VIEW

A

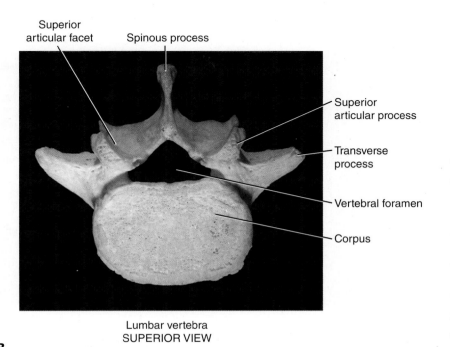

Lumbar vertebra
SUPERIOR VIEW

B

Figure 2–10. **A.** Lumbar vertebrae articulated with sacrum and coccyx (*left*). Upper right shows the superior view of lumbar vertebra, and lower right shows the lateral view. **B.** Superior view of lumbar vertebra. *Source:* From Seikel/Drumright/King. *Anatomy & Physiology for Speech, Language, and Hearing, 5th Ed.* ©Cengage, Inc. Reproduced by permission.

Spinal Cord Injury

The spinal cord is well protected by the osseous vertebral column, in that the vertebrae fit together in a partial lock-and-key fashion to inhibit motion. The vertebral column is richly bound together by ligaments and surrounded by muscles of the back.

Despite this degree of redundant protection, the spinal cord is frequently traumatized. The most frequent cause of spinal cord injury is vehicle accidents, especially those in which the occupant is not properly restrained. When a person is ejected from a vehicle, the vertebral column can undergo rotatory stresses that can tear the spinal cord, and the impact can compress the vertebral column, resulting in distention of the spinal cord. Both ejection and whiplash injuries can result in hyperextension of the cervical vertebrae, which can cause damage to the odontoid process, compress and distend the disc, and stretch or tear the spinal cord. Typically the compression occurs in the corpus. Significant transverse forces can cause a shearing of the spinal cord as well.

The result of spinal cord injury is frequently the loss of motor and sensory function to the area below the spinal cord injury, with subsequent paraplegia (legs paralyzed) or quadriplegia (both arms and legs paralyzed). For an exhaustive review of spinal cord injury, see Mackay, Chapman, and Morgan (1997).

pelvic girdle: the area comprised of the ilium, sacrum, pubic bone, and ischium

pectoral: L., pertaining to the chest

The lower extremities are attached to this axis by means of the **pelvic girdle**, and the upper extremities are attached through the **pectoral girdle**.

The pelvic girdle is comprised of the ilium, sacrum, pubis (pubic bone), and ischium (Figure 2–11). The combination provides an extremely strong structure capable of bearing a great deal of translated weight from the use of the legs. The pectoral girdle is the superior counterpart of the pelvic girdle.

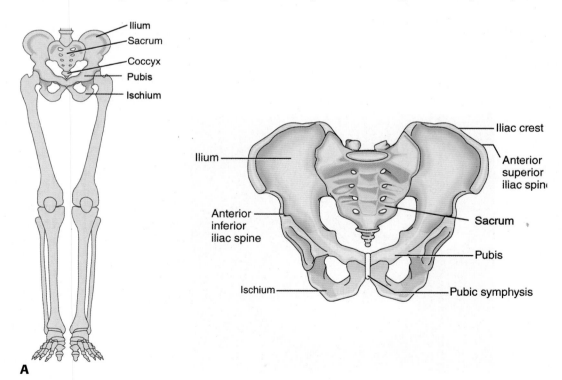

Figure 2–11. A. Pelvic girdle, consisting of the ilium, pubis, and ischium. *Source:* From Seikel/Drumright/King. *Anatomy & Physiology for Speech, Language, and Hearing, 5th Ed.* ©Cengage, Inc. Reproduced by permission.

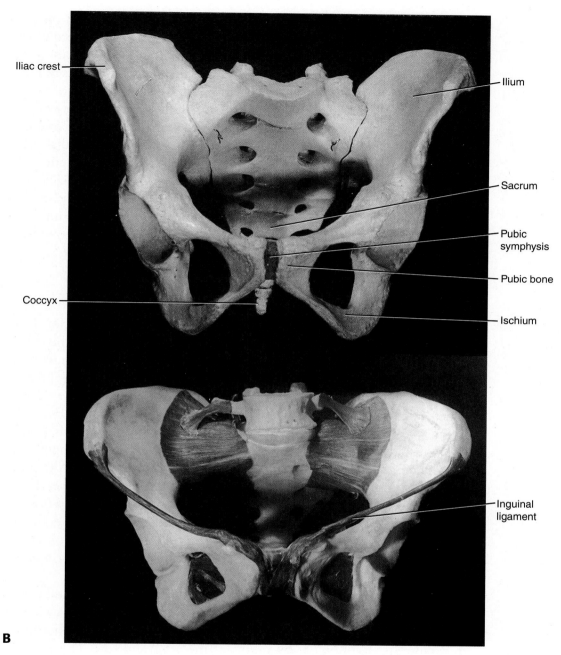

Iliac crest

Ilium

Sacrum

Pubic symphysis

Pubic bone

Coccyx

Ischium

Inguinal ligament

B

Figure 2–11. *continued* **B.** Anterior view of pelvis. Lower view shows location of the inguinal ligament. *Source:* From Seikel/Drumright/King. *Anatomy & Physiology for Speech, Language, and Hearing, 5th Ed.* ©Cengage, Inc. Reproduced by permission.

Pelvic Girdle

The pelvic girdle provides a strong structure for attaching the legs to the vertebral column (see Figure 2–11). Forces generated through movement of the legs are distributed across a mass of bone, which, in turn, is attached to the vertebral column (Whitmore, Willan, Gosling, & Harris, 2002).

The pelvic girdle, as mentioned earlier, is made up of the ilium, sacrum, pubic bone, and ischium. The **ilium** is a large, wing-like bone (similar in

ilium: one of the bones of the pelvic girdle

scapula: the major structure of the pectoral girdle

pubic symphysis: the joint between the paired pubic bones

shoulder girdle: another term for pectoral girdle

clavicle: L., clavicula, little key

this way to the **scapula** or shoulder blade of the upper body) that provides the bulk of the support for the abdominal musculature and the prominent hip bone on which many parents carry their children. The iliac crest of the superior-lateral surface is an important landmark: The anterior-superior iliac spine (ASIS) marks the termination of the crest as well as the superior point of attachment for the inguinal ligament. The inguinal ligament runs from the ASIS of the iliac crest to the **pubic symphysis**, which is the point of union between the two pubic bones. Deep to the ilium is the massive medial structure, the sacrum. The sacrum articulates with the fifth lumbar vertebra. The iliac bones articulate with the sacrum laterally, forming the sacroiliac joints. The coccyx is the inferior-most segment of the spinal column, consisting of four fused vertebrae articulating at the inferior aspect of the sacrum. The structure comprised of the iliac, ischium, and pubis bones is referred to as the **innominate** or *hip bone; innominate* means, literally, *unnamed.*

Pectoral Girdle

The pectoral or **shoulder girdle** includes the scapula and **clavicle**, bones that support the upper extremities. The clavicle, also known as the collarbone, is attached to the superior sternum, running laterally to join with the wing-like scapula. The clavicle provides the anterior support for the shoulder (Figure 2–12). The scapula has its only skeletal attachment via the clavicle, which in turn has its only skeletal attachment at the sternum. From the scapula are slung several muscles that hold it in a dynamic tension that facilitates flexible upper-body movement without compromising strength. The downside of this precarious arrangement is the vulnerability of the junction of the scapula and clavicle. Disarticulation of these two bones causes a collapse of the structure so that the shoulder rotates forward and inward.

The physical arrangement of the pectoral girdle provides an "A-frame" of support to distribute force through relatively solid articulation at the scapula and through muscular attachment in the form of the massive muscles of the thorax and back.

When taken together, one can view the human skeleton as a tube with two A-frames attached at the ends. The tube provides flexible yet strong support for the trunk, even as the A-frames give that trunk the opportunity to explore its environment by means of the arms and legs. The A-frame design provides maximum strength for these extremities with a minimum of bone mass and weight.

ⓥ To summarize:

- The bony support structure of the respiratory system is composed of the **rib cage** and **vertebral column**.
- At the base of the vertebral column is the **pelvic girdle**, composed of the **ilium**, **sacrum**, **pubic bone**, and **ischium**.
- The **pectoral girdle** is composed of the **scapula** and **clavicle**, which attach to the **sternum**.

- These structures provide the points of attachment for the lower and upper extremities.

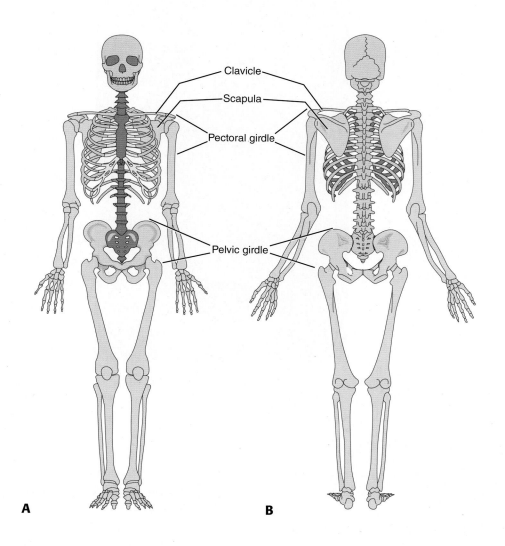

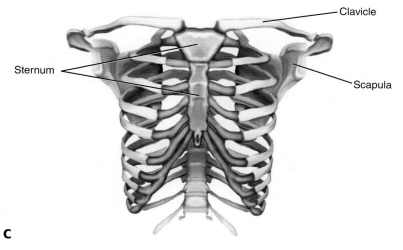

Figure 2–12. **A.** Anterior view of skeleton, showing components of pelvic and pectoral girdles. **B.** Posterior view. **C.** Isolated pectoral girdle. *Source:* From Seikel/ Drumright/King. *Anatomy & Physiology for Speech, Language, and Hearing, 5th Ed.* ©Cengage, Inc. Reproduced by permission. *continues*

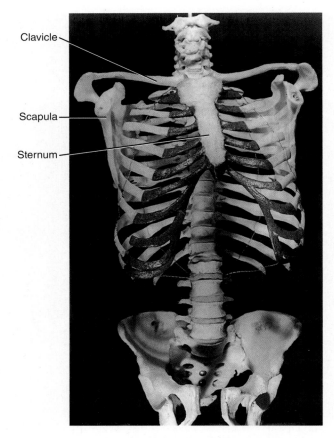

Clavicle

Scapula

Sternum

D   PELVIC AND PECTORAL GIRDLES

Figure 2–12. *continued*
D. Photograph of articulated thorax with pelvic and pectoral girdles. *Source:* From Seikel/ Drumright/King. *Anatomy & Physiology for Speech, Language, and Hearing, 5th Ed.* ©Cengage, Inc. Reproduced by permission.

Ribs and Rib Cage

Ribs are capable of a degree of movement so that the rib cage can rock up in front and flare out via lateral rotation, being hinged on the vertebral articulation with the rib cage. The rib cage is made up of 12 ribs, with all but the lowest two attached by means of cartilage to the sternum in the front aspect. Figure 2–13 shows that the sternum provides a focal point for the rib cage, and the sternum turns out to be a significant structure in respiration.

Another thing you might notice in Figure 2–13 is that the rib cage tends to slant down in front. With the mobility of the rib cage granted by the articulation of the vertebrae and ribs, the rib cage can elevate during inspiration to increase the size of the thorax.

Ribs

There are 12 pairs of ribs in the human **thorax**, with each rib generally consisting of five components; the **head, neck, tubercle, shaft**, and **angle** (Figure 2–14). The tubercle and the head provide the articulating surfaces with the vertebral column, and the angle represents the point at which the rib begins the significant curve in its course forward. The barrel shape of

shaft of rib: the long, relatively straight component of a rib, between the neck and the angle of the rib

angle of rib: the portion of the rib between the head and shaft, at which the direction of the rib takes an acute turn

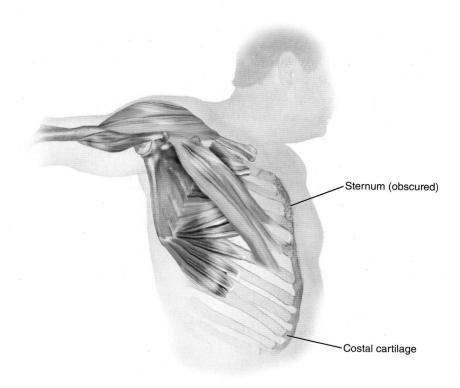

Sternum (obscured)

Costal cartilage

Figure 2–13. Lateral view of rib cage showing relationship between ribs and sternum. Note that the rib cage slants down in the front. *Source:* From Seikel/Drumright/ King. *Anatomy & Physiology for Speech, Language, and Hearing, 5th Ed.* ©Cengage, Inc. Reproduced by permission.

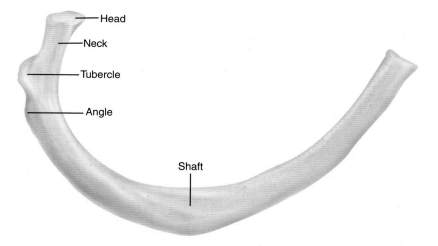

Head

Neck

Tubercle

Angle

Shaft

A

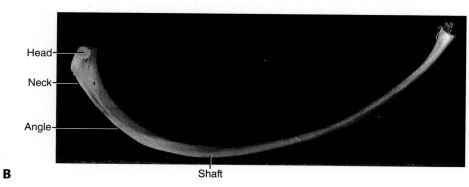

Head

Neck

Angle

Shaft

B

Figure 2–14. A. Schematic of second rib with landmarks. **B.** Photograph of rib. *Source:* From Seikel/Drumright/ King. *Anatomy & Physiology for Speech, Language, and Hearing, 5th Ed.* ©Cengage, Inc. Reproduced by permission.

the thorax is created by the relatively small superior and inferior ribs as compared to the longer middle ribs. The rib cage provides attachment for numerous muscles that provide strength, rigidity, continuity, and mobility to the rib cage.

Ribs are of three general classes: **true ribs**, **false ribs**, and **floating ribs**. The true (or vertebrosternal) ribs consist of the upper ribs (1 through 7), all of which form a more or less direct attachment with the sternum. Their actual attachment is by means of a cartilaginous union through the **chondral** (i.e., cartilaginous) portion of the rib (Figure 2–15). The false, or vertebro-chondral, ribs (8, 9, and 10) are also attached to the sternum by means of cartilage, although this chondral portion must run superiorly to attach to the sternum. The floating or vertebral ribs (11 and 12) articulate only with the vertebral column.

While we like to think of the rib cage as being constant and consistent across humans, it really is not. Most of us have 12 pairs of ribs, but fully 8% of adults reveal a 13th rib pair. That 8% is in good company, as both chimpanzees and gorillas sport the full complement of 13 rib pairs. Similarly, 1% of the human population may have neck ribs attached to the cervical verte-brae. This rare phenomenon can cause problems with the vascular supply.

The elastic properties of cartilage permit the ribs to be twisted (torqued) on the long axis without breaking. Thus, the rib cage is quite strong (being made up predominantly of bone), but capable of movement (being well endowed with resilient cartilage).

The rib cage gives significant protection to the heart and lungs. The rib cage also provides the basis for respiration, and the general structure of the barrel deserves some attention at this juncture.

true ribs: a.k.a. vertebrosternal ribs, consisting of those ribs making direct attachment with the sternum (ribs 1 through 7)

false ribs: a.k.a. vertebrochondral ribs, consisting of those ribs making indirect attachment with the sternum (ribs 8, 9, and 10)

floating ribs: those ribs that do not articulate with the sternum (ribs 11 and 12)

chondral: Gr., chondros, cartilaginous

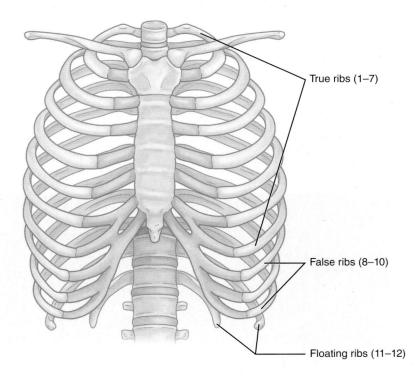

True ribs (1–7)

False ribs (8–10)

Floating ribs (11–12)

Figure 2–15. Schematic of relationships among true, false, and floating ribs. *Source: From Seikel/Drumright/King. Anatomy & Physiology for Speech, Language, and Hearing, 5th Ed.* ©Cengage, Inc. Reproduced by permission.

As you can see in Figure 2–16, the ribs make their posterior attachment along the vertebral column. If a fly were to walk along the superior surface of a rib, beginning from the tip of the head and walking to the point of attachment at the sternum, it would start out by walking in a posterolateral direction, but would quickly round a curve that would aim it toward the front. Its hike would be along a great, sweeping arc ending when it reached the cartilaginous portion of the sternal attachment. In short, the rib's course—running posterolateral and then arching around to the anterior aspect of the body—provides the bony structure for most of the posterior, lateral, and anterior aspects of the thorax. In addition, the fly would have hiked downhill, because the ribs slope downward when the rib cage is inactive and at equilibrium. The beauty of the rib cage, the vertebral attachments, and the chondral (cartilaginous) portion of the sternal attachment is that the rib cage can elevate, providing an increase in lung capacity for respiration.

The posterior attachment of the rib is made through a gliding (arthrodial) articulation with the thoracic vertebrae, thus permitting the rib to rock up in both lateral and anterior aspects during inspiration. As mentioned, most of the ribs actually attach to two vertebrae.

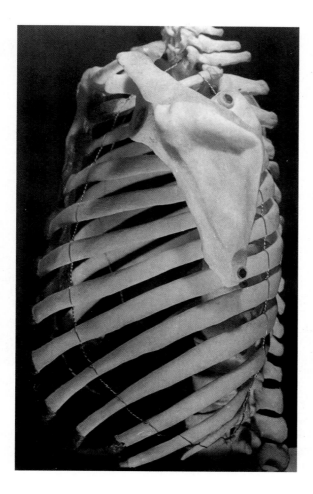

Figure 2–16. Lateral view of the rib cage. The downward tilt of the rib cage in front provides one of the mechanisms for increasing the volume of the thorax during respiration. *Source:* From Seikel/Drumright/King. *Anatomy & Physiology for Speech, Language, and Hearing, 5th Ed.* ©Cengage, Inc. Reproduced by permission.

Sternum

manubrium sterni: L., handle of sternum

ensiform: L., ensi, sword; sword-like

xiphoid: Gr., sword

manubrosternal angle: the point of articulation of manubrium sterni and corpus sterni

The sternum has three components: the **manubrium sterni**, the **corpus sterni** (body), and the **ensiform** or **xiphoid** process (Figure 2–17). The sternum has articular cavities for costal attachment, with the manubrium sterni providing the attachment for the clavicle and first rib, and the second rib articulating at the juncture of the manubrium and corpus, known as the **manubrosternal angle**. The corpus provides articulation for five more ribs by means of relatively direct costal cartilage, and the remaining (false) ribs 8, 9, and 10 are attached by means of costal cartilage as well.

The sternum provides an excellent opportunity to investigate anatomy with your own hands. As you look at Figure 2–17 of the sternum, you can palpate your own sternal structures. First, find your Adam's apple, which will

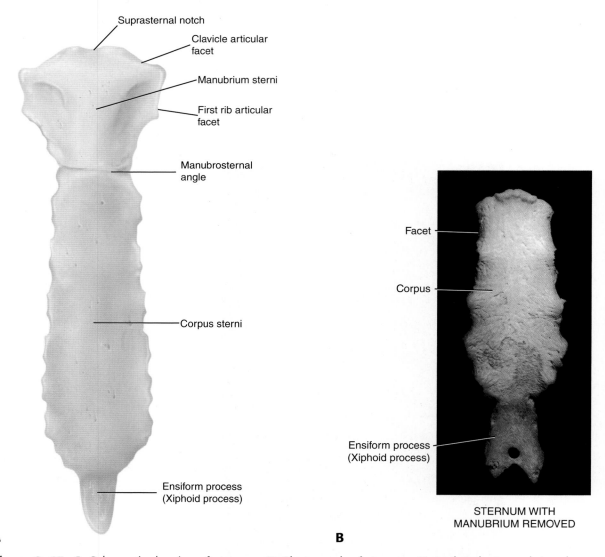

A

Suprasternal notch

Clavicle articular facet

Manubrium sterni

First rib articular facet

Manubrosternal angle

Corpus sterni

Ensiform process (Xiphoid process)

B

Facet

Corpus

Ensiform process (Xiphoid process)

STERNUM WITH MANUBRIUM REMOVED

Figure 2–17. A. Schematic drawing of sternum. **B.** Photograph of sternum. Note that the manubrium has been removed from the sternum. *Source:* From Seikel/Drumright/King. *Anatomy & Physiology for Speech, Language, and Hearing, 5th Ed.* ©Cengage, Inc. Reproduced by permission.

be quite a bit less pronounced in females for reasons we will talk about in the next unit. This prominence is actually a landmark of the thyroid cartilage of the larynx. Now bring your finger downward until you reach the significant plateau at about the level of your shoulders. This is the superior surface of the manubrium sterni and is known as the **suprasternal** or **sternal notch**. Ignoring the tendon that you can feel on either side, palpate the bone that is directed laterally. This is the clavicle. If you can feel the place where the clavicle articulates with the manubrium, you can probably find the articulation of the first rib immediately inferior to it. If you once again find the sternal notch and draw your finger downward about 2 inches, you may feel a very prominent bump, which is the manubrosternal angle or junction. Now if you draw your finger downward another 4 or 5 inches, you can find the point at which the sternum and xiphoid process articulate, an important landmark for individuals performing cardiopulmonary resuscitation (CPR). At that point, you have also found the anterior-most attachment of your diaphragm.

⊘ *To summarize:*

- The **rib cage** is composed of 12 ribs (7 true ribs, 3 false ribs, and 2 floating ribs).

- The **cartilaginous attachment** of the ribs to the sternum permits the ribs to rotate slightly during respiration, allowing the rib cage to elevate.

- The construction of the rib provides the characteristic curved barrel shape of the rib cage.

- At rest, the ribs slope downward, but they elevate during inspiration.

Soft Tissue of the Thorax and Respiratory Passageway

Deep to the rib cage lies the core of respiration. Gas exchange for life occurs within the lungs, which are made up of spongy, elastic tissue that is richly perfused with vascular supply and air sacs. Healthy, young lungs are pink, whereas older lungs that have undergone the stresses of modern, polluted life are distinctly gray. Communication between the lungs and the external environment is by means of the respiratory passageway, which includes the oral and nasal cavities, larynx, trachea, and bronchial tubes.

The **trachea** is a flexible tube, approximately 11 cm in length and composed of a series of 16 to 20 hyaline cartilage rings that are open in the posterior aspect. This tube runs from the inferior border of the larynx for about 11 cm, where it bifurcates (divides) to become the left and right **mainstem bronchi** (or **bronchial tubes**), which serve the left and right lungs, respectively (Figure 2–18). Note that within this bifurcation is the carina tracheae. The **carina** is the inner cartilaginous edge of the bifurcation, and the epithelial lining overlying the carina is extremely sensitive to contact by foreign bodies, providing a last line of defense through the cough reflex.

suprasternal notch: a.k.a. sternal notch. the notch on the superior aspect of the manubrium sterni

ANAQUEST LESSON ▶

trachea: Gr., tracheia, rough; cartilaginous tube connecting larynx and bronchial passageways

bronchi: Gr., bronchos, air passageway

bronchial tubes: another name for mainstem bronchi, the cartilaginous tubes connecting the trachea to the lungs

carina: L., keel of boat

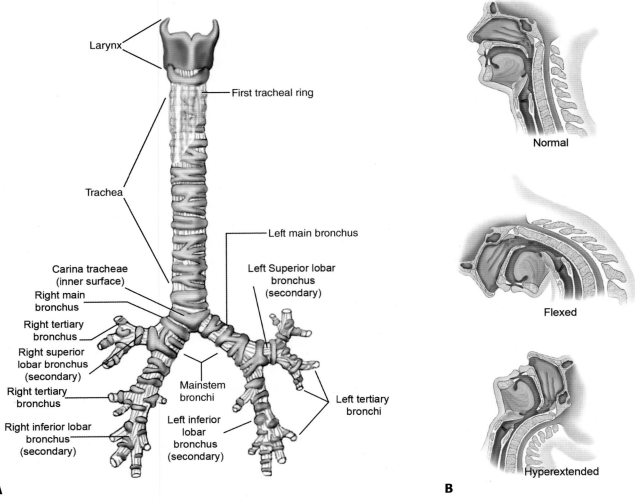

Figure 2–18. A. Bronchial passageway, including trachea, mainstem bronchi, lobar (secondary) bronchi, and segmental (tertiary) bronchi. *Source:* From Seikel/Drumright/King. *Anatomy & Physiology for Speech, Language, and Hearing, 5th Ed.* ©Cengage, Inc. Reproduced by permission. **B.** Effect of head posture on airway patency. Note that both flexion and hyperextension narrow the airway, compromising respiration in unconscious patients. *Source:* From Seikel/Drumright/King. *Anatomy & Physiology for Speech, Language, and Hearing, 5th Ed.* ©Cengage, Inc. Reproduced by permission. *continues*

Keeping the Airway Open in Respiratory Emergency

In times of respiratory emergency, it sometimes becomes necessary to ensure that the respiratory pathway remains patent (open). In a conscious patient, the normal head and neck orientation places the mouth at a 90° angle with the airway above the larynx and the pharyngeal space. If an unconscious individual's head flexes forward (see Figure 2–18B), the airway may become occluded and limit respiration. In the case of hyperextension, the airway is also narrowed. Both hyperextension and flexion can reduce or occlude the airway in an unconscious patient.

In some cases, there may be concern that the vocal folds or airway above the larynx will not remain open, so an emergency tracheostomy is performed (*trachea*, trachea; *stoma*, mouth). This medical procedure involves opening an artificial passageway into the trachea, typically 1 to 3 cm below the cricoid cartilage.

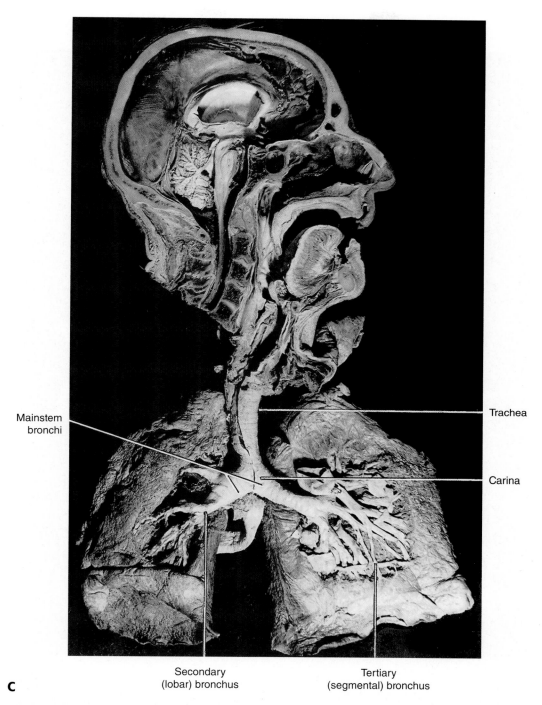

Mainstem
bronchi

Trachea

Carina

Secondary
(lobar) bronchus

Tertiary
(segmental) bronchus

C

Figure 2–18. *continued* **C.** Respiratory passageway from oral cavity to segmental bronchi. Note that lungs have been dissected to reveal the bronchi within. *Source:* From Seikel/Drumright/King. *Anatomy & Physiology for Speech, Language, and Hearing, 5th Ed.* ©Cengage, Inc. Reproduced by permission. *continues*

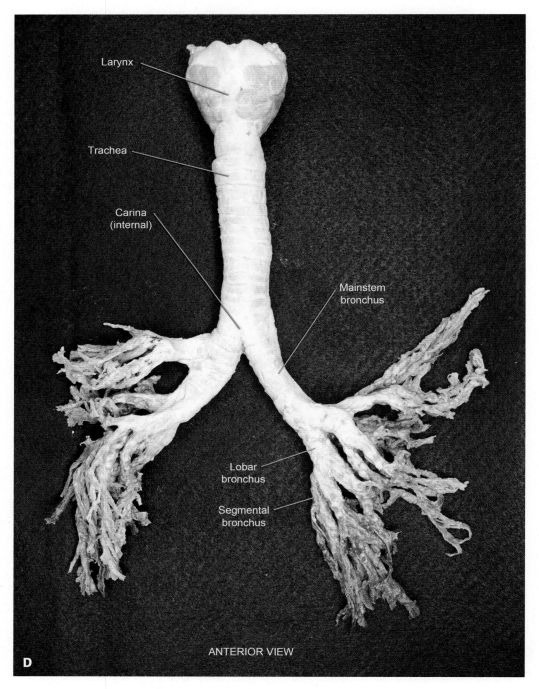

Figure 2–18. *continued* **D.** Anterior view of bronchial tree. *continues*

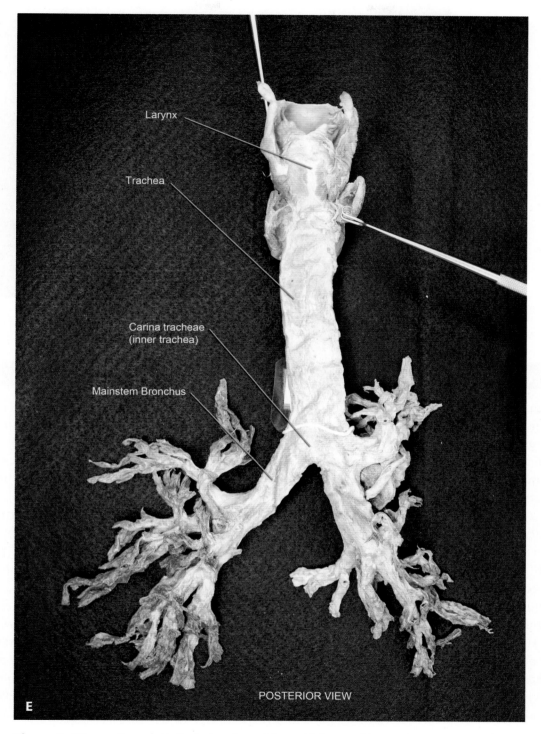

Larynx

Trachea

Carina tracheae
(inner trachea)

Mainstem Bronchus

POSTERIOR VIEW

E

Figure 2–18. *continued* **E.** Posterior view of bronchial tree with esophagus removed.
continues

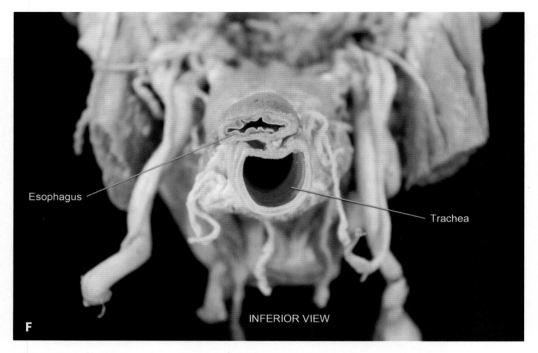

Esophagus

Trachea

INFERIOR VIEW

F

Figure 2–18. *continued*   **F.** Inferior view of relationship between trachea and esophagus.

Congenital Thorax Deformities

A number of congenital (present at birth) problems may occur within the thoracic wall. **Pectus excavatum** is a condition in which the sternum and costal cartilages are depressed relative to the rib cage. This depression may be bilateral or asymmetrical, providing the individual with costal flaring, a broad-but-thin chest and hook-shoulder deformity. The deformity can be repaired surgically but may reoccur, especially during the period of rapid growth in puberty. The opposite deformity, **pectus carinatum**, involves protrusion of the sternum anteriorly. Surgical repair is typically successful.

Poland's syndrome is a congenital condition in which both the pectoralis major and minor muscles are absent, and the child has fusion of the fingers or toes (syndactyly). The muscles may be partially or completely absent, and the breast is typically involved. In significantly affected individuals, the anterior and cartilaginous portions of ribs 2 through 5 may be absent as well. Although the muscle cannot be restored, surgery can correct the defect of the rib cage to establish thoracic symmetry.

Cleft sternum is a rare congenital deformity that can have devastating consequences. In the simple and more benign case, the sternum has a simple cleft as a result of failure of the sternal bars during gestation. The cleft is covered with skin, and the heart and diaphragm are normal. *Ectopia cordis* is a life-threatening form of cleft sternum, in which the infant is born with the heart exposed extrathoracically. Repair of this condition is extremely difficult.

You may wish to examine the thorough discussion of these disorders in Schamberger (2000).

The tracheal rings are 2 to 2.5 cm in diameter, and 0.4 to 0.5 cm wide. They are connected by a continuous mucous membrane lining, which provides both continuity and flexibility. The ring is discontinuous in the posterior aspect, allowing for increase and decrease of the diameter of the ring, an action largely controlled by the trachealis muscle. The gap between the rings is spanned by smooth muscle that is in a steady state of contraction until oxygen needs of an individual increase, at which time the muscle relaxes. That is, the tube is in a state of slight constriction until oxygen needs are sufficiently great that the muscle action is inhibited, at which time the diameter of the trachea increases to improve air delivery to the lungs. The inner mucosal lining of the trachea is infused with submucosal glands that assist in cleaning the trachea.

The cartilaginous rings of the trachea are particularly well suited for the task of air transport. Because the process involves drawing air into the lungs and expelling it, pressures (negative and positive) must be generated to get that gas moving. Pressure tends to collapse or expand cavities that are not reinforced for strength. Yet, a strictly rigid tube would not permit the degree of flexibility dictated by an active life (i.e., differential head and thorax movement). Thus, the trachea must be both rigid and flexible. In response to this need, the trachea is built of hyaline cartilage rings connected by fibroelastic membrane. The cartilage provides support, while the membrane permits freedom of movement.

Posterior to the trachea is the **esophagus**. The esophagus is a long, collapsed tube running parallel to and behind the trachea, providing a conduit to the digestive system. It retains its collapsed condition except when occupied with a **bolus** of food being propelled by gravity and peristaltic contractions to the waiting stomach.

The trachea bifurcates to form the right and left mainstem (or main) bronchi. The right side forms a 20° to 30° angle relative to the trachea, and the left forms a 45° to 55° angle. (This difference explains why the right lung is most often the landing site for the errant peanut that makes it past the protective laryngeal structure.)

The lungs are a composite of blood, arterial and venous network, connective tissue, respiratory pathway, and tissue specialized for gas exchange. The **bronchial tree** is characterized by increasingly smaller tubes as it progresses into the depths of the lungs, but the total surface area at any given level of the tree is greater than that of the level before it. There are 14 generations of the bronchial tree in the left lung and 28 generations in the right lung, beginning with the single trachea. The left and right mainstem bronchi bifurcate off the trachea to serve the left and right lungs, respectively, while **lobar** (secondary or intermediate) bronchi supply the lobes of the lungs (see Figure 2–18). **Tertiary** branches arise from the lobar branches, serving each segment of a lobe. Below this level of segmental branching there are numerous sub-segmental branchings, ending with the final **terminal respiratory bronchioles**. This division process is shown in Table 2–2 and Figure 2–19. Within the cartilaginous passageway, there are 1 trachea, 2 mainstem bronchi, 5 lobar bronchi, 19 segmental bronchi, and so forth. The essential concept to grasp is that each branch provides rapidly increasing volume of air passageway.

esophagus: the tube connecting the laryngopharynx with the stomach, through which food passes during swallowing

bolus: L., lump

lobar bronchi: secondary bronchial passageways connecting the mainstem bronchi with individual lobes of the lungs

segmental (tertiary) bronchi: segmental bronchial passageways connecting the lobar (secondary) bronchi with individual segments of each lobe

terminal respiratory bronchioles: the last bronchioles in the respiratory tree, connecting the respiratory tree to the alveoli

Table 2–2

Divisions of the Bronchial Tree						
	Generation From					
	Trachea	**Segmental Bronchus**	**Terminal Bronchiole**	**Number**	**Diameter**	**Cross-Section**
Trachea	0			1	2.5 cm	5.0 cm^2
Main bronchi	1			2	11–19 mm	3.2 cm^2
Lobar bronchi	2–3			5	4.5–13.5	2.7 cm^2
Segmental	3–6	0		19	4.5–6.5 mm	3.2 cm^2
Subsegmental bronchi	4–7	1		38	3–6 mm	6.6 cm^2
Bronchi		2–6		Variable	Variable	Variable
Terminal bronchi		3–7		1,000	1.0 mm	7.9 cm^2
Bronchioles		5–14		Variable	Variable	Variable
Terminal bronchioles		6–15	0	35,000	0.65 mm	116 cm^2
Respiratory bronchioles			1–8	Variable	Variable	Variable
Terminal respiratory bronchioles			2–9	630,000	0.45 mm	1,000 cm^2
Alveolar ducts and sacs			4–12	14 × 10^6	0.40 mm	1.71 m^2
Alveoli				300 × 10^6	0.24–0.3 mm	70 m^2

From *Respiratory Emergencies* by K. M. Moser & R. G. Spragg, 1982, p. 15. St. Louis, MO: C. V. Mosby. Copyright 1982 C. V. Mosby Co. Reprinted with permission.

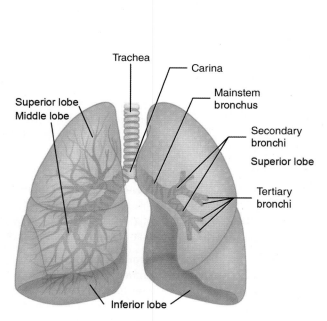

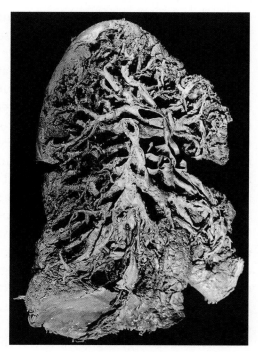

Figure 2–19. A. Bronchial tree. **B.** Lung dissected to reveal bronchial passageway. *Source:* From Seikel/Drumright/King. *Anatomy & Physiology for Speech, Language, and Hearing, 5th Ed.* ©Cengage, Inc. Reproduced by permission.

Nanotechnology and the Body

As technology advances, our susceptibility to design errors increases. Nanotechnology is the field involved in the production of nanoscale devices that include micromotors, molecule-sized robots, and chemical delivery systems. The nanoscale devices are proliferating as production abilities develop, but there remain questions about the body's response to them. The fact that the lungs are not capable of eliminating pollutants that are very small has prompted research into the impact of airborne nanoscale particles on respiration.

Recent evidence indicates that the effects of nanoscale particles may extend to the vascular supply as well. We know that particulate pollution from automobiles in the 2.5 micrometer (called PM2.5 particles, or 2.5 parts per million) range is related to increases in heart disease. Recent evidence reveals that particles 1/10 the size (PM0.25) cause increases in the buildup of atherosclerotic plaque.

These particles enter the lungs as pollution and, because of their minute size, are able to enter the bloodstream. There they act like "cement," closing off the arteries of the vascular system. While the causal link has been proven only in mice (Araujo et al., 2008), there remains the distinct probability that what you cannot see will hurt you. That having been said, dust-level products have existed for some time (e.g., erionite and quartz dust), and much research is needed into the nature of their toxicology as well (Donaldson & Seaton, 2012).

On the flip side of the "nano-coin" is use of technology as filters. Nanoscale materials are being developed that absorb specific toxins within the body and are being designed to greatly enhance our ability to image cancer and even to treat diseases (Sargent, 2011). Nanoscale technology has the potential for being an exceptionally powerful societal force in the coming years.

The lobar or secondary divisions serve the lobes of the lungs. The right lung is composed of three lobes, separated by fissures. The left lung has only two lobes (see Figure 2–19). Space on the left is taken up by the heart and **mediastinal** or "middle space" structures. The right mainstem bronchus divides to supply the superior, middle, and inferior lobes of the right lung. The left mainstem bronchus bifurcates to serve the superior and inferior lobes of the left lung, although there is a vestigial middle lobe (called the **lingula**). The space of the missing lobe is taken up by the heart on the left side (Figure 2–20).

The third level of branching serves the segments of each lobe. At this third level of division, the bronchi divide repeatedly into smaller and smaller cartilaginous tubes, with the final tube being the **terminal** (end) **bronchiole** (Figure 2–21).

This repeated branching has an important effect on respiratory function. There are up to 28 generations of subdivisions in the respiratory tree, with between 14 and 17 of these being involved in gas exchange (Phalen & Oldham, 1983). This branching provides a truly amazing amount of surface area for respiration (Spector, 1961). Although the cross-sectional area of the trachea is about 5 cm^2 (about the size of a quarter), the cross-sectional area of the 300,000,000 alveoli would equal 70 m^2, or the area of a rug large enough to cover a 10 × 24 room.

The first nine divisions of the bronchial tree (trachea through terminal bronchioles) are strictly conductive and cartilaginous, being designed only to transport gas between the environment and the lungs (see Table 2–2).

Right lung		Left lung	
Superior lobe		Superior lobe	
Apical	1	Upper division	
Posterior	2	Apical/Posterior	1 & 2
Anterior	3	Anterior	3
Middle lobe		Lower division (lingular)	
Lateral	4	Superior lingula	4
Medial	5	Inferior lingula	5
Inferior lobe		Inferior lobe	
Superior	6	Superior	6
Medial basal	7	Anterior medial basal	7 & 8
Anterior basal	8	Lateral basal	9
Lateral basal	9	Posterior basal	10
Posterior basal	10		

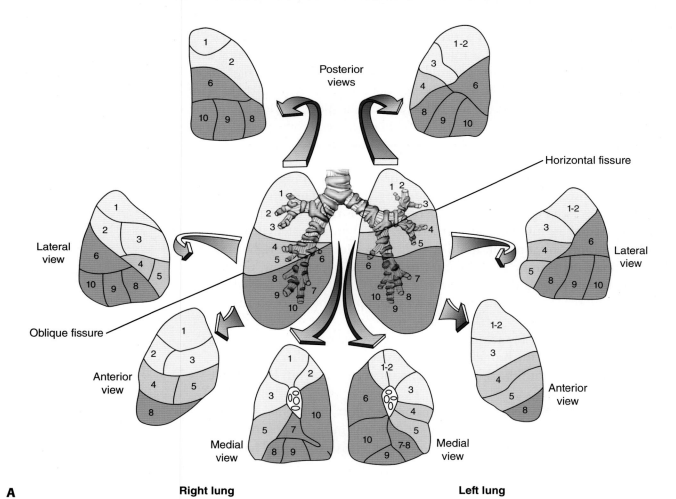

A   **Right lung**   **Left lung**

Figure 2–20. A. Schematic representation of lungs, showing lobes and segments. *Source:* From Seikel/Drumright/King. *Anatomy & Physiology for Speech, Language, and Hearing, 5th Ed.* ©Cengage, Inc. Reproduced by permission. *continues*

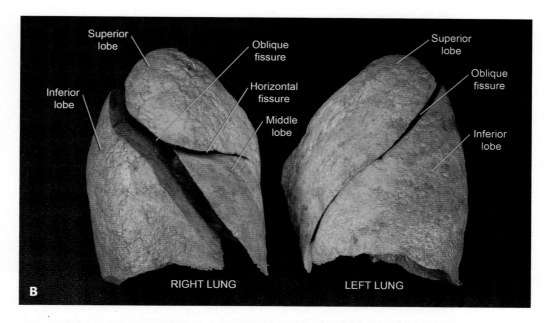

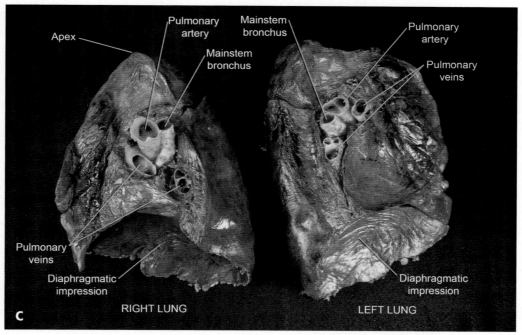

Figure 2–20. *continued* **B.** Lobes and fissures of the lungs. **C.** Root of the lungs shown through medial view. Note pulmonary artery and veins. *continues*

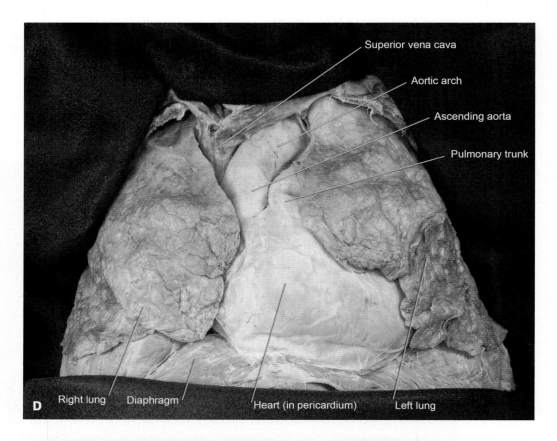

D

Superior vena cava

Aortic arch

Ascending aorta

Pulmonary trunk

Right lung   Diaphragm   Heart (in pericardium)   Left lung

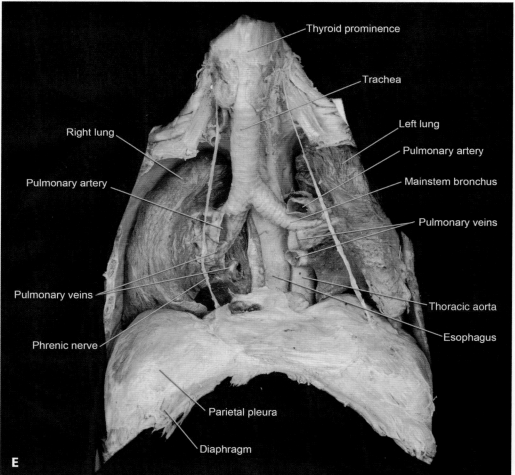

E

Thyroid prominence

Trachea

Right lung   Left lung

Pulmonary artery   Pulmonary artery

Mainstem bronchus

Pulmonary veins

Pulmonary veins

Thoracic aorta

Esophagus

Phrenic nerve

Parietal pleura

Diaphragm

Figure 2–20. *continued* **D.** Heart and lungs in situ. Note relationship of heart and lungs with diaphragm. **E.** Bronchial tree. Note diaphragm and phrenic nerve that innervates it. *continues*

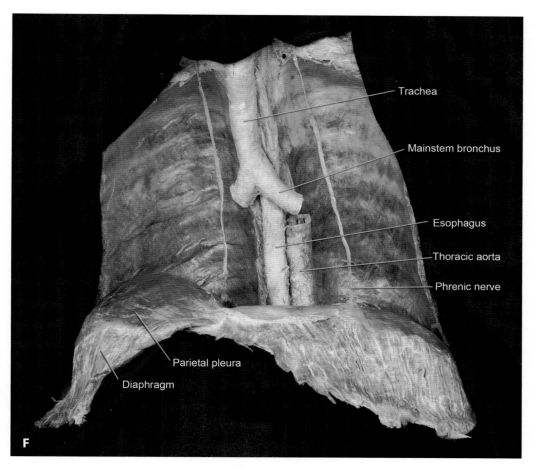

Figure 2–20. *continued* **F.** Thoracic cavity.

Labels in figure: Trachea, Mainstem bronchus, Esophagus, Thoracic aorta, Phrenic nerve, Parietal pleura, Diaphragm, F

Gastroesophageal Reflux

The esophageal orifice is situated in the inferior laryngopharynx and is enveloped by the musculature of the inferior pharyngeal constrictors. The cricopharyngeus muscle, which is actually part of the inferior constrictor, controls the size of the orifice by contracting to constrict the opening.

Gastroesophageal reflux refers to the reintroduction of gastrointestinal contents into the esophagus and respiratory passageway. This condition may be found in the newborn and very young child who has a weak esophageal sphincter or hypersensitivity of the esophageal sphincter, resulting in reflux, inability to retain nourishment, and life-threatening malnutrition. It is not uncommon among children with cerebral palsy, typically resulting in frequent vomiting, loss of nutrition, and aspiration pneumonia (see clinical note "Aspiration").

The size of the esophageal opening may be reduced surgically through a procedure known as **Nissen fundoplication** ("sling"), thereby inhibiting regurgitation of stomach contents. Nissen fundoplication involves surgical narrowing of the esophageal opening by releasing a flap of tissue from the stomach, followed by elevation and suturing of the flap to the esophageal orifice. The individual may receive nutrition through a nasogastric tube (*naso,* nose; *gastric,* stomach) run through the nasal cavity into the esophagus or through orogastric feeding (oral feeding, a.k.a. gavage), again via tube.

Surgical placement of a gastronomy tube may be required if reflux cannot be controlled adequately to guarantee nutrition. This procedure, referred to as **gastronomy**, results in surgical placement of a feeding tube into the stomach wall. Similarly, **jejunostomy** is the placement of a feeding tube into the small intestine. For a more detailed discussion of these problems in cerebral palsy, see Langley and Lombardino (1991).

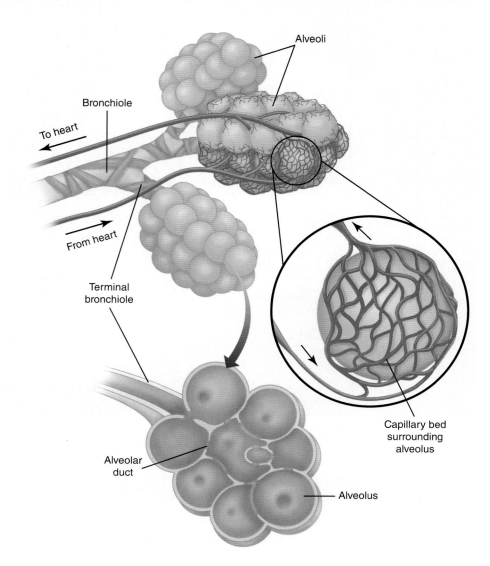

Figure 2–21. Schematic representation of cluster of alveoli with capillary bed. Lower portion shows a cross-section through alveoli and terminal bronchiole. *Source:* From Seikel/Drumright/ King. *Anatomy & Physiology for Speech, Language, and Hearing, 5th Ed.* ©Cengage, Inc. Reproduced by permission.

Successive divisions of the noncartilaginous airway (respiratory bronchioles) reach a minimal diameter of 1 mm. This conducting zone, which includes the conducting regions of both the upper and lower respiratory tracts and terminates with the terminal bronchioles, makes up approximately 150 mL in the adult, a volume known as *dead air* because air that does not descend below the space cannot undergo gas exchange with the blood. The final divisions are actual respiratory zones composed of the respiratory bronchioles, alveolar ducts, and alveoli. The respiratory bronchioles ("little bronchi") are the terminal bronchioles, serving the alveoli.

The terminal bronchiole is small (about 1 mm in diameter) and at its end becomes the alveolar duct, which in turn communicates with the alveolus. The alveoli are extremely small (approximately 1/4 mm in diameter), but extremely plentiful, with approximately 300 million in the mature lungs.

You might think of the final respiratory exchange region as a series of apartment houses. As you can see in Figure 2–21, the respiratory bronchioles

thorax almost impervious to the outside world, were it not for the respiratory passageway. The only way air can enter or leave the lungs is by means of the tubes connected to them (the bronchial tree, continuous with the upper respiratory passageway).

Now comes the tricky part. The lungs are simply placed inside this cavity, not held to the walls by ligaments or cartilage. It is as if you placed a too-small sponge in a too-large bottle, because the thoracic volume is *greater* than that of the lungs at rest.

The lungs and inner thoracic wall are each completely covered with a **pleural lining** (Figure 2–22) that provides a means of smooth contact for rough tissue, as well as a mechanism for translating the force of thorax enlargement into inspiration. The lungs are encased in linings referred to as the **visceral pleurae** and the thoracic linings are the **parietal pleurae**. The regions of the parietal pleurae are identified by location: mediastinal, pericardial (not shown in figure), diaphragmatic, parietal, and apical pleurae. The **mediastinal pleura** covers the mediastinum and the **diaphragmatic pleura** covers the diaphragm. The **costal pleurae** cover the inner surface of the rib cage. The **apical pleurae** cover the superior-most region of the rib cage.

The pleural membranes are composed of elastic and fibrous tissue and are endowed with **venules** and lymphocytes. Although it is convenient to think of the pleural linings as being separate entities, the visceral and parietal pleurae are actually continuous with each other. These wrappings completely encase both the lungs and the inner thorax, with the reflection point being the hilum (root of lung, at about the level of T4 or T5). This continuous sheet provides the airtight seal required to permit the lungs to follow the movement of the thorax.

pleural: Gr., pleura, a side

visceral pleurae: pleural linings encasing the lungs

parietal pleurae: pleural linings of the thoracic cavity

mediastinal pleura: parietal pleural lining covering the mediastinum

diaphragmatic pleura: parietal pleural lining covering the diaphragm

costal: L., costae, coast

costal pleurae: pleural lining of the inner rib cage.

apical pleurae: parietal pleural linings covering the lung superior aspect

venules: L., venula, tiny veins

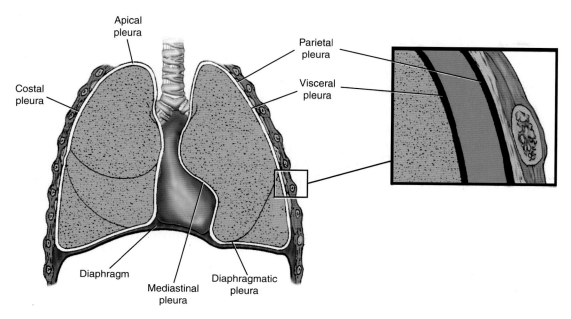

Figure 2–22. Pleural linings of the lungs and thorax. Parietal pleurae include costal, diaphragmatic, mediastinal, and apical pleurae. Visceral pleurae line the surface of the lungs. *Source:* From Seikel/Drumright/King. *Anatomy & Physiology for Speech, Language, and Hearing, 5th Ed.* ©Cengage, Inc. Reproduced by permission.

Pleurisy

Pleurisy is a condition in which the pleural linings of the thoracic cavity are inflamed. When the inflammation results in dry pleurisy, the patient experiences extreme pain upon breathing as a result of the loss of lubricating quality of the intrapleural fluid. Adhesions may result, in which portions of the parietal pleurae adhere to the visceral pleurae. (The patient may experience "breaking up" of these adhesions for quite some time following a bout with pleurisy.) Pleurisy may be unilateral or bilateral and may result in excessive fluid (potentially purulent) in the pleural space.

When you contract the **diaphragm**, the pleural lining of the diaphragm maintains its contact with the visceral pleurae of the two lungs above it, causing the lungs to expand. Likewise, if you expand the thorax transversely by elevating the rib cage, you find that the lungs follow faithfully. In this manner, the lungs are able to follow the action of the muscles without actually being attached to them.

The pleural linings serve another function as well. Because the mating surfaces of the two linings are infused with a serous secretion, the friction of movement of the two linings is greatly reduced, making respiration much more efficient. When this fluid is lost or reduced, as in the disorder known as dry pleurisy, the friction is greatly increased and pain results. As a protection, each lung is separately endowed with a pleural lining. If the lining of one lung is damaged through disease or trauma, we still have the other lung in reserve.

diaphragm: the primary, unpaired muscle of respiration that completely separates the abdomen and thorax

Understanding how these pleurae help us breathe takes a little thought. You have probably experienced the difficulty involved in separating two pieces of plastic food wrap, especially if there is fluid between the two sheets. There is a degree of surface tension arising from the presence of fluid and highly conforming surfaces that helps keep the sheets together. Cuboidal cells within the pleural lining produce a mucous solution that is released in the space between the parietal and visceral pleurae. This surfactant reduces the surface tension in the lungs and provides a slippery interface between the lungs and the thoracic wall, permitting easy, low-friction gliding of the lungs within the thorax. The presence of surfactant keeps the two sheets from clinging to each other. The two surfaces conform to each other as a result of the fluid bond between them, and a negative pressure is maintained by lack of contact with the outside atmosphere. (If you puncture the membrane, the bond is broken.)

We have discussed the lungs and hinted at the second most important muscle of the body (the diaphragm), but have glossed over the fact that the most important muscle of the body (the heart) is located deep within the thorax, in a region known as the **mediastinum**. The heart is encased in the mediastinal pleurae, along with nerves, blood vessels, lymphatic vessels, and the esophagus (Figure 2–23).

mediastinum: L., medius, middle; middle space

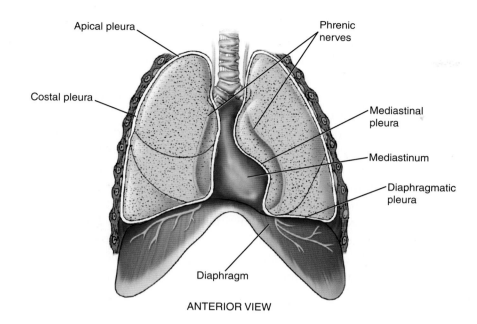

Apical pleura

Phrenic nerves

Costal pleura

Mediastinal pleura

Mediastinum

Diaphragmatic pleura

Diaphragm

ANTERIOR VIEW

Figure 2–23. Relationship among pleural linings of mediastinum, diaphragm, and lungs. Note the phrenic nerve innervation of the diaphragm. *Source:* From Seikel/Drumright/King. *Anatomy & Physiology for Speech, Language, and Hearing, 5th Ed.* ©Cengage, Inc. Reproduced by permission.

The mediastinum is the most protected region of the body. This space is occupied primarily by the heart, as well as by the trachea, the major blood vessels, nerves, the thymus gland, lymph nodes, and the conducting portion of the gastrointestinal tract known as the esophagus.

The mediastinum lies deep to the bony thorax and its muscular coverings and is nestled deep in the lungs. Its central location in the body betrays its importance to all regions, and its critical placement surrounded by lung tissue guarantees efficient transfer of gas to (and from) the blood pumped by the heart.

Because the heart is such an important muscle, it is located deep within several layers of thick muscle and bone. In the posterior are the vertebrae and the massive muscles of the back, and the anterior-lateral aspect of the thorax is a strong wall of bone and muscle. The heart is well protected against most trauma, with the exception of romantic disappointment!

The organs and structures of the mediastinum are encased by a continuation of the parietal pleurae. This lining provides a low-friction mating surface between the lungs and the middle space. The visceral pleural lining of the lungs adjacent to the mediastinum is termed the **mediastinal pleura.** The left and right phrenic nerves serving the diaphragm pass anterior to the root structures of the lungs, coursing along the lateral surfaces of the pericardium (the membranous sac enclosing the heart) to innervate the diaphragm. The left and right vagus nerves enter the posterior mediastinum to innervate the heart, first passing behind the root structures of the lung, coursing inferiorly to the anterior and posterior surfaces of the esophagus. They descend through the diaphragm adjacent to the esophagus through the esophageal **hiatus** to innervate the abdominal viscera. The vagal pulmonary branches provide a parasympathetic nerve supply for the lungs, with nerve fibers found even in the smallest bronchioles. The vagus mediates the cough reflex and controls the airway diameter.

hiatus: L., an opening

Movement of the rib cage for inspiration requires muscular effort. Muscles of respiration may be divided into muscles of inspiration and expiration (Table 2–3). Before delving into these muscles, we should give you a word of caution. The primary muscles of respiration are relatively easy to identify, but we will inevitably make some assumptions about function of secondary muscle groups based on muscle attachment. It is also wise to explain at the start that expiration can be either forced or passive but is much more often a passive process. Thus, the muscles of expiration are not always active and depend on some other forces to help us eliminate carbon dioxide–laden air. A second, very important note is that *identification of origin and insertion are determined by function.* Remember that our speech mechanisms are built on nonspeech functions: Sometimes we use muscles for speech in a manner that is different from the basic function, which means that *the origin and insertion may be different from what you might find in basic anatomy texts.* This reality reflects just how ingenious we humans have been at making the basic human physiology work for speech, language, and hearing.

Table 2–3

Muscles of Respiration

Inspiration	Expiration
Muscles of trunk	**Muscles of trunk**
Primary of thorax	**Muscles of thorax, back, and upper limb anterior**
Diaphragm	Internal intercostal (interosseous portion)
Accessory of thorax anterior	Transversus thoracis
External intercostal	**Posterior**
Inner intercostal, interchondral portion	Subcostal
Posterior	Serratus posterior inferior
Levatores costarum (brevis and longis)	Innermost intercostal
Serratus posterior superior	Latissimus dorsi
Muscles of neck	**Abdominal muscles anterolateral**
Sternocleidomastoid (superficial neck)	Transversus abdominis
Scalenus (anterior, middle, posterior)	Internal oblique abdominis
Trapezius	External oblique abdominis
Muscles of thorax, back, and upper limb	Rectus abdominis
Pectoralis major	**Posterior**
Pectoralis minor	Quadratus lumborum
Serratus anterior	
Subclavius	
Levator scapulae	
Rhomboideus major	
Rhomboideus minor	

✅ *To summarize:*

- The lungs are covered with **pleural linings**, which, in conjunction with the thoracic wall, provide the mechanism for air movement through muscular action.

- When the diaphragm contracts, the lungs are pulled down because of the association between the pleurae and the diaphragm.

- **Diaphragmatic contraction** expands the lungs, drawing air into them through the bronchial passageway.

- Origins and insertions are based on the function of the muscle as used for speech, and this may result in reversal of these functional descriptions with those found in classical anatomy.

Muscles of Inspiration

As with many voluntary bodily functions, inspiration is a graded activity. Depending on the needs of your body, you are capable of **quiet inspiration**, which involves primarily the diaphragm, and **forced inspiration**, which calls on many more muscles. We enlist the help of increasingly larger numbers of muscles as our respiratory needs increase. You may wish to refer to Appendix C for a summary of the muscles of respiration.

If the lungs are to expand and fill with air, the thorax must increase in size as well. As mentioned, there are only two ways this can happen. The first way to expand the thorax is to increase its vertical (superior-inferior) dimension, a process that occurs for both quiet and forced inspiration. Picture the lungs encased in bone around the barrel-shaped midsection of the rib cage

ANAQUEST LESSON

quiet inspiration: inspiration that involves minimal muscular activity, primarily that of the diaphragm

forced inspiration: inspiration that involves both diaphragm and accessory muscles of inspiration

Muscle:	Diaphragm, Sternal head
Origin:	Xiphoid process of sternum
Course:	Superiorly and medially
Insertion:	Central tendon
Innervation:	Phrenic nerve arising from cervical plexus of spinal nerves C3, C4, and C5
Function:	Depresses central tendon of diaphragm; enlarges vertical dimension of thorax; distends abdomen and compresses abdominal viscera
Muscle:	Diaphragm, Costal head
Origin:	Inferior margin of ribs 7 through 12
Course:	Superiorly and medially
Insertion:	Central tendon
Innervation:	Phrenic nerve arising from cervical plexus of spinal nerves C3, C4, and C5
Function:	Depresses central tendon of diaphragm; enlarges vertical dimension of thorax; distends abdomen and compresses abdominal viscera

Muscle:	Diaphragm, Vertebral head
Origin:	Transverse processes of L1, corpus of L1 through L4
Course:	Superiorly and medially
Insertion:	Central tendon
Innervation:	Phrenic nerve arising from cervical plexus of spinal nerves C3, C4, and C5
Function:	Depresses central tendon of diaphragm; enlarges vertical dimension of thorax; distends abdomen and compresses abdominal viscera

and bounded above by the clavicle and first rib. Remember that the rib cage is open at the bottom.

A thin but strong muscle placed across the bottom margin of the rib cage, configured like a drumhead, would be an economical means of expanding the size of the rib cage without having to manipulate the bony portion at all. The thorax and abdominal cavity below are separated by one of the most important muscles of the body, the diaphragm.

The diaphragm takes the form of an inverted bowl, with its attachments along the lower margin of the rib cage, sternum, and vertebral column. It forms a complete separation between the upper (thoracic) and lower (abdominal) chambers; and when it contracts, the force of contraction is directed downward toward the abdominal viscera. This contraction results in elongation of the cavity formed by the ribs, so that the lungs expand and air enters through the respiratory passageway.

Primary Inspiratory Muscle of the Thorax: The Diaphragm

The primary muscle of inspiration is the diaphragm. As seen in Figure 2–24, the diaphragm completely separates the abdominal and thoracic cavities (with the exception of vascular and esophageal hiatuses). The edges attach along the inferior boundary of the rib cage, to the xiphoid process, and to the vertebral column in the posterior aspect. The intermediate region is made up of a large, leafy aponeurosis called the **central tendon**. When the muscle contracts, muscle fibers shorten and the diaphragm pulls the central tendon down and forward. Let us look at this extremely important muscle in detail.

The muscle fibers of the diaphragm radiate from the central tendon, forming the sternal, costal, and vertebral attachments. The anterior-most sternal attachment is made at the xiphoid process, with fibers coursing up and back to insert into the anterior central tendon. Lateral to the xiphoid, the fibers of the diaphragm attach to the inner border of ribs 7 through 12 and to the costal cartilages to form the costal attachment. In the posterior aspect, the vertebral diaphragmatic attachment is made with the corpus of L1 through L4 and transverse processes of L1.

central tendon: large aponeurosis making up the central portion of the diaphragm

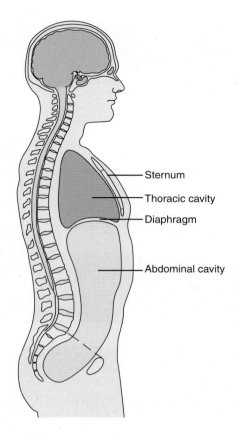

- Sternum
- Thoracic cavity
- Diaphragm
- Abdominal cavity

A

Figure 2–24. A. Lateral-view schematic of the diaphragm and thorax. Notice that the diaphragm courses markedly down from the sternum to the vertebral attachment, completely separating the thorax from the abdomen. *Source:* From Seikel/Drumright/King. *Anatomy & Physiology for Speech, Language, and Hearing, 5th Ed.* ©Cengage, Inc. Reproduced by permission. *continues*

The fibers from these attachments course upward and inward to insert into the central tendon (Figure 2–25). The posterior vertebral attachment also provides support for the esophageal hiatus. The vertebral attachment is accomplished by means of two **crura**. The right crus arises from attachment at L1 through L4, in which the fibers ascend and separate to encircle the esophageal hiatus. Fibers of the left crus also arise from L1 through L4, passing to the left of the hiatus.

Although the diaphragm separates the thorax from the abdomen, the need for nutrients dictates that there be communication between the oral cavity and abdominal region. The region below the diaphragm also has vascular needs, and these require supply routes through the diaphragm. There are three openings (diaphragmatic hiatuses) through which structures pass. As seen in Figure 2–25, the descending abdominal aorta passes through the aortic hiatus located adjacent and lateral to the vertebral column. The *esophageal hiatus*, through which the esophagus passes, is found immediately anterior to the aortic hiatus, while the inferior vena cava traverses these two cavities by means of the foramen vena cava (which is in the right-central aspect of the diaphragm as viewed from above).

The actual muscle fibers of the diaphragm radiate from the imperfect center formed by the central tendon. Careful examination of the forces of muscular contraction will be most helpful in later discussion of muscular

crus: L., cross (plural: crura)

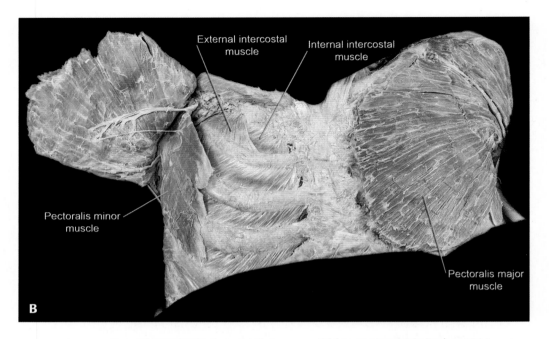

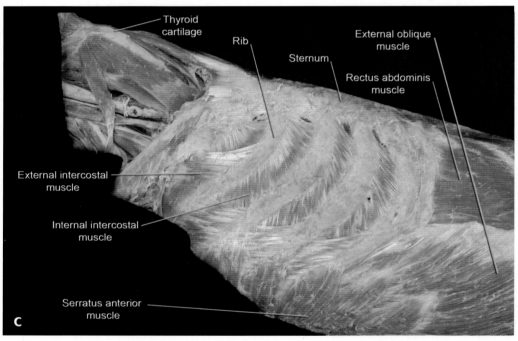

Figure 2–24. *continued* **B.** Anterior view of rib cage, showing accessory thorax muscles of respiration. **C.** Lateral view of thorax, in supine position.

contraction and action. Realize, again, that muscle can perform only one task, and that is to shorten. If a muscle is attached to two points, shortening will tend to bring those two points closer together, or simply tense the muscle if neither point is capable of moving. The basic muscle function

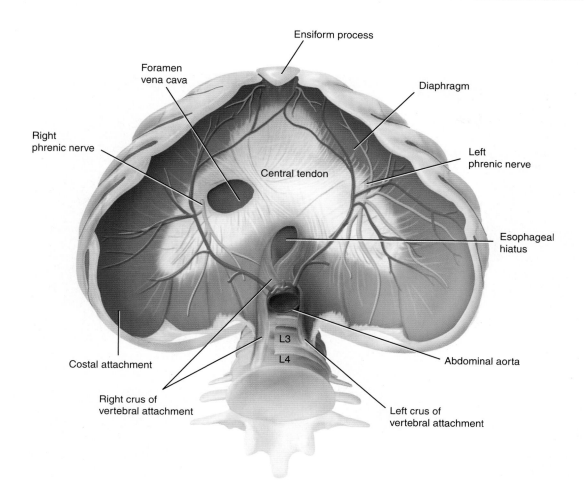

A INFERIOR VIEW

Figure 2–25. A. Inferior-view schematic of diaphragm, as seen from the abdominal cavity. *Source:* From Seikel/Drumright/King. *Anatomy & Physiology for Speech, Language, and Hearing, 5th Ed.* ©Cengage, Inc. Reproduced by permission. *continues*

of the diaphragm is somewhat more complex. Movement of the diaphragm will not make a great deal of sense, although the principles of muscle action and resulting shortening of the muscle still hold, until you realize where the points of attachment really are.

Figure 2–26 is a schematic drawing of the diaphragm and central tendon. First, look at the upper portion of the figure. If you choose some subset of those fibers and shorten them, the end result will be that the central tendon moves toward the point of firm attachment, the origin. But when the diaphragm contracts, all fibers contract together, which means that all fibers pull equally on the central tendon. Now look at the second part of the figure and trace the same effect. If you contract (shorten) one fiber, the central tendon moves down toward the origin of the fiber. If you contract the entire diaphragm, the net result is that the diaphragm is pulled down as a

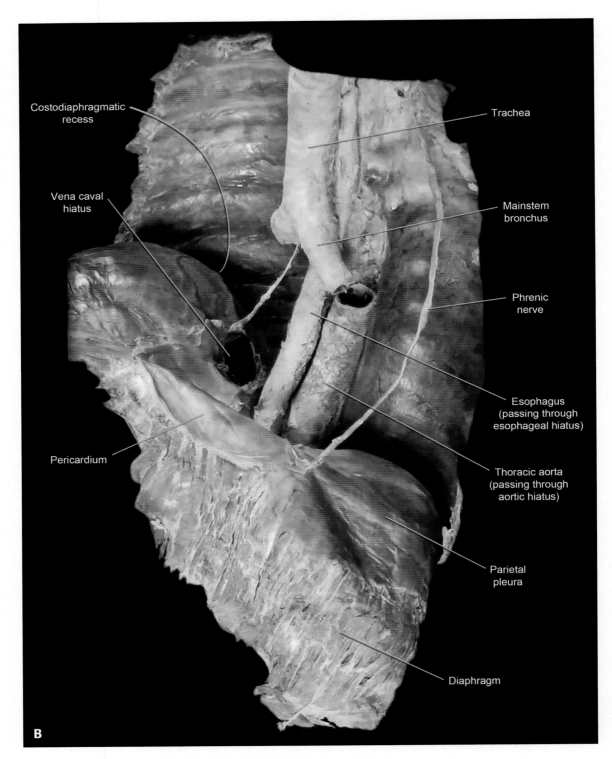

Figure 2–25. *continued* **B.** Photograph of superior view of diaphragm.

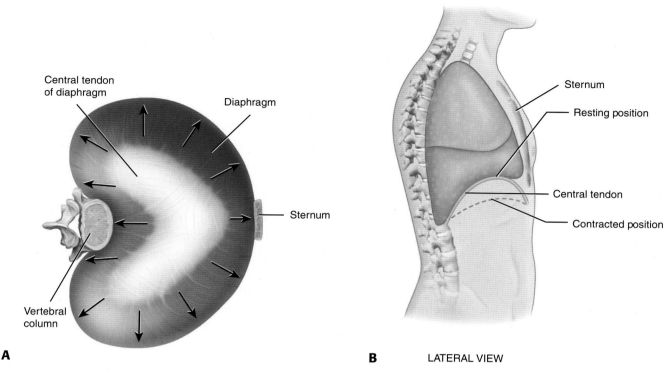

Figure 2–26. A. Schematic of transverse view of the diaphragm with central tendon. The arrows depict the direction of force upon contraction of the diaphragm. **B.** This lateral view of the diaphragm shows that contractions of the diaphragm pull the central tendon downward. *Source:* From Seikel/Drumright/King. *Anatomy & Physiology for Speech, Language, and Hearing, 5th Ed.* ©Cengage, Inc. Reproduced by permission.

unit. The fibers in the front are longer than those in the back. *Contraction of the diaphragm has the result of pulling the central tendon downward and forward.* This contraction is directly analogous to placing someone in the middle of a blanket while a host of friends pull on all of the corners of the blanket. When the friends pull together, the person in the middle flies up. Because the diaphragm has the shape of an inverted bowl, pulling on the edges (muscular contraction) draws the center down, but (gravity notwithstanding) the analogy holds.

The prominent central tendon is the last element of the diaphragm that we need to consider. Look again at Figure 2–26 and notice that the central tendon is a crescent-shaped aponeurosis that is white and translucent. The tendon tends to conform to the prominence of the vertebral column in the thoracic cavity, so its shape mimics the curvature of the transverse thoracic cavity. It has the flexibility of an aponeurosis, but has no contractile qualities. It depends on the radiating fibers of the diaphragm for movement. Above the central tendon is the heart, and this tendon provides a strong and secure floor for that mediastinal organ.

Innervation of the diaphragm is by means of the **phrenic nerves** (see Figure 2–23). The diaphragm can be placed under voluntary control (you can hold your breath), but it is primarily under the control of the autonomic

phrenic nerves: the nerve arising from the cervical plexus that innervates muscular activity of the diaphragm

cervical plexus: group of nerves that anastomoses from the spinal nerves C1, C2, C3, and C4

system (you have no choice but to breathe eventually). Nature has provided bilateral innervation of the diaphragm, supporting the notion that this is an exceptionally important unpaired muscle. The phrenic nerves originate in the **cervical plexus** (a *plexus* is a group of nerves coming together for a common purpose) from spinal nerves C3, C4, and C5 on both sides of the spinal cord (Kuehn, Lemme, & Baumgartner, 1989; Miller, Bianchi, & Bishop, 1997).

Each phrenic nerve descends deep to the omohyoid and sternocleidomastoid muscles and superficial to the anterior scalenus muscle, into the mediastinal space on the left and right sides of the heart. The nerve fibers descend and divide to innervate the superior surface of the diaphragm. One branch (the left and right phrenicoabdominal) descends deep to innervate the inferior surface. The left branch is longer than the right, because it has a greater distance to travel around the mediastinum. The phrenic nerves mediate both motor and sensory information. The lower intercostal nerve serves the inferior-most boundary of the diaphragm.

One final comment is warranted on the diaphragm and its action. Throughout this description we have ignored the abdominal viscera; beneath the diaphragm are numerous organs that undergo continual cycles of compression during respiration, a fact that will work to the advantage of anyone wishing to forcefully exhale (or perform the Heimlich maneuver, as we shall see).

✔ To summarize:

- The primary muscle of inspiration is the **diaphragm**, the dividing line between the thorax and the abdomen.
- The fibers of the diaphragm pull on the **central tendon**, resulting in the downward motion of the diaphragm during inspiration. This movement expands the lungs in the **vertical dimension**.

ANAQUEST LESSON

Accessory Muscles of Inspiration

Although the diaphragm is the major contributor to inspiration, it needs help to meet the needs of your body for forced inspiration. If you take a look at Figure 2–27, you can see the rib cage from the side. Direct your attention first to the way the ribs run: They are directed distinctly downward as they make their path to the front of the skeleton. Next, imagine raising the ribs in front, and realize that when you do that, the front of the rib cage expands. Swinging those ribs up means that they will swing out a bit in both anterior and lateral aspects, thereby increasing the volume of the rib cage.

For a demonstration of this function in everyday terms, look at Figure 2–27 showing venetian blinds from the side. When they are closed, they are similar to the rib cage at rest, and when they are tilted, so that you can see through them, they are similar to the point of elevation of the ribs. That elevation brings the ribs more nearly horizontal, just like the blinds, which increases the overall front-back dimension.

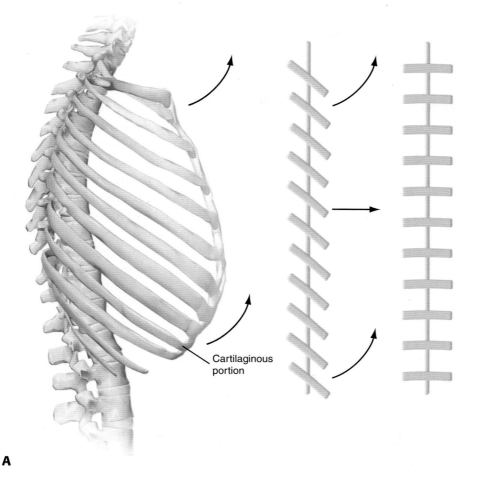

A

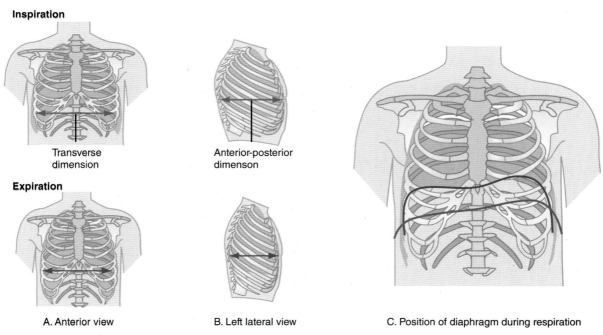

Inspiration

Transverse
dimension

Anterior-posterior
dimenson

Expiration

A. Anterior view · · · B. Left lateral view · · · C. Position of diaphragm during respiration

B

Figure 2–27. A. Schematic of rib cage from the side. Notice that the ribs slant down as they run forward. During inspiration, the rib cage elevates, as shown by the arrows. On the right side, the "Venetian blinds" shown from the side demonstrate the change in volume achieved by elevation of the rib cage. **B.** Schematic showing changes in thoracic dimensions during inspiration and at expiration to the resting state. *Source:* From Seikel/Drumright/King. *Anatomy & Physiology for Speech, Language, and Hearing, 5th Ed.* ©Cengage, Inc. Reproduced by permission.

Because the goal is to raise all of the ribs, we rely on the muscles attached to broad areas of the ribs to achieve this. The **external intercostal** muscles (Figure 2–28) are positioned so that when they contract, the entire rib cage elevates, with most of the distance moved being in the front aspect.

By labeling these muscles as accessory muscles of inspiration, we are acknowledging the simple fact that we could perform the respiratory act without them. They provide a significant increase in the amount of air we are able to process, but one is capable of surviving on diaphragmatic support alone, in the absence of the accessory muscles. You most likely are using little of the accessory muscles as you quietly read this text, but you would probably invoke them to help you discuss this chapter in front of a class. We differentiate these muscles based on the region of the body: anterior and posterior thoracic muscles, neck muscles, and muscles of the arm and shoulder.

Anterior Thoracic Muscles of Inspiration

External Intercostal and Interchondral Portion, Internal Intercostal Muscles

The external intercostal muscles are among the most significant accessory respiratory muscles for speech. They not only provide a significant proportion of the total respiratory capacity, but they also perform functions that are uniquely speech-related.

As you can see in Figure 2–28, the 11 external intercostal muscles reside between the 12 ribs of the thorax, providing the ribs with both unity and mobility. The external intercostal muscles originate in the lower surface of

Figure 2–28. A. Rib cage with external and internal intercostal muscles. External intercostals are absent near the sternum, and thus one can see the deeper internal intercostals within that region. *Source:* From Seikel/Drumright/King. *Anatomy & Physiology for Speech, Language, and Hearing,* 5th Ed. ©Cengage, Inc. Reproduced by permission. *continues*

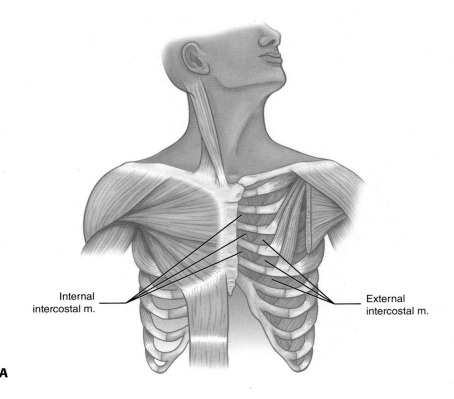

Internal intercostal m.

External intercostal m.

A

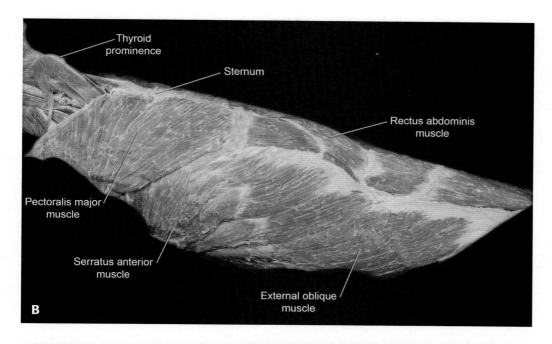

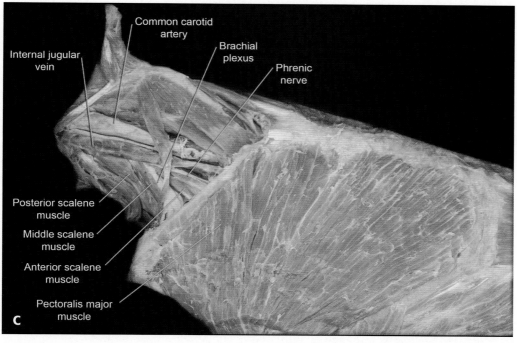

Figure 2–28. *continued* **B.** Photograph showing some accessory muscles of inspiration and expiration, including rectus abdominis, external oblique, serratus anterior, and pectoralis major muscles. **C.** Accessory muscles of respiration of the thorax and neck. Note the presence of brachial plexus *continues*

each rib (except rib 12) and course downward and inward to insert into the upper surface of the rib immediately below. These muscles provide a unified surface of diagonally slanting striated muscle on all costal surfaces of the rib cage with the exception of the region near the sternum, because contraction

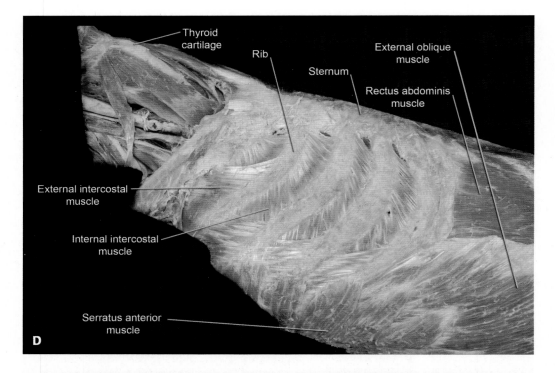

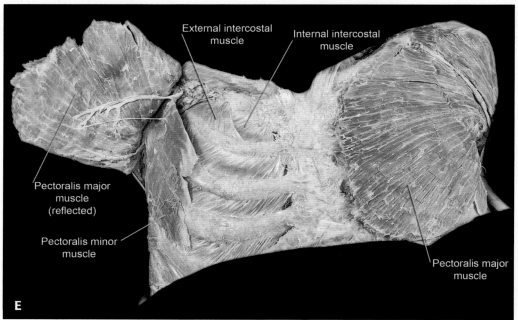

Figure 2–28. *continued* **D.** Intercostal muscles. **E.** Pectoral muscles.

of external intercostal fibers in that region would provide little benefit (and perhaps some negative effect) to the job of increasing cavity size.

The external intercostal muscles are covered with the translucent intercostal membrane that separates them from the internal intercostal muscles.

The internal intercostal muscles are predominantly muscles of expiration, with the exception of the interchondral (cartilaginous) component. The

parasternal (near the sternum) portion of the internal intercostal muscles encompassing the chondral aspect of the ribs is active during forced inspiration. The musculature is capable of segmental activation, so that one portion of this muscle can contract while contraction of the rest of the muscle is inhibited. The cross-laced effect of external and internal intercostal muscles forms a strong protective barrier for the lungs and heart and an impervious cavity for the forces of gas exchange.

Functionally, the external intercostal muscles elevate the rib cage. When the rib cage is elevated, the flexible coupling of the costo-sternal attachment permits the chondral portion of the ribs to rotate as they elevate. The net result is that the sternum remains relatively parallel to the vertebral column even as the rib cage expands, increasing the anterior dimension and thus the volume of the lungs (see Figure 2–27).

Innervation of the external intercostal muscles is achieved by the anterior divisions of the 11 pairs of thoracic spinal nerves, identified by the location of the region they innervate. The thoracic intercostal nerves arise from T1 through T6, and the thoracoabdominal intercostal nerves that pass into the abdominal wall arise from T7 through T11. These intercostal nerves supply not only the intercostal muscles but also several other muscles of respiration located in the anterior abdominal wall (Figure 2–29).

Although the external intercostals account for most of the second dimensional change (the anterior-posterior dimension), there are other

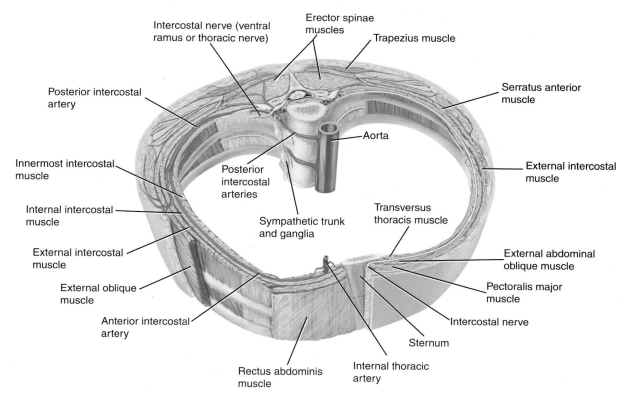

Figure 2–29. Schematic of intercostal nerves as seen from within the thoracic cavity.

Muscle:	External intercostal muscles
Origin:	Inferior surface of ribs 1 through 11
Course:	Down and obliquely in
Insertion:	Upper surface of rib immediately below
Innervation:	Intercostal nerves: thoracic intercostal nerves arising from T1 through T6 and thoracoabdominal intercostal nerves from T7 through T11
Function:	Elevate rib cage

Muscle:	Internal intercostal muscles, interchondral portion
Origin:	Upper margin of ribs 2 through 12
Course:	Up and in
Insertion:	Lower surface of rib above
Innervation:	Intercostal nerves: thoracic intercostal nerves arising from T1 through T6 and thoracoabdominal intercostal nerves from T1 through T11
Function:	Elevate ribs 2 through 12

muscles that, by virtue of their arrangement, are assumed to be of help. Any muscle that attaches to the rib cage or sternum, and could feasibly elevate either, could assist in the process of inspiration.

Some other possible assistants in respiration are the **levatores costarum** (brevis and longis) and **serratus posterior superior**, shown in Figure 2–30. They elevate the rib cage on contraction.

serratus: L., serratus, toothed; notched

Posterior Thoracic Muscles of Inspiration

- Levatores Costarum (Brevis and Longis)
- Serratus Posterior Superior
- Erector Spinae (Sacrospinal Muscles)
- Lateral (Illiocosto Cervicalis) Bundle
- Intermediate (Longissimus) Bundle
- Medial (Spinalis) Bundle

Levator Costarum (Brevis and Longis). If you examine the course of the levator costarum (*levator*, elevator; *costarum*, of the rib) shown in Figure 2–30A you will see that shortening these muscles tends to elevate the rib cage. Although these muscles may appear to be muscles of the back, they are considered to be thoracic muscles. The **brevis** (brief) portions of the levator costarum originate on the transverse processes of vertebrae C7 through T11, for a total of 12 levator costarum brevis muscles. Fibers course obliquely down and out to insert into the tubercle of the rib below (McMinn, Hutchings & Logan, 1994).

The **longis** portions originate on the transverse processes of T7 through T11, with fibers coursing down and obliquely out. The fibers bypass the rib

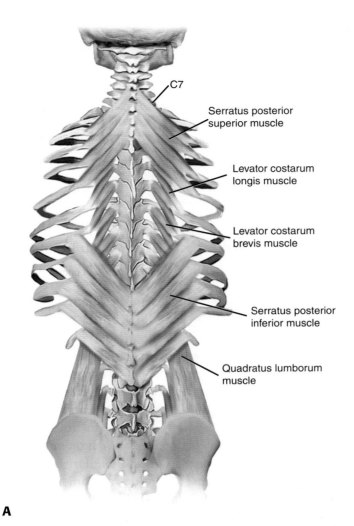

C7

Serratus posterior
superior muscle

Levator costarum
longis muscle

Levator costarum
brevis muscle

Serratus posterior
inferior muscle

Quadratus lumborum
muscle

A

Figure 2–30. A. Posterior thoracic muscles of inspiration. Note that the levatores costarum are present on all ribs, but in the superior aspect they are deep to the serratus posterior muscles. *Source: From Seikel/Drumright/ King. Anatomy & Physiology for Speech, Language, and Hearing, 5th Ed.* ©Cengage, Inc. Reproduced by permission. *continues*

below the point of origin, inserting rather into the next rib. You can see that the longis portion will have a greater effect on the elevation of the rib cage.

Much like the intercostal muscles, the levatores costarum take their innervation from the dorsal rami (branches) of the intercostal nerves. Upon exiting the spinal column, the dorsal rami course abruptly back, dividing into medial and lateral branches. The lateral branch of the dorsal ramus provides innervation of the levatores costarum.

Muscle:	Levator costarum, brevis
Origin:	Transverse processes of vertebrae C7 through T11
Course:	Obliquely down and out
Insertion:	Tubercle of the rib below
Innervation:	Dorsal rami (branches) of the intercostal nerves arising from spinal nerves C7 through T11
Function:	Elevate rib cage

Lateral (iliocosto cervicalis) bundle: Subdivided into iliocostalis lumborum, iliocostalis thoracis, and iliocostalis cervicis.

Muscle:	Iliocostalis lumborum of the lateral (iliocosto cervicalis) bundle
Origin:	Sacral crest, L1 through L5, T11 through T12 vertebrae
Course:	Up
Insertion:	Angles of ribs 6 through 12
Innervation:	Dorsal rami of lower cervical nerves and thoracic and lumbar nerves
Function:	Stabilizes and moves the vertebral column

Muscle:	Iliocostalis thoracis of the lateral (iliocosto cervicalis) bundle
Origin:	Ribs 6 through 12
Course:	Up
Insertion:	Ribs 1 through 6 and C7 vertebra
Innervation:	Dorsal rami of lower cervical nerves and thoracic and lumbar nerves
Function:	Stabilizes and moves the vertebral column

Muscle:	Iliocostalis cervicis of the lateral (iliocosto cervicalis) bundle
Origin:	Ribs 3 through 6
Course:	Up
Insertion:	C4 through C6 vertebrae
Innervation:	Dorsal rami of lower cervical nerves and thoracic and lumbar nerves
Function:	Stabilizes and moves the vertebral column

and C4, to insert into the posterior mastoid process of the temporal bone. Together, these muscles provide great support for the vertebral column and become major players in neck extension during development (Bly, 1994).

Medial (Spinalis) Bundle. This bundle consists of three muscles as well: spinalis thoracis, spinalis cervicis, and spinalis capitis. The spinalis thoracis is medial to the longissimus thoracis, arising from the posterior spines of the 11th and 12th thoracic vertebrae and L1 through L3. It inserts into the upper fourth through eighth thoracic vertebrae (T4–T8). The muscle spinalis cervicis is often absent, but if it is present, it courses from the nuchal ligament and posterior spine of C7 to insert into C2. Spinalis capitis is often indistinct from the semispinalis capitis, which arises from the posterior spine of T1 through T6 and C7, as well as the articular processes of C4 through C6, by means of a tendinous slip. The muscle inserts into the nuchal line of the skull and aids in neck extension and hyperextension.

Accessory Muscles of the Neck

- Sternocleidomastoid (Sternomastoid)
- Scalenes (Anterior, Middle, Posterior)

Muscle:	Longissimus thoracis of the intermediate (longissimus) bundle
Origin:	L1 through L5 transverse processes and thoracolumbar fascia
Course:	Up
Insertion:	T1 through T12 vertebrae, transverse processes and ribs 3 through 12
Innervation:	Dorsal rami of lower cervical nerves and thoracic and lumbar nerves
Function:	Stabilize and move vertebral column

Muscle:	Longissimus cervicis of the intermediate (longissimus) bundle
Origin:	T1 through T5 vertebrae
Course:	Up
Insertion:	C2 through C6 vertebrae, transverse processes
Innervation:	Dorsal rami of lower cervical nerves and thoracic and lumbar nerves
Function:	Stabilize and move vertebral column

Muscle:	Longissimus capitis of the intermediate (longissimus) bundle
Origin:	C1 through C5 vertebrae
Course:	Up
Insertion:	Posterior mastoid process of temporal bone
Innervation:	Dorsal rami of lower cervical nerves and thoracic and lumbar nerves
Function:	Stabilize and move vertebral column

Muscle:	Spinalis thoracis of the medial (spinalis) bundle
Origin:	T11 and T12, L1 through L3 vertebrae
Course:	Up
Insertion:	T1 through T8
Innervation:	Dorsal rami of lower cervical nerves and thoracic and lumbar nerves
Function:	Stabilize and move vertebral column

Muscle:	Spinalis cervicis of the medial (spinalis) bundle
Origin:	Nuchal ligament and C7 vertebra
Course:	Up
Insertion:	C2 vertebra
Innervation:	Dorsal rami of lower cervical nerves and thoracic and lumbar nerves
Function:	Stabilize and move vertebral column

Muscle:	Spinalis capitis of the medial (spinalis) bundle
Origin:	T1 through T6, C4 through C7 vertebrae
Course:	Up
Insertion:	Nuchal line of skull
Innervation:	Dorsal rami of lower cervical nerves and thoracic and lumbar nerves
Function:	Stabilize and move vertebral column

Several neck muscles assist in inspiration (Figure 2–31). The **sternocleido-mastoid** (alternately sternomastoid) muscle makes a direct attachment to the sternum and elevates that structure and the rib cage with it. Other potential muscles of inspiration are the **scalenus anterior**, **medius**, and **posterior** muscles, which are muscles of the neck. When they contract, they elevate the first and second ribs.

As with virtually all anatomical structures involved in speech, the muscles of the neck serve double duty. Although the muscles discussed in this section are important for respiration, they are also sources of stability and control for neck flexion and extension. As an infant develops, it is the early control of neck musculature that marks the shift from the neonatal flexion position to one of balance between flexion and extension. When flexion and extension are balanced, the infant is well on the road toward whole-body stability required for speech.

Sternocleidomastoid. The sternocleidomastoid courses from its origin on the mastoid process of the temporal bone to its insertion at the sternum

Muscle:	Sternocleidomastoid (sternomastoid)
Origin:	Mastoid process of temporal bone
Course:	Down
Insertion:	Sternal head: superior manubrium sterni
Clavicular head:	Superior surface of clavicle
Innervation:	XI accessory, spinal branch arising from spinal cord in the regions of C2 through C4 or C5
Function:	Elevates sternum and, by association, rib cage

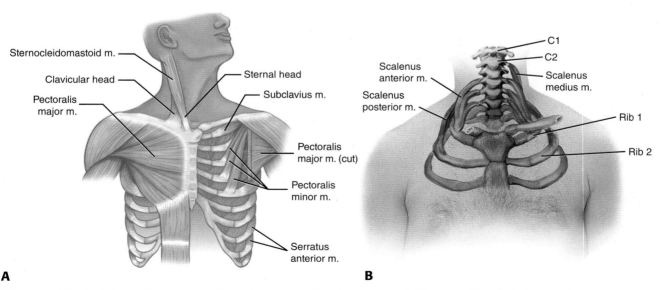

A   B

Figure 2–31. A. Schematic of pectoralis major, pectoralis minor, sternocleidomastoid, subclavius, and serratus anterior muscles. **B.** Schematic of scalenus anterior, medius, and posterior muscles. *Source:* From Seikel/Drumright/King. *Anatomy & Physiology for Speech, Language, and Hearing, 5th Ed.* ©Cengage, Inc. Reproduced by permission.

(sterno) and clavicle (cleido) (see Figure 2–31). This muscle is prominent, and its outline is easily visible on an individual, especially when the head is turned toward one side. When contracted separately, the sternocleidomastoid rotates the head toward the side of contraction. When both left and right sternocleidomastoid muscles are simultaneously contracted, the sternum and the anterior rib cage elevate.

The sternocleidomastoid and trapezius muscles derive their innervation from the 11th cranial nerve, spinal branch XI accessory. The spinal portions of the accessory nerves originate from rootlets that arise from the side of the spinal cord in the regions of C2 through C4 or C5. These fibers join to become the spinal root, ascending within the vertebral column behind the denticulate ligament. The spinal root enters the skull via the foramen magnum, where it joins with the cranial root to exit the skull through the jugular foramen. The spinal and cranial branches separate, with the spinal branch coursing to innervate the sternocleidomastoid. This is supported in this by its interconnection with C2 spinal nerve, which also innervates the muscle. This branch continues, descending deep to the trapezius muscle and above the clavicle, finally communicating with C3 and C4 to form a pseudoplexus, subsequently innervating the trapezius. The fibers of the cranial parts of the accessory nerve join the X vagus to be distributed among skeletal muscles as vagal fibers.

Scaleni Anterior, Middle, Posterior. The **scaleni** (or *scalenes*, as they also are called) are muscles of the neck that provide stability to the head and facilitate rotation; by virtue of their attachment to the first and second ribs, they also increase the vertical dimension of the thorax (Gray, Bannister, Berry, & Williams, 1995; Kang, Jeong, & Choi, 2016) (see Figure 2–31).

The anterior scaleni originate on the transverse processes of vertebrae C3 through C6, with fibers coursing down to insert into the superior surface of the first rib. The middle scaleni take their origin on transverse processes

scalenus: L., uneven

Clavicular Breathing

Clavicular breathing is a form of respiration in which thorax expansion arises primarily through the elevation of the rib cage via contraction of the accessory muscles of inspiration, most notably the sternocleidomastoid. Clavicular breathing is often an adaptive response by an individual to some previous or present pathological condition, such as chronic obstructive pulmonary disease, which prohibits use of other means to expand the thorax. Because elevation of the sternum results in only a small increase in thorax size, clavicular breathing is a less-than-perfect solution to the problem of respiration.

Use of accessory muscles of inspiration to augment diminished respiratory support most typically includes the anterior, middle, and posterior scalene muscles (to elevate the first and second ribs) and the sternocleidomastoid (to elevate the sternum and increase the anterior-posterior dimension of the rib cage). You may have seen patients with severe respiratory difficulties stretch out their arms and hold onto the back of a chair to breathe: When they do this, they give the pectoralis major muscles something to work against, thus allowing these muscles to increase the anterior-posterior dimension. You may have also seen a shrugging action by these patients, a sure sign that the trapezius muscle is in use to raise the rib cage.

Muscle:	Scalenus anterior
Origin:	Transverse processes of vertebrae C3 through C6
Course:	Down
Insertion:	Superior surface of rib 1
Innervation:	Cervical plexus and brachial plexus, derived from C3 through C8
Function:	Elevates rib 1

Muscle:	Scalenus medius
Origin:	Transverse processes of vertebrae C2 through C7
Course:	Down
Insertion:	Superior surface of the first rib
Innervation:	Cervical plexus and brachial plexus, derived from C3 through C6
Function:	Elevates rib 1

Muscle:	Scalenus posterior
Origin:	Transverse processes of C5 through C7
Course:	Down
Insertion:	Second rib
Innervation:	Cervical plexus and brachial plexus, derived from C3 through C8
Function:	Elevates rib 2

of vertebrae C2 through C7, also inserting into the first rib. The posterior scaleni insert into the second rib, having coursed from the transverse processes of C5 through C7.

The scaleni anterior are innervated by spinal nerves C3 through C8. The middle scaleni are innervated primarily by the cervical plexus and brachial plexus, derived from C3 through C6.

Accessory Muscles of the Upper Arm and Shoulder

- Pectoralis Major
- Pectoralis Minor
- Serratus Anterior
- Subclavius
- Levator Scapulae
- Rhomboideus Major
- Rhomboideus Minor
- Trapezius

The accessory muscles of the arm may assist the external intercostals in elevation of the thorax by virtue of their attachment to the sternum and ribs. Although not all have been confirmed through physiological study, the action of each of the following muscles has been thought to have the potential to increase the anterior–posterior dimension of the thorax.

Pectoralis Major and Minor. The pectoralis major is a large, fan-shaped muscle that originates from two heads (see Figure 2–31). The sternal head attaches along the length of the sternum at the costal cartilages, while the clavicular head arises from the anterior surface of the clavicle. The pectoralis major runs from the sternal and clavicular origins up and out to insert into the greater tubercle of the humerus. The muscle converges at the crest of the greater tubercle of the humerus. In respiration, the pectoralis major elevates the sternum and thus increases the transverse dimension of the rib cage (Cerqueira & Garbellini, 1999; Rohen, Yokochi, Lutjen-Drecoll, & Romrell, 2002). The pectoralis minor originates on the anterior surface of ribs 2 through 5, with fibers coursing up to converge on the coracoid process of the scapula. As with the pectoralis major, respiratory function involves elevation of the rib cage (Nepomuceno, Nepomuceno, Regalo, Cerqueira, & Souza, 2014).

Innervation of the pectoralis major and pectoralis minor is by the pectoral nerves arising from the medial and lateral cords of the brachial plexus, a formation of C5 through C8 and T1 spinal nerves (Figure 2–32).

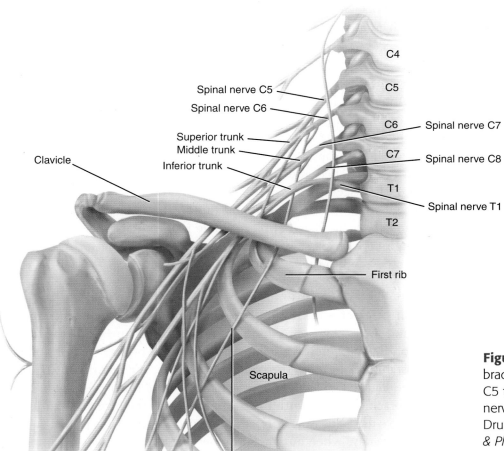

Figure 2–32. Schematic of brachial plexus arising from C5 through C8 and T1 spinal nerves. *Source:* From Seikel/Drumright/King. *Anatomy & Physiology for Speech, Language, and Hearing, 5th Ed.* ©Cengage, Inc. Reproduced by permission.

Muscle:	Pectoralis major
Origin:	Sternal head: length of sternum at costal cartilages; Clavicular head: anterior clavicle
Course:	Fan out laterally, converging at humerus
Insertion:	Greater tubercle of humerus
Innervation:	Superior branch of the brachial plexus (spinal nerves C5 through C8 and T1)
Function:	Elevates sternum and, subsequently, increases transverse dimension of rib cage

Muscle:	Pectoralis minor
Origin:	Anterior surface of ribs 2 through 5 near chondral margin
Course:	Up and laterally
Insertion:	Coracoid process of scapula
Innervation:	Superior branch of the brachial plexus (spinal nerves C5 through C8 and T1)
Function:	Increases transverse dimension of rib cage

Muscle:	Subclavius
Origin:	Inferior surface of clavicle
Course:	Oblique and medial
Insertion:	Superior surface of rib 1 at chondral margin
Innervation:	Brachial plexus, lateral branch, from C5 and C6
Function:	Elevates rib 1

Serratus Anterior. The saw-like fingers of this muscle give it its name (*serratus* as in serrated knife). Fibers of the serratus anterior arise from ribs 1 through 9 along the side of the thorax, coursing up to converge on the inner vertebral border of the scapula. Contraction of the muscle may elevate the ribs to which it is attached and subsequently the rib cage (Carlson, Hunt, & Johnson, 2017) (see Figure 2–31).

As with the pectoralis major and minor, the serratus anterior receives innervation from the brachial plexus. The long thoracic nerve arises from C5 through C7 and passes between the middle and posterior scalene neck muscles to descend to the level of the serratus anterior.

Subclavius. The subclavius muscle courses under the clavicle, as the name implies. It originates on the inferior margin of the clavicle and takes an oblique and medial course to insert into the superior surface of the first rib at the chondral margin. It is a small muscle with the primary responsibility of scapular stability, but it has the potential to elevate the first rib during inspiration (see Figure 2–31). The subclavius muscle is innervated by branches from the brachial plexus, with fibers originating in the fifth and sixth spinal nerves. The subclavius is not present in all people and is most likely a holdover from the days when our ancestors were quadrupeds.

Levator Scapulae. The levator scapulae provides neck support secondarily as a result of its function as an elevator of the scapula. This muscle originates

Muscle:	Serratus anterior
Origin:	Ribs 1 through 9, lateral surface of thorax
Course:	Up and back
Insertion:	Inner vertebral border of scapula
Innervation:	Brachial plexus, long thoracic nerve from C5 through C7
Function:	Elevates ribs 1 through 9

Muscle:	Levator scapulae
Origin:	Transverse processes of C1 through C4
Course:	Down
Insertion:	Medial border of scapula
Innervation:	C4 through C5
Function:	Neck support: elevates scapula

from the transverse processes of C1 through C4, and courses down to insert into the medial border of the scapula (Figure 2–33). As with the scaleni anterior, middle, and posterior, the levator scapulae derives its innervation from C4 through C5. Its respiratory component may well be postural, in that maintenance of forward head posture in respiration diminishes vital capacity,

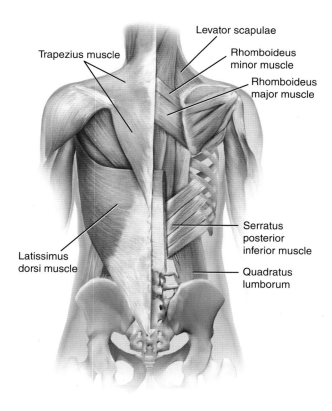

Levator scapulae

Trapezius muscle

Rhomboideus minor muscle

Rhomboideus major muscle

Latissimus dorsi muscle

Serratus posterior inferior muscle

Quadratus lumborum

POSTERIOR VIEW

Figure 2–33. Accessory muscles of respiration: trapezius, levator scapulae, rhomboideus minor, rhomboideus major, serratus posterior inferior, latissimus dorsi, and quadratus lumborum. *Source:* From Seikel/Drumright/King. *Anatomy & Physiology for Speech, Language, and Hearing, 5th Ed.* ©Cengage, Inc. Reproduced by permission.

and the levator scapulae is a significant contributor to neck extension (Han, Park, Kim, Choi, & Lyu, 2016).

Rhomboideus Major and Minor. The rhomboids (major and minor) lie deep to the trapezius, originating on the spinous processes of T2 through T5 (**rhomboideus** major) and from C7 and T1. The muscle courses down and laterally to insert into the medial border of the scapula. The primary speech function of the rhomboids is the support they provide for the upper body, and especially for the stability of the shoulder girdle (De Freitas & Vitti, 1980).

rhomboideus: L., rhombus, parallelogram; oid, like

The rhomboids receive their innervation from the dorsal scapular nerves off the upper roots of the brachial plexus (C4, C5). The dorsal scapular nerves pass through the scaleni medius muscles in their course to the rhomboids.

Trapezius. The trapezius muscle (see Figure 2–33) is a massive muscle making up the superficial upper back and neck, originating along the spinous processes of C2 to T12 by means of fascial connection. (The trapezius is alternately considered a muscle of the arm.) Fibers of this muscle fan laterally to insert into the acromion of the scapula and the superior surface of the clavicle. Contraction of this muscle clearly plays a significant role in elongation of the neck and for head control (Turgut, Duzgun, & Baltaci, 2016).

For respiration, support is the primary function of the back muscles, although there are distinct respiratory actions. Back muscles provide a dense, multilayered mass of tissue that supports and protects (see Figure 2–33). Perhaps the most important function of these muscles is the maintenance of the delicate balance of upper body mobility in the face of required stability.

Muscle:	Rhomboideus major
Origin:	Spinous processes of T2 through T5
Course:	Down and laterally in
Insertion:	Scapula
Innervation:	Spinal C4 and C5 from the dorsal scapular nerve of upper root of brachial plexus
Function:	Stabilizes shoulder girdle
Muscle:	Rhomboideus minor
Origin:	Spinous processes of C7 and T1
Course:	Down and laterally in
Insertion:	Medial border of scapula
Innervation:	Spinal C4 and C5 from the dorsal scapular nerve of upper root of brachial plexus
Function:	Stabilizes shoulder girdle

To experience this firsthand, place both feet firmly on the ground while sitting erect, and then with one arm reach straight ahead as if you were about to grasp an object beyond your reach. You will need to overextend when you do this, but if you attend to the musculature of your head, shoulders, and back, you will feel them tighten to support your efforts. Your shoulders rotate while the rest of your trunk remains relatively stable.

In the big picture of trunk control, certain back muscles are key players. The trapezius and levator scapulae muscles serve clear roles in neck elongation and head stability. Support for the vertebral column is provided by the trapezius muscle and the rhomboideus major and minor muscles, and this support serves respiration in a stabilizing manner. The erector spinae, discussed earlier, play a vital role in head, neck, and trunk stability. The clinical note "Trunk Stability and Upper Body Mobility," on the development of motor coordination, emphasizes the importance of trunk and back muscle development from an oral motor perspective.

Muscle:	Trapezius
Origin:	Spinous processes of C2 through T12
Course:	Fan laterally
Insertion:	Acromion of scapula and superior surface of clavicle
Innervation:	XI accessory, spinal branch arising from spinal cord in the regions of C3 and C4
Function:	Elongates neck: controls head

Trunk Stability and Upper Body Mobility

Infant motor development is a process of increasing the control of motor function: Control of speech musculature depends in large part on the development of trunk control. It is truly a "for want of a nail" situation: If the infant fails to develop neck extension, the ability to balance neck extensors and flexors will not develop. Once the normal extension begins development, the back muscles begin to come under control, again becoming dynamically opposed by anterior trunk muscles. Through this interplay of antagonist and agonist trunk muscles, the infant develops the ability to rotate the trunk, stabilize the hips (and, of course, walk), and elevate the head in preparation for speech. Once controlled, the infant can rotate the head, differentiate mandible movement from head movement and tongue from mandible. All the while, the infant is developing the dynamic aspects of laryngeal control that permit the larynx to descend and the tongue to become controlled.

This is a long-winded way of saying that, although the respiratory function of the back muscles is open to question, the absence of controlled use of the back muscles would most certainly result in loss of head control for speech, reduced differentiation of facial muscle control, and lack of laryngeal control due to the tonic imbalance of the torso. The indirect effects of muscle imbalance within the trunk are innumerable.

(✓) *To summarize:*

- The **diaphragm** is an exceptionally important muscle of inspiration, but there are many **accessory muscles** of inspiration and expiration that also serve respiration.
- Generally, muscles of the thorax and neck that elevate the rib cage serve some accessory function for inspiration.

In the next section we see that muscles that compress the abdomen or pull down on the rib cage also assist in expiration.

 ANAQUEST LESSON (▶)

Muscles of Forced Expiration

Active expiration requires that musculature act on the lungs indirectly to "squeeze" the air out of them. This is achieved in two ways. Because the rib cage expands in two dimensions, it makes sense that its volume can be reduced through manipulation of those two dimensions as well. The front-to-back dimension is expanded by elevating the rib cage, so active expiration should reduce that dimension. The rib cage can be pulled down by the internal intercostal muscles, the innermost intercostal muscles, and the transversus thoracis muscles. Remember that the second means of expanding the volume of the thorax is by increasing the vertical dimension through contraction of the diaphragm (Figure 2–34) and relaxing the diaphragm returns it to its original position, and no farther. If you note the viscera of the abdomen below the diaphragm, you can see the second means of active

Figure 2–34. Lateral-view schematic of diaphragm showing relative position during inspiration (contracted position) and passive expiration (resting position). *Source:* From Seikel/Drumright/King. *Anatomy & Physiology for Speech, Language, and Hearing, 5th Ed.* ©Cengage, Inc. Reproduced by permission.

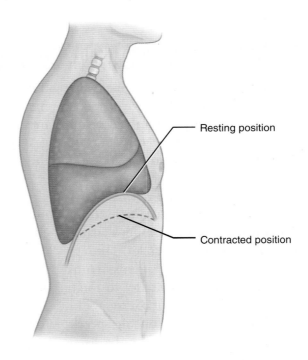

Resting position

Contracted position

LATERAL VIEW

expiration. If you can somehow squeeze your abdominal viscera, you will be able to push your diaphragm higher into the thorax and remove more air from your lungs. (If you want to verify this, have one of your friends perform a gentle version of the Heimlich maneuver on you and feel what happens with your respiration. Do you inhale or exhale?)

We can forcefully expire by contracting the muscles of the abdominal region, which, in turn, squeeze the abdomen and force the viscera upward, reducing the size of the thorax. This is half of the reason you get the wind knocked out of you when someone punches you in the abdomen. See the clinical note "Getting the Wind Knocked Out of You" for the other half of that story.

If you examine the abdominal muscles of expiration (Figure 2–35), you see that they are very much like a cummerbund, wrapping the abdomen into a neat package in the front, side, and back. The major players in the anterior abdomen are the internal and external oblique abdominis, transversus abdominis, and the **rectus** abdominis muscles. In the posterior abdomen, the quadratus lumborum, iliacus, and psoas major and minor muscles serve this function (Cala et al., 1992). If you look at Figure 2–33, you can see that the latissimus dorsi muscles appear to be useful in maintaining an open, expanded thorax during respiration for professional singers and could well have that function in everyday speaking as well, particularly if the speaker is projecting the voice (Watson, Williams, & James, 2012).

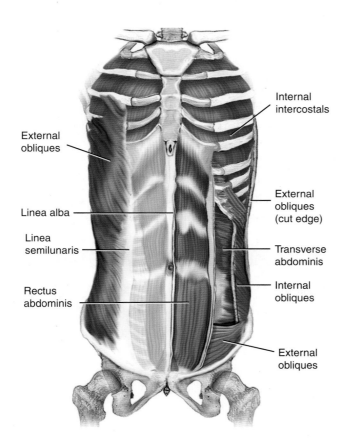

Figure 2–35. Accessory muscles of expiration and landmarks of the abdominal aponeurosis. *Source:* From Seikel/Drumright/King. *Anatomy & Physiology for Speech, Language, and Hearing, 5th Ed.* ©Cengage, Inc. Reproduced by permission.

The layers of abdominal muscles provide excellent support for the rib cage during lifting and similar actions, such as pushing a heavy object. These actions virtually demand fixing the thorax by inflating the lungs and closing off the vocal folds, and the abdominal muscles help to compress the viscera while simultaneously stabilizing the thorax.

Muscles of the Thorax: Anterior and Lateral Thoracic Muscles

- Internal Intercostal (Interosseous Portion)
- Innermost Intercostals
- Transversus Thoracis

Internal Intercostal (Interosseous Portion)

The interosseous portion of the internal intercostal muscles is a significant contributor to forced expiration (Wallbridge et al., 2018). As seen earlier in Figure 2–28, the internal intercostal muscles are pervasive in the thorax, originating on the superior margin of each rib (except the first) and running up and medially to insert into the inferior surface of the rib above. They are conspicuously absent in the posterior aspect of the rib cage near the vertebral column. Because the external intercostal muscles run at nearly right angles to the internals, these two sets of muscles provide significant support for the rib cage and protection for the ribs within, as well as maintenance of rib spacing.

The course of the muscle fibers is constant from the front to side to back of the rib cage. That is, while the fibers run up and medially in front, that translates to running up and laterally in the dorsal aspect.

Besides their support function, the internal intercostal muscles also provide a mechanism for depressing the rib cage. As you can see from the schematic in Figure 2–36, when the interosseous portion of the internal intercostals contracts and shortens, the direction of movement is downward, and the expanded rib cage becomes smaller.

Innermost Intercostal (Intercostales Intimi)

The innermost intercostal muscles are the deepest of the intercostal muscles, with fibers coursing between the inner costal surfaces of adjacent ribs. The

Muscle:	Internal intercostal, interosseous portion
Origin:	Superior margin of ribs 2 through 12
Course:	Up and in
Insertion:	Inferior surface of the rib above
Innervation:	Intercostal nerves: thoracic intercostal nerves arising from T2 through T6 and thoracoabdominal intercostal nerves from T7 through T11
Function:	Depresses ribs 1 through 11

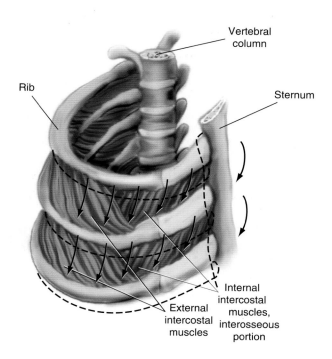

Vertebral column

Rib

Sternum

Internal intercostal muscles, interosseous portion

External intercostal muscles

Figure 2–36. Effect of contraction of the interosseous portion of the internal intercostals is depression of the rib cage, thereby decreasing the volume of the lungs. *Source:* From Seikel/Drumright/King. *Anatomy & Physiology for Speech, Language, and Hearing, 5th Ed.* ©Cengage, Inc. Reproduced by permission.

Getting the Wind Knocked Out of You

Why *does* a blow to the abdomen result in your losing your breath? Logic would dictate that you would lose your breath from being hit in the chest.

Try to recall what happened the last time you had the wind knocked out of you. First, something hit you in the abdominal region. From what you now know, forced expiration depends in large part on the contraction of the abdominal muscles, which, in turn, causes the abdominal viscera to push the diaphragm upward and pull the thorax down. Both these gestures remove air forcefully from the lungs.

This does not explain the agony you experience trying to regain respiratory control, however. When those muscles are passively moved (stretched), a stretch reflex is triggered, which causes the muscle to contract involuntarily. This contraction serves only to increase the effect of being hit in the abdomen, because it is essentially doing the same thing the blunt force did. To cap it all, your attempts to contract your diaphragm add a third dimension to the problem, because that will once again stretch the abdominal muscles and promote further reflexive contraction.

innermost intercostals have a course parallel to those of the internal intercostal muscles, with fibers originating on the superior surface of the lower rib and coursing obliquely up to insert into the rib above. As with the external intercostals, the innermost intercostals are absent in the chondral portion of the ribs, first becoming apparent in the lateral aspect of the inner rib cage. The innermost intercostals are absent near the vertebral and sternal borders, are sparse in the upper thorax, and parallel the morphology of the internal intercostals. The innermost intercostals interdigitate with the subcostal muscles (see Figure 2–29) and are considered muscles of forced expiration.

Muscle:	Innermost intercostals
Origin:	Superior margin of ribs 1 through 11; sparse or absent in superior thorax
Course:	Upward and in
Insertion:	Inferior surface of the rib above
Innervation:	Intercostal nerves: thoracic intercostal nerves arising from T2 through T6 and thoracoabdominal intercostal nerves from T7 through T11
Function:	Depresses ribs 1 through 11

Use of Abdominal Muscles for Childbirth and Other Biological Functions

Nature has a way of getting the most use out of structures, and the abdominal muscles are a great example. Clearly, we use the abdominal muscles to force air out of the lungs, but they serve several other worthwhile (even vital) functions. The act of vomiting requires evacuation of the gastric or even intestinal contents and doing so necessitates forceful action from the abdominal muscles.

A less obvious function has to do with thoracic fixation. For the muscles of the upper body to gain maximum benefit, they need to pull against a relatively rigid structure. The thorax can be made rigid by inhaling and then capturing the respiratory charge by closing off the vocal folds. To demonstrate this process, take a very deep breath and hold it: To do this, you must close off the vocal folds.

This thoracic fixing gives leverage for lifting, but it also gives leverage for expulsion in the other direction. Notice that you may grunt when you lift because some air is escaping past the vocal folds, having been compressed by your muscular effort. Defecation is facilitated by compression of the abdomen and an increase in abdominal pressure, and that process also demands thoracic fixation for efficiency.

Another not immediately obvious use for abdominal muscle contraction is childbirth. Although you may not have experienced this directly, you are probably familiar with midwives, nurses, or partners whose job it is to remind the mother-to-be to breathe. It shouldn't surprise you to realize that the mother has not forgotten this basic biological process, but rather she has an overwhelming, deep biological urge to push. Besides providing supportive encouragement, the person who is cheerleading is doing so to synchronize breathing with contractions and to keep the mother from closing the vocal folds (you can't breathe through closed folds), because if she does, she will start pushing the baby to its new home before the time has come (Creasy, 1997).

Transversus Thoracis

The transversus thoracis muscles (transverse muscles of the thorax) are found on the inner surface of the rib cage. The muscles originate on the margin of the sternum, with fibers coursing to the inner chondral surface of ribs 2 through 6. As seen in Figure 2–37, contraction of the muscles would tend to resist elevation of the rib cage and decrease the volume of the thoracic cavity.

Considering the proximity of the transversus thoracis to the internal intercostal muscles, it should not be surprising that the transversus thoracis takes its innervation from the same source (the thoracic intercostal nerves), as well as from the thoracoabdominal intercostal nerves and subcostal nerves derived from T2 through T1 spinal nerves.

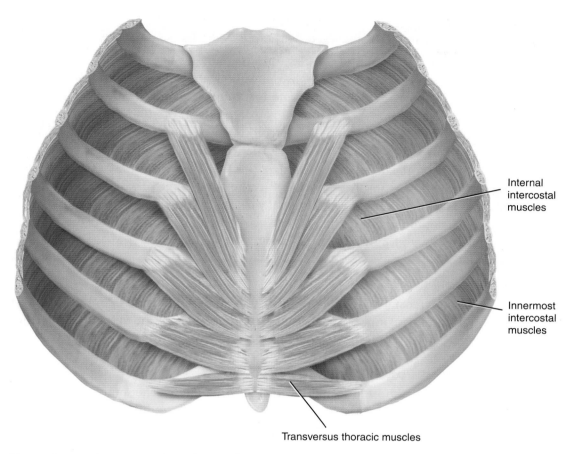

Internal
intercostal
muscles

Innermost
intercostal
muscles

Transversus thoracic muscles

Figure 2–37. Transversus thoracis muscles, as viewed from within the thoracic cavity. *Source:*
From Seikel/Drumright/King. *Anatomy & Physiology for Speech, Language, and Hearing, 5th Ed.*
©Cengage, Inc. Reproduced by permission.

Muscle:	Transversus thoracis
Origin:	Inner thoracic lateral margin of sternum
Course:	Laterally
Insertion:	Inner chondral surface of ribs 2 through 6
Innervation:	Thoracic intercostal nerves, thoracoabdominal intercostal nerves, and subcostal nerves derived from T2 through T6 spinal nerves
Function:	Depresses rib cage for expiration

Posterior Thoracic Muscles

- Subcostals
- Serratus Posterior Inferior

Subcostals

The subcostals are widely variable but generally take a course parallel to the
internal intercostals and thus have the potential of aiding forced expiration.
The subcostals are found on the inner posterior wall of the thorax. Unlike

Palpation of the Rib Cage

Although you cannot palpate your diaphragm, you can identify its margins easily enough. First, find your xiphoid process. This point marks part of the origin of the rectus abdominis, but the diaphragm attaches on the inner surface. Place your fingers on the xiphoid process and the muscle below and breathe deeply in and out once. You can feel the rectus abdominis being stretched during inspiration. Now place the fingers of both hands at the bottom of the rib cage on either side of the sternum so that your fingers press into your abdominal muscles. Breathe out as deeply as you can and hold that posture while you bend slightly forward. Your fingers are marking the margin of the diaphragm, although you are palpating abdominal muscles.

Bring your fingers up to feel your ribs. Place your fingers between the ribs, with your little finger of each hand on the abdominal muscles below the rib cage. Breathe in a couple of times and feel the abdominal muscles first draw in and then tighten up as you reach maximum inspiration. Feel your rib cage elevate as you do this.

the intercostal muscles, the subcostals may span more than one rib. The subcostals are innervated by the intercostal nerves of the thorax, arising from the ventral rami of the spinal nerves.

Serratus Posterior Inferior

The serratus posterior inferior muscles originate on the spinous processes of the T11, T12, and L1 through L3 and course up and laterally to insert into the lower margin of the lower five ribs. Contraction of these muscles would tend to pull the rib cage down, supporting expiratory effort, although neither anatomical (Loukas et al., 2008) nor physiological (Vilensky et al., 2001) studies have found evidence of this (see Figure 2–33). The serratus posterior inferior derives its innervation from the intercostal nerves arising from T9 through T11 and the subcostal nerve from T12.

Muscle:	Subcostal
Origin:	Inner posterior thorax; sparse in upper thorax; from inner surface of rib near angle
Course:	Down and lateral
Insertion:	Inner surface of second or third rib below
Innervation:	Intercostal nerves of thorax, arising from the ventral rami of the spinal nerves
Function:	Depresses thorax
Muscle:	Serratus posterior inferior
Origin:	Spinous processes of T11, T12, L1 through L3
Course:	Up and laterally
Insertion:	Lower margin of ribs 7 through 12
Innervation:	Intercostal nerves from T9 through T11 and subcostal nerve from T12
Function:	Contraction of these muscles tends to pull the rib cage down, supporting expiratory effort

Abdominal Muscles of Expiration

If you once again examine the skeleton in Figure 2–3 and imagine placing muscles in the region between the rib cage and the pelvis, you may realize that there are few places from which muscles can originate. Clearly one could attach muscles to the rib cage, vertebral column, and the pelvic girdle to give some structure, but that leaves a great deal of territory to cover in the anterior aspect. To deal with this, nature has provided a tendinous structure, the **abdominal aponeurosis**. Let us examine how it is constructed and then attach some muscles to that structure. Figure 2–38 shows a schematic representation of the abdominal aponeurosis from the front, as well as in transverse view.

abdominal aponeurosis: the aponeurotic complex of the anterior abdominal wall that forms points of origination for abdominal musculature

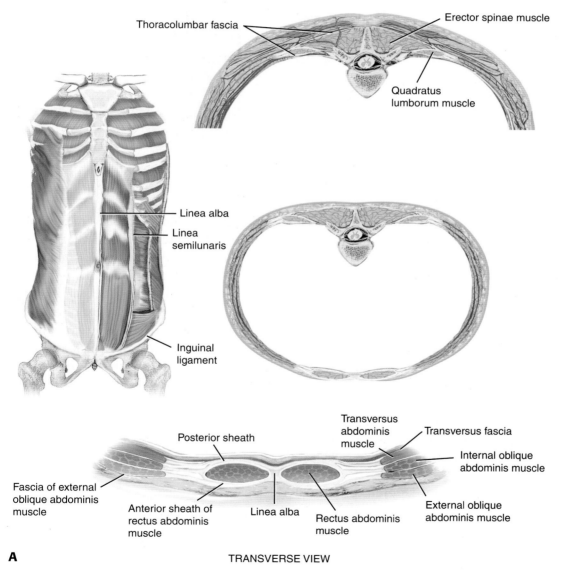

Thoracolumbar fascia

Erector spinae muscle

Quadratus lumborum muscle

Linea alba

Linea semilunaris

Inguinal ligament

Posterior sheath

Transversus abdominis muscle

Transversus fascia

Internal oblique abdominis muscle

Fascia of external oblique abdominis muscle

Anterior sheath of rectus abdominis muscle

Linea alba

Rectus abdominis muscle

External oblique abdominis muscle

A

TRANSVERSE VIEW

Figure 2–38. A. Schematic of abdominal aponeurosis as related to the abdominal muscles of expiration. *Source:* From Seikel/Drumright/King. *Anatomy & Physiology for Speech, Language, and Hearing, 5th Ed.* ©Cengage, Inc. Reproduced by permission. *continues*

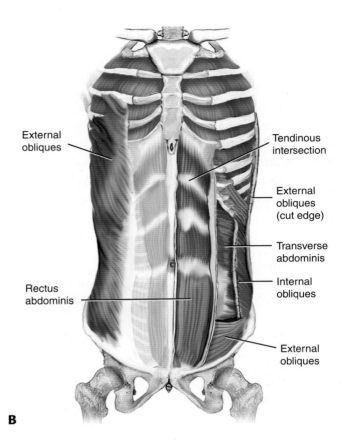

Figure 2–38. *continued*
B. Transversus abdominis, rectus abdominis, external and internal oblique abdominis muscles. *Source:* From Seikel/ Drumright/King. *Anatomy & Physiology for Speech, Language, and Hearing, 5th Ed.* ©Cengage, Inc. Reproduced by permission.

linea alba: L., white line

The **linea alba** (white line) runs from the xiphoid process to the pubic symphysis, forming a midline structure for muscular attachment. As the linea alba progresses laterally, it differentiates into two sheets of aponeurosis, between which is found the rectus abdominis. This aponeurotic wrapping comes back together to form another band of tendon, the linea semilunaris. This tendon once again divides, but this time into three sheets of aponeurosis, which provide a way to attach three more muscles to this structure.

In the posterior aspect, the fascia of the abdominal muscles joins to form the lumbodorsal fascia. This structure provides for the union of three abdominal muscles (transversus abdominis, internal oblique abdominis, and external oblique abdominis) with the vertebral column.

The external oblique aponeurosis communicates directly with the fascia covering the rectus abdominis, forming a continuous layer of connective tissue from the linea alba to the external oblique muscle.

Anterior-Lateral Abdominal Muscles

The abdominal muscles of expiration function by compressing the abdominal viscera. This compression function is not only useful in respiration but also aids in defecation, vomiting, and childbirth (with vocal folds tightly adducted).

- Transversus Abdominis
- Internal Oblique Abdominis

- External Oblique Abdominis
- Rectus Abdominis

Transversus Abdominis. Lateral to the rectus abdominis is the transversus abdominis, the deepest of the anterior abdominal muscles (see Figure 2–38). The transversus abdominis runs laterally (that is, horizontally; hence the name *transversus*), originating in the posterior aspect of the vertebral column via the thoracolumbar fascia of the abdominal aponeurosis. The transversus abdominis muscle attaches to the transversus abdominis aponeurosis in the anterior aspect, as well as to the inner surface of ribs 6 through 12, interdigitating at that point with the fibers of the diaphragm. Its inferior-most attachment is at the pubis. Contraction of the transversus significantly reduces the volume of the abdomen (Misuri et al, 1997).

Innervation of the transversus abdominis is via the thoracic and lumbar nerves, specifically from the lower thoracoabdominal nerves (derived from T7 to T12) and first lumbar nerve, iliohypogastric and ilioinguinal branches.

Internal Oblique Abdominis. The internal oblique abdominis is located between the external oblique abdominis and the transversus abdominis. As seen in Figure 2–38, this muscle fans out from its origin on the inguinal ligament and iliac crest to the cartilaginous portion of the lower ribs and the portion of the abdominal aponeurosis lateral to the rectus abdominis, and thus, by association, inserts into the linea alba. Contraction of the internal oblique abdominis assists in the rotation of the trunk, if unilaterally

Muscle:	Transversus abdominis
Origin:	Posterior abdominal wall at the vertebral column via the thoracolumbar fascia of the abdominal aponeurosis
Course:	Lateral
Insertion:	Transversus abdominis aponeurosis and inner surface of ribs 6–12, interdigitating at that point with the fibers of the diaphragm; inferior-most attachment is at the pubis
Innervation:	Thoracic and lumbar nerves from the lower spinal intercostal nerves (derived from T7 through T12) and first lumbar nerve, iliohypogastric and ilioinguinal branches
Function:	Compresses abdomen
Muscle:	Internal oblique abdominis
Origin:	Inguinal ligament and iliac crest
Course:	Fans medially
Insertion:	Cartilaginous portion of lower ribs and the portion of the abdominal aponeurosis lateral to the rectus abdominis
Innervation:	Thoracic and lumbar nerves from the lower spinal intercostal nerves (derived from T7 through T12) and first lumbar nerve, iliohypogastric and ilioinguinal branches
Function:	Rotates trunk; flexes trunk; compresses abdomen

contracted, or flexion of the trunk, when bilaterally contracted, and participates in forced expiration (Kera & Maruyama, 2005). The internal oblique abdominis is innervated by the first eight intercostal nerves, as well as the ilioinguinal and iliohypogastric nerves.

External Oblique Abdominis. The external oblique abdominis are the most superficial of the abdominal muscles, as well as the largest of this group. These muscles originate along the osseous portion of the lower seven ribs and fan downward to insert into the iliac crest, inguinal ligament, and abdominal aponeurosis (lateral to the rectus abdominis). Bilateral contraction of these muscles flexes the vertebral column, while unilateral contraction results in trunk rotation. The external oblique abdominis muscles are important muscle of forced expiration (Misuri et al., 1997). They receive innervation from the thoracoabdominal nerve arising from T7 through T11 and the subcostal nerve from T12.

Rectus Abdominis. The rectus abdominis muscles are the prominent midline muscles of the abdominal region, and they originate at the pubis inferiorly (see Figure 2–35). The superior attachment is at the xiphoid process of sternum and the cartilage of the last true rib (rib 7) and the false ribs (ribs 8, 9, & 10).

rectus: L., straight (not crooked)

    These "rectangular" (i.e., **rectus**) muscles are manifest in a series of four or five segments connected (and separated) by tendinous slips known as **tendinous intersections**. Use of this muscle is a must if you are to succeed at your sit-ups, because contraction draws the chest closer to the knees, and

Muscle:	External oblique abdominis
Origin:	Osseous portion of the lower seven ribs
Course:	Fan downward
Insertion:	Iliac crest, inguinal ligament, and abdominal aponeurosis lateral to rectus abdominis
Innervation:	Thoracoabdominal nerve arising from T7 through T11 and subcostal nerve from T12
Function:	Bilateral contraction flexes vertebral column and compresses abdomen; unilateral contraction results in trunk rotation
Muscle:	Transversus abdominis
Origin:	Posterior abdominal wall at the vertebral column via the thoracolumbar fascia of the abdominal aponeurosis
Course:	Lateral
Insertion:	Transversus abdominis aponeurosis and inner surface of ribs 6 through 12, interdigitating at that point with the fibers of the diaphragm; inferior-most attachment is at the pubis
Innervation:	Thoracic and lumbar nerves from the lower spinal intercostal nerves (derived from T7 through T12) and first lumbar nerve, iliohypogastric and ilioinguinal branches
Function:	Compresses abdomen

the only way to do this is to bend. Contraction of the rectus abdominis, which is the dominant action of forced expiration, also compresses the abdominal contents.

Innervation is by T5 through T11 intercostal (thoracoabdominal) nerves and the subcostal nerve from T12. This segmented muscle is segmentally innervated as well: T7 supplies the uppermost segment, T8 supplies the next section, and the remaining portions are supplied by T9 through T12.

Posterior Abdominal Muscle: Quadratus Lumborum

As seen in Figures 2–30 and 2–33, the quadratus lumborum is in the dorsal aspect of the abdominal wall. These muscles originate along the iliac crest and fan up and inward to insert into the transverse processes of the lumbar vertebrae and inferior border of the 12th rib. Unilateral contraction of the quadratus lumborum assists in lateral movement of the trunk, whereas bilateral contraction fixes the abdominal wall in support of abdominal compression. This muscle is innervated by the lowest thoracic nerve T12 and the first four lumbar nerves.

There are other abdominal muscles supporting abdominal wall fixation. The psoas major and minor muscles and the iliacus may also provide abdominal support for forced expiration.

Respiratory Muscle of the Upper Limb: Latissimus Dorsi

The **latissimus** dorsi muscle (see Figure 2–33) originates from the lumbar, sacral, and lower thoracic vertebrae, with fibers rising fanlike to insert into the humerus. Its primary role is in assisting the movement of the upper extremity, but it clearly plays a role in chest stability, and perhaps expiration.

latissimus: L., widest

Muscle:	Rectus abdominis
Origin:	Originates as four or five segments at the pubis inferiorly
Course:	Up to segment border
Insertion:	Xiphoid process of sternum and the cartilage of ribs 5 through 7
Innervation:	T5 through T11 intercostal (thoracoabdominal) nerves, subcostal nerve from T12 (T5 supplies upper segment, T8 supplies the second, T9 through T12 supply remainder)
Function:	Flexion of vertebral column
Muscle:	Quadratus lumborum
Origin:	Iliac crest
Course:	Fan up and inward
Insertion:	Transverse processes of the lumbar vertebrae and inferior border of rib 12
Innervation:	Thoracic nerve T12 and L1 through L4 lumbar nerves
Function:	Bilateral contraction fixes abdominal wall in support of abdominal compression

Muscle:	Latissimus dorsi
Origin:	Lumbar, sacral, and lower thoracic vertebrae
Course:	Up fanlike
Insertion:	Humerus
Innervation:	Brachial plexus, posterior branch; fibers from the regions C6 through C8 form the long subscapular nerve
Function:	For respiration, stabilizes posterior abdominal wall for expiration

With the arm immobilized, contraction of the latissimus dorsi stabilizes the posterior abdominal wall, performing a function similar to that of the quadratus lumborum.

Innervation for this muscle arises from the posterior branch of the brachial plexus. Fibers from the regions C6 through C8 of this plexus form the long subscapular nerve to supply the latissimus dorsi.

✓ To summarize:

- To inflate the lungs, you need to expand the cavity that holds them so air can rush in.

- To do this, you can either increase the long dimension, fairly easily, by contracting the **diaphragm**, or you can elevate the rib cage with just a little bit more effort.

- **Forced expiration** reverses this process by pulling the thorax down and in and by forcing the diaphragm higher into the thorax.

- The next chapter provides insight into the details of inspiration, expiration, and respiration for speech.

Chapter Summary

Respiration is the process of gas exchange between an organism and its environment. The **rib cage**, made up of the **spinal column** and **ribs**, houses the lungs, which are the primary machinery of respiration. By means of the cartilaginous **trachea** and **bronchial tree**, air enters the lungs for gas exchange within the minute **alveolar sacs**. Oxygen enters the blood and carbon dioxide is removed by expiration.

Air enters the lungs through muscular effort. The **diaphragm**, placed between the thorax and abdomen, contracts during inspiration. The **lungs** expand when the diaphragm contracts, drawn by **pleurae** linked through surface tension and negative pressure. When lungs expand, the air pressure within the lungs becomes negative with respect to the outside atmosphere, and **Boyle's law** dictates that air flows from the region of higher pressure to fill the lungs. **Accessory muscles** also provide for added expansion of the rib cage for further inspiration.

Expiration may occur passively through the forces of **elasticity** and **gravity** acting on the ribs and rib cage. Expiration may also be **forced**, using muscles of the abdomen and those that depress the rib cage to evacuate the lungs.

❓ Chapter 2 Study Questions

1. _____ is defined as force distributed over area.

2. _____ pressure causes air to enter a chamber that has expanded until the pressure is equalized.

3. How many of each of the following vertebrae are there?

   A. _____ cervical vertebrae

   B. _____ thoracic vertebrae

   C. _____ lumbar vertebrae

   D. _____ sacral vertebrae (fused)

4. On the figure below, identify the landmarks indicated.

   A. _____ process

   B. _____ process

   C. _____

   D. _____ facet

   E. _____ facet

   F. _____ facet

   G. _____ foramen

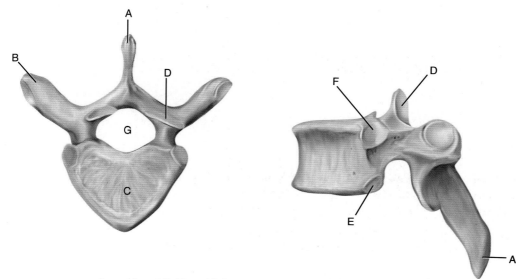

Source: From Seikel/Drumright/King. *Anatomy & Physiology for Speech, Language, and Hearing, 5th Ed.* ©Cengage, Inc. Reproduced by permission.

5. The _____ passes through the vertebral foramen.

6. On the following figures, identify the landmarks indicated.

A. _____ (bone)

B. _____ (bone)

C. _____ (bone)

D. _____

E. _____

F. _____

G. _____ (bone)

H. _____ (bone)

I. _____ (bone)

J. _____

K. _____

L. _____

M. _____

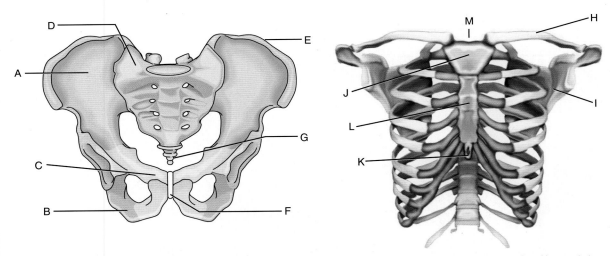

Source: From Seikel/Drumright/King. *Anatomy & Physiology for Speech, Language, and Hearing, 5th Ed.* ©Cengage, Inc. Reproduced by permission.

7. On the figure that follows, identify the landmarks indicated.

A. _____

B. _____

C. _____

D. _____

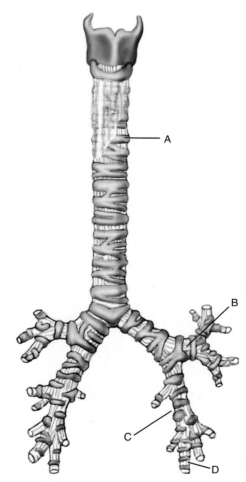

Source: From Seikel/Drumright/King.. *Anatomy & Physiology for Speech,*
Language, and Hearing, 5th Ed. ©Cengage, Inc. Reproduced by permission.

8. On the following figure, identify the muscles and structures indicated.

A. _____

B. _____

C. _____

D. _____

E. _____

F. _____ ligament

G. _____

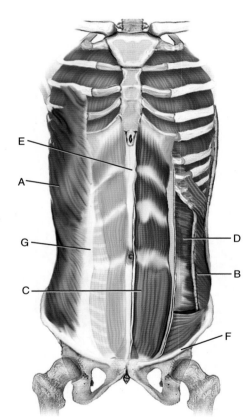

Source: From Seikel/Drumright/King. *Anatomy & Physiology for Speech, Language, and Hearing, 5th Ed.* ©Cengage, Inc. Reproduced by permission.

9. On the following figure, identify the muscles indicated.

A. _____

B. _____

C. _____

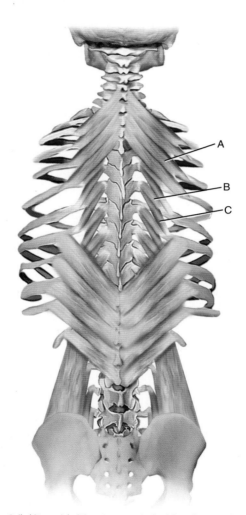

Source: From Seikel/Drumright/King. *Anatomy & Physiology for Speech, Language, and Hearing, 5th Ed.* ©Cengage, Inc. Reproduced by permission.

10. Identify the muscles indicated on the following figure.

    A. _____

    B. _____

    C. _____

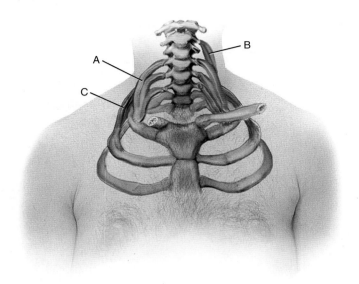

Source: From Seikel/Drumright/King. *Anatomy & Physiology for Speech, Language, and Hearing, 5th Ed.* ©Cengage, Inc. Reproduced by permission.

11. Identify the muscles and portions of muscles indicated in the figure below.

    A. _____

    B. _____ head

    C. _____ head

    D. _____

    E. _____

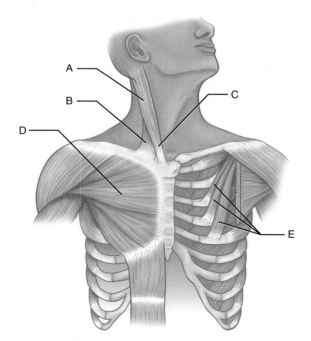

Source: From Seikel/Drumright/King. *Anatomy & Physiology for Speech, Language, and Hearing, 5th Ed.* ©Cengage, Inc. Reproduced by permission.

12. Contraction of the diaphragm increases the _____ dimension of the thorax.

13. Contraction of the accessory muscles of inspiration increases the _____ dimension of the thorax.

14. Contraction of the muscles of expiration _____ the volume of the thorax.

15. Emphysema results in a breakdown of the alveolar wall, resulting in enlargement of alveolar clusters and consequent enlargement of the thorax known as *barrel chest*. The result of this condition is that the diaphragm is pulled down at rest. Discuss the implications of the muscular action of inspiration and expiration on this altered system.

Chapter 2 Study Question Answers

1. **PRESSURE** is defined as force distributed over area.

2. **NEGATIVE** pressure causes air to enter a chamber that has expanded until the pressure is equalized.

3. A. **7** cervical vertebrae; B. **12** thoracic vertebrae; C. **5** lumbar vertebrae; D. **5** sacral vertebrae (fused)

4. The landmarks are as follows:

    A. **SPINOUS** process

    B. **TRANSVERSE** process

    C. **CORPUS**

    D. **SUPERIOR ARTICULAR** facet

    E. **INFERIOR COSTAL** facet

    F. **SUPERIOR COSTAL** facet

    G. **VERTEBRAL** foramen

5. The **SPINAL CORD** passes through the vertebral foramen.

6. The landmarks indicated are as follows:

    A. **ILIUM**

    B. **ISCHIUM**

    C. **PUBIC BONE**

    D. **SACRUM**

    E. **ILIAC CREST**

    F. **PUBIC SYMPHYSIS**

    G. **COCCYX**

    H. **CLAVICLE**

    I. **SCAPULA**

    J. **MANUBRIUM STERNI**

    K. **XIPHOID** or **ENSIFORM PROCESS**

    L. **CORPUS STERNI**

    M. **STERNAL NOTCH**

7. The landmarks indicated are as follows:

    A. **TRACHEA**

    B. **MAINSTEM BRONCHUS**

    C. **SECONDARY BRONCHUS**

    D. **TERTIARY BRONCHUS**

8. The muscles and structures indicated are as follows:

    A. **EXTERNAL OBLIQUE ABDOMINIS**

    B. **INTERNAL OBLIQUE ABDOMINIS**

    C. **RECTUS ABDOMINIS**

    D. **TRANSVERSUS ABDOMINIS**

    E. **LINEA ALBA**

    F. **INGUINAL LIGAMENT**

    G. **LINEA SEMILUNARIS**

9. The muscles indicated are as follows:

    A. **SERRATUS POSTERIOR SUPERIOR**

    B. **LEVATOR COSTARUM BREVIS**

    C. **LEVATOR COSTARUM LONGIS**

10. The muscles indicated are as follows.

    A. **SCALENUS ANTERIOR**

    B. **SCALENUS MEDIUS**

    C. **SCALENUS POSTERIOR**

11. The muscles and portions of muscles indicated are as follows:

    A. **STERNOCLEIDOMASTOID**

    B. **CLAVICULAR** head

    C. **STERNAL** head

    D. **PECTORALIS MAJOR**

    E. **PECTORALIS MINOR**

12. Contraction of the diaphragm increases the **VERTICAL** dimension of the thorax.

13. Contraction of the accessory muscles of inspiration increases the **TRANSVERSE** dimension of the thorax.

14. Contraction of the muscles of expiration **DECREASES** the volume of the thorax.

15. In advanced emphysema, the diaphragm is pulled down and stretched relatively flat by the flaring of the rib cage. In normal inspiration, contraction of the diaphragm causes the central tendon to pull down, causing air to enter the lungs (Boyle's law dictates that a drop in alveolar pressure causes air to flow in). When the diaphragm of an individual

with advanced emphysema contracts, it pulls the ribs closer together because they were distended by the barrel chest. As a result, the alveoli are compressed, causing an increase in alveolar pressure and causing air to leave the lungs. Thus, the inspiratory movement of the diaphragm causes expiration. The single inspiratory avenue left to the individual is to elevate the sternum and clavicle using clavicular breathing.

Bibliography

Araujo, J. A., Barajas, B., Kleinman, M., Wang, X., Bennett, B. J., Gong, K. W., . . . Nel, A. E. (2008). Ambient particulate pollutants in the ultrafine range promote early atherosclerosis and systemic oxidative stress. *Circulation Research, 102*(5), 589–596. https://doi.org/10.1161/CIRCRESAHA.107.164970

Bly, L. (1994). *Motor skills acquisition in the first year.* Tucson, AZ: Therapy Skill Builders.

Cala, S. J., Edyvean, J., & Engel, L. A. (1992). Chest wall and trunk muscle activity during inspiratory loading. *Journal of Applied Physiology, 73*(6), 2373–2381.

Carlson, S., Hunt, W., & Johnson, J. (2017). Pulmonary recovery positions increase EMG activity in accessory respiratory muscles. *Physical Therapy Scholarly Projects, 552.* Retrieved from https://commons.und.edu/pt-grad/552

Cernak, I., & Noble-Haeusslein, L. J. (2010). Traumatic brain injury: An overview of pathobiology with emphasis on military populations. *Journal of Cerebral Blood Flow Metabolism, 30*(2), 255–266.

Cerqueira, E. P., & Garbellini, D.(1999). Electromyographic study of the pectoralis major, serratus anterior, and external oblique muscles during respiratory activity in humans. *Electromyography Clinical Neurophysiology, 39*(3), 131–137.

Creasy, R. K. (1997). *Management of labor and delivery.* Malden, MA: Blackwell Science.

De Freitas, V., & Vitti, M. (1980). Electromyographic study of the trapezius (pars media) and rhomboideus major during respiration. *Electromyography Clinical Neurophysiology, 20*(6), 503–507.

Des Jardins, T., & Burton, G. G. (2015). *Clinical manifestation and assessment of respiratory disease* (7th ed.). Chicago, IL: C. V. Mosby.

Donaldson, K., & Seaton, A. (2012). A short history of toxicology of inhaled products. *Particle and Fiber Toxicology, 9*(13), 2–12.

Ganong, W. F. (2003). *Review of medical physiology* (21st ed.). New York, NY: McGraw-Hill/Appleton & Lange.

Gilroy, A. M., MacPherson, B. R., & Ross, L. M. (2012). *Atlas of anatomy.* New York, NY: Thieme.

Gray, H., Bannister, L. H., Berry, M. M., & Williams, P. L. (Eds.). (1995). *Gray's anatomy.* London, UK: Churchill Livingstone.

Han, J., Park, S., Kim, Y., Choi, Y., & Lyu, H. (2016). Effects of forward head posture on forced vital capacity and respiratory muscles activity. *Journal of Physical Therapy Science, 28*(1), 128–131.

Kang, J. I., Jeong, D. K., & Choi, H. (2016). The effect of feedback respiratory exercise on muscle activity, craniovertebral angle, and neck disability index of the neck flexors of patients with forward head posture. *Journal of Physical Therapy Science, 28*(9), 2477–2481.

Kera, T., & Maruyama, H. (2005). The effect of posture on respiratory activity of the abdominal muscles. *Journal of Physiological Anthropology and Applied Human Science, 24*(4), 259–265.

Kuehn, D. P., Lemme, M. L., & Baumgartner, J. M. (1989). *Neural bases of speech, hearing, and language.* Boston, MA: Little, Brown.

Langley, M. B., & Lombardino, L. J. (Eds.). (1991). *Neurodevelopmental strategies for managing communication disorders in children with severe motor dysfunction.* Austin, TX: Pro-Ed.

Loukas, M., Louis, R. G. Jr., Wartmann, C. T., Tubbs, R. S., Gupta, A. A., Apaydin, N., & Jordan, R. (2008). An anatomic investigation of the serratus posterior superior and serratus posterior inferior muscles. *Surgical & Radiological Anatomy, 30*(2), 119–123.

Mackay, L. E., Chapman, P. E., & Morgan, A. S. (1997). *Maximizing brain injury recovery: integrating critical care and early rehabilitation.* New York, NY: Aspen.

McMinn, R. M. H., Hutchings, R. T., & Logan, B. M. (1994). *Color atlas of head and neck anatomy.* London, UK: Mosby-Wolfe.

Miller, A. D., Bianchi, A. L., & Bishop, B. P. (1997). *Neural control of the respiratory muscles.* Boca Raton, FL: CRC Press.

Misuri, G., Colagrande, S., Gorini, M., Iandelli, I., Mancini, M., Duranti, R., & Scano, G. (1997). In vivo ultrasound assessment of respiratory function of abdominal muscles in normal subjects. *European Respiratory Journal, 10*(12), 2861–2867.

Moser, K. M., & Spragg, R. G. (1982). *Respiratory emergencies.* St. Louis, MO: C. V. Mosby.

Nepomuceno, V. R., Nepomuceno, E. M., Regalo, S. C. H., Cerqueira, E. P., & Souza, R. R. (2014). Electromyographic study on the sternocleidomastoid and pectoralis major muscles during respiratory activity in humans. *Journal of Morphological Sciences, 31*(02), 98–102.

Phalen, R. F., & Oldham, M. J. (1983). Tracheobronchial airway structure as revealed by casting techniques. *American Review of Respiratory Disease, 128*(2 Pt. 2), S1–S4.

Rohen, J. W., Yokochi, C., Lutjen-Drecoll, E., & Romrell, L. J. (2002). *Color atlas of anatomy* (5th ed.). Philadelphia, PA: Williams & Wilkins.

Sargent, J. R. (2011). Nanotechnology and environmental, health, and safety: Issues for consideration. *Congressional Research Service,* 7-5700, RL34614.

Schamberger, R. C. (2000). Chest wall deformities. In T. W. Shields, J. LoCicero, III, & R. B. Ponn (Eds.). *General thoracic surgery* (5th ed., pp. 535–569). Philadelphia, PA: Lippincott Williams & Wilkins.

Shaffer, R. E., & Rengasamy, S. (2009). Respiratory protection against airborne nanoparticles: A review. *Journal of Nanoparticle Research, 11*(7), 1661–1672.

Spector, W. S. (1961). *Handbook of biological data.* Philadelphia, PA: W. B. Saunders.

Turgut, E., Duzgun, I., & Baltaci, G. (2016). Effect of trapezius muscle strength on three-dimensional scapular kinematics. *Journal of Physical Therapy Science, 28*(6), 1864–1867.

Vilensky, J. A., Baltes, M., Weikel. L., Fortin, J. D., & Fourie, L. J. (2001). Serratus posterior muscles: Anatomy, clinical relevance, and function. *Clinical Anatomy, 14*(4), 237–241.

Wallbridge, P., Parry, S. M., Das, S., Law, C., Hammerschlag, G., Irving, L., . . . Steinfort, D. (2018). Parasternal intercostal muscle ultrasound in chronic obstructive pulmonary disease correlates with spirometric severity. *Scientific Reports, 8*(1), 15274.

Watson, A. H., Williams, C., & James, B. V. (2012). Activity patterns in latissimus dorsi and sternocleidomastoid in classical singers. *Journal of Voice, 26*(3), e-95–e-105.

Whitmore, I., Willan, P. L. T., Gosling, J. A., & Harris, P. F. (2002). *Human anatomy: Color atlas and text* (4th ed.). St. Louis, MO: C. V. Mosby.

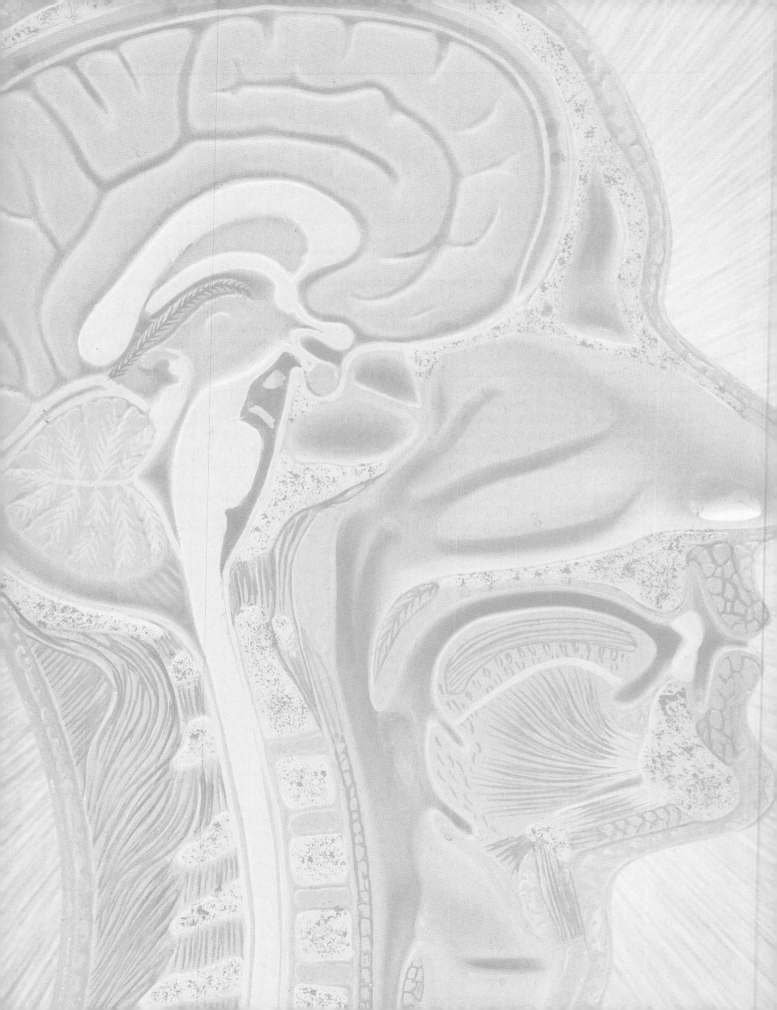

CHAPTER 3

Physiology of Respiration

Respiration requires muscular effort, and the degree to which an individual can successfully activate and control the musculature determines, in large part, the efficiency of respiration itself. Respiratory function (physiology) changes as we exercise, age, or suffer setbacks in health. Considering its importance in speech, it is no wonder that as the respiratory system goes, so goes communication.

We are capable of both **quiet** and **forced inspiration**. There is a parallel to this in expiration, because we are capable of **passive** and **active expiration**. In passive expiration, we let the elastic forces of the tissues restore the system to a resting position after inspiration. In active expiration, we use muscular effort to push just a little farther. Let us examine these forces.

ANAQUEST LESSON ▶

The process of expiration is one of eliminating the waste products of respiration. Attend to your own respiratory cycle to learn an important aspect of quiet expiration. Close your eyes while you breathe in and out 10 times, quietly and in a relaxed manner. Pay particular attention to the area of your body around your diaphragm, including your rib cage and your abdomen.

What you experienced is the active contraction of the diaphragm, followed by a simple relaxing of the musculature. You actively contract to breathe in, and then simply let nature take its course for expiration. You may liken this to blowing up a balloon. The balloon expands when you blow and deflates as soon as you let go of your grip. The forces on the balloon that cause it to lose its air are among those that cause your lungs to deflate. The forces we need to talk about are elasticity and gravity.

Recall that the lungs are highly elastic, porous tissue. They are sponge-like, and when they are compressed, they expand as soon as the compression is released. Likewise, if you grab a sponge by its edges and stretch it, the sponge tends to return to its original shape and size when you release it.

You can think of the lungs as small sponges in a large bottle. The lungs truly will not fill up that "bottle" of the chest cavity when they are left to their own devices (i.e., permitted to deflate to their natural resting condition). In the adult body, the lungs are actually stretched beyond their resting position, but this is not so with the infant.

During early development, the lungs completely fill the thorax. As the child develops, the rib cage grows faster than the lungs, and the pleural linings and increased negative intrapleural pressure provide a means for the lungs to be stretched out to fill that space.

The result of this stretching is greatly increased capacity and reserve in adults, but not in infants. Because the thorax and lungs are of the same size in infants, they must breathe two to three times as often as an adult for adequate respiration. The adult's lungs are stretched out and are never completely compressed, so there is always a reserve of air within them that is not undergoing gas exchange.

Upon increasing the thorax size, the lungs expand just as if you had grabbed them and stretched them out. When the muscles that are expanding the rib cage relax, the lungs tend to return to their original shape and size. In addition, when you inhale and your abdomen protrudes, you are stretching the abdominal muscles. Relaxing the inspiratory process lets those muscles return to their original length. That is, the abdominal muscles tend to push your abdominal viscera back in and force the diaphragm up.

A second force acting in support of passive expiration is gravity. When standing or sitting erect, gravity acts on the ribs to pull them back after they have been expanded through the effort of the accessory muscles of inspiration. Gravity also works in favor of maximizing overall capacity, because it pulls the abdominal viscera down, leaving more room for the lungs. We will talk about gravity more later in this chapter, because body position becomes a significant issue in the efficiency of respiration.

There is one final force that bears attention. For years, speech scientists acknowledged the triad of torque, elasticity, and gravity as the forces driving passive expiration. It was believed that expansion of the rib cage during inspiration twisted the cartilaginous portion of the rib cage, thereby storing a restoring force that would cause the rib cage to return to rest upon relaxation. The reality, as identified by Hixon in his 2006 paper, is that the rib cage is under a negative torque at relaxation (i.e., it is pulled toward the lungs) and that inspiration, which increases the thoracic volume, serves only to move the rib cage to a neutral condition during normal respiration. Only after one has achieved upward of 60% of vital capacity (i.e., taken a significantly deep inspiration) does the rib cage assist in expiration. It is worth noting that inhalation above 60% does occur, particularly when shouting, so torque could continue to have a role in respiration.

✔ *To summarize:*

- We are capable of quiet respiration as well as forced inspiration and expiration.

- Expiration may be passive, driven by the forces of **elasticity** and **gravity**.

- We may also use muscles that reduce the size of the thorax by compressing the **abdomen** or pulling the rib cage down, and this forces air out of the lungs beyond that which is expired in passive expiration.

The Flow of Respiration

The quantity of air processed through respiration is dictated primarily by bodily needs, and speech physiology operates within these limits. We discuss respiration in terms of rate of flow in respiration, volume and lung capacities, and pressure.

Instruments in Respiration

Respiratory flow, volumes, and capacities are measured using a **spirometer** (Figure 3–1). The classic wet spirometer consists of a tube connected to a container opened at the bottom. This container is placed inside another container that is full of water.

spirometer: device used to measure respiratory volume

To measure lung volume, an individual breathes into the tube, causing a volume of water to be displaced. The amount of water displaced gives an accurate estimate of the air that was required to displace it. (For now, we are ignoring the *pressure* required to raise the container and the effort involved in this process.)

In reality, spirometers take many forms. A whole-body plethysmograph is a chamber in which a subject sits. As the person's chest wall moves during respiration, the volume of the chamber changes, so volumes and capacities can be estimated more accurately than using a wet spirometer. (Biologists use a version of the whole-body plethysmograph, a micro-spirometer, to measure

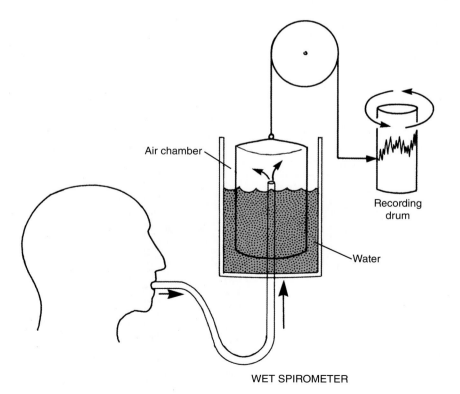

Air chamber

Recording drum

Water

WET SPIROMETER

Figure 3–1. Wet spirometer used to measure lung volumes. When the individual exhales into the tube, gas entering the air chamber displaces the water, causing the chamber to rise. These changes are charted on the recording drum. *Source:* From Seikel/Drumright/King. *Anatomy & Physiology for Speech, Language, and Hearing, 5th Ed.* ©Cengage, Inc. Reproduced by permission.

respiration in animals and insects, by placing the organism in an enclosure and reading the volume changes.) A portable spirometer outfitted with a windmill blade makes measurement of forced capacity readily available in any clinical site.

A pneumotachograph is a spirometer that can measure the rate of airflow, and this instrument comes in a variety of designs. One of the most reliable types uses a small turbine held within the mouthpiece: The harder an individual blows, the faster the turbine blades turn. The turning relates directly to how much flow has occurred, so volume over time can easily be calculated. Pneumotachographs are particularly useful for characterizing ongoing respiratory function and have the added benefit over the old wet spirometers of having fresh air for the subject to breathe. The wet spirometer was a closed system, in that you really had only one respiratory cycle before you were recycling your own breath.

The classic U-tube **manometer** is one means of measuring pressure, as shown in Figure 3–2. A subject is asked to place the tube between the lips and to blow. The force of the subject's expiration is exerted on a column of water that rises as a result. The more force the person uses, the higher the column rises. We can measure the effects of that force in inches or in centimeters of water displaced (barometric pressure is often reported in millimeters of mercury, which refers to how many millimeters of mercury were elevated by the pressure). Because water is considerably less dense than mercury, the same amount of pressure elevates a column of water much higher than a similar column of mercury. For this reason, we measure the rather small pressures of respiration with the water standard.

As with spirometers, there exists an array of pressure-sensing devices that can be used for the measurement of human respiration. Portable manometers allow reliable clinical and field measurement of respiratory function,

manometer: device for measuring air pressure differences

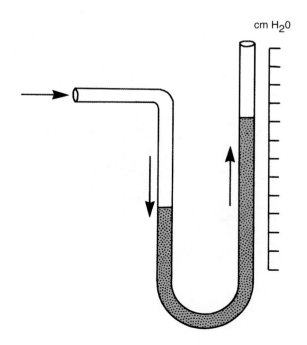

Figure 3–2. U-tube manometer for measurement of respiratory pressure. *Source:* From Seikel/Drumright/ King. *Anatomy & Physiology for Speech, Language, and Hearing, 5th Ed.* ©Cengage, Inc. Reproduced by permission.

cm H$_2$0

and manometers with alarms are used by respiratory therapists to monitor ventilation of patients. Similarly, inflation manometers are used to determine pressure for endotracheal cuff inflation, but these tend to be mechanical rather than electronic. We're going to see that the relationship between pressure and volume come into play as we look at issues such as the lung's ability to be distended, also known as *compliance*.

Breathing requires that gas be exchanged on an ongoing basis. The body has specific life-function needs that must be met continually, so we need to discuss respiration in terms of the **rate of flow** of air in and out of the lungs (measured as cubic centimeters per second or minute). We also need to speak of the quantities or **volumes** that are involved in this gas exchange (measured in liters [L], milliliters [mL], cubic centimeters [cc], or on occasion, cubic inches).

Respiration for Life

What is obvious is that respiration is vital. If you are a swimmer, you probably remember staying under water a little too long, discovering the limits of your respiratory system, and feeling panic when you reached those limits. Let us examine why those limits are reached and how we work within those limits for speech.

When you breathe in, you are engaged in a simple gesture with very complex results. The goal of respiration is oxygenation of blood and elimination of carbon dioxide. This basic process of gas exchange has four stages: ventilation, distribution, perfusion, and diffusion. **Ventilation** refers to the actual movement of air in the conducting respiratory pathway. This air is distributed to the 300 million alveoli where the oxygen-poor vascular supply from the right pulmonary artery is perfused to the 6 billion capillaries that supply those alveoli. **Perfusion** refers to the migration of gas or liquid through a barrier. The actual gas exchange across the alveolar-capillary membrane is referred to as **diffusion**.

ventilation: air inhaled

perfusion: migration of fluid or gas through a barrier

diffusion: migration or mixing of one material (e.g., liquid) through another

The ventilation process is a direct result of the action of the diaphragm and muscles of respiration. As discussed in Chapter 2, contraction of muscles of inspiration causes expansion of the alveoli that results in a negative alveolar pressure and air being drawn into the lungs. Understanding the pressure changes in this process is critical.

Effects of Turbulence on Respiration

When lungs expand, pressure throughout the system drops, expanding the alveoli. Air courses through the large-diameter conducting bronchi, which, being comprised of cartilage, resist the negative pressure to collapse. In healthy lungs, this results in relatively low resistance and laminar flow of air. The term *laminar flow* refers to air or fluid with molecules that flow in parallel to one another. *Turbulent flow* is the condition in which the molecules are moving in a nonlaminar fashion, similar to eddies. Some slight turbulence occurs at bifurcations such as where the trachea splits to become the right and left main stem bronchi, but generally the flow is unimpeded.

Turbulence is not a trivial condition, because even a small irregularity in the airway (such as mucus) greatly increases the resistance to airflow and also the difficulty in respiration.

Respiratory Cycle

During quiet respiration, adults complete between 12 and 18 cycles of respiration per minute (Figure 3–3). A cycle of respiration is defined as one inspiration and one expiration. We refer to this cycle of respiration as tidal respiration, with a tidal inspiration and tidal expiration. The actual volume of tidal respiration varies dependent upon the amount of effort exerted. This quiet breathing pattern, known as **quiet tidal** respiration (because it can be visualized as a tidal flow of air into and out of the lungs), involves about 500 mL (1/2 liter) of air with each cycle. You can visualize this by imagining a 2-liter bottle of soda being one quarter full. A quick calculation reveals that we process something on the order of 6,000 to 8,000 mL (6–8 liters) of air every minute. The volume of air involved in 1 minute of respiration is referred to as the **minute volume.**

Because these values are based on quiet, sedentary breathing, it should not surprise you to learn that they increase during strenuous work. An adult male increases his oxygen requirements by up to a factor of 20 during strenuous work. As you can see in Table 3–1, as work increases, the ventilation requirements are met by increased respiratory flow. As shown in the table, an increase in work performed (kilograms moved over 1 meter per minute) from

quiet tidal volume: the volume of air exchanged during one cycle of quiet respiration

minute volume: the volume of air exchanged by an organism in 1 minute

Turbulence and Respiration

The respiratory passageway offers relatively low resistance to airflow, a fact that works in favor of efficient respiration with little effort. As resistance to airflow increases, the effort required to draw air into the lungs increases as well, which causes rapid fatigue. You may remember the exhaustion you felt the last time you had a respiratory infection that caused excessive secretions in your respiratory passageway. Part of the fatigue you felt was the product of the turbulence produced by the mucus within the passageway. The extra drag caused by these elements has to be overcome to keep the body oxygenated, and the muscles of respiration have to work overtime to do the task.

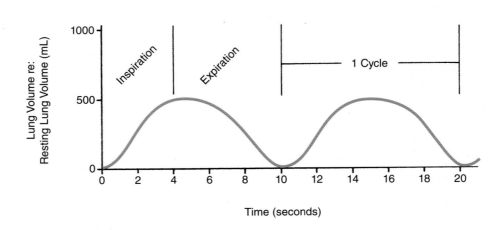

Figure 3–3. Volume display of two cycles of quiet respiration. *Source:* From Seikel/ Drumright/King. *Anatomy & Physiology for Speech, Language, and Hearing, 5th Ed.* ©Cengage, Inc. Reproduced by permission.

Table 3–1

Respiratory Volume as a Function of Work Intensity		
	Work intensity (kg m/min)	Ventilation (mL)
Female	600	3470
	900	5060
Male	900	4190
	1200	5520
	1500	7090

Source: Data from *Handbook of Biological Data* by W. S. Spector, 1956, pp. 162, 176–180, 353. Philadelphia, PA: W. B. Saunders.

900 kg m/min to 1200 kg m/min results in an increased ventilator requirement of 1330 mL of air during that same period of time. A corresponding increase to 1500 kg m/min adds another 1570 mL or air, so that the total increase of 600 kg m/min requires 2900 mL increase in ventilation. This reflects a linear increase in ventilation, which is a proxy for the oxygenation requirements of the increased effort.

Developmental Processes in Respiration

There are developmental effects on the physical structures of respiration, with functional implications in respiratory cycle and respiratory volumes. The lungs undergo a great deal of prenatal development, as seen in Figure 3–4. By the time the infant is born, the cartilaginous conducting airway is complete, although the number of alveoli will increase from about 25 million at birth to more than 300 million by 8 years of age. We retain that number throughout life.

The conducting airways grow steadily in diameter and length until thorax growth is complete, although the thorax expands to a greater degree than the lungs. As the thorax expands, the lungs are stretched to fill the cavity, a fact that helps to explain two differences between adults and children. As we mentioned earlier, adults breathe between 12 and 18 times per minute while at rest, but the newborn breathes between 40 and 70 cycles per minute. By 5 years, the child is down to about 20 breaths per minute (bpm), and this number drops to about 18 bpm at 15 years of age (Table 3–2). The adult has a considerable volume of air that is never expelled, but the infant does not have this reserve. In essence, the thorax expands during growth and development and stretches the lungs beyond their natural volume.

As a result of this expansion, there is a volume of air in the adult lung that cannot be expelled (residual volume), and this volume helps to account for the reserve capacity of adults relative to infants. Infant lungs have yet to undergo the proliferation of the alveoli seen during childhood, and thus infants must breathe more frequently to meet their metabolic needs.

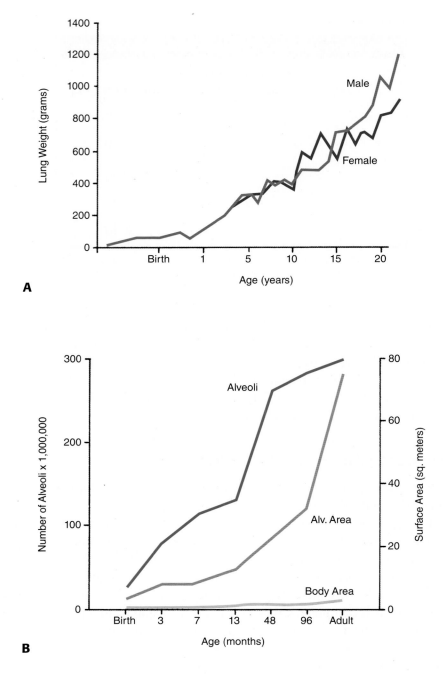

Figure 3–4. A. Changes in lung weight as a function of age. Notice that males and females are essentially equivalent in lung weight until puberty, at which time the increased thoracic cavity size of the male is reflected in larger lung weight. **B.** Changes in lung tissue with age. The number of alveoli increases radically through the fourth year of life, and the total alveolar area stabilizes around puberty when the thorax approximates its adult volume. *Source:* From Seikel/Drumright/King. *Anatomy & Physiology for Speech, Language, and Hearing, 5th Ed.* ©Cengage, Inc. Reproduced by permission. (Data from *Physiology of Respiration* by J. H. Comroe, 1965. Chicago: Year Book Medical Publishers.)

ANAQUEST LESSON

Lung Volumes and Capacities

Respiration is the product of several forces and structures, and for us to make sense of them, we need to define some volumes and capacities of the lungs. When we refer to volumes, we are partitioning off the respiratory system so that we may get an accurate estimate of the amount of air each compartment can hold. For instance, we could conceivably talk about the volume of a single alveolus, which is about 250 microns in diameter, or about 250 millionths of a meter, although that might not produce a very

Table 3–2

Respiration Rate in Breaths Per Minute as a Function of Age	
Age	**Respiration Rate (bpm)**
Newborn	60
1 year	30
2 years	25
3 years	24
5 years	20
10 years	18
15 years	18
20 years	17

Source: Data from *Physical Growth and Development* by J. Valadian & D. Porter, 1977, p. 311. Boston, MA: Little, Brown, & Co.

useful number. We also might speak of capacities, which are more functional units. **Capacities** refer to combinations of volumes that express physiological limits. Volumes are discrete, whereas capacities represent functional combinations of volumes.

Both volumes and capacities are measured in milliliters (mL, which are thousandths of a liter) or cubic centimeters (cc, which is another name for the same thing). To get an idea of what these volumes and capacities really amount to, use a 2-liter soda bottle as a reference. One liter is 1000 mL, which is also 1000 cc.

In respiration, there are five volumes that we should consider. Refer to Tables 3–3 and 3–4, as well as to Figure 3–5 as we discuss these.

Lung Volumes

Tidal Volume (TV)

The volume of air that we breathe in during a respiratory cycle is referred to as *tidal volume*. The definition of TV makes precise measurement difficult, because it varies as a function of physical exertion, body size, and age. **Quiet tidal volume** (or Resting tidal volume, TV at rest) has an average for adult males of around 600 cc and for adult females of approximately 450 cc. This works out to an average of 525 cc for adults, or approximately one-quarter of the volume of a 2-liter soda bottle every 5 seconds. So the volume of air we breathe at rest fills up three of these bottles every minute. As shown in Table 3–1, TV increases markedly as effort increases.

Quiet tidal volume: the volume of air exchanged during one cycle of quiet respiration.

Table 3–3

Respiratory Volumes and Capacities
Volumes
Tidal volume (TV): The volume of air exchanged in one cycle of respiration
Inspiratory reserve volume (IRV): The volume of air that can be inhaled after a tidal inspiration
Expiratory reserve volume (ERV): The volume of air that can be expired following passive, tidal expiration; also known as **resting lung volume**
Residual volume (RV): The volume of air remaining in the lungs after a maximum exhalation
Dead space air: The volume of air within the conducting passageways that cannot be involved in gas exchange (included as a component of residual volume)
Capacities
Vital capacity (VC): The volume of air that can be inhaled following a maximal exhalation; includes inspiratory reserve volume, tidal volume, and expiratory reserve volume (VC = IRV + TV + ERV)
Functional residual capacity (FRC): The volume of air in the body at the end of passive exhalation; includes expiratory reserve and residual volumes (FRC = ERV + RV)
Total lung capacity (TLC): The sum of inspiratory reserve volume, tidal volume, expiratory reserve volume, and residual volume (TLC = IC + FRC)
Inspiratory capacity (IC): The maximum inspiratory volume possible after tidal expiration (IC = TV + IRV)

Table 3–4

Typical Respiratory Volumes and Capacities in Adults			
Volume/capacity	**Males (in cc)**	**Females (in cc)**	**Average (in cc)**
Tidal volume	600	450	525
Inspiratory reserve volume	3000	1950	2475
Expiratory reserve volume	1200	800	1000
Residual volume	1200	1000	1100
Dead space air (included in Residual Volume)	150	125	138
Vital capacity	4800	3200	4000
Functional residual capacity	2400	1800	2100
Total lung capacity	6000	4200	5100
Inspiratory capacity	3600	2400	3000

Note: Volumes and capacities vary as a function of body size, gender, age, and body height. These volumes represent approximate values for healthy adults between 20 and 30 years of age. Vital capacity is estimated by accounting for age (in years) and height (in cm):

Males:
VC in mL = (27.63 − [0.112 × age in yrs]) X height in cm

Females:
VC in mL = (21.78 − [0.101 × age in yrs]) X height in cm

Source: Data from Baldwin, Cournand, & Richards (1948) as cited in *An Introduction to Respiratory Physiology* by F. F. Kao, 1972, p. 39. Amsterdam, The Netherlands: Excerpta Medica; and *The Mechanical Basis of Respiration* by R. M. Peters, 1969, p. 49. Boston, MA: Little, Brown, & Co.

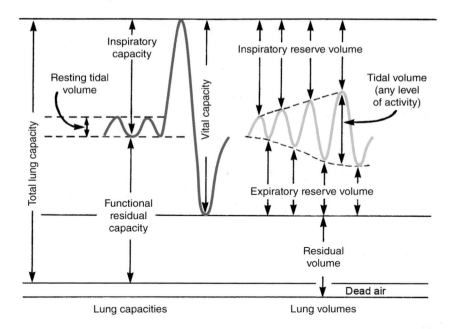

Figure 3–5. Lung volumes and capacities as displayed on a spirogram. *Source:* From Seikel/Drumright/King. *Anatomy & Physiology for Speech, Language, and Hearing, 5th Ed.* ©Cengage, Inc. Reproduced by permission. (Modified from Pappenheimer et al., 1950.)

Inspiratory Reserve Volume (IRV)

The second volume of interest is **inspiratory reserve volume** (IRV). IRV is the volume that can be inhaled after a tidal inspiration. It is the volume of air that is in reserve for use *beyond* the volume you would breathe in tidally.

To help remember the IRV, do the following exercise. Sit quietly and breathe in and out tidally until you become aware of your breath, and tag each breath mentally with the words *in* and *out*. After a few ins and outs, stop breathing at the end of one of your inspirations. This is the peak of the tidal inspiration. Instead of breathing out (which is what you want to do), breathe in as deeply as you can. The amount you inspired after you stopped is the IRV, and if you are an average adult, the volume is about 2475 cc (2.475 liters).

inspiratory reserve volume: the volume of air that can be inhaled after a tidal inspiration

Expiratory Reserve Volume (ERV)

The parallel volume for expiration is the **expiratory reserve volume** (ERV). ERV is the amount of air that can be expired following passive, tidal expiration. To experience this, breathe as you did before, but this time stop following expiration, before you breathe in. This point is easier to reach, because you can just *relax* your muscles and air will flow out without muscular effort. Expire as completely as you can, and you experience ERV: It is the amount of air you expire after that tidal expiration, amounting to about 1000 cc (1.0 liter). This volume is also referred to as **resting lung volume** (RLV), because it is the volume present in the resting lungs after a passive exhalation.

expiratory reserve volume: the volume of air that can be expired after a tidal expiration

Residual Volume (RV)

A fourth volume of interest is **residual volume** (RV), the volume remaining in the lungs after a maximum exhalation. No matter how forcefully or

residual volume: in respiration, the volume of air remaining after a maximum exhalation

completely you exhale, there is a volume of air (about 1.1 liters) that cannot be eliminated. This volume exists because the lungs are stretched as a result of the relatively expanded thorax, so it should come as no shock to know that it is not present in the newborn. You might think of it as an acquired space. By the way, this does not mean we do not use that air, but rather simply that it is a *volume* that is not eliminated during expiration. The residual volume does undergo gas exchange.

Dead Space Air

We have accommodated the major volumes, but we must deal with the volume that cannot be involved in gas exchange. The air in the conducting passageways cannot be involved in gas exchange because there are no alveoli. Recall that the conducting passageways of the lungs are constructed largely of cartilage, and the upper respiratory passageway (consisting of the mouth, pharynx, and nose) certainly does not have alveoli. The volume that cannot undergo gas exchange in the respiratory system is referred to as **dead space air** and in the adult has a volume of about 150 cc. This varies also with age and weight, but is approximately equal (in cc) to your weight in pounds. The volume associated with dead space air is included in RV, because both are volumes associated with air that cannot be expelled.

The concept of dead space air (and its importance) may become more vivid if you consider a swimmer using a tube or snorkel to breathe from underwater. This person has additional dead space air associated with the tube: The longer the tube is, the greater the volume needed to be inhaled to pull air from the surface into the lungs. In pathological conditions, the term "dead space air" takes on new meaning. In the healthy individual, **anatomical dead space air** (described previously) and **physiological dead space air** (wasted ventilation) are the same. As you found in the clinical note on Emphysema in Chapter 2, there are conditions that contribute to increased physiological dead space air; that is, pathological conditions of the respiratory system often result in wastage of respiratory effort and air.

dead space air: the air within the conducting passageways that cannot be involved in gas exchange

Lung Capacities

ANAQUEST LESSON

The volumes may be combined in a number of ways to characterize physiological needs. The following four capacities are useful combinations of volumes.

Vital Capacity (VC)

Of the capacities, **vital capacity** (VC) is the most often cited in speech and hearing literature, because it represents the capacity available for speech (Figure 3–6). Vital capacity is the combination of IRV, ERV, and TV. That is, VC represents the total volume of air that can be inspired after a maximal expiration. Resting Tidal Volumeis approximately 4000 cc in the average adult. Based on normative data (Needham, Rogan & McDonald, 1954), expiratory reserve volume (resting lung volume) is about 29% of vital capacity.

vital capacity: the total volume of air that can be inspired after a maximal expiration

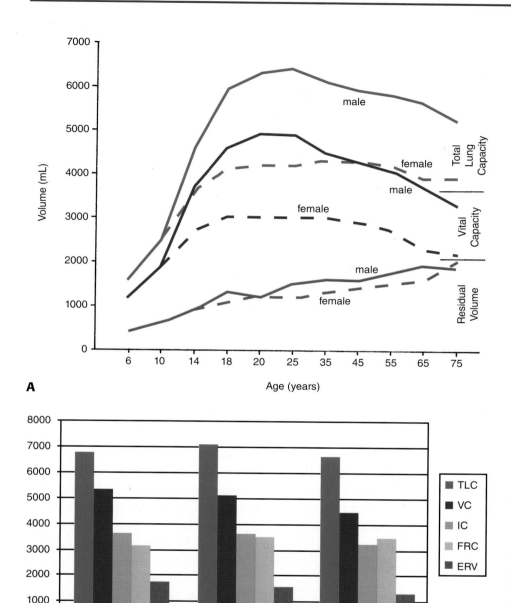

Figure 3–6. A. Vital capacity, total lung capacity, and residual volume as a function of age. *Source:* From Seikel/Drumright/King. *Anatomy & Physiology for Speech, Language, and Hearing, 5th Ed.* ©Cengage, Inc. Reproduced by permission. (From data of Hoit, J. D. & Hixon, T. J. (1987). Age and speech breathing. *Journal of Speech and Hearing Research, 30,* p. 357.) **B.** Effect of age on selected volumes and capacities in healthy males. Note that the total lung capacity (TLC) remains the same across the adult life-span, but vital capacity (VC), inspiratory capacity (IC), and expiratory reserve volume (ERV) diminish. Functional residual capacity (FRC) increases as one ages because it reflects the loss of inspiratory capacity of aging. *Source:* From Seikel/Drumright/King. *Anatomy & Physiology for Speech, Language, and Hearing, 5th Ed.* ©Cengage, Inc. Reproduced by permission. (Data from *Handbook of Biological Data* by W. S. Spector, 1956, p. 267. Philadelphia: W. B. Saunders.)

Functional Residual Capacity (FRC)

Functional residual capacity is the volume of air remaining in the body after a passive exhalation (FRC = ERV + RV). In the average adult, this comes to approximately 2100 mL.

functional residual capacity: the volume of air remaining in the body after a passive exhalation

Total Lung Capacity (TLC)

Total lung capacity is the sum of all the volumes (TLC = TV + IRV + ERV + RV), totaling approximately 5100 cc. Note that this is different from VC, which represents the volume of air that is involved in a maximal respiratory cycle, whereas TLC includes RV. RV serves as a buffer in respiration

total lung capacity: sum of tidal volume, inspiratory reserve volume, expiratory reserve volume, and residual volume

because it is not immediately involved in interaction with the environment. Oxygen-rich air is diluted by mixing with the air of the RV, so that during brief periods of fluctuating air quality, relatively constant oxygenation occurs.

Inspiratory Capacity (IC)

inspiratory capacity: the maximum inspiratory volume possible after tidal expiration

Inspiratory capacity is the maximum inspiratory volume possible after tidal expiration (IC = TV + IRV). This refers to the capacity of the lungs for inspiration and represents a volume of approximately 3000 cc in the adult.

Effect of Age on Volumes and Capacities

As we age, tissue changes. What may surprise us is how rapidly our body reaches its peak function and how steady the decline is. VC is a function of body weight, age, and height—a relationship that can be expressed mathematically, as seen in Table 3–4 and graphically in Figures 3–6 and 3–7.

What you can see from these figures is that as age increases, VC decreases by about 100 mL per year in adulthood. Figure 3–6 also shows that VC increases steadily with body growth up to about 20 years of age, holds constant through about age 25, and then begins a steady decline. Females have smaller VC throughout the life span, as reflected in the height element (males tend to be taller). As you can see in Figure 3–6B, age also has an effect on the other capacities. Hoit and Hixon (1987) showed that TLC remained essentially unaltered across the life span for healthy Caucasian males. What can be seen, however, is a reflection of the mathematically produced curve of Figure 3–7: VC shows a clear decline with age. In addition, IC and ERV decrease. Take a look at Figure 3–6A and notice that residual volume increases with age. We maintain the same lung capacity (TLC) throughout life, but we have a marked reduction in function as we age. As individuals age, compliance of the lungs decreases, which results in reduced ability to inflate the

Figure 3–7. Mathematically predicted changes in vital capacity based on age and gender. *Source:* From Seikel/Drumright/King. *Anatomy & Physiology for Speech, Language, and Hearing, 5th Ed.* ©Cengage, Inc. Reproduced by permission.

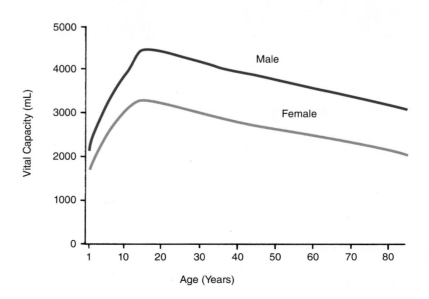

Muscle Weakness and Respiratory Function

Many disease processes reduce respiratory function, which can have a remarkable effect on other systems as well. Diseases that produce spasticity can result in paradoxical contraction of the muscles of expiration during inspiration, greatly reducing the VC. Likewise, individuals may have flaccid or hypotonic (low muscle tone) conditions that reduce the degree and strength of muscular contraction. When you think about it, it makes perfect sense that diseases that cause muscular weakness could reduce **respiratory capacity**.

We have a warning about quickly blaming the muscles of respiration for apparent deficits in vital capacity, inspiratory reserve, and so on. When testing an individual with a compromised motor system, remember that you are testing the whole system. An individual being evaluated in our clinic had weak labial muscles that caused her to have difficulty getting an adequate seal around the mouthpiece of the spirometer. Readings from this instrument thus implied respiratory deficit when, in reality, the problem was with the articulatory system. Likewise, insufficiency of the soft palate, whether due to muscular weakness or inadequate tissue, can result in nasal leakage during respiratory tasks. Again, this can masquerade as an apparent respiratory deficit.

respiratory capacities: combinations of volumes that express physiological limits

lungs. The lung volume is constant, but you see a *steady growth in the volume that is unavailable for direct gas exchange*, residual volume. Lung compliance is a measure of lung distensibility, or the ability of a lung to be distended. Lung tissue is elastic, but as tissue is damaged through some disease states such as emphysema, the lungs become more distended and so the lungs become more compliant. In contrast, diseases that increase airway resistance result in less distension, and thus have less compliance.

Compliance is expressed as the change in volume (liters) divided by the change in pressure (cm H_2O). Essentially, an efficient lung is one in which there is maximal volume inhaled or exhaled for a given pressure change. If you have to increase the pressure to move a given volume, lung compliance drops. Normal lung compliance for an adult is about 100 cc per cm of H_2O pressure. Reduced compliance, such as that found with pulmonary edema, requires greater pressure for a given volume of air. In contrast, increased compliance is seen in diseases in which the alveoli have collapsed, such as emphysema. In this case, the increased compliance in the lungs reflects reduced useable volume. Too much compliance and there will be too little volume displaced for a given pressure, while too great a compliance requires a great deal of pressure to make a volume change.

☑ *To summarize:*

- There are several volumes and capacities of importance to your study of respiration.

- The volumes, which indicate arbitrary partitioning of the respiratory system, include **tidal volume** (the volume inspired and expired in a cycle of respiration), **inspiratory reserve volume** (air inspired beyond tidal inspiration), **expiratory reserve volume** (air expired beyond tidal expiration), **residual volume** (air that remains in the lungs after maximal expiration), and **dead space air** (air that does not undergo gas exchange).
- Capacities are combinations of volumes that reflect functional limits. **Vital capacity** is the volume of air that can be inspired after a maximal expiration, while **Functional residual capacity** is the air that remains in the body after passive exhalation. **Total lung capacity** represents the sum of all lung volumes. **Inspiratory capacity** is the volume that can be inspired from resting lung volume.

ANAQUEST LESSON

Pressures of the Respiratory System

There are five specific pressures for nonspeech and speech functions: alveolar pressure, intrapleural pressure, subglottal pressure, intraoral pressure, and atmospheric pressure (Figure 3–8).

The atmosphere surrounding the earth and within which we live exerts a sizable pressure on the surface of the earth (760 mm Hg; i.e., sufficient pressure to elevate a column of mercury 760 mm against gravity). **Atmospheric pressure** (P_{atm}) is actually our reference in discussions of the respiratory system, and so we will treat it as a constant zero against which to compare respiratory pressures. **Intraoral**, or **mouth pressure** (P_m) is the pressure that could be measured within the mouth, while **subglottal pressure** (P_s) is the pressure below the vocal folds. During normal respiration with open vocal folds, we may assume that subglottal and intraoral pressures are equal to alveolar pressure. As we progress more deeply into the lungs, we can estimate **alveolar** or **pulmonic pressure** (P_{al}), the pressure that is present within the individual alveolus. If we were to measure the pressure in the space between parietal and visceral pleurae, we would refer to it as **intrapleural pressure** or **pleural** (P_{pl}). Intrapleural pressure is negative throughout respiration. Recall that the lungs, inner thorax, and diaphragm are wrapped in a continuous

atmospheric pressure: Pressure exerted by the weight of the atmosphere

subglottal pressure: Pressure measured below the level of the vocal folds

intraoral (mouth) pressure: air pressure measured within the mouth

alveolar (pulmonic) pressure: air pressure measured at the level of the alveolus in the lung

intrapleural (pleural) pressure: pressure in the space between parietal and visceral pleurae

Pneumothorax

Pneumothorax (*pneumo* = air) is aggregation of air in the pleural space between the lungs and the chest wall, with subsequent loss of the negative intrapleural pressure. This condition can arise through one of several means, but the product is always a collapsed lung. In *open* pneumothorax, air is introduced into the space through a breach of the thoracic wall, typically by means of a puncture wound (e.g., knife wound, automobile accident).

Recall that this pressure maintains the close bond between the visceral pleural lining of the lungs and that of the inner thorax. When that bond is broken by the open wound, the lungs will collapse, putting them in a state of constant outward distension arising from the difference between adult thorax size and adult lung size (see the section on Developmental Processes in Respiration, above).

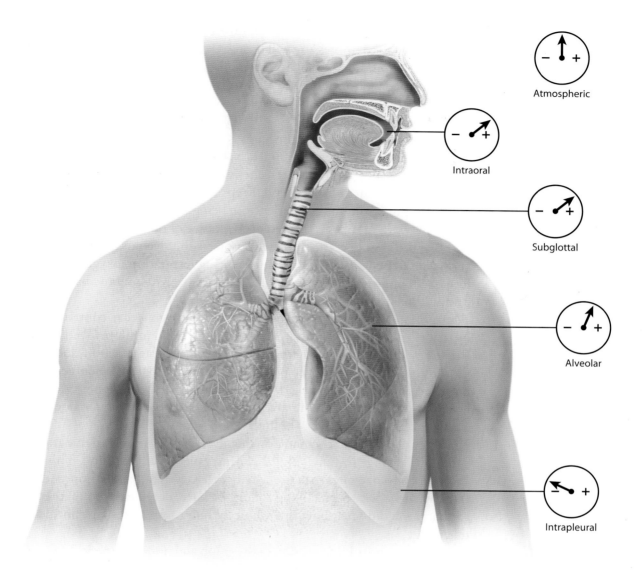

Atmospheric

Intraoral

Subglottal

Alveolar

Intrapleural

Figure 3–8. Pressures of respiration. *Source:* From Seikel/Drumright/King. *Anatomy & Physiology for Speech, Language, and Hearing, 5th Ed.* ©Cengage, Inc. Reproduced by permission.

sheet of pleural lining. When one attempts to separate the visceral from parietal pleurae, a negative pressure ensues.

These pressure measurements are all made relative to atmospheric pressure. When we refer to alveolar pressure as being, for instance, +3 cm H_2O, it means that, through muscular effort, we have generated +3 cm H_2O pressure *above and beyond* atmospheric pressure (e.g., if atmospheric pressure is 1033 cm H_2O, then alveolar pressure would be 1036 cm H_2O). Alveolar pressure may be indirectly estimated by having an individual swallow a balloon and breathe. Because the trachea and esophagus are adjacent structures sharing a common wall, the pressure changes within the trachea produce analogous changes in the esophagus, and a pressure sensor in the balloon will permit estimation of air pressure below the level of the vocal folds.

When the diaphragm is pulled down for tidal inspiration, Boyle's law predicts that alveolar pressure will drop (relative to atmospheric pressure). In quiet tidal inspiration, alveolar pressure drops to approximately -2 cm H_2O until equalized with atmospheric pressure by inspiratory flow. Likewise, during expiration, the pressure at the alveolar level becomes positive with reference to the atmosphere, increasing to $+2$ cm H_2O during quiet tidal breathing.

The work of expanding the lungs is one of overcoming resistance within the lungs. Surface active solution (surfactant) is released into the alveoli, and the result is greatly reduced surface tension. This decrease in surface tension reduces the pressure of the alveoli, keeps the alveolar walls from collapsing, and keeps fluid from the capillaries from being drawn into the lungs. Pressure in any network of tubes is greatest at the source of the pressure, which in this case is at the alveolus. The surfactant protects the alveolus, promotes airflow, and facilitates effort-free respiration. During respiration, oxygen is perfused into the bloodstream across the alveolar–capillary membrane barrier, while carbon dioxide is perfused into the alveolus.

When the thorax is expanded by means of muscular contraction, the lungs will follow faithfully, expanding the 300 million alveoli within the lungs. Secreting cells within the visceral pleurae release a lubricating fluid into the potential space between visceral and parietal pleurae, and the presence of this fluid lets the lungs and thorax make a slippery, extremely low-friction contact. At the alveolus, oxygen and carbon dioxide diffuse across the alveolus–capillary boundary.

Figure 3–9 is a schematic of the alveolar pressures, intrapleural pressures, and change in lung volume during quiet tidal breathing. This figure shows the alveolar pressure associated with a cycle of respiration and illustrates what we have been talking about. We have placed markers on the figure so that we can discuss how this whole system of pressures and flows works together.

Look at the volume portion of the graph and notice the periodic function representing tidal respiration. Point A represents the peak of that inspiration, and the lungs have about 500 cc of air in them. Point B represents the end of the expiratory cycle, where our subject has relaxed the forces of inspiration, and the lungs have passively evacuated down to resting lung volume. The point marked C represents the electromyographic activity recorded from the diaphragm as it contracts. Putting these volume and EMG traces together, you can see that as the diaphragm contracts, the volume increases to a maximum, ending at the point where the diaphragmatic contraction is complete.

Let us examine the flow component. As the diaphragm contracts, there is a fairly steady flow of air into the lungs (measured in mL/second), indicated by point D. When the inspiratory effort is completed (represented by termination of the diaphragm activity and the volume peak at A), the flow of air into the lungs ends. That is, when the diaphragm stops contracting, air stops flowing. As air leaves the lungs, the airflow becomes negative at point E (which simply means that the air is flowing in a different direction). Alveolar pressure goes positive ($+2$ cm H_2O) during expiration, a change you

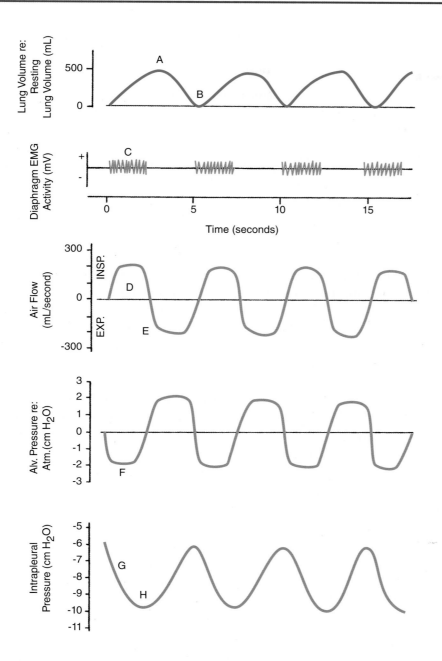

Figure 3–9. Relationships of pressures, flows, and volumes to diaphragm activity. Contraction of the diaphragm causes a drop in intrapleural pressure, which results in an increase in airflow and lung volume. The letters on the figure are explained in the text. *Source:* From Seikel/Drumright/King.. *Anatomy & Physiology for Speech, Language, and Hearing, 5th Ed.* ©Cengage, Inc. Reproduced by permission. (Data from *Physiology of Respiration* by J. H. Comroe, 1965. Chicago, IL: Year Book Medical Publishers.)

would predict from what you know about the lungs. To summarize, when the diaphragm contracts, airflow begins and is fairly steady throughout the inspiratory cycle; when the diaphragm stops contracting, the air begins to flow out of the lungs.

This is a good point to examine the pressures driving this process. Recall that contraction of the diaphragm causes the alveolar pressure to drop; then the point marked F will make sense: When the diaphragm is active (C), pressure deep within the lungs drops. Alveolar pressure reaches its maximum negativity during this tidal inspiration (–2 cm H_2O relative to atmospheric pressure), because the negative pressure is responsible for airflow into the lungs. Looking at G will explain why that pressure drops. Recall that intrapleural pressure is constantly negative relative to atmospheric pressure, arising from the fact that the lungs are in a state of continued expansion within the thoracic cavity. Because of this constant state of expansion, intrapleural pressure never goes positive.

When the diaphragm contracts, the intrapleural pressure becomes even more negative as the diaphragm attempts to pull the diaphragmatic pleurae away from the visceral pleurae. During the entire period of contraction of the diaphragm, the pressure continues to drop: The diaphragm is pulling farther away from its resting point, and the pressure between the pleurae increases proportionately. As the diaphragm reaches the end of its contraction, intrapleural pressure reaches a maximum negativity (H) that reverses upon relaxation of the diaphragm. When the diaphragm contracts, the volume (space) between the two pleural linings increases; Boyle's law dictates that pressure will drop, and it does. Depression of the diaphragm for quiet tidal inspiration results in an intrapleural pressure of approximately -10 cm H_2O, but relaxing the diaphragm during quiet expiration does not return the pressure to atmospheric, but rather returns it to a constant rest pressure of -6 cm H_2O. In the normal, healthy individual, intrapleural pressure remains negative at all times, becoming increasingly negative as muscles of inspiration act on the lungs.

The fact that this intrapleural pressure remains negative underscores two important notions. First, the lungs are in a state of continual expansion because the thorax is larger than the lungs that fill it. Second, the lungs are never completely deflated under normal circumstances, because of the residual volume discussed earlier.

During inspiration and expiration, two more pressures are of interest to us. Subglottal pressure is the pressure measured beneath the level of the vocal folds (*glottis* refers to the space between the vocal folds). Above the vocal folds, the respiratory pressure measured within the oral cavity is referred to as **intraoral pressure**. When the vocal folds are open, intraoral pressure, subglottal pressure, and alveolar pressure are the same.

The pressure beneath and above the vocal folds is directly related to what is happening in the lungs, as long as the vocal folds are open for air passage. If the lungs are drawing in air, there will be a negative pressure at both of these locations. If the lungs are in expiration, the pressure will be relatively positive. Things get more complicated when the vocal folds are closed.

When we close the vocal folds for phonation (voicing), we place a significant blockage in the flow of air through the upper respiratory pathway. Closing the vocal folds causes an immediate increase in the pressure below the vocal folds (subglottal air pressure) as the lungs continue expiration. At the same time, closing the vocal folds causes the pressure above the vocal folds (intraoral pressure) to drop to near atmospheric, resulting in a large difference in pressure between the supraglottal (above vocal folds) and subglottal regions. If this *transglottal pressure* exceeds 3 to 5 cm H_2O, the vocal folds will be blown open and voicing will begin. This level of pressure is critical, because it marks the minimal requirement of respiration for speech (Netsell & Hixon, 1978). We are going to revisit this 3 to 5 cm H_2O pressure when we discuss checking action later in this chapter.

The requirements for speech and nonspeech breathing are markedly different. Nonspeech respiration mandates a specific level of gas exchange to meet metabolic requirements. Respiration for speech requires, in addition, maintenance of a relatively steady flow of air at a relatively steady pressure. This is a tall order for a system that is designed for cycling air in and out of a cavity. Because we are inherently efficient creatures, we work very hard to avoid working very hard. The most efficient range of respiration in terms of energy outlay is to maintain VC at approximately resting lung volume. Recall that as you inflate your lungs to greater and greater values above RLV, you must use increasingly more muscle activity. Frankly, we do not like to spend a lot of time in these extremes, because it takes a lot of energy. Instead, we tend to keep our VC near the RLV regions for conversational speech, ranging from 35% to 60% of VC. Because RLV is 38% of VC, you can see that we work a small bit in ERV and considerably more in IRV, but we stay away from the extremes. Loud speech requires greater inspiration, using lung volumes upward of 80% of VC.

Having drawn these conclusions about volume, what can we say about maintenance of subglottal pressure? Pressure is obviously a direct function of the forces of expiration, which are generally passive above 38% of VC. Because we operate almost exclusively within the region above 38% of VC, generation of subglottal pressure is mostly a function of the forces of expiration, specifically elasticity and gravity. We must use the muscles of inspiration to check that outflow of air, so the muscular effort in speech beyond the initial inspiration is dominated by using the muscles of inspiration *again* to impede the outflow of air. By delicate manipulation of these muscles, we are able to maintain a constant subglottal pressure that can be used for the fine control of phonation by the larynx. In the section on pressures and volumes of speech we examine the effects of tissue characteristics on respiration, particularly as they relate to maintaining constant subglottal pressure.

While we readily manipulate the respiratory mechanism for speech, there is ample evidence that we take specific care to prepare for this act. Hixon, Goldman, and Mead (1973) showed that when individuals prepare for speech, they expand and "set" the thorax to a greater extent than in nonspeech for a given volume of air. The authors hypothesize that this preparatory act provides the optimum thoracic positioning for production of respiratory pulses needed for speech suprasegmental aspects.

You can now view these critical pressures as a system. We are continually playing the respiratory system against the relatively stable **atmospheric pressure**. Contraction of the diaphragm and muscles of inspiration causes the intrapleural pressure to decrease markedly, which in turn causes the lungs to expand. When the lungs expand, alveolar pressure drops relative to atmospheric pressure, causing air to enter the lungs. Relaxing the muscles of inspiration permits the natural recoil of the lungs and cartilage to draw the chest back to its original position, and the relaxed diaphragm again returns to its relatively elevated position in the thorax. When this happens, intrapleural pressure increases (but still stays negative) and alveolar pressure becomes positive relative to atmospheric pressure. Air leaves the lungs.

✅ *To summarize:*

- Volumes and pressures vary as a direct function of the forces acting on the respiratory system.

- With the vocal folds open, **oral pressure**, **subglottal pressure**, and **alveolar pressure** are roughly equivalent.

- **Intrapleural pressure** is always negative, increasing in negativity during inspiration.

- These pressures are all measured relative to **atmospheric pressure**.

- During inspiration, expansion of the thorax decreases the already negative intrapleural pressure, and the increased lung volume results in a **negative alveolar pressure**.

- Air from outside the body will flow into the lungs as a result of the pressure difference between the lungs and the atmosphere.

- During expiration, this pressure differential is reversed, with air escaping the lungs to equalize the **positive alveolar pressure** with the relatively negative atmospheric pressure.

Pressures Generated by the Tissue

At this point, we should address the forces of expiration in earnest. The process of inspiration is one of exerting force to overcome gravity and the elastic forces of tissue. Inspiration is generally active, requiring muscular action to complete it.

Expiration capitalizes on elasticity and gravity to reclaim some of the energy expended during inspiration. When muscles of inspiration contract, they stretch tissue and cause the abdomen to distend. When these muscles relax during expiration, the stretched tissues tend to return to their original dimension due to their elastic nature, and gravity works to depress the rib cage. To breathe in, you have to move all of these muscles and bones, and as you relax, they return to their original positions.

These restoring forces actually generate pressures themselves. Recoil of the chest during exhalation obeys the laws applying to any elastic material: The greater you distend or distort the material, the greater is the force required to hold it in that position and the greater is the force with which it returns to rest.

You can get common-sense validation of this recoil force if you recall loading a stapler with staples. As you pull back the spring that holds the staples, you reach a point where the spring almost wins. The force required to hold the spring back is much greater as it gets farther from its point of rest. You know also the force with which your finger can get whacked if you do not get out of the way in time; the farther you have pushed the spring, the more it hurts when it is inadvertently released.

The same elastic forces govern how much effort is required to inhale. Close your eyes and breathe in as deeply as you can and hold it for a few seconds. Feel how much pressure you are fighting to hold your chest in that position. Next, take in a quiet breath and hold it. Do you feel the difference in pressure?

This relationship is described in the curve of Figure 3–10, which shows the result of pressure generated by all that force (remember that pressure is force exerted over an area). The farther the rib cage is expanded, the greater the force that is trying to return the rib cage to rest.

This curve is called the *relaxation pressure curve*, and it was generated by asking people to do what you just did with your eyes closed. The subjects were told to inhale to some percentage of their VC and then to relax their muscu-lature while their intraoral pressure (which approximates both subglottal and alveolar pressures) was measured using a manometer. Repeated measures of this sort at various percentages of VC resulted in the upper positive portion of the curve. The curve is positive because the tissue is attempting to return to rest. This is a measure of the strength of those physical restoring forces. Note that you are capable of generating some reasonably large forces with this tissue recoil. Pressures on the order of 60 cm H_2O are fairly significant, considering that phonation requires only about 5 cm H_2O.

The bottom half of the curve is produced in much the same way, only this time the subjects were asked to exhale down to a percentage of their VC. The horizontal line at 38% is a true relaxation point, because it is the point where no pressure is generated and all parts of the system are at equilibrium. (Breathe out and then do not breathe in again: This relaxation point *before you inhale a new breath* is one of three times during a respiratory cycle when atmospheric pressure equals alveolar pressure.) The relaxation point of zero pressure represents about 29% of VC. When you relax entirely with open airway, the lungs still have about 29% of the total directly exchangeable

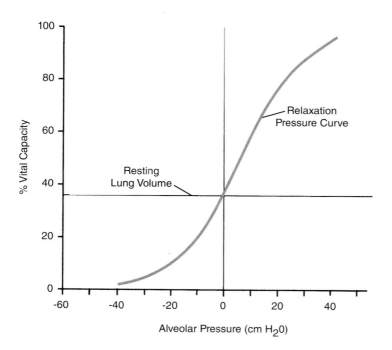

Figure 3–10. Relaxation pressure curve representing pressures generated by the passive forces of the respiratory system. *Source:* From Seikel/Drumright/King. *Anatomy & Physiology for Speech, Language, and Hearing, 5th Ed.* ©Cengage, Inc. Reproduced by permission.

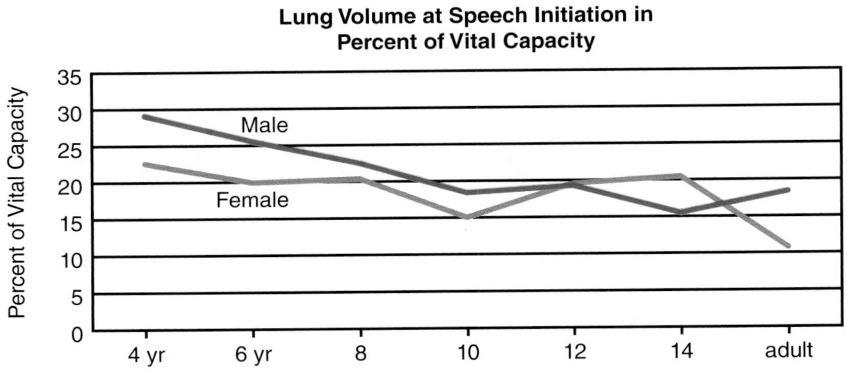

Figure 3–14. Lung volume in percent of vital capacity for low-intensity speech. *Source:* From Seikel/Drumright/King. *Anatomy & Physiology for Speech, Language, and Hearing, 5th Ed.* ©Cengage, Inc. Reproduced by permission. (From data of Stathopoulos, E. T. & Sapienza, C. M. (1997). Developmental changes in laryngeal and respiratory function with variations in sound pressure level. *Journal of Speech, Language and Hearing Research, 40,* 595–614.)

of air. This process is called **checking action**. That is, you check (impede) the flow of air out of your inflated lungs by means of the muscles that got it there in the first place—the muscles of inspiration.

Checking action is extremely important for respiratory control of speech, because it directly addresses the ability to restrain the flow of air. When people have a deficit associated with checking action (as in paralysis), they are at a tremendous disadvantage, because they are restricted to extremely short bursts of speech.

Checking action permits us to maintain the constant flow of air through the vocal tract, which in turn lets us accurately control the pressure beneath vocal folds that have been closed for phonation. We will see in Chapter 5 that this is very important when it comes to maintaining constant vocal intensity and frequency of vibration.

If you take a look at Figure 3–15A, you will see the relaxation pressure curve that we talked about earlier, but with some additions. Remember that 3 to 5 cm H_2O is the critical pressure required to sustain vocal fold vibration for speech. We have marked off the diagram so you can see how that pressure relates to relaxation pressures.

Recall that relaxation pressure is the pressure exerted by the tissues of the respiratory system on the lungs. As you inhale to your maximum (100% of vital capacity), your lung and chest recoil generates a great deal of positive pressure that is working hard to exhale air. As you exhale as much air as you can (approaching 0% of vital capacity), your lungs are trying very hard to inhale. Now, look at what happens when you superimpose the requirements of speech on this same breathing (the 5 cm H_2O line) (Figure 3–15B). In the area on the right of the figure, the forces of expiration *easily* give adequate pressure to drive the vocal folds. Not until you have exhausted down to about 50% of vital capacity do you need to think about using muscular force to *increase* subglottal pressure. In fact, in the region above 50% of VC, we have

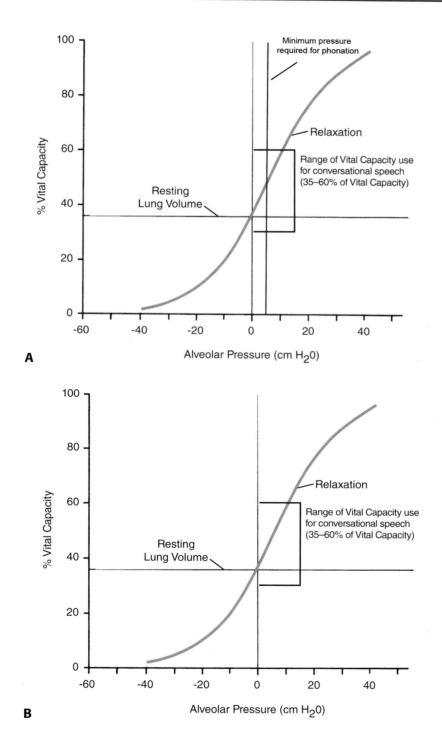

Figure 3–15. A. Relationship between relaxation pressure and minimum driving force required for phonation. The vocal folds require 5 cm H_2O pressure for onset and sustained vibration. At about 50% of vital capacity, the muscles of inspiration must be used to control outflow of air in order to maintain a constant 5 cm H_2O pressure (checking action). Below that point, increasing use of the muscles of expiration is required to maintain the 5 cm H_2O pressure for phonation. **B.** The typical volume use range for conversational speech is 35% to 60% of vital capacity. *Source:* From Seikel/Drumright/King. *Anatomy & Physiology for Speech, Language, and Hearing, 5th Ed.* ©Cengage, Inc. Reproduced by permission.

to use muscular activity as a brake to impede the expiratory forces, and this is called *checking action.* You are *checking* or *impeding* the outflow of air by using the muscles of inspiration. More importantly for this discussion, you are impeding the pressure-generation so as not to exceed the 5 cm H_2O point. To do so will result in louder speech, which may not necessarily be your goal.

Notice also that once the relaxation pressure generated by the tissue is not enough to generate that 5 cm H_2O pressure, we enlist muscles of expiration

Chronic Obstructive Pulmonary Disease

There are two major subtypes of chronic obstructive pulmonary disease (COPD): chronic bronchitis and emphysema. Chronic bronchitis is most often caused by tobacco smoking and affects about 5% of adults and 6% of children globally. Worldwide, there are about 2.9 million deaths annually from chronic bronchitis. An individual is considered to have chronic bronchitis if that person has a productive cough that lasts for 3 months or longer and occurs twice in 1 year for 2 years. The cause is inflammation of the bronchial passageway, and the result is excessive mucus production, coughing, wheezing, and shortness of breath. The disease may lead to rib fractures or even consciousness loss due to shortness of breath. The diagnostic indicators of chronic bronchitis are poor lung function, including reduced capacity, cough, and mucus secretion. A patient with chronic bronchitis may experience shortness of breath and even fevers and chills. The disease is often treated using bronchodilators, steroids to reduce the inflammation, long-term oxygen therapy, and even lung transplant. The effect on speech is reduced vocal intensity, short phrasing, and fatigue during speech.

Emphysema is the second form of COPD, resulting in loss of continuity of the alveoli. Essentially, in emphysema the inner alveolar walls break down so that alveolar surface area is diminished. The walls weaken and rupture, resulting in reduced oxygen transfer. Emphysema is most often caused by tobacco smoking, second-hand smoke, or environmental pollutants, and symptoms include shortness of breath and fatigue. Symptoms typically develop between 40 and 60 years of age, and complications include pneumothorax (collapsed lung), heart problems due to the increased workload on the heart, and physical changes. The most striking physical change is a barrel chest. We talked about paradoxical respiration in Chapter 2 as a component of chronic obstructive pulmonary disease (COPD). In emphysema, when the alveolus walls break down, the result is loss of surface area for gas exchange, but also expansion of the end-cluster of alveoli at the alveolar duct. The breakdown of the alveolar walls results in an expanded thorax, seen as a barrel-shaped chest. With this distension of the thorax, the rib cage is expanded laterally, stretching the diaphragm so that it is flat instead of its inverted bowl shape. The paradoxical part is that when a person inhales, the diaphragm contracts and actually pulls the ribs closer together, causing expiration. In speech, emphysema causes short phrasing, limited phonatory ability, and significant fatigue upon speaking.

Sleep Apnea

There are three types of sleep apnea: obstructive, central, and complex. Obstructive sleep apnea comes from having a flaccid pharynx, which results in the airway collapsing during sleep. Central sleep apnea is a neurological issue, in which the brain doesn't alert the body to breathe. Complex sleep apnea is a combination of central and obstructive apnea. Signs and symptoms of apnea include loud snoring, episodes reported by another in which a person stops breathing during sleep, gasping during sleep, awakening with dry mouth, and excessive daytime sleepiness. The patient may be treated using continuous positive airway pressure (CPAP), in which continuous positive air pressure presented nasally during sleep results in the airway remaining open.

Pulmonary Fibrosis

In pulmonary fibrosis, lung tissue—particularly the alveolar walls—becomes scarred and thickened. The disease can arise from several conditions, including pneumonia), genetic conditions such as cystic fibrosis, or from unknown (idiopathic) etiology. There are occupational risk factors, including working with silica or asbestos or working in grain or coal dust. People who have radiation therapy or undergo some types of chemotherapy may also be at risk. The fibrosis is seen more often in men than in women, and smokers are more likely to develop it. Signs and symptoms of pulmonary fibrosis are shortness of breath, presence of a dry cough, fatigue, aching muscles and joints, and clubbing of the tips of the fingers and toes (widening and rounding of the fingers and toes, downward rounding of the nails). Speech signs with pulmonary fibrosis include short phrasing, reduced vocal intensity, and fatigue during speech.

Asthma

In the chronic condition of asthma, the bronchial passageway narrows, there is overproduction of mucus, and the bronchi are inflamed. This condition may be life threatening. Signs and symptoms of asthma are shortness of breath, chest pain or tightness, sleep disturbance, wheezing, and coughing. Asthma may result from exercise, occupational irritants, cold air, some medications, emotional stress, gastroesophageal reflux, or allergy. When people experience rapidly increasing symptoms, they may require emergency treatment, but long-term treatment is typically use of an inhaled bronchial dilator. Besides short phrasing, low vocal intensity, weakness, and fatigue, people undergoing an asthma attack can have paradoxical vocal fold movement (PVFM), which is involuntary adduction of vocal folds during inspiration. PVFM can co-occur with asthma or occur separately from asthma.

Lung Cancer

Lung cancer is the leading cause of cancer deaths in the United States, with the primary risk factor being smoking tobacco. Tobacco smoke contains carcinogens, and a person who resides in a high-radon environment and who is a smoker has an even greater risk of cancer. It was originally hoped that e-cigarettes would be a means of facilitating smoking cessation, but this has not come to fruition (Grana, Benowitz, & Glantz, 2014) and has, in fact, increased the problems.

Chapter 3 Study Questions

1. Passive expiration involves the forces of _____ and
   _____.

2. Identify the indicated volumes and capacities described below.

   A. _____ volume: The volume of air that we breathe in during a
      respiratory cycle.

   B. _____ volume: The volume that can be inhaled after a tidal
      inspiration.

   C. _____ volume: The volume that can be exhaled after a tidal
      expiration.

   D. _____ volume: The volume remaining in the lungs after a maximal
      exhalation.

   E. _____ capacity: The combination of inspiratory reserve volume,
      expiratory reserve volume, and tidal volume.

   F. _____ capacity: The volume of air remaining in the body after a
      passive exhalation.

   G. _____ capacity: The sum of all the volumes.

3. _____ is the volume of air that cannot undergo gas exchange.

4. _____ pressure is the air pressure measured within the oral cavity.

5. _____ pressure is the air pressure measured below the vocal folds.

6. _____ pressure is the pressure within the alveolus.

7. _____ pressure is the pressure between the visceral and parietal pleural
   membranes.

8. When the diaphragm contracts, pressure within the alveolus _____
   (increases/decreases).

9. When air pressure within the lungs is lower than that of the atmosphere, air will
   _____ (enter/leave) the lungs.

10. When the body is placed in a reclining position, the resting lung volume
    _____ (increases/decreases).

11. Use of the muscles of inspiration to impede the outward flow of air during speech is
    termed _____.

12. Coordination of muscular activity is largely the responsibility of the cerebellum of the
    brain. An individual with neuropathology involving the cerebellum will have a deficit in
    coordination of motor function. What impact would this deficit have on speech function?

Chapter 3 Study Question Answers

1. Passive expiration involves the forces of **ELASTICITY** and **GRAVITY**.

2. Volumes and capacities:

    A. **TIDAL VOLUME:** The volume of air that we breathe in during a respiratory cycle.

    B. **INSPIRATORY RESERVE** volume: The volume that can be inhaled after a tidal inspiration.

    C. **EXPIRATORY RESERVE** volume: The volume that can be exhaled after a tidal expiration.

    D. **RESIDUAL** volume: The volume remaining in the lungs after a maximal exhalation.

    E. **VITAL** capacity: The combination of inspiratory reserve volume, expiratory reserve volume, and tidal volume.

    F. **FUNCTIONAL RESIDUAL** capacity: The volume of air remaining in the body after a passive exhalation.

    G. **TOTAL LUNG** capacity: The sum of all the volumes.

3. **DEAD SPACE AIR** is the volume of air that cannot undergo gas exchange.

4. **INTRAORAL** pressure is the air pressure measured within the oral cavity.

5. **SUBGLOTTAL** pressure is the air pressure measured below the vocal folds.

6. **ALVEOLAR** or **PULMONIC** pressure is the pressure within the alveolus.

7. **INTRAPLEURAL** or **PLEURAL** pressure is the pressure between the visceral and parietal pleural membranes.

8. When the diaphragm contracts, pressure within the alveolus **DECREASES**.

9. When air pressure within the lungs is lower than that of the atmosphere, air will **ENTER** the lungs.

10. When the body is placed in a reclining (supine) position, the resting lung volume **DECREASES**.

11. Use of the muscles of inspiration to impede the outward flow of air during speech is termed **CHECKING ACTION**.

12. Neuromuscular conditions that affect cerebellar function can result in loss of coordination of diaphragm contraction, difficulty maintaining constant subglottal pressure due to a deficit in checking action, and difficulty coordinating the respiratory effort with phonation, among other problems.

Bibliography

Agostoni, E., & Mead, J. (1964). Statics of the respiratory system. In W. Fenn & H. Rahn (Eds.), *Handbook of physiology, Section 3: Respiration* (Vol. 2). Baltimore, MD: Williams & Wilkins.

Comroe, J. H. (1965). *Physiology of respiration.* Chicago, IL: Year Book Medical Publishers.

Grana, R., Benowitz, N., & Glantz, S. A. (2014). E-cigarettes: A scientific review. *Circulation, 129*(19), 1972–1986.

Hixon, T. J. (2006). Rib torque does not assist resting tidal expiration or most conversational speech expiration. *Journal of Speech, Language, and Hearing Research, 49,* 213–214.

Hixon, T. J., Goldman, M. D., & Mead, J. (1973). Kinematics of the chest wall during speech production: Volume displacement of the rib cage, abdomen, and lung. *Journal of Speech, Language, and Hearing Research, 16,* 78–115.

Hixon, T. J., & Weismer, G. (1995). Perspectives on the Edinburgh study of speech breathing. *Journal of Speech, Language, and Hearing Research, 38,* 42–60.

Hoit, J. D., & Hixon, T. J. (1987). Age and speech breathing. *Journal of Speech, Language, and Hearing Research, 30,* 351–366.

Kao, F. F. (1972). *An introduction to respiratory physiology.* Amsterdam, The Netherlands: Exerpta Medica.

Needham, C. D., Rogan, M. C., & McDonald, I. (1954). Normal standards for lung volumes, intrapulmonary gas-mixing, and maximum breathing capacity. *Thorax, 9*(4), 313.

Netsell, R., & Hixon, T. J. (1978). A noninvasive method of clinically estimating subglottal air pressure. *Journal of Speech and Hearing Disorders, 43,* 323–330.

Pappenheimer, J. R., Comroe, J. H., Cournand, A., Ferguson, J. K. W., Filley, G. F., Fowler, W. S., . . . Riley, R. L. (1950). Standardization of definitions and symbols in respiratory physiology. *Federation Proceedings, 9*(3), 602–605.

Peters, R. M. (1969). *The mechanical basis of respiration.* Boston, MA: Little, Brown, & Co.

Rahn, H., Otis, A., Chadwick, L. E., & Fenn, W. (1946). The pressure–volume diagram of the thorax and lung. *American Journal of Physiology, 146,* 161–178.

Roychowdhury, P., Pramanik, T., Prajapati, R., Pandit, R., & Singh, S. (2011). In health—vital capacity is maximum in supine position. *Nepal Medical College Journal, 13*(2), 131–132.

Spector, W. S. (1956). *Handbook of biological data.* Philadelphia, PA: W. B. Saunders.

Stathopoulos, E. T., & Sapienza, C. M. (1997). Developmental changes in laryngeal and respiratory function with variations in sound pressure level. *Journal of Speech, Language, and Hearing Research, 40,* 595–614.

Winkworth, A. L, Davis, P. J., Adams, R. D., & Ellis, E. (1995). Breathing patterns during spontaneous speech. *Journal of Speech and Hearing Research, 38,* 124–144.

Anatomy of Phonation

Spoken communication uses both voiceless and voiced sounds, and this chapter is concerned with that critical distinction. As you'll remember from your phonetics course, the term *phoneme* refers to the sounds of speech. **Voiceless** phonemes are produced without the use of the vocal folds, such as the phonemes /s/ or /f/. **Voiced** phonemes are produced by the action of the vocal folds, as in /z/ and /v/. **Phonation**, or voicing, is the product of vibrating vocal folds, and this occurs within the larynx. Remember from Chapter 3 that we referred to respiration as the source of *energy* for speech. Phonation is the source of *voice* for speech. Respiration is the energy source that permits phonation to occur; and without respiration there would be no voicing.

The vocal folds are made up of five layers of tissue, with the deepest layer being muscle. The space between the vocal folds is termed the **glottis** (or **rima glottidis**), and the area below the vocal folds is the **subglottal** region. The vocal folds are located within the course of the airstream at the superior end of the trachea. As the airstream passes between the vocal folds, they may be made to vibrate, much as a flag flaps in the wind. Try this: Place your hand on the side of your neck and hum. You should feel a tickling vibration. This is the mechanical correlate of the sound you hear. If you alternately produce /a/ and /h/, you should feel your vocal folds start vibrating and stop, because /a/ is a voiced sound and /h/ is voiceless sound.

When you felt the vibrations of the vocal folds, you might also have noted a very important aspect of phonation. You were able to turn your voice on and off to produce the alternating voiced and voiceless sounds. When you alternated those two sounds, you were actually moving the vocal folds into and out of the airstream to cause them to start and then stop vibrating. The vocal folds are bands of tissue that can be set into vibration. Now we are ready to look at the structure of the vocal mechanism (Figure 4–1).

ANAQUEST LESSON

rima glottidis: L., slit of the glottis

Framework of the Larynx

ANAQUEST LESSON

The larynx is a musculo-cartilaginous structure located at the superior (upper) end of the trachea. It is composed of three unpaired and three paired cartilages bound by ligaments and lined with mucous membrane. Take a look at Figure 4–1. In this figure you can see the relationship between the trachea

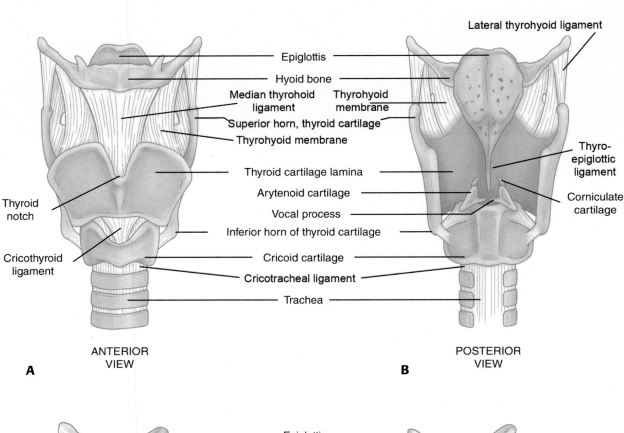

A. ANTERIOR VIEW

Epiglottis
Hyoid bone
Median thyrohoid ligament
Thyrohyoid membrane
Thyrohyoid membrane
Superior horn, thyroid cartilage
Thyroid cartilage lamina
Arytenoid cartilage
Vocal process
Inferior horn of thyroid cartilage
Cricoid cartilage
Cricotracheal ligament
Trachea
Thyroid notch
Cricothyroid ligament

B. POSTERIOR VIEW

Lateral thyrohyoid ligament
Thyro-epiglottic ligament
Corniculate cartilage

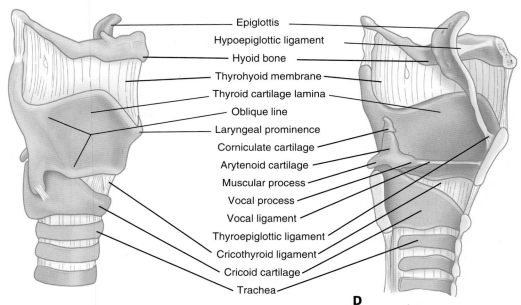

C.

Epiglottis
Hypoepiglottic ligament
Hyoid bone
Thyrohyoid membrane
Thyroid cartilage lamina
Oblique line
Laryngeal prominence
Corniculate cartilage
Arytenoid cartilage
Muscular process
Vocal process
Vocal ligament
Thyroepiglottic ligament
Cricothyroid ligament
Cricoid cartilage
Trachea

D.

Figure 4–1. A. Larynx in anterior view. **B.** Posterior view of larynx. **C.** Lateral view of larynx. **D.** View of the relationship of cricoid and arytenoids cartilages, as seen in larynx that has been cut sagittally at midline. *continues*

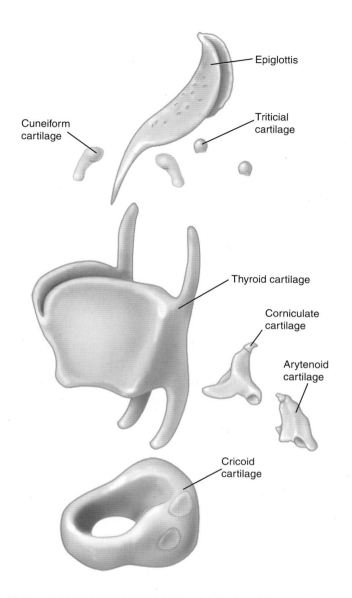

Epiglottis

Cuneiform
cartilage

Triticial
cartilage

Thyroid cartilage

Corniculate
cartilage

Arytenoid
cartilage

Cricoid
cartilage

E

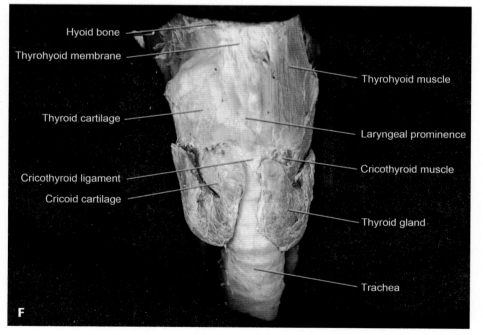

Hyoid bone

Thyrohyoid membrane

Thyrohyoid muscle

Thyroid cartilage

Laryngeal prominence

Cricothyroid muscle

Cricothyroid ligament

Cricoid cartilage

Thyroid gland

Trachea

F

Figure 4–1. *continued*
E. Exploded view of disarticulated laryngeal cartilages. *Source:* From Seikel/Drumright/King. *Anatomy & Physiology for Speech, Language, and Hearing, 5th Ed.* ©Cengage, Inc. Reproduced by permission. **F.** Photograph of anterior larynx.

Biological Functions of the Larynx

Although we capitalize on the larynx for phonation, it has a much more important function in nature. The larynx is an exquisite sphincter in that the vocal folds are capable of a very strong and rapid clamping of the airway in response to the threat of intrusion by foreign objects. As evidence of this function, there are three pairs of laryngeal muscles directly responsible for either approximating or tensing the vocal folds, although there is only one pair of muscles responsible for opening them. The vocal folds are wired to close immediately on stimulation by outside agents, such as food or liquids, a response that is followed quickly by the rapid and forceful exhalation of a cough. This combination of actions is designed to stop intrusion by foreign matter and to rapidly expel it from the opening of the airway.

The larynx has other important functions as well. Because the vocal folds provide an excellent seal to the respiratory system, they permit you to hold your breath, thus capturing a significant respiratory charge for such activities as swimming.

Holding your breath serves other functions. Lifting heavy objects requires you to *fix* your thorax by inspiring and clamping your laryngeal sphincter (vocal folds). This gives the muscles of the upper body a solid framework with which to work. You should also note from the margin notes in Chapter 2 that tightly clamping the vocal folds plays an important part in childbirth and defecation.

---

and larynx. Remember that the trachea is composed of a series of cartilage rings, connected and separated by a fibroelastic membrane. The larynx sits as an oddly shaped box atop the last ring of the trachea. It is adjacent to cervical vertebrae 4 through 6 in the adult, but the larynx of an infant is located higher. The average length of the larynx in adult males is 44 mm; in females it is 36 mm.

The **cricoid cartilage** is a complete ring resting atop the trachea and is the most inferior of the laryngeal cartilages. From the side, the cricoid cartilage takes on the appearance of a signet ring, with its back arching up relative to the front. The cricoid and thyroid cartilages articulate at the cricothyroid joint. The **thyroid cartilage** is the largest of the laryngeal cartilages, articulating with the cricoid cartilage below by means of paired processes that let it rock forward and backward at that joint. With this configuration, the paired **arytenoid cartilages** ride on the high-backed upper surface of the cricoid cartilage, forming the posterior point of attachment for the vocal folds. The **corniculate cartilages** ride on the superior surface of each arytenoid and are prominent landmarks in the aryepiglottic folds. The cuneiform cartilage, residing within the aryepiglottic folds, provides a degree of rigidity to the folds.

The thyroid cartilage articulates with the **hyoid bone** by means of a pair of superior processes. Medial to the hyoid bone and thyroid cartilage is the **epiglottis**, a leaflike cartilage. The epiglottis is a protective structure in that it drops to cover the **orifice** of the larynx during swallowing. There have been questions about its function in protection of the airway during swallowing, but the fact is that people who have had surgical removal of the epiglottis (e.g., to treat laryngeal or lingual cancer) are much more likely to have swallowing problems than those who retain the epiglottis. Indeed, reduced movement of the epiglottis after cancer surgery increases aspiration during swallowing (Halczy-Kowalik et al., 2012).

cricoid: Gr., krikos, ring; ring-form

arytenoid: Gr., arytaina, ladle; ladle-form

corniculate: L., cornu, horn; little horn

epiglottis: Gr., epi, over; over glottis

Laryngectomy

Patients who undergo **laryngectomy** (surgical removal of the larynx) lose the voicing source for speech. The larynx is removed and the oral cavity is sealed off from the trachea and lower respiratory passageway as a safeguard because the protective function of the larynx is also lost. **Laryngectomees** (individuals who have undergone laryngectomy) must alter their activities because they now breathe through a **tracheostoma**, an opening placed in the trachea through a surgical procedure known as a **tracheostomy**.

Loss of the ability to phonate is but one of the difficulties facing the laryngectomee. This patient will have difficulty with **expectoration** (elimination of phlegm from the respiratory passageway) and coughing, and will no longer be able to enjoy swimming or other activities that would expose the **stoma** to water or pollutants. The air entering the patient's lungs is no longer humidified or filtered by the upper respiratory passageway, and a filter must be kept over the stoma to prevent introduction of foreign objects. The patient may be restricted from having house pets that shed hair, as the hair can work its way into the unprotected airway. The flavor of foods is greatly reduced, because the patient may no longer breathe through the nose; and our perception of food relies heavily on the sense of smell. Depending on pre- and postoperative treatment, patients may experience extreme dryness of oral tissues (xerostomia) arising from damage to the salivary glands from radiation therapy. One result of this dryness may be a swallowing dysfunction (dysphagia). Recognize that because the trachea has been completely separated from the esophagus, the risk of aspiration is reduced after healing occurs, although the stoma always will have to be protected from intrusion of foreign bodies or liquids.

⊘ To summarize:

- The **larynx** is a musculo-cartilaginous structure located at the upper end of the trachea. It is composed of the **cricoid, thyroid,** and **epiglottis cartilages**, as well as the paired **arytenoid, corniculate,** and **cuneiform cartilages**.
- The thyroid and cricoid cartilages articulate by means of the **cricothyroid joint** that lets the two cartilages come closer together in front.
- The **arytenoid** and **cricoid cartilages** also articulate with a joint that permits a wide range of arytenoid motion.
- The **corniculate cartilages** rest on the upper surface of the arytenoids, while the **cuneiform cartilages** reside within the **aryepiglottic folds**.
- The epiglottis protects the airway during swallowing.

Inner Larynx

When these cartilages are combined with the trachea and the airway above the larynx, the result is a rough tube-like space with a constriction caused by the cartilages. This construction is unique, however, in that it is an *adjustable valve*. The vocal folds are bands of mucous membrane, connective tissue, and thyrovocalis muscle that are slung between the arytenoid cartilages

Valleculae and Swallowing

The valleculae are "little valleys" formed by the membrane between the tongue and the epiglottis. During a normal swallow, the larynx elevates and the epiglottis folds down to protect the airway from food and liquid. The food and liquid pass over the back of the tongue, through the valleculae, into the pyriform sinuses, and finally into the esophagus (this process will be discussed in detail in Chapter 8). When swallowing is compromised, as in the deficit arising from cerebrovascular accident (see Chapter 12), the larynx may not elevate properly (Dejaeger, Pelemans, Ponette, & Joosten, 1997), or the tongue movement may be inadequate, and food can accumulate in the valleculae. Based on this condition, you can presume that malodorous breath in an individual who is neurologically compromised may be a significant indicator of a dangerous swallowing dysfunction, because if the epiglottis is not covering the airway, there is a good chance that the vocal folds are not doing their job in protecting the lungs and that the lungs are being exposed to food and drink.

and the thyroid cartilage so that they may be moved into and out of the airstream. (Alternately, some anatomists consider the vocal folds as the mucous membrane and connective tissue only, excluding the thyrovocalis muscle.) Muscles attached to the arytenoids provide both adductory and abductory functions, with which we control the degree of airflow by means of muscular contraction.

ANAQUEST LESSON

triticeal: L., triticeus, wheat; wheat-like

Laryngeal Membranes

The cavity of the larynx is a constricted tube with a smooth and reasonably aerodynamic surface (see Figures 4–1 and 4–2). This tube is created by developing a deep structure of cartilages; connecting those cartilages through sheets and cords of ligaments and membrane; and lining the entire structure with a wet, smooth mucous membrane. The extrinsic ligaments provide attachment between the hyoid or trachea and the cartilage of the larynx. As seen in Figure 4-1A, the **thyrohyoid membrane** stretches across the space between the greater cornu of the hyoid and the lateral thyroid. Posterior to this is the **lateral thyrohyoid ligament**, which runs from the superior cornu of the thyroid to the posterior tip of the greater cornu hyoid. A small **triticeal cartilage** (not shown: also known as the tritiate cartilage) may or may not be found here, as it is present in only 33% of the population (Wilson et al., 2017). In front, running from the corpus hyoid to the upper border of the anterior thyroid, is the **median thyrohyoid ligament**. Together, the median thyrohyoid ligament, thyrohyoid membrane, and lateral thyrohyoid ligament connect the larynx and the hyoid bone. There are other extrinsic ligaments. The **hyoepiglottic ligament** (Figure 4–2C) and **thyroepiglottic ligament** (Figure 4–2A) attach the epiglottis to the corpus hyoid and the inner thyroid cartilage, just below the notch, respectively (not shown). The epiglottic attachment to the tongue is made by means of the **lateral** and **median glossoepiglottic ligaments** (Figure 4–2E), and the overlay of the mucous membrane on these ligaments produces the "little valleys" or **valleculae** (see Figure 4–2E) between the tongue and the epiglottis. The trachea

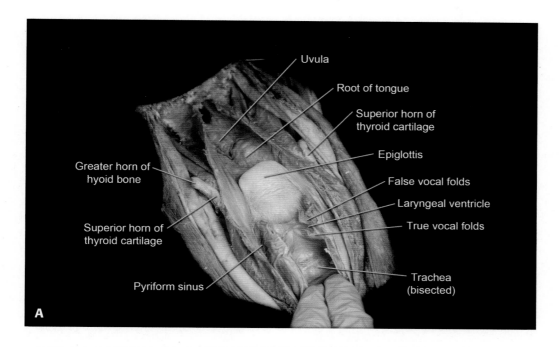

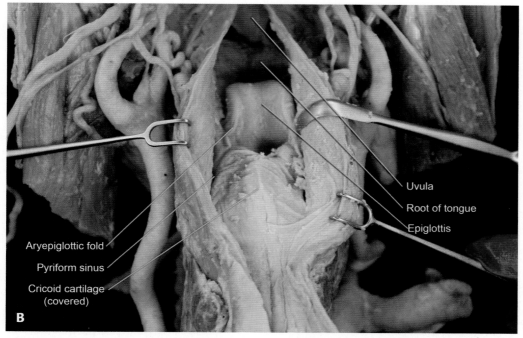

Figure 4–2. A. Cavity of the larynx with landmarks, as viewed from behind. Note that the laryngeal space has been revealed by a sagittal incision, and the posterior laryngeal wall has been spread for access to the structure. *Source:* From Seikel/Drumright/King. *Anatomy & Physiology for Speech, Language, and Hearing, 5th Ed.* ©Cengage, Inc. Reproduced by permission. **B.** Posterior view elevated to reveal aryepiglottic folds and pyriform sinuses. *continues*

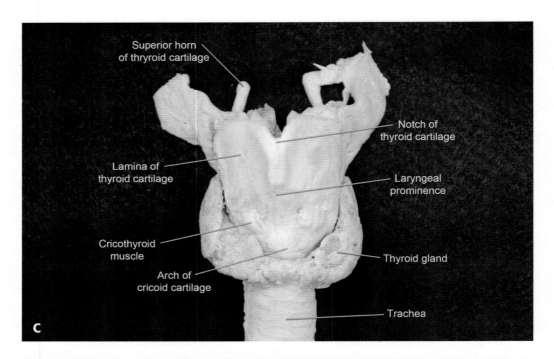

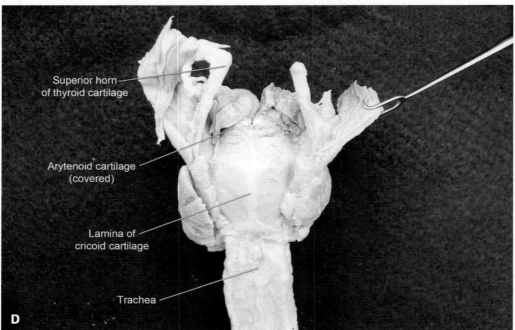

Figure 4–2. *continued* **C.** Excised anterior larynx with trachea. **D.** Excised posterior larynx with trachea. *continues*

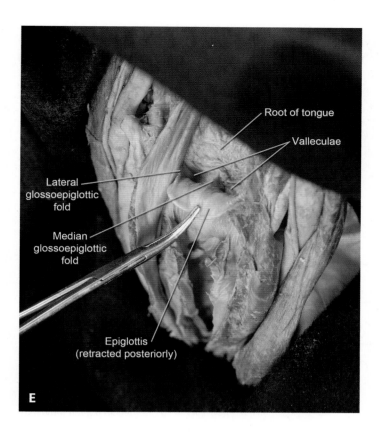

Root of tongue

Valleculae

Lateral glossoepiglottic fold

Median glossoepiglottic fold

Epiglottis (retracted posteriorly)

E

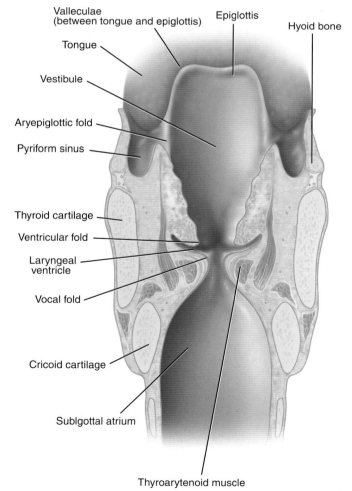

Valleculae (between tongue and epiglottis)

Epiglottis

Hyoid bone

Tongue

Vestibule

Aryepiglottic fold

Pyriform sinus

Thyroid cartilage

Ventricular fold

Laryngeal ventricle

Vocal fold

Cricoid cartilage

Sublgottal atrium

Thyroarytenoid muscle

F

Figure 4–2. *continued* **E.** Posterior larynx with epiglottis deflected to reveal valleculae. **F.** Drawing of cavity of landmark with larynx, as viewed from behind through coronal section. *continues*

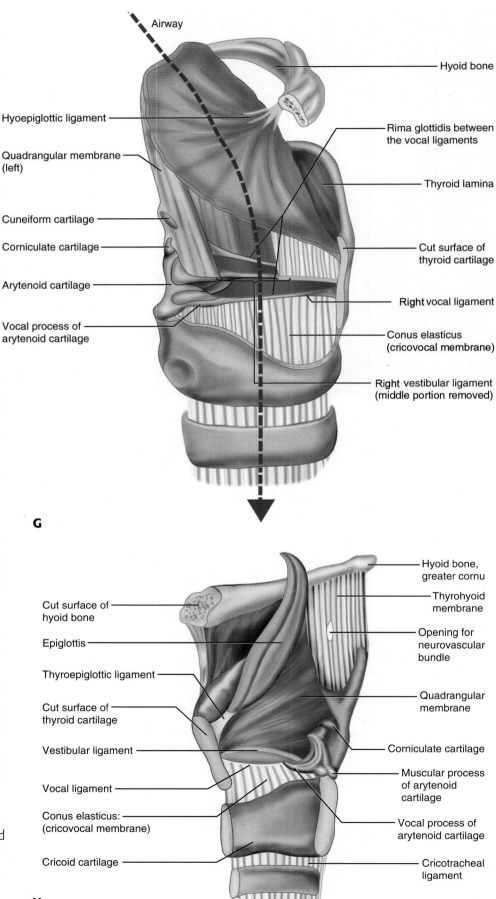

Airway

Hyoid bone

Hyoepiglottic ligament

Rima glottidis between the vocal ligaments

Quadrangular membrane (left)

Thyroid lamina

Cuneiform cartilage

Cut surface of thyroid cartilage

Corniculate cartilage

Arytenoid cartilage

Right vocal ligament

Vocal process of arytenoid cartilage

Conus elasticus (cricovocal membrane)

Right vestibular ligament (middle portion removed)

G

Hyoid bone, greater cornu

Cut surface of hyoid bone

Thyrohyoid membrane

Epiglottis

Opening for neurovascular bundle

Thyroepiglottic ligament

Cut surface of thyroid cartilage

Quadrangular membrane

Vestibular ligament

Corniculate cartilage

Vocal ligament

Muscular process of arytenoid cartilage

Conus elasticus: (cricovocal membrane)

Vocal process of arytenoid cartilage

Cricoid cartilage

Cricotracheal ligament

H

Figure 4–2. *continued*
G. Membranes and ligaments of the larynx. Note particularly the hyoepiglottic ligament, conus elasticus (cricovocal membrane), quadrangular membrane, and vocal ligament. **H.** Membranes and ligaments of the larynx, viewed after sagittal cut. Note the thyrohyoid membrane, quadrangular membrane, conus elasticus, and vocal ligament.

must attach to the larynx as well, and this is achieved through the **cricotracheal ligament** (see Figure 4–2A).

The **intrinsic ligaments** connect the cartilages of the larynx and form the support structure for the cavity of the larynx, as well as that of the vocal folds. The **fibroelastic membrane** of the larynx is composed of the upper **quadrangular membranes** and **aryepiglottic folds**, the lower **conus elasticus**, and the **vocal ligament**, which is actually the upward free extension of the conus elasticus. The conus elasticus is also referred to as the cricovocal membrane or the cricothyroid ligament (McHanwell, 2008). The conus elasticus is the dominant membranous lining that is situated below the vocal folds and that attaches to the lower thyroid cartilage and upper surface of the cricoid cartilage and tip of the vocal process of the arytenoid. The upper edge of the conus elasticus between the vocal process and the angle of the thyroid cartilage forms the vocal ligament within the vocal folds (Figure 4–3). The conus elasticus (Figure 4–2D) has the shape and form of a vortex and is believed to reduce resistance to airflow.

The quadrangular membranes are the undergirding layer of connective tissue running from the arytenoids to the epiglottis and thyroid cartilage, and

quadrangular: L., quadri, four; angulus, right; right-angled

conus elasticus: L., elastic cone

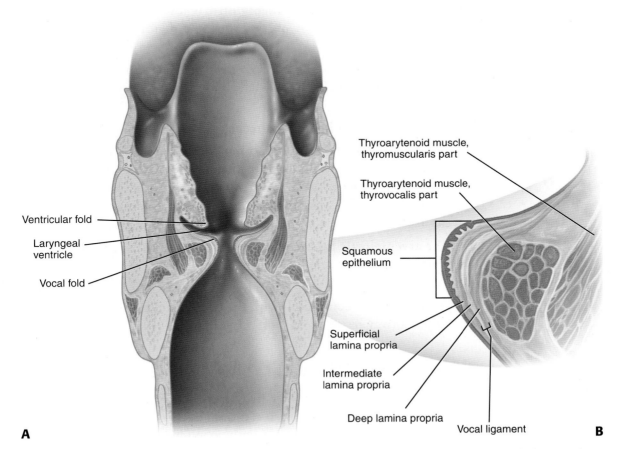

Thyroarytenoid muscle, thyromuscularis part

Thyroarytenoid muscle, thyrovocalis part

Ventricular fold

Laryngeal ventricle

Vocal fold

Squamous epithelium

Superficial lamina propria

Intermediate lamina propria

Deep lamina propria

Vocal ligament

A

B

Figure 4–3. A. Transverse section through the larynx revealing the vocal folds. **B.** Expanded view of the vocal folds, showing layers. *Source:* From Seikel/Drumright/King. *Anatomy & Physiology for Speech, Language, and Hearing, 5th Ed.* ©Cengage, Inc. Reproduced by permission.

forming the false vocal folds. They originate at the inner thyroid angle and sides of the epiglottis and form an upper cone that narrows as it terminates in the free margin of the arytenoid and corniculate cartilages. The **aryepiglottic muscles** course from the side of the epiglottis to the arytenoid apex, forming the upper margin of the quadrangular membranes and laterally, the aryepiglottic folds. These folds are simply the ridges marking the highest elevation of these membranes and muscles slung from the epiglottis to the arytenoids. The **pyriform sinus** is the space between the aryepiglottic folds and the thyroid cartilage, marking an important point of transit for food and liquid during a swallow, as will be discussed in Chapter 8.

✓ To summarize:

- The **cavity** of the **larynx** is a constricted tube with a smooth surface.
- Sheets and cords of ligaments connect the cartilages, while a smooth **mucous membrane** covers the medial-most surface of the larynx.
- The **thyrohyoid membrane**, **lateral thyrohyoid ligament**, and **median thyrohyoid ligament** cover the space between the hyoid bone and the thyroid.
- The **hyoepiglottic** and **thyroepiglottic ligaments** attach the epiglottis to the corpus hyoid and the inner thyroid cartilage, respectively.
- The **valleculae** are found between the tongue and the epiglottis, within folds arising from the lateral and median glossoepiglottic ligaments.
- The **cricotracheal ligament** attaches the trachea to the larynx.
- The **fibroelastic membrane** is composed of the upper **quadrangular membranes** and **aryepiglottic folds**, the lower **conus elasticus**, and the **vocal ligament**, which is actually the upward free extension of the conus elasticus. The **pyriform sinus** is the space between the fold of the aryepiglottic membrane and the thyroid cartilage laterally.
- The **aryepiglottic folds** course from the side of the epiglottis to the arytenoid apex.
- The conus elasticus is the membranous cover beneath the level of the vocal folds. It is continuous with the vocal ligament and is thought to reduce airway resistance leading to the glottis.

Fine Structure of the Vocal Folds

The vocal folds are composed of five layers of tissue, as can be seen in Figure 4–3. The most superficial is a protective layer of squamous epithelium, approximately 0.1 mm thick, with an underlying layer of basement membrane to bind it to the next layer. This epithelial layer gives the vocal folds the glistening white appearance seen during **laryngoscopic** examination (use of a **laryngoscope**, a device typically used by laryngologists or speech-language pathologists to view the larynx). This protective layer aids in keeping the delicate tissues of the vocal folds moist by assisting in fluid retention.

The next layer is the superficial lamina propria (SLP) made up of elastin fibers, so named because of their physical qualities that allow them to be extensively stretched. The fibrous and elastic elements of the SLP cushion the vocal folds. The elastin fibers of the SLP are cross-layered with the intermediate lamina propria (ILP), which is deep to the SLP. The ILP is approximately 1 to 2 mm thick and is also composed of elastin fibers running in an anterior-posterior direction, making them cross-layered with the SLP. The combination of these two layers provides both elasticity and strength. The deep lamina propria (DLP) is approximately 1 to 2 mm thick and primarily supportive, being made up of collagen fibers that prohibit extension. The ILP and DLP combine to make up the vocal ligament.

Deep to the lamina propria is the fifth layer of the vocal folds, the thyro-arytenoid muscle (thyrovocalis and thyromuscularis). This layer makes up the bulk of the vocal fold. Because the muscle course is anterior-posterior, the fibers are arranged in this orientation. This combination of tissues provides both active and passive elements. The thyroarytenoid is the active element of the vocal folds, while the passive elements consist of the layers of lamina propria that provide strength, cushioning, and elasticity.

The **mucosal lining of the vocal folds** is actually a combination of the epithelial lining and the disorganized first lamina propria layer. The second and third layers (elastin and collagen) constitute the **vocal ligament**, a structure giving a degree of stiffness and support to the vocal folds. Some authors refer alternately to the layers as the **cover** of the vocal folds (superficial epithelium, primary and secondary layers of lamina propria) and the **body** (third layer of lamina propria and thyroarytenoid muscle) of the vocal folds.

Cavities of the Larynx

If you look at the profile of the larynx in Figure 4–4, you will appreciate some of the relationships among the structures. The **aditus laryngis** or **aditus** (Figure 4–4D) is the entry to the larynx from the pharynx above. (Some anatomists define the aditus as the first space of the larynx; others view it simply as the entryway to the first cavity—the vestibule—to be discussed shortly.) You may think of the aditus as the doorframe through which you would pass when entering a house. The anterior boundary of the frame of the aditus is the epiglottis, with the folds of membrane and muscle slung between the epiglottis and the arytenoids (the **aryepiglottic folds**) comprising the lateral margins of the aditus. In Figure 4–5A you can see two "bumps" under the aryepiglottic folds. These are caused by the cuneiform cartilages embedded within the folds. The second set of prominences posterior to the first two are from the corniculate prominences of the corniculate cartilages on the arytenoids.

aditus laryngis: L., entrance; laryngeal entrance

aditus: entry to the larynx from the pharynx

aryepiglottic: ary(tenoid) epiglottis

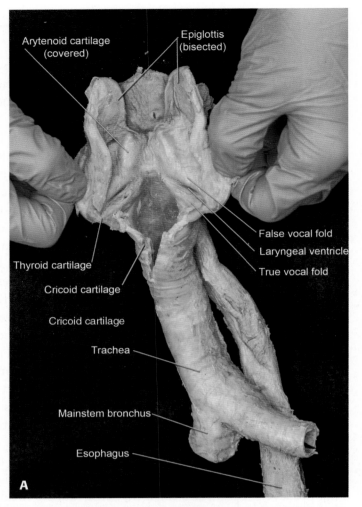

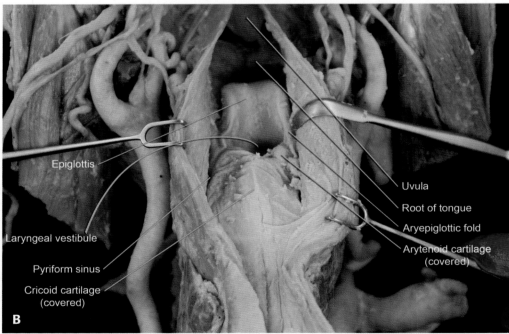

Figure 4–4. A. Larynx that has been cut sagittally with the sides reflected, revealing the false folds, true folds, and laryngeal ventricle. Note trachea and orientation of esophagus. **B.** Larynx, as seen from behind and above. *continues*

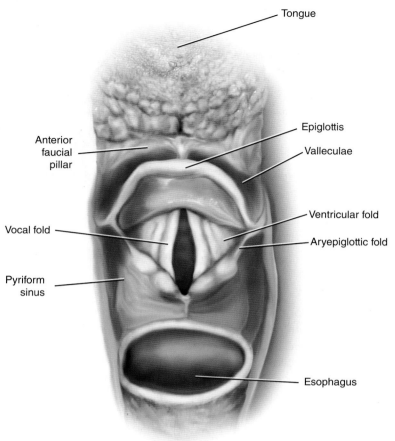

Tongue

Epiglottis

Valleculae

Anterior
faucial
pillar

Ventricular fold

Vocal fold

Aryepiglottic fold

Pyriform
sinus

Esophagus

C

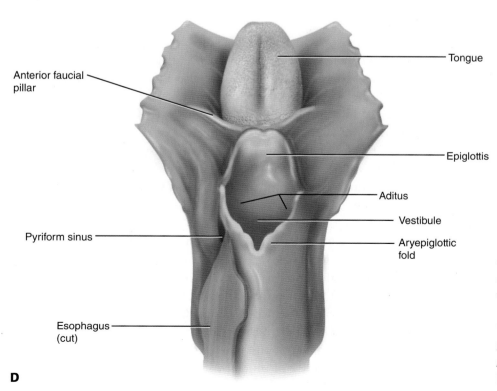

Tongue

Anterior faucial
pillar

Epiglottis

Aditus

Vestibule

Pyriform sinus

Aryepiglottic
fold

Esophagus
(cut)

D

Figure 4–4. *continued*
C. Drawing showing landmarks
of superior larynx. **D.** Drawing
of posterior view of larynx
with esophagus cut. *Source:*
From Seikel/Drumright/
King. *Anatomy & Physiology
for Speech, Language, and
Hearing, 5th Ed.* ©Cengage,
Inc. Reproduced by permission.

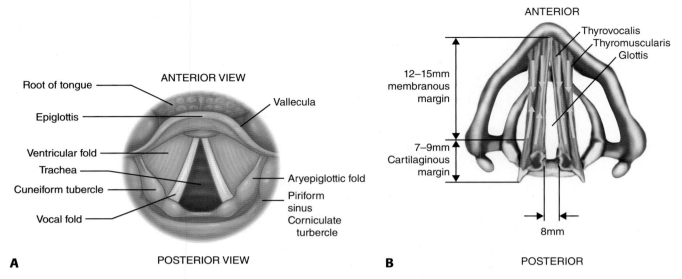

Figure 4–5. A. Vocal folds as seen from above. Note that true vocal folds appear white upon examination as a result of the superficial layer of squamous epithelial tissue. Seen immediately superior to the true vocal folds are the ventricular or false folds. Note the corniculate and cuneiform tubercles. These prominences arise from the presence of the corniculate and cuneiform cartilages deep in the aryepiglottic folds. **B.** Same view of vocal folds, but with the membranous lining and supportive muscle of larynx removed, to reveal only cartilages and the thyroarytenoid muscle (thyrovocalis and thyromuscularis). The membranous margin of the vocal folds is approximately 12 to 15 mm long in adults, while the cartilaginous margin is approximately 7 to 9 mm long. The space between the vocal folds (glottis) at rest is approximately 8 mm. *Source:* From Seikel/Drumright/King. *Anatomy & Physiology for Speech, Language, and Hearing, 5th Ed.* ©Cengage, Inc. Reproduced by permission.

rima vestibuli: L., slit of the vestibule

The first cavity of the larynx is the **vestibule**, or entryway. The vestibule is the space between the entryway or aditus and the **ventricular** (or **vestibular**) folds. The ventricular folds are also known as the **false vocal folds** because they are not used for phonation except in rare (and clinically significant) cases. The vestibule is wide at the aditus but narrows at the ventricular folds. The lateral walls are comprised of the aryepiglottic folds, and the posterior walls are made up of the membrane covering the arytenoid cartilages, which project superiorly to the false folds. The false vocal folds are made up of a mucous membrane and a fibrous **vestibular ligament**, but not muscular tissue. The space between the false vocal folds is termed the **rima vestibuli**.

The middle space of the larynx lies between the margins of the false vocal folds and the true vocal folds below. This space is the **laryngeal ventricle** (or **laryngeal sinus**), and the anterior extension of this space is the **laryngeal saccule** (also known as the appendix of the ventricle). The saccule (or pouch) is endowed with more than 60 mucous glands that secrete lubricating mucus into the laryngeal cavity. The thyroepiglottic muscle passes between the saccule and the thyroid cartilage, and when this muscle contracts it squeezes on the saccule, causing release of mucus onto laryngeal tissue. There are, in reality, mucous glands throughout the larynx, including the surface of the epiglottis and aryepiglottic folds. These glands secrete mucus periodically to

Saccular Cysts and Laryngoceles

The saccule of the laryngeal ventricle is a fibrous pouch that encapsulates the mucus to be secreted into the airway for lubrication and to entrap foreign particles. The fibrous wall can break down and weaken, allowing a herniation of the saccule, which is termed a laryngocele and is a rare occurrence (Gulia, Yadav, Khaowas, Basur, & Agrawal, 2012). The saccule will enlarge, expanding beyond its location in the ventricle. An internal laryngocele may expand under the aryepiglottic fold, ultimately reaching the valleculae. If it reaches the thyrohyoid membrane it may emerge superficial to the membranes, becoming an external laryngocele, which may be palpated at the neck. External laryngoceles may be quite slow in developing. Internal laryngoceles can interfere with the airway, causing hoarseness, swallowing problems (dysphagia), and laryngeal stridor (noisy inhalations and exhalations because of airway obstruction).

Saccular cysts are growths that can occur if the opening of the saccule is obstructed, for instance as a result of growth of a tumor. The saccule will enlarge and often become inflamed and infected. The expansion will take the same form as a laryngocele. Saccular cysts and laryngoceles can become health-threatening in youngsters, as they can expand to obstruct the airway, and infection of any internal tissue or organ is a significant issue.

lubricate the vocal folds, because the folds themselves do not have mucous glands (McHanwell, 2008). The secretions are important for maintaining the health of the vocal folds and reducing airway resistance (Fujiki, Chapleau, Sundarrajan, McKenna, & Sivasankar, 2017). The mucus also assists in eliminating errant food particles that enter the airway by encapsulating them, thereby enabling them to be eliminated through coughing.

The glottis is the space between the vocal folds, inferior to the ventricle and superior to the conus elasticus. This is the most important laryngeal space for speech, because it is defined by the *variable sphincter* that permits voicing. The length of the glottis at rest is approximately 20 mm in adults from the **anterior commissure** (anterior-most opening posterior to the angle of the thyroid cartilage) to the **posterior commissure** (between the arytenoid cartilages). The glottis area is variable, depending upon the moment-by-moment configuration of the vocal folds. At rest the posterior glottis is approximately 8 mm wide, although that dimension will double during times of forced respiration.

The lateral margins of the glottis are the vocal folds and the arytenoid cartilage. The anterior three fifths of the vocal margin is made up of the soft tissue of the vocal folds. (You will see this referred to as the **membranous glottis**, because some anatomists define the glottis as the entire vocal mechanism. Physicians sometimes refer to this as the phonatory glottis [Merati & Rieder, 2003].) In adult males, the free margin of the vocal folds is approximately 15 mm in length, and in females it is approximately 12 mm. This free margin of the vocal folds is the vibrating element that provides voice. The posterior two fifths of the vocal folds is comprised of the cartilage of the arytenoids. (This portion is often referred to as the **cartilaginous glottis**, because *glottis* is sometimes used to refer to the entire vocal mechanism. Physicians sometimes refer to it as the respiratory glottis [e.g., Gaffey, Sun, & Richter, 2018]). This portion of the vocal folds is between 4 and 8 mm

Reinke's Edema

The larynx is lined with mucous membrane, designed to retain moisture and provide a low-resistance surface for the airway. The membrane is reasonably loose throughout, allowing movement of laryngeal structures. The exception is at the vocal ligament: At this location, the mucous membrane is fixed, and therein lies the problem. When tissue is irritated, extracellular fluid accumulates, causing swelling (edema). In the case of the larynx, that accumulation of fluid can't go anywhere because the lining is bound to the vocal ligament. The result is that the inner lining of the larynx expands, and particularly the vocal folds become swollen. The swelling is maintained because of the poor lymphatic swelling of the space. This condition is known as Reinke's edema, because the space deep to the superficial lamina propria is called Reinke's space. The condition can arise from vocal abuse, but most often is seen in people who smoke (Móz, Domingues, Castilho, Branco, & Martins, 2013), because smoking irritates tissue.

Vocal Fold Hydration

The vocal folds are extremely sensitive to the internal and external environment. Although cigarette smoke and other pollutants are known to cause irritation to the tissues of the vocal folds, the internal environment appears to have an impact as well.

When the vocal folds are subject to abuse, several problems may arise, among them contact ulcers and vocal nodules. Hydration therapy is a frequent prescription to counteract the problems of irritated tissue. Dry tissue does not heal as well as moist tissue, so the client will be told to increase the environmental humidity, drink fluids, or even take medications to promote water retention. This type of therapy makes more than medical sense. Verdolini, Titze, and Fennell (1994) found that the *effort* of phonation increased as individuals became dehydrated and decreased when they were hydrated beyond normal levels. Indeed, the airflow required to produce the same phonation is greatly increased by a poorly lubricated larynx. When lubricated, the vocal folds vibrate much more periodically (they have greatly reduced perturbation, or cycle-by-cycle variation). When the relative periodicity of the vocal folds decreases, the voice sounds hoarse, a perception that you will agree with if you think of the last time you had laryngitis.

long, depending on gender and body size. The conus elasticus begins at the margins of the true vocal folds and extends to the inferior border of the cricoid cartilage, widening from the vocal folds to the base of the cricoid.

✅ *To summarize:*

- The **vocal folds** consist of five layers of tissue.
- Deep to the thin **epithelial layer** is the **lamina propria**, made up of two layers of elastin and one layer of collagen fibers. The thyroarytenoid muscle is the deepest of the layers.
- The **vocal ligament** is made of elastin. The **aditus** is the entryway of the larynx, marking the entry to the **vestibule**.
- The **ventricular** and **vocal folds** are separated by the laryngeal **ventricle**.
- The glottis is the variable space between the vocal folds.

Cartilaginous Structure of the Larynx

Cartilage has the precise qualities needed for the larynx, in that it is flexible but also provides the structure needed to withstand negative and positive pressures. A simple epithelial tube such as the esophagus would collapse as pressure within it dropped, and a bony structure wouldn't allow a person to flex and bend the neck.

Cricoid Cartilage

The unpaired cricoid cartilage can be viewed as an expanded tracheal cartilage (Figure 4–6). As the most inferior cartilage of the larynx, the cricoid cartilage is the approximate diameter of the trachea. It is higher in the back than in the front.

There are several important landmarks on the cricoid. The low, anterior cricoid arch provides clearance for the vocal folds that will pass over

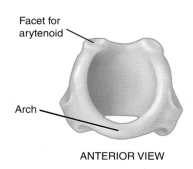

Facet for arytenoid

Arch

ANTERIOR VIEW

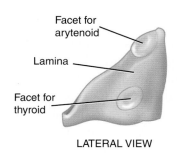

Facet for arytenoid

Lamina

Facet for thyroid

LATERAL VIEW

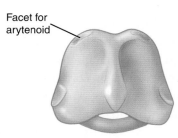

Facet for arytenoid

POSTERIOR VIEW

A

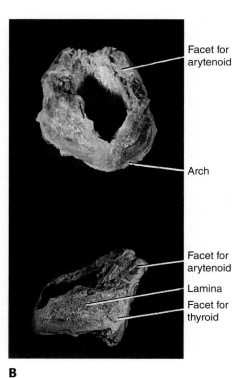

Facet for arytenoid

Arch

Facet for arytenoid

Lamina

Facet for thyroid

B

Figure 4–6. A. Cricoid cartilage and landmarks. **B.** Photograph of cricoid cartilage, superior and lateral views. *Source:* From Seikel/Drumright/King. *Anatomy & Physiology for Speech, Language, and Hearing, 5th Ed.* ©Cengage, Inc. Reproduced by permission.

that point, while the posterior elevation, the superior surface of the **posterior quadrate lamina**, provides the point of articulation for the arytenoid cartilages. On the lateral surfaces of the cricoid are articular facets or *faces*, marking the point of articulation for the inferior horns of the thyroid cartilage. This **cricothyroid joint** is a synovial, pivoting joint that permits the rotation of the two articulating structures. The joint is encased in a capsular ligament that allows rotation of the thyroid cartilage relative to the cricoid. Anterior, posterior, and lateral ceratocricoid ligaments provide reinforcement to the capsule.

One more note on the cricoid. The figures and photographs are quite misleading concerning the size of laryngeal structures. For perspective, your cricoid cartilage would fit loosely upon your little finger, which is about the diameter of your trachea. The laryngeal structures are *small*. Indeed, subglottic stenosis (narrowing of the area below the glottis) is a frequent laryngeal problem following endotracheal intubation (ventilation by means of a tube placed into the airway through the larynx) and its subsequent scarring.

Thyroid Cartilage

The unpaired thyroid cartilage is the largest of the laryngeal cartilages. As you can see in Figure 4–7, the thyroid cartilage has a prominent anterior surface made up of two plates called the thyroid laminae, joined at the midline at the **thyroid angle**. At the superior-most point of that angle you will see the **thyroid notch**, which you can palpate if you do the following. Place your finger under your chin and on your throat, and bring it downward to the point you might refer to as your Adam's apple (in adult males, the two lamina meet at about a 90-degree angle, while the angle for females is more like 120 degrees. This acute angle in males results in a more prominent Adam's apple.). When you have found the top of that structure, you have identified the thyroid notch. Look at the drawing as you feel the indentation in your own thyroid. Now draw your finger down the midline a little until you feel the angle. If you put your index finger on the angle and your thumb and second finger on the sides, you will have digits on the angle and both laminae. Do take a moment to discover these regions on yourself, because they provide you with a reference that is near and dear to you. Incidentally, with your finger on the notch, you are as close as you can be to touching your vocal folds, because they attach to the thyroid cartilage just behind that point.

Drawing your attention back to Figure 4–7, on the lateral superficial aspect of the thyroid laminae you will see the **oblique line**. This marks the point of attachment for two muscles we will talk about shortly.

The posterior aspect of the thyroid is open and is characterized by two prominent sets of **cornu** or horns. The inferior cornua project downward to articulate with the cricoid cartilage, while the superior cornua project superiorly to articulate with the hyoid. In some individuals a small **triticeal** cartilage (*cartilago triticea*) may be found between the superior cornu of the thyroid cartilage and the hyoid bone.

cornu: L., horn (as in cornucopia, the "horn of plenty")

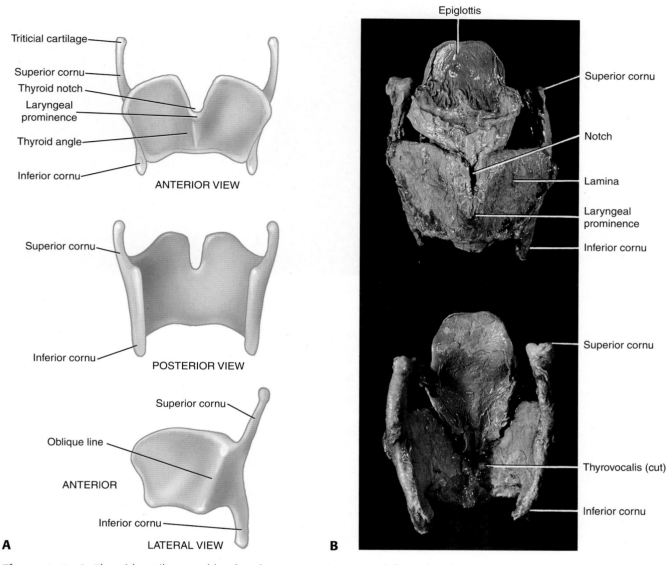

Figure 4–7. A. Thyroid cartilage and landmarks. **B.** Posterior view of thyroid and epiglottis cartilages. *Source:* From Seikel/Drumright/King. *Anatomy & Physiology for Speech, Language, and Hearing, 5th Ed.* ©Cengage, Inc. Reproduced by permission. *continues*

Arytenoid and Corniculate Cartilages

The paired arytenoid cartilages are among the most important of the larynx. They reside on the superior posterolateral surface of the cricoid cartilage and provide the mechanical structure that permits onset and offset of voicing. The form of the arytenoid may be likened to a pyramid to aid in visualization (Figure 4–8). Each cartilage has two processes and four surfaces.

The apex is the truncated superior portion of the pyramidal arytenoid cartilage, and on the superior surfaces of each arytenoid is a **corniculate cartilage**, projecting posteriorly to form the peak of the distorted pyramid. The inferior surface of the cartilage is termed the **base**, and its concave

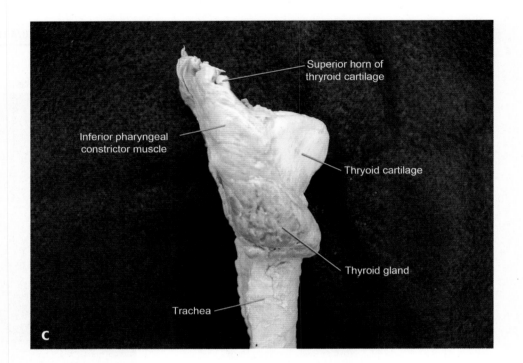

Figure 4–7. *continued* C. Lateral view of larynx and trachea.

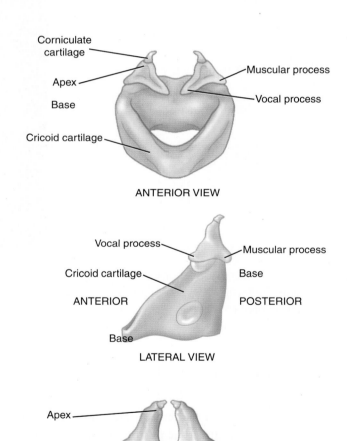

ANTERIOR VIEW

LATERAL VIEW

Figure 4–8. Arytenoid cartilages articulated with cricoid cartilage. *Source:* From Seikel/ Drumright/King. *Anatomy & Physiology for Speech, Language, and Hearing, 5th Ed.* ©Cengage, Inc. Reproduced by permission.

surface is the point of articulation with the convex arytenoid facet of the cricoid cartilage.

The names of the two processes of the arytenoid give a hint as to their function. The **vocal processes** project anteriorly toward the thyroid notch, and it is these processes to which the posterior portion of the vocal folds themselves attach. The **muscular process** forms the lateral outcropping of the arytenoid pyramid and, as its name implies, is the point of attachment for muscles that adduct and abduct the vocal folds.

Epiglottis

The unpaired epiglottis is a leaflike structure that arises from the inner surface of the angle of the thyroid cartilage just below the notch, being attached there by the thyroepiglottic ligament. The sides of the epiglottis are joined with the arytenoid cartilages via the aryepiglottic folds, which are the product of the membranous lining being draped over muscle and connective tissue.

The epiglottis projects upward beyond the larynx and above the hyoid bone and is attached to the root of the tongue by means of the median and lateral glossoepiglottic ligaments, with the overlying epithelium that produces the **glossoepiglottic fold**. This juncture produces the valleculae, a landmark that will become important in your study of swallowing and swallowing deficit. During swallowing, food passes over the epiglottis and, from there, laterally to the **pyriform** (also piriform) sinuses, which are small fossae or indentations between the aryepiglottic folds medially and the mucous lining of the thyroid cartilage. Together, the pyriform sinuses and valleculae are called the **pharyngeal recesses** (see Figure 4–5).

The epiglottis is attached to the hyoid bone via the **hyoepiglottic ligament**. The surface of the epiglottis is covered with a mucous membrane lining, and beneath this lining, on the posterior concave surface, may be found branches of the internal laryngeal nerve of the X **vagus** that conduct sensory information from the larynx.

vagus: L., wandering

See Chapter 11 for a discussion of the X vagus nerve.

Cuneiform Cartilages

The **cuneiform** cartilages are small cartilages embedded within the aryepiglottic folds. They are situated above and anterior to the corniculate cartilages and cause a small bulge on the surface of the membrane that looks white under illumination. These cartilages apparently provide support for the membranous laryngeal covering.

cuneiform: L., cuneus, wedge; wedge-shaped

Hyoid Bone

Although not a bone of the larynx, the hyoid forms the union between the tongue and the laryngeal structure. This unpaired small bone articulates loosely with the superior cornu of the thyroid cartilage and has the distinction of being the only bone of the body that is not attached to another bone (Figure 4–9). It is a good idea to pay close attention to this structure, as it will

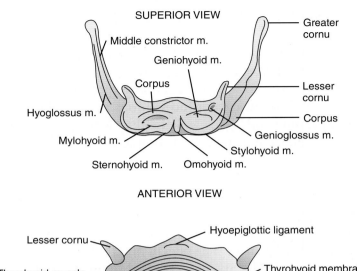

Figure 4–9. Hyoid bone as seen from above (**A**) and behind (**B**). Points of attachment of muscles and membranes are indicated. *Source:* From Seikel/ Drumright/King. *Anatomy & Physiology for Speech, Language, and Hearing, 5th Ed.* ©Cengage, Inc. Reproduced by permission.

come back into prominence in Chapter 8, where we discuss swallowing function! This is a significant radiographic landmark in assessment of swallowing.

As you can see from the view of the hyoid bone from above, this structure is U-shaped, being open in the posterior aspect. There are three major elements of the hyoid bone. The corpus or body of the hyoid is a prominent shield-like structure forming the front of the bone and is a structure you can palpate. If you place your finger on your thyroid notch and push *lightly* back toward your vertebral column, you can feel the hard structure of the corpus near your fingernail. As you are doing this, take one more look at Figure 4–1, showing the structures together, to become acquainted with the relationship of these structures.

Infant Larynx

Infants have different anatomy from adults, particularly as it relates to the larynx. The larynx is markedly narrow and is higher than the adult larynx. The top of the epiglottic cartilage is visible over the back of the tongue, and all the laryngeal cartilages are softer and more pliable than those of adults. Indeed, laryngomalacia (audible breathing, or *stridor*) is frequently caused by the airway being so pliant and collapsing on itself in infants, as well as the fact that the mucous membrane lining of the larynx is more loosely bound to the larynx than in adults. The thyroid cartilage is proportionately closer to the hyoid bone than in adults (the infant larynx is one third the size of an adult's larynx). The vocal folds are around 4.5 mm long, and the laryngeal saccule is relatively larger in infants than in adults (Standring, 2008). Because of the small size of the larynx, any conditions that cause swelling of the tissues of the airway place the infant at significant risk. By 3 years of age, sex differences begin to emerge with the male larynx being larger than that of the female, but these changes come to full bloom during puberty.

The front of the corpus is convex, and the inner surface is concave. The corpus is the point of attachment for six muscles—no small feat for such a small structure.

The **greater cornu** arises on the lateral surface of the corpus, projecting posteriorly. At the junction of the corpus and greater cornu you can see the **lesser cornu**. Three additional muscles attach to these two structures.

Movement of the Cartilages

The cricothyroid and cricoarytenoid joints are the only functionally mobile points of the larynx, and both of these joints serve extremely important laryngeal functions.

The cricothyroid joint is the junction of the cricoid cartilage and the inferior cornu of the thyroid cartilage, as mentioned earlier. These are synovial (diarthrodial) joints that permit the cricoid and thyroid to rotate and glide relative to each other. As seen in Figure 4–10, rotation at the cricothyroid joint permits the thyroid cartilage to rock down in front, and the joint also permits the thyroid to glide forward and backward slightly, relative to the cricoid. This joint provides the major adjustment for change in vocal pitch.

The **cricoarytenoid joint** is the articulation formed between the cricoid and arytenoid cartilages. Recall that the base of the arytenoid cartilage is concave, mating with the smooth convex superior surface of the cricoid cartilage. These synovial joints permit rocking, gliding, and perhaps even minimal rotation. The arytenoid facet of the cricoid is a convex, oblong

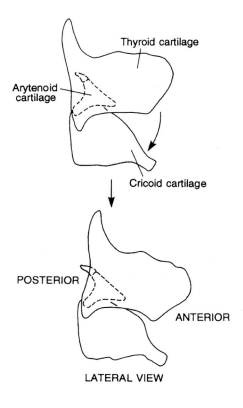

Figure 4–10. Movement of the cricoid and thyroid cartilages about the cricothyroid joint. When the cricoid and thyroid move toward each other in front, the arytenoid cartilage moves farther away from the thyroid cartilage, tensing the vocal folds. *Source:* Redrawn from Seikel/Drumright/King. *Anatomy & Physiology for Speech, Language, and Hearing, 5th Ed.* ©Cengage, Inc. Reproduced by permission.

surface, and the axis of motion is around a line projecting back along the superior surface of the arytenoid and converging at a point above the arytenoid (Figure 4–11). This rocking action brings the two vocal processes toward each other, permitting the vocal folds to **approximate** (make contact). The arytenoids are also capable of gliding on the long axis of the facet, facilitating changes in vocal fold length. The arytenoids also appear to rotate upon a vertical axis drawn through the apex of the arytenoid, but this motion may be limited to extremes of abduction (Fink & Demarest, 1978). Evidence produced through the study of cadaver specimens supports the role of arytenoid rotation during phonation (Storck et al., 2012).

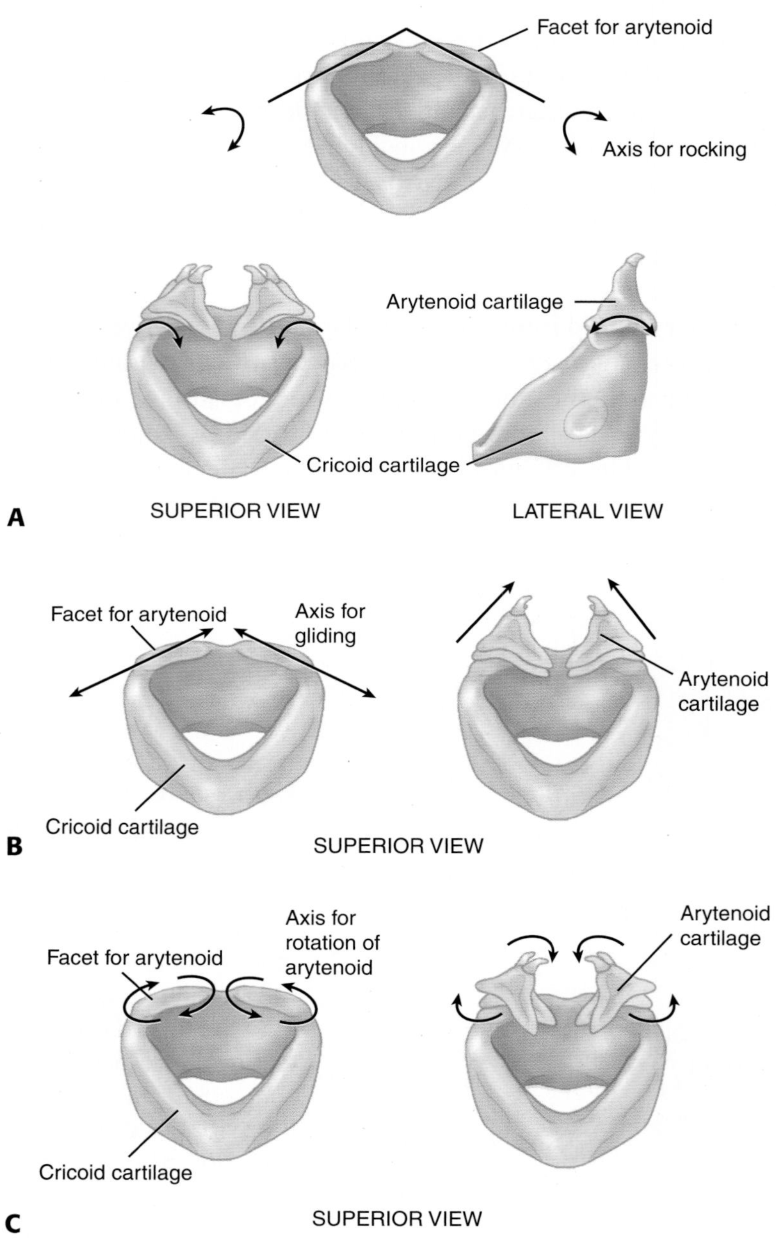

Figure 4–11. The articular facet for the arytenoid cartilage permits rocking, gliding, and rotation. **A.** The shape of the articular facet for the arytenoid cartilage promotes inward rocking of the arytenoid cartilage and vocal folds, as shown by the arrows. **B.** The long axis of the facet permits limited anterior-posterior gliding. **C.** The arytenoids may also rotate as shown, although evidence of functional movement through rotation is conflicting. *Source: From Seikel/Drumright/ King. Anatomy & Physiology for Speech, Language, and Hearing, 5th Ed.* ©Cengage, Inc. Reproduced by permission. (Based on data of Broad, 1973; Fink & Demarest, 1978)

Palpation of the Larynx

To palpate the larynx, first identify the prominent thyroid notch or Adam's apple (see Figure 4–7). Once you have found it, place your index finger on the notch itself, with your thumb and second finger on either side. Your thumb and second finger should feel a fairly flat surface, the thyroid lamina. Now bring your index finger straight down a little bit; you should feel the prominent thyroid angle. Bring your finger back up to the top of the notch; when your finger is on top of the notch, the hard region contacting your fingernail is the corpus of the hyoid bone. In some people, this is very difficult to differentiate from the thyroid.

Palpate lateral to the notch on the superior surface, and you should feel the superior cornu of the thyroid. With a little discomfort, you may feel the articulation of the hyoid and thyroid. If you draw your finger down the angle again, you can find the lower margin of the thyroid and feel the cricoid beneath. After carefully placing your thumb at the junction of the cricoid and thyroid, you can hum up and down the scale and feel the thyroid and cricoid moving closer together and farther apart as you do this. You should also feel the entire larynx elevate as you reach the upper end of your range. Finally, draw your finger to find the lower margin of the cricoid, marking the beginning of the trachea. Palpate the tracheal rings.

The combination of these movements provides the mechanism for vocal fold approximation and abduction. Your understanding of the movement of these cartilages in relation to one another will provide a valuable backdrop for understanding the laryngeal physiology presented in Chapter 5.

✓ To summarize:

- The laryngeal cartilages have a number of important landmarks to which muscles are attached.
- The **cricoid** cartilage is shaped like a signet ring, higher at the back.
- The **arytenoid** cartilages ride on the superior surface of the cricoid, with the cricoarytenoid joint permitting rotation, rocking, and gliding.
- The **muscular** and **vocal processes** provide attachment for the **thyromuscularis** and **thyrovocalis** muscles.
- The **corniculate** cartilages attach to the upper margin of the arytenoids.
- The **thyroid** cartilage has two prominent laminae, superior and inferior horns, and a prominent thyroid notch.
- The **hyoid bone** attaches to the superior cornu of the thyroid, while the **cricoid** cartilage attaches to the inferior horn via the cricothyroid joint.
- The **epiglottis** attaches to the tongue and thyroid cartilage, dropping down to cover the larynx during swallowing.
- The **cuneiform** cartilages are embedded within the aryepiglottic folds.

ANAQUEST LESSON

Laryngeal Musculature

As summarized in Table 4–1, muscles of the larynx may be conveniently divided into those that have both origin and insertion on laryngeal cartilages (**intrinsic laryngeal muscles**) and those with one attachment on a laryngeal

Table 4–1

Muscles Associated With Laryngeal Function
Intrinsic Muscles of Larynx
Adductors Lateral cricoarytenoid muscles Transverse arytenoid muscles Oblique arytenoid muscles
Abductor Posterior cricoarytenoid muscles
Glottal tensors Cricothyroid muscles, pars recta, and pars oblique Thyrovocalis (medial thyroarytenoid) muscles
Relaxers Thyromuscularis (lateral thyroarytenoid) muscles
Auxiliary musculature Thyroarytenoid muscles Superior thyroarytenoid muscles Aryepiglotticus muscles Thyroepiglotticus muscles*
Extrinsic Muscles of Larynx (suprahyoid and infrahyoid muscles)
Hyoid and laryngeal elevators Digastricus anterior and posterior muscles Stylohyoid muscles Mylohyoid muscles Geniohyoid muscles Hyoglossus muscles Genioglossus muscles Thyropharyngeus muscles Inferior pharyngeal constrictor muscles
Hyoid and laryngeal depressors Sternothyroid muscles Omohyoid muscles Sternohyoid muscles Thyrohyoid muscles

*Note that the thyroepiglottic muscle is included here by virtue of its relevance to the swallowing function.

Referral in Voice Therapy

The phonatory mechanism is extremely sensitive, and vocal signs can be indicators for a broad range of problems. We must always refer an individual to a physician when we identify vocal dysfunction, even though we may be fairly certain that the problem is behavioral in nature. When a client comes to us with a hoarse voice, we may find out that the person is abusing the phonatory mechanism by spending too much time in loud, smoky settings that require raising the voice when speaking. What we don't know from this information is whether there is a vocal pathology, perhaps secondary to the same behavioral conditions, that is developing on the vocal folds. Although we suspect vocal nodules, the client could also be showing early signs of laryngeal cancer.

In a similar vein, a client who comes to us with a voice that is progressively weaker during the day, and for whom muscular effort of any sort is extremely difficult as the day wears on, will easily merit a referral, although it will be to a neurologist. Myasthenia gravis is a myoneural disease that results in a complex of speech disorders, including progressive weakening of phonation, progressive degeneration of articulatory function, and progressive hypernasality, all arising from the use of the speech mechanism over the course of a day or briefer time. The condition is quite treatable, but often the speech-language pathologist is the individual to first recognize the signs because the client sees it primarily as a speech problem.

cartilage and the other attachment on a nonlaryngeal structure (**extrinsic laryngeal muscles**). The extrinsic muscles make major adjustments to the larynx, such as elevating or depressing it, while the intrinsic musculature makes fine adjustments to the vocal mechanism itself. Extrinsic muscles tend to work in concert with the articulatory motions of the tongue, and many are important in swallowing and some are variably active during respiration. Intrinsic muscles assume responsibility for opening, closing, tensing, and relaxing the vocal folds. We begin with a discussion of the intrinsic muscles. The summary information of Appendix D may be helpful to your studies.

Intrinsic Laryngeal Muscles

ANAQUEST LESSON

Adductors

- Lateral cricoarytenoid
- Transverse arytenoid
- Oblique arytenoid

Lateral Cricoarytenoid Muscles

This extremely important muscle is one of the more difficult laryngeal muscles to visualize. The **lateral cricoarytenoid muscles** attach to the cricoid and the muscular processes of the arytenoids, causing the muscular processes to move forward and medially (Figure 4–12). The origin of the lateral cricoarytenoid muscles is on the superior-lateral surfaces of the cricoid cartilage. The muscles course up and back to insert into the muscular processes of the arytenoid cartilage. As you can see from this figure, the course of the muscles dictates that when the muscles are contracted, the muscular process are drawn

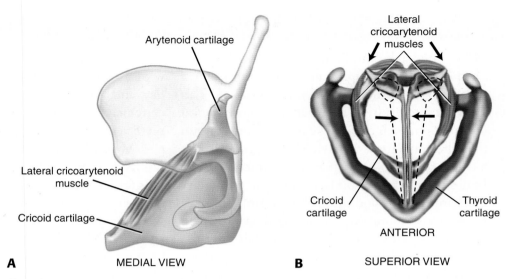

Figure 4–12. A. Course and effect of lateral cricoarytenoid muscle. **B.** Contraction of the lateral cricoarytenoid muscle pulls the muscular process forward, adducting the vocal folds (seen from above). *Source:* From Seikel/Drumright/King. *Anatomy & Physiology for Speech, Language, and Hearing, 5th Ed.* ©Cengage, Inc. Reproduced by permission.

forward, and the motion rocks the arytenoid inward and downward. This inward-and-downward rocking is the major adjustment associated with the adduction of the vocal folds. In addition, this movement may lengthen the vocal folds (Hirano, Kiyokawa, & Kurita, 1988). Contraction of the lateral cricoarytenoid is the primary means of moving the arytenoid cartilages medially and adducting the cartilaginous portion of the vocal folds, although, as we will see, the thyrovocalis (the medial muscle of the vocal fold) appears to be responsible for adduction of the membranous portion of the vocal folds (Chhetri, Neubauer, & Berry, 2012).

Innervation of all intrinsic muscles of the larynx is by means of the X vagus nerve. The vagus is a large, wandering nerve with multiple responsibilities for sensation and motor function in the thorax, neck, and abdomen. The vagus arises from the nucleus ambiguus of the medulla oblongata and divides into two major branches: the recurrent (inferior) laryngeal nerve (RLN) and the superior laryngeal nerve (SLN). The RLN is so named because of its course. The left RLN *re-courses* beneath the aorta, after which it ascends to

Muscle:	Lateral cricoarytenoid
Origin:	Superior-lateral surface of the cricoid cartilage
Course:	Up and back
Insertion:	Muscular process of the arytenoids
Innervation:	X vagus, recurrent laryngeal nerve
Function:	Adducts vocal folds; increases medial compression

innervate the larynx. The right RLN courses under the subclavian artery before ascending to the larynx. This close association to the vascular supply may cause voice problems arising from vascular disease, because **aneurysm** or enlargement of the aorta or subclavian artery may compress the left RLN and cause vocal dysfunction. See Matteucci, Rescigno, Capestro, and Torracca (2012) for a case study of Ortner's syndrome.

aneurysm: Gr., aneurysma, widening

Transverse Arytenoid Muscle

The **transverse arytenoid muscle** may also be called the **transverse inter-arytenoid** muscle. This unpaired muscle is a band of fibers spanning the posterior surface of both the arytenoid cartilages. Figure 4–13 shows the transverse arytenoid. The muscle runs from the lateral margin of the posterior surface of one arytenoid to the corresponding surface of the other arytenoid. Its function is to pull the two arytenoids closer together and, by association, to approximate the vocal folds; but its adductory force is considerably less than the lateral cricoarytenoid (McHanwell, 2008) and even less than the oblique arytenoid muscle (to be discussed later in this section). The transverse arytenoid muscle provides additional support for tight occlusion or closing of the vocal folds and is a component force in generating medial compression. **Medial compression** refers to the degree of force that may be applied by the vocal folds at their point of contact. Increased medial compression is a function of increased force of adduction, and this is a vital element in vocal intensity change. Motor innervation of the transverse arytenoid muscles is by means of the inferior branch of the RLN arising from the X vagus.

Oblique Arytenoid Muscles

The **oblique arytenoid muscles** are also known as the **oblique interarytenoid muscles**. The oblique arytenoid muscles are immediately superficial to the transverse arytenoid muscles and perform a similar function. The

Muscle:	Transverse arytenoid
Origin:	Lateral margin of posterior arytenoids
Course:	Laterally
Insertion:	Lateral margin of posterior surface, opposite arytenoids
Innervation:	X vagus, recurrent laryngeal nerve
Function:	Adducts vocal folds
Muscle:	Oblique arytenoids
Origin:	Posterior base of the muscular processes
Course:	Obliquely up
Insertion:	Apex of the opposite arytenoids
Innervation:	X vagus, recurrent laryngeal nerve
Function:	Pulls the apex medially

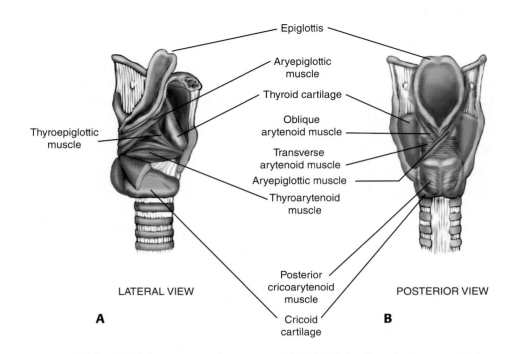

LATERAL VIEW

A

POSTERIOR VIEW

B

Figure 4–13. A. Schematic illustrating the relationship among thyroarytenoid, aryepiglottic and thyroepiglottic muscles. **B.** Schematic of posterior cricoarytenoid muscle, transverse and oblique arytenoid muscles, and aryepiglottic muscles. Contraction of the transverse and oblique arytenoid muscles pulls the arytenoids closer together, thereby supporting adduction. Contraction of the posterior cricoarytenoid muscle pulls the muscular process back, abducting the vocal folds. *Source:* From Seikel/Drumright/King. *Anatomy & Physiology for Speech, Language, and Hearing, 5th Ed.* ©Cengage, Inc. Reproduced by permission. **C.** Photo of posterior larynx showing transverse arytenoid, oblique arytenoid, posterior cricoarytenoid, and trachealis muscles.

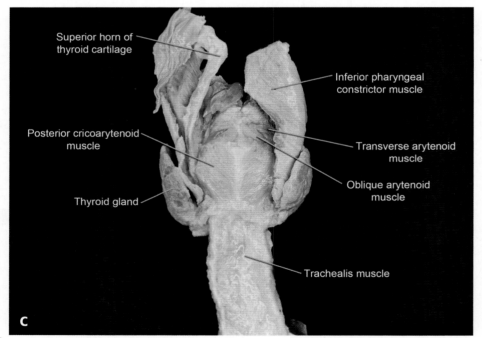

paired oblique arytenoid muscles take their origins at the posterior base of the muscular processes to course obliquely up to the apex of the opposite arytenoid. This course results in a characteristic X arrangement of the muscles, as well as in the ability of these muscles to pull the apex medially. This action promotes adduction, enforces medial compression, and rocks the arytenoid and vocal folds down and in. This action generates more adductory force than the transverse arytenoid, but still considerably less than the lateral cricoarytenoid (McHanwell, 2008). Working in concert with the aryepiglottic muscle, the oblique arytenoid muscle aids in pulling the epiglottis to cover the opening to the larynx as it also serves tight adduction. Innervation of the oblique arytenoid muscles is the same as that for the transverse arytenoid muscles.

Abductor

- Posterior cricoarytenoid

Posterior Cricoarytenoid Muscle

The **posterior cricoarytenoid muscles** are the sole abductors of the vocal folds. They are small but prominent muscles of the posterior larynx. As you can see from Figure 4–13, the posterior cricoarytenoid muscles originate on the posterior cricoid lamina. Fibers project up and out to insert into the posterior aspect of the muscular process of the arytenoid cartilages. By virtue of their attachments to the muscular processes, the posterior cricoarytenoid muscles are direct antagonists to the lateral cricoarytenoids (Figure 4–14), a function confirmed by Chhetri et al. (2012).

Contraction of this muscle pulls the muscular process posteriorly, rocking the arytenoid cartilage out on its axis and abducting the vocal folds. This muscle is quite active during physical exertion, broadly abducting the vocal folds to permit greater air movement into and out of the lungs. The muscle is also active during production of voiceless consonants. The posterior cricoarytenoid is innervated by the RLN, a branch of the X vagus.

Muscle:	Posterior cricoarytenoid
Origin:	Posterior cricoid lamina
Course:	Superiorly
Insertion:	Posterior aspect of the arytenoids
Innervation:	X vagus, recurrent laryngeal nerve
Function:	Rocks arytenoid cartilage laterally; abducts vocal folds

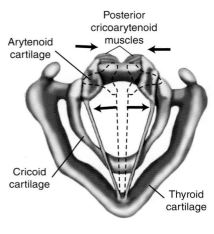

SUPERIOR VIEW

Figure 4–14. Superior view of action of the posterior cricoarytenoid muscles. *Source:* From Seikel/Drumright/King. *Anatomy & Physiology for Speech, Language, and Hearing, 5th Ed.* ©Cengage, Inc. Reproduced by permission.

Glottal Tensors

- Cricothyroid
- Thyrovocalis

Cricothyroid Muscle

The primary tensor of the vocal folds achieves its function by rocking the thyroid cartilage forward relative to the cricoid cartilage. The **cricothyroid muscle** is composed of two heads, the pars recta and pars oblique, as seen in Figure 4–15.

The **pars recta** is the medial-most component of the cricothyroid muscle, originating on the anterior surface of the cricoid cartilage immediately beneath the arch. The pars recta courses up and out to insert into the lower surface of the thyroid lamina. The **pars oblique** arises from the cricoid cartilage lateral to the pars recta, coursing obliquely up to insert into the point of juncture between the thyroid laminae and inferior horns. The angle of incidence of these two segments speaks of their relative functions. Although both tense the vocal folds, individually these muscles have differing effects on the motion of the thyroid. Let us look at both of them.

By virtue of its more directly superior course, contraction of the pars recta rocks the thyroid cartilage downward, which rotates upon the cricothyroid joint. Due to the flexibility of the loosely joined tracheal cartilages below, the cricoid also rises to meet the thyroid. This is a good time to remind you that the points of attachment of the vocal folds are the inner margin of the thyroid cartilage and the arytenoid cartilages and that the arytenoid cartilages are attached to the posterior cricoid cartilage. The effect of rocking the thyroid cartilage forward is that the vocal folds, slung between the posterior cricoid and anterior thyroid, *are stretched*. That is, rocking the thyroid and cricoid closer together in front makes the posterior cricoid more distant from the thyroid. The cricothyroid is largely responsible for stiffening the vocal folds (Chhetri, Berke, Lotfizadeh & Goodyer, 2009). It is worth special note that the cricothyroid is innervated by the superior laryngeal nerve, in contrast

pars recta: L., pars, part; recta, straight

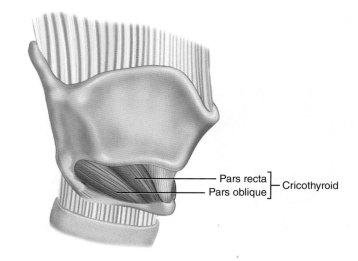

Figure 4–15. Cricothyroid muscle, pars recta, and pars oblique. *Source:* From Seikel/ Drumright/King. *Anatomy & Physiology for Speech, Language, and Hearing, 5th Ed.* ©Cengage, Inc. Reproduced by permission.

Pars recta ⎤
Pars oblique ⎦ Cricothyroid

Muscle:	Cricothyroid
Origin:	Pars recta: anterior surface of the cricoid cartilage beneath the arch Pars oblique: cricoid cartilage lateral to the pars recta
Course:	Pars recta: up and out Pars oblique: obliquely up
Insertion:	Pars recta: lower surface of the thyroid lamina Pars oblique: thyroid cartilage between laminae and inferior horns
Innervation:	X vagus, external branch of superior laryngeal nerve
Function:	Depresses thyroid relative to cricoid; tenses vocal folds

Vocal Hyperfunction

We have emphasized the notion that the larynx is a *small* structure, but we should add that even small muscles are capable of being misused. **Vocal hyperfunction** refers to using excessive adductory force, often resulting in **laryngitis**, which is inflammation of the vocal folds. Excessively forceful contraction of the lateral cricoarytenoid and arytenoid muscles is undoubtedly the primary contributor to this problem, although it is also likely that laryngeal tension arising from the contraction of the thyroarytenoid (thyromuscularis and thyrovocalis) and cricothyroid (with support from the posterior cricoarytenoid) are contributors to this extraordinary force. In case you did not notice, these muscles include virtually all the significant intrinsic laryngeal musculature, which should emphasize the notion that vocal hyperfunction is the result of general laryngeal tension. Vocal hyperfunction can result in laryngitis, vocal nodules, contact ulcers, vocal polyps, and vocal fatigue, and is usually behavioral in etiology.

Treatment typically requires a significant behavioral change in the client, but this is not without a cost. The voice is an extremely personal entity and is very tightly woven into an individual's self-concept. Approaching clients to change their voice is a delicate and challenging task for a clinician.

to all the other intrinsic laryngeal muscles, which are innervated by the recurrent laryngeal nerve. This innervation has a direct impact on diagnosis of neurogenic voice disorders (Aronson, 1985; Baken & Orlikoff, 1999).

The cricothyroid joint also permits the thyroid to slide forward and backward. The forward sliding motion is a function of the pars oblique, and the result is to tense the vocal folds as well. Together, the pars recta and oblique are responsible for the major laryngeal adjustment associated with pitch change. The cricothyroid is innervated by the external branch of the SLN of the X vagus. This branch courses lateral to the inferior pharyngeal constrictor to terminate on the cricothyroid muscle.

Thyrovocalis Muscle

The **thyrovocalis muscle** is actually the medial muscle of the vocal folds. Many anatomists define a singular muscle coursing from the posterior surface of the thyroid cartilage to the arytenoid cartilages, labeling it as the

Muscle:	Thyrovocalis (medial thyroarytenoid)
Origin:	Inner surface, thyroid cartilage near notch
Course:	Back
Insertion:	Lateral surface of the arytenoid vocal process
Innervation:	X vagus, recurrent laryngeal nerve
Function:	Tenses vocal folds

thyroarytenoid. There is ample *functional* evidence to support the differentiation of the thyroarytenoid into two separate muscles, the thyromuscularis and the thyrovocalis, although its anatomical support is questionable. Although the thyromuscularis is discussed as a glottal relaxer, contraction of the thyrovocalis distinctly tenses the vocal folds, especially when contracted in concert with the cricothyroid muscle. It is specifically responsible for adduction of the membranous portion of the vocal folds (Chhetri et al., 2012).

The thyrovocalis (often abbreviated as vocalis) originates from the inner surface of the thyroid cartilage near the thyroid notch. The muscle courses back to insert into the lateral surface of the arytenoid vocal process. Contraction of this muscle draws the thyroid and cricoid cartilages farther apart in front, making this muscle a functional antagonist of the cricothyroid muscle (which draws the anterior cricoid and anterior thyroid closer together). This antagonistic function has earned the thyrovocalis the classification as a glottal tensor, because contraction of the thyrovocalis (in conjunction with contraction of the cricothyroid muscle) tenses the vocal folds. The thyrovocalis is innervated by the RLN, a branch of the X vagus.

Relaxers

- Thyromuscularis

Thyromuscularis Muscles

The paired **thyromuscularis muscles** (or simply, muscularis) are considered the muscle masses immediately lateral to each thyrovocalis, and which, with the thyrovocalis, make up the thyroarytenoid muscle. The **thyromuscularis** or **external (lateral) thyroarytenoid** muscles originate on the inner surface of the thyroid cartilage, near the notch and lateral to the origin of the thyrovocalis. They run back to insert into the arytenoid cartilage at the muscular process and base.

Although there are questions about whether these muscles are truly differentiated from the vocalis, functional differences are clearly seen. As you can see from Figure 4–16, the forces exerted on the arytenoid from pulling differentially on the vocal or muscular process would produce markedly different effects. Contraction of the thyromuscularis has essentially the same effect on the vocal folds as that of the lateral cricoarytenoid. The vocal folds adduct and lengthen (Hirano et al., 1988; Zhang, 2011).

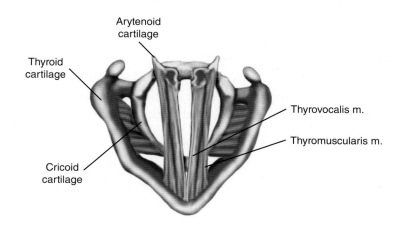

Thyroid cartilage

Arytenoid cartilage

Thyrovocalis m.

Thyromuscularis m.

Cricoid cartilage

SUPERIOR VIEW

Figure 4–16. The thyromuscularis muscle is the lateral muscular component of the vocal folds; the thyrovocalis is the medial-most muscle of the vocal folds. Together they are often referred to as the thyroarytenoid muscle. *Source:* From Seikel/Drumright/ King. *Anatomy & Physiology for Speech, Language, and Hearing, 5th Ed.* ©Cengage, Inc. Reproduced by permission.

Muscle:	Thyromuscularis (lateral thyroarytenoid)
Origin:	Inner surface of thyroid cartilage near the notch
Course:	Back
Insertion:	Base and muscular process of arytenoid cartilage
Innervation:	X vagus, recurrent laryngeal nerve
Function:	Relaxes vocal folds

Contraction of the medial fibers of the thyromuscularis may relax the vocal folds as well. By virtue of their attachment on the anterior surface of the arytenoid, these fibers pull the arytenoids toward the thyroid cartilage without influencing medial rocking. Thus, the pair of thyromuscularis muscles is classically considered to be a laryngeal relaxer. The thyromuscularis is innervated by the RLN.

Auxiliary Musculature

- Thyroarytenoid
- Superior thyroarytenoid
- Aryepiglotticus
- Thyroepiglotticus

Thyroarytenoid Muscle

As discussed previously, the thyroarytenoid muscle (see Figure 4–16), which consists of the thyrovocalis and thyromuscularis muscles, arises from the lower thyroid angle. The thyroarytenoid courses back to insert into the anterolateral surface of the arytenoid cartilages. The medial fibers of the thyroarytenoid constitute the thyrovocalis muscle, while the superior fibers are continuous with the thyroepiglotticus superiorly.

Superior Thyroarytenoid Muscle

The superior thyroarytenoid is inconsistently present, arising from the inner angle of the thyroid cartilage and coursing to the muscular process of the arytenoid. When present it is lateral to the thyromuscularis. It is assumed that the superior thyroarytenoid, like the thyroarytenoid, serves as a relaxer of the vocal folds, although this has not been demonstrated.

Aryepiglotticus Muscle

The aryepiglottic muscle (Figure 4–17) arises from the superior aspect of the oblique arytenoid muscle (i.e., the arytenoid apex) and continues as the muscular component of the aryepiglottic fold as it courses to insert into the lateral epiglottis.

Thyroepiglotticus Muscle

The thyroepiglotticus dilates the laryngeal opening, while the aryepiglotticus assists in protecting the airway during swallowing by deflecting the epiglottic cartilage over the laryngeal aditus (Gray, Bannister, Berry, & Williams, 1995).

Muscle:	Thyroarytenoid
Origin:	Inner angle of thyroid cartilage
Course:	Back
Insertion:	Muscular process of arytenoids
Innervation:	Recurrent laryngeal nerve, X vagus
Function:	Presumably relaxes vocal fold
Muscle:	Superior thyroarytenoid
Origin:	Inner angle of thyroid cartilage
Course:	Back
Insertion:	Muscular process of arytenoids
Innervation:	Recurrent laryngeal nerve, X vagus
Function:	Perhaps relaxes vocal fold
Muscle:	Aryepiglottic muscle
Origin:	Continuation of oblique arytenoid muscle from arytenoid apex
Course:	Back and up as muscular component of aryepiglottic fold
Insertion:	Lateral epiglottis
Innervation:	Recurrent laryngeal nerve, X vagus
Function:	Constricts laryngeal opening
Muscle:	Thyroepiglottic muscle
Origin:	Inner surface of thyroid at angle
Course:	Back and up
Insertion:	Lateral epiglottis
Innervation:	Recurrent laryngeal nerve, X vagus
Function:	Dilates airway, compresses laryngeal saccule for mucus secretion

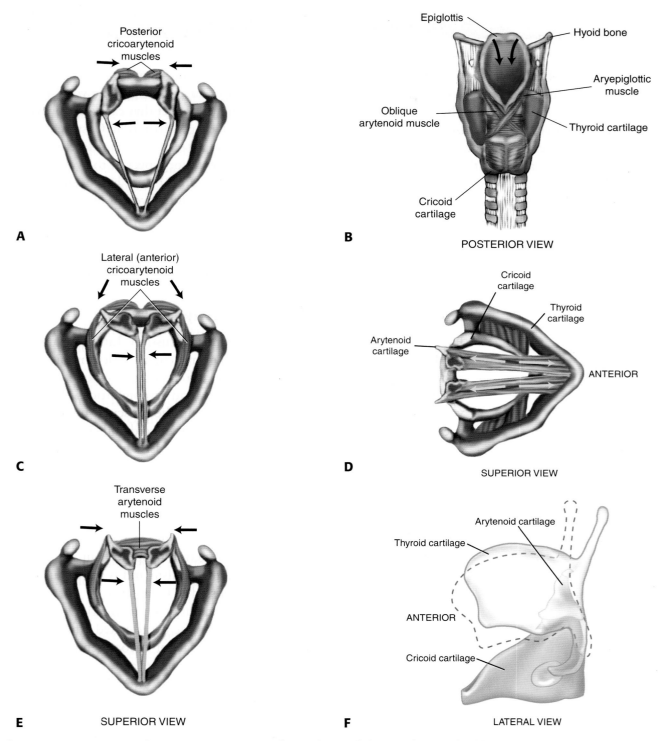

Figure 4–17. A. Action of posterior cricoarytenoid muscles in abducting the vocal folds. **B.** View of posterior intrinsic muscles of the larynx. **C.** Action of lateral cricoarytenoid muscles in adducting the vocal folds. **D.** Contraction of the thyromuscularis relaxes the vocal folds. **E.** Contraction of the transverse arytenoid muscles moves the vocal folds toward midline, as does contraction of the lateral cricoarytenoid muscles. **F.** Contraction of the cricothyroid muscle rocks the thyroid down in the anterior aspect, tensing the vocal folds. *Source:* From Seikel/Drumright/King. *Anatomy & Physiology for Speech, Language, and Hearing, 5th Ed.* ©Cengage, Inc. Reproduced by permission.

- Mylohyoid
- Geniohyoid
- Genioglossus
- Hyoglossus
- Thyropharyngeus
- Inferior pharyngeal constrictor

Digastricus Anterior and Posterior Muscles

As seen in Figure 4–18, the **digastricus muscle** is actually composed of two separate bellies. The anterior and posterior bellies of the digastricus muscle converge at the hyoid bone, and their paired contraction elevates the hyoid. The **digastricus anterior** originates on the inner surface of the mandible at the digastricus fossa, near the point of fusion of the two halves of the mandible, the symphysis. The muscle courses medially and down to the level of the hyoid, where it joins with the posterior digastricus by means of an **intermediate tendon**. The **posterior digastricus** originates on the mastoid process of the temporal bone, behind and beneath the ear. The intermediate tendon passes through and separates the fibers of another muscle, the stylohyoid, as it inserts into the hyoid at the juncture of the hyoid corpus and greater cornu.

The structure and attachment of the digastricus bellies define their function. Contraction of the anterior component results in the hyoid being drawn up and forward, whereas contraction of the posterior belly causes the hyoid to be drawn up and back. Simultaneous contraction results in hyoid

digastricus: L., two; belly

In apes, the laryngeal saccules are so well developed that they contribute to the resonance of the voice.

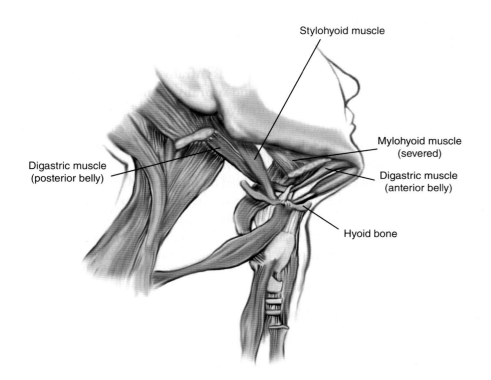

Stylohyoid muscle

Mylohyoid muscle (severed)

Digastric muscle (anterior belly)

Digastric muscle (posterior belly)

Hyoid bone

Figure 4–18. Schematic of digastricus, stylohyoid, and mylohyoid muscles. *Source:* From Seikel/Drumright/King. *Anatomy & Physiology for Speech, Language, and Hearing, 5th Ed.* ©Cengage, Inc. Reproduced by permission.

Muscle:	Digastricus, anterior and posterior
Origin:	Anterior: inner surface of the mandible, near symphysis
	Posterior: mastoid process of temporal bone
Course:	Medial and down
Insertion:	Hyoid, by means of intermediate tendon
Innervation:	Anterior: V trigeminal nerve, mandibular branch, via the mylohyoid branch of the inferior alveolar nerve
	Posterior: VII facial nerve, digastric branch
Function:	Anterior belly: draws hyoid up and forward
	Posterior belly: draws hyoid up and back
	Together: elevate hyoid

elevation without anterior or posterior migration. You see a great deal of activity in the digastricus during swallowing.

At this point, it is wise to mention that the muscles attached to the mandible, such as the digastricus, may also be depressors of the mandible. That is, the digastricus anterior could help to pull the mandible down if the musculature *below* the hyoid were to fix it in place. You will want to retain this notion for our discussion of the role of hyoid musculature in oral motor development and control in Chapter 5. The anterior belly is innervated by the mandibular branch of the V **trigeminal** nerve via the mylohyoid branch of the inferior alveolar nerve. This branch courses along the inner surface of the mandible in the mylohyoid groove and exits to innervate the mylohyoid (to be discussed shortly) and the anterior digastricus. The posterior belly is supplied by the digastric branch of the VII facial nerve.

trigeminal: L., tres, three; gemina, twin

Stylohyoid Muscle

The **stylohyoid muscle** originates on the prominent styloid process of the temporal bone, a point medial to the mastoid process (see Figure 4–18). The course of this muscle is medially down, such that it crosses the path of the posterior digastricus (which actually passes through the stylohyoid) and inserts into the corpus of hyoid.

Muscle:	Stylohyoid muscle
Origin:	Styloid process of temporal bone
Course:	Down and anteriorly
Insertion:	Corpus of hyoid
Innervation:	Motor branch of the VII facial nerve
Function:	Move hyoid posteriorly

Contraction of the stylohyoid elevates and retracts the hyoid bone. The stylohyoid and posterior digastricus are closely allied in development, function, and innervation. Both the stylohyoid and posterior belly of the digastricus are innervated by the motor branch of the VII facial nerve.

Mylohyoid Muscle

As with the digastricus anterior, the **mylohyoid muscle** originates on the underside of the mandible and courses to the corpus hyoid. Unlike the digastricus, the mylohyoid is fanlike, originating along the lateral aspects of the inner mandible on a prominence known as the mylohyoid line. The anterior fibers converge at the median fibrous raphe (ridge), a structure that runs from the **symphysis menti** (the juncture of the fused paired bones of the mandible) to the hyoid. The posterior fibers course directly to the hyoid. Taken together, the fibers of the mylohyoid form the floor of the oral cavity. The relationship between the digastricus and the mylohyoid muscles may be seen in Figure 4–19. As may be derived from the examination of its fiber course, the mylohyoid elevates the hyoid and projects it forward, or alternately depresses the mandible, in much the manner of the digastricus anterior. Unlike the digastricus, the mylohyoid muscle is responsible for the elevation of the floor of the mouth during the first stage of deglutition.

The mylohyoid is allied with the anterior belly of the digastricus, through proximity, development, and innervation. As with the anterior

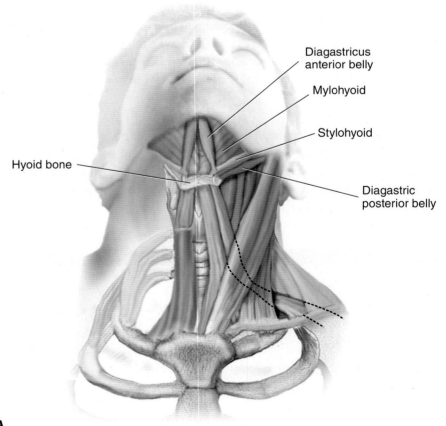

Figure 4–19. A. Schematic of the relationship among mylohyoid, digastricus, and stylohyoid muscles. *continues*

A

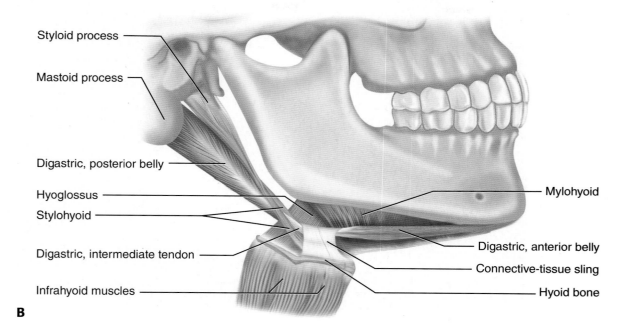

Styloid process
Mastoid process
Digastric, posterior belly
Hyoglossus
Stylohyoid
Digastric, intermediate tendon
Infrahyoid muscles

Mylohyoid
Digastric, anterior belly
Connective-tissue sling
Hyoid bone

B

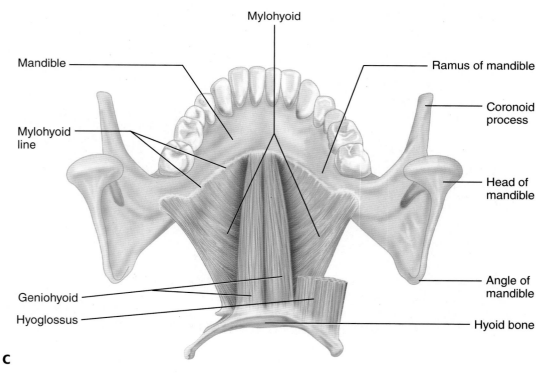

Mylohyoid
Mandible
Ramus of mandible
Coronoid process
Mylohyoid line
Head of mandible
Angle of mandible
Geniohyoid
Hyoglossus
Hyoid bone

C

Figure 4–19. *continued* **B.** Relationship among digastricus anterior, digastricus posterior, hyoglossus, mylohyoid, and stylohyoid. **C.** View of the floor of the mouth from above. Note particularly the relationship between geniohyoid and mylohyoid. *Source:* From Seikel/Drumright/King. *Anatomy & Physiology for Speech, Language, and Hearing, 5th Ed.* ©Cengage, Inc. Reproduced by permission. *continues*

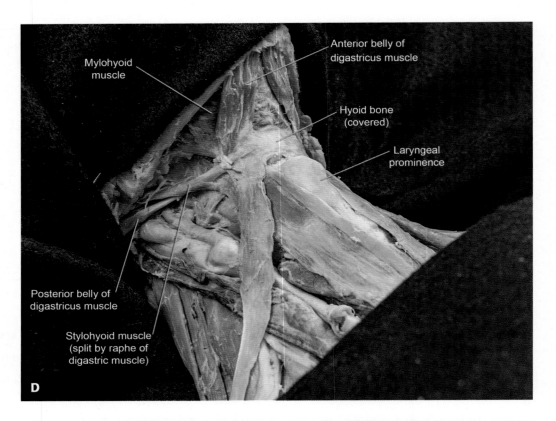

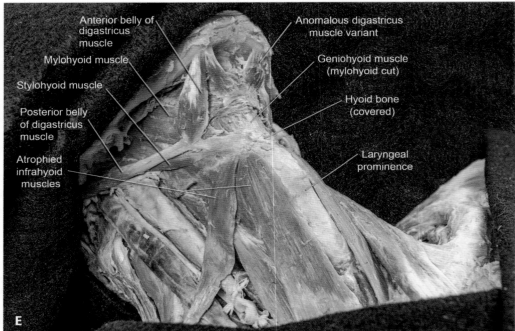

Figure 4–19. *continued* **D.** Photograph showing the relationship among mylohyoid, anterior and posterior digastricus, and stylohyoid muscles. Note the muscle atrophy of the infrahyoid muscles, likely due to cerebrovascular accident or other disease process. **E.** Photograph showing relationship among mylohyoid, geniohyoid, digastricus and stylohyoid muscles. Note that the stylohyoid is split by the digastricus raphe. Compare the digastricus anterior origin of both D and E to recognize the digastricus variant in Figure D (see De-Ary-Pires, Ary-Pires, & Pires-Neto, 2003 for a discussion of digastricus variations).

digastricus, the mylohyoid is innervated by the alveolar nerve, arising from the V trigeminal nerve, mandibular branch. As stated for the digastricus anterior, this nerve courses within the mylohyoid groove of the inner surface of the mandible, branches, and innervates the mylohyoid.

Geniohyoid Muscle

The **geniohyoid muscle** is superior to the mylohyoid, originating at the **mental spines** of the inner mandible, projecting in a course parallel to the anterior belly of the digastricus from the inner mandibular surface (see Figure 4–19). Fibers of this narrow muscle course back and down to insert into the hyoid bone at the corpus. When contracted, the geniohyoid elevates the hyoid and draws it forward. It may also depress the mandible if the hyoid is fixed. The geniohyoid is innervated by the XII **hypoglossal** nerve and C1 spinal nerve. Although most of the hypoglossal originates in the hypoglossal nucleus of the medulla oblongata of the brain stem, those fibers innervating the geniohyoid arise from the first cervical spinal nerve.

mental spines: Spinous processes on the inner surface of the anterior mandible; these prominences provide a means for muscles to attach to bones

hypoglossal: L., glossa, tongue; under, tongue

Hyoglossus Muscle

The **hyoglossus** and genioglossus provide another example of the interrelatedness of musculature. These muscles are also lingual (tongue) depressors (see Figure 6–38 in Chapter 6), because they have attachments on both of these structures. Speech-language pathologists concerned with oral motor control are painfully aware of these relationships and studying them will benefit you as well. The hyoglossus is a laterally placed muscle. It arises from the entire superior surface of the greater cornu and corpus of the hyoid and courses up to insert into the side of the tongue. The point of insertion in the tongue is near that of the styloglossus, a muscle we will discuss in Chapter 6. The

hyoglossus: L., hyo, hyoid; glossus, tongue

Muscle:	Mylohyoid
Origin:	Mylohyoid line, inner surface of mandible
Course:	Fanlike to median fibrous raphe and hyoid
Insertion:	Corpus of hyoid
Innervation:	V trigeminal, mandibular branch, alveolar nerve
Function:	Elevates hyoid or depresses mandible

Muscle:	Geniohyoid
Origin:	Mental spines, inner surface of mandible
Course:	Back and down
Insertion:	Corpus hyoid bone
Innervation:	XII hypoglossal nerve and C1 spinal nerve
Function:	Elevates hyoid bone; depresses mandible

muscle has a quadrilateral appearance and is a lingual depressor or hyoid elevator. The hyoglossus muscle is innervated by the XII hypoglossal.

Genioglossus Muscle

See Chapters 2 and 11 for discussion of spinal nerves.

Although the **genioglossus muscle** is appropriately considered a muscle of the tongue (see Figure 6–38), it definitely is a hyoid elevator as well. The genioglossus originates on the inner surface of the mandible at the symphysis and courses up, back, and down to insert into the tongue and anterior surface of the hyoid corpus. We will discuss the lingual function of this muscle in Chapter 6, but note that the attachment at the hyoid guarantees that this muscle will elevate the hyoid. The genioglossus muscle is innervated by the motor branch of the XII hypoglossal.

Inferior Pharyngeal Constrictor

Orifice: an opening

The **thyropharyngeus** and **cricopharyngeus muscles** constitute the **inferior pharyngeal constrictor**. The cricopharyngeus is the sphincter muscle at the **orifice** of the esophagus. (Note that Mu and Sanders [2008] offered evidence that the sphincter function in humans may arise from a newly discovered muscle, the cricothyropharyngeus.) The thyropharyngeus is involved in propelling food through the pharynx. Its attachment to the thyroid provides an opportunity for laryngeal elevation (see Figure 6–43 in Chapter 6). Innervation of the thyropharyngeus follows that of the other

Muscle:	Hyoglossus
Origin:	Hyoid bone, greater cornu, and corpus
Course:	Down
Insertion:	Sides of tongue
Innervation:	XII hypoglossal
Function:	Elevates hyoid; depresses tongue
Muscle:	Genioglossus
Origin:	Mental spines, inner surface of mandible
Course:	Up, back, and down
Insertion:	Tongue and corpus hyoid
Innervation:	Motor branch of XII hypoglossal
Function:	Elevates hyoid
Muscle:	Thyropharyngeus of inferior pharyngeal constrictor
Origin:	Thyroid lamina and inferior cornu
Course:	Up, medially
Insertion:	Posterior pharyngeal raphe
Innervation:	X vagus, pharyngeal branch, and IX glossopharyngeal nerve, pharyngeal branch
Function:	Constricts pharynx and elevates larynx

constrictors. The X vagus, pharyngeal branch, is responsible for the outer, faster layer of fibers, while the IX glossopharyngeal nerve, pharyngeal branch, innervates the inner, slower fibers (Mu & Sanders, 2007).

The thyropharyngeus arises from the thyroid lamina and inferior cornu, coursing up medially to insert into the posterior pharyngeal raphe. Contraction of this muscle promotes elevation of the larynx while constricting the pharynx. The inferior constrictors are innervated by branches from the X vagi, including the RLN and SLN.

Hyoid and Laryngeal Depressors

- Sternohyoid
- Omohyoid
- Sternothyroid
- Thyrohyoid

Laryngeal depressors depress and stabilize the larynx via attachment to the hyoid, but also stabilize the tongue by serving as antagonists to the laryngeal elevators. The interconnectedness of the laryngeal and tongue musculature may at first be daunting, but take heart. Mastery of the components will greatly enhance your clinical competency because oral motor control has its foundation in these interactions.

Sternohyoid Muscle

As the name implies, the **sternohyoid** runs from sternum to the hyoid. It originates from the posterior-superior region of the manubrium sterni as well as from the medial end of the clavicle. It courses superiorly to insert into the inferior margin of the hyoid corpus.

Contraction of the sternohyoid depresses the hyoid or, if suprahyoid muscles are in contraction, fixes the hyoid and larynx. The lowering function is clearly evident following the pharyngeal stage in swallowing. The sternohyoid is innervated by the ansa cervicalis (*ansa* = loop; i.e., cervical loop), arising from C1 through C3 spinal nerves.

Omohyoid Muscle

As you can see in Figure 4–20, the **omohyoid** is a muscle with two bellies. The superior belly terminates on the side of the hyoid corpus, while the

Muscle:	Sternohyoid
Origin:	Manubrium sterni and clavicle
Course:	Up
Insertion:	Inferior margin of hyoid corpus
Innervation:	Ansa cervicalis from spinal C1 through C3
Function:	Depresses hyoid

inferior belly has its origin on the upper border of the scapula. The bellies are joined at an intermediate tendon. As you can see from this figure, the omohyoid passes deep to the sternocleidomastoid, which, along with the deep cervical fascia, restrains the omohyoid muscle to give it its characteristic dogleg angle. When contracted, the omohyoid depresses the hyoid bone and larynx. The superior belly is innervated by the superior ramus of the ansa cervicalis arising from the C1 spinal nerve, whereas the inferior belly is innervated by the main ansa cervicalis, arising from C2 and C3 spinal nerves.

Muscle:	Omohyoid, superior and inferior heads
Origin:	Superior: Intermediate tendon
	Inferior: upper border, scapula
Course:	Superior: down
	Inferior: Up and medially
Insertion:	Superior: lower border, hyoid
	Inferior: intermediate tendon
Innervation:	Superior belly: superior ramus of ansa cervicalis from C1
	Inferior belly: ansa cervicalis, spinal C2 and C3
Function:	Depresses hyoid

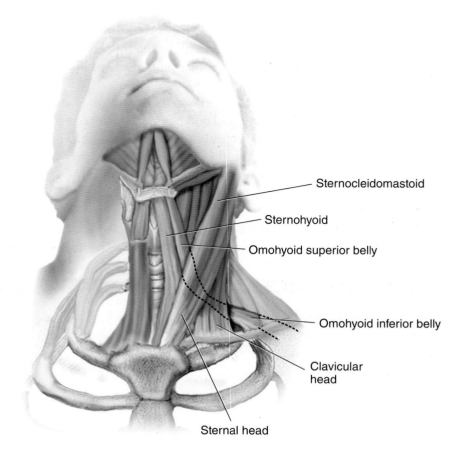

Figure 4–20. Schematic of the relationship among omohyoid, sternocleidomastoid, and sternohyoid muscles. Clavicle on left side of the image has been removed for clarity. *Source:* From Seikel/Drumright/King. *Anatomy & Physiology for Speech, Language, and Hearing, 5th Ed.* ©Cengage, Inc. Reproduced by permission.

Sternothyroid Muscle

As shown in Figure 4–21, contraction of the **sternothyroid muscle** depresses the thyroid cartilage. This muscle originates at the manubrium sterni and first costal cartilage, coursing up and out to insert into the oblique line of the thyroid cartilage. It is active during swallowing, drawing the larynx downward following elevation for the pharyngeal stage of deglutition. The sternothyroid is innervated by fibers from the spinal nerves C1 and C2 that pass into the hypoglossal nerve.

Thyrohyoid Muscle

This muscle is easily seen as the superior counterpart to the sternothyroid (see Figure 4–21). Coursing from the oblique line of the thyroid cartilage to the

Muscle:	Sternothyroid
Origin:	Manubrium sterni and first costal cartilage
Course:	Up and Out
Insertion:	Oblique line, thyroid cartilage
Innervation:	XII hypoglossal and spinal nerves C1 and C2
Function:	Depresses thyroid cartilage

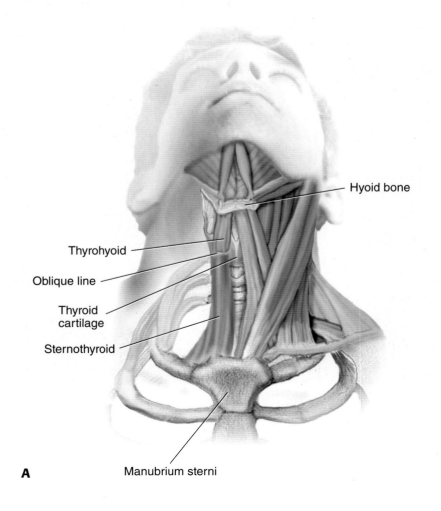

A

Hyoid bone

Thyrohyoid

Oblique line

Thyroid cartilage

Sternothyroid

Manubrium sterni

Figure 4–21. A. Sternothyroid and thyrohyoid muscles. Clavicle on left side of the image has been removed for clarity. *Source:* From Seikel/Drumright/King. *Anatomy & Physiology for Speech, Language, and Hearing, 5th Ed.* ©Cengage, Inc. Reproduced by permission. *continues*

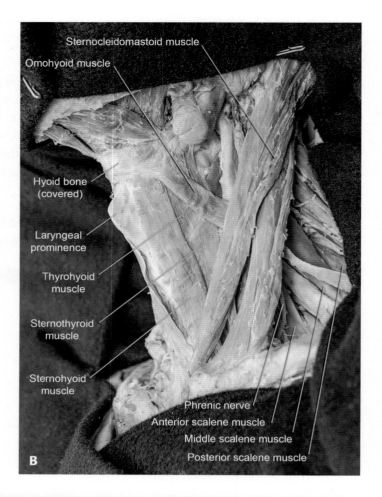

Sternocleidomastoid muscle

Omohyoid muscle

Hyoid bone
(covered)

Laryngeal
prominence

Thyrohyoid
muscle

Sternothyroid
muscle

Sternohyoid
muscle

Phrenic nerve

Anterior scalene muscle

Middle scalene muscle

Posterior scalene muscle

B

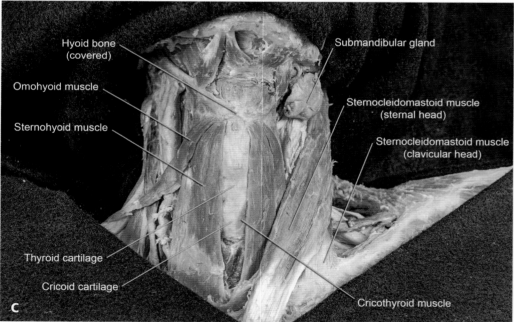

Hyoid bone
(covered)

Submandibular gland

Omohyoid muscle

Sternohyoid muscle

Sternocleidomastoid muscle
(sternal head)

Sternocleidomastoid muscle
(clavicular head)

Thyroid cartilage

Cricoid cartilage

Cricothyroid muscle

C

Figure 4–21. *continued* **B.** Lateral view of neck musculature showing superior omohyoid, sternothyroid, thyrohyoid andsternocleidomastoid muscles. The phrenic nerve can be seen as well. **C.** Anterior view of neck, showing sternohyoid, sternocleidomastoid and cricothyroid muscles.

inferior margin of the greater cornu of the hyoid bone, the **thyrohyoid muscle** either depresses the hyoid or raises the larynx. The thyrohyoid is innervated by the fibers from spinal nerve C1 that course along with the hypoglossal nerves.

Laryngeal Stability

Laryngeal stability is the key to laryngeal control, and this stability is gained through the development of the infra- and suprahyoid musculature. You can think of the larynx as a box connected to a flexible tube at one end (trachea) and loosely bound above. This box has liberal movement in the vertical dimension and has some horizontal movement as well, but there must be a great deal of control in the contraction of all this musculature for this arrangement to work.

The larynx is intimately linked, via the hyoid bone, to the tongue so that movement of the tongue is translated to the larynx. During development, an infant begins to gain control of neck musculature as early as 4 weeks, as seen in the ability to elevate the neck in the prone position. This ability to extend the previously flexed neck heralds the beginning of oral motor control because the ability to balance neck extension with flexion permits the child to control the gross movement of the head. During this stage, the larynx is quite elevated, so much so that you can easily see the superior tip of the epiglottis behind the tongue of a 2-year-old. In the early stages, the elevated larynx facilitates the anterior tongue protrusion required in infancy for nursing.

As the child develops, the larynx descends, starting a process of muscular differentiation between the tongue and the larynx. In the nursing position of the tongue, laryngeal stability is not as important, but the ability to move semihard and hard food around in the oral cavity is quite important as the child begins to eat solid foods. Now the child develops the ability to move the tongue and larynx independently, permitting a much wider set of oral movements. With this differentiation comes the control needed for accurate speech production. For information on head and neck control in children with motor dysfunction, you may wish to examine Jones-Owens (1991), and certainly you will want to read the work of Bly (1994) for insight into the development of muscle control.

See the Clinical Note "Trunk Stability and Upper Body Mobility" in Chapter 2 for a discussion of trunk stability and upper body mobility.

Muscle:	Thyrohyoid
Origin:	Oblique line, thyroid cartilage
Course:	Up
Insertion:	Greater cornu, hyoid
Innervation:	XII hypoglossal nerve and fibers from spinal C1
Function:	Depresses hyoid or elevates larynx

✅ *To summarize:*

- The **extrinsic muscles** of the larynx include the **infrahyoid** and **suprahyoid** muscles.
- The **digastricus** anterior and posterior elevate the hyoid, whereas the **stylohyoid** retracts it.
- The **mylohyoid** and **hyoglossus** elevate the hyoid, and the **geniohyoid** elevates the hyoid and draws it forward.
- The **thyropharyngeus** and **cricopharyngeus** muscles elevate the larynx, and the **sternohyoid, sternothyroid, thyrohyoid,** and **omohyoid** muscles depress the larynx.

Interaction of Musculature

The larynx is virtually suspended from a broad sling of muscles that must work in concert to achieve the complex motions required for speech and nonspeech functions. Movement of the larynx and its cartilages requires both gross and fine adjustments. It appears that the gross movements associated with laryngeal elevation and depression provide the background for the fine adjustments of phonatory control. The supra- and infrahyoid muscles

Vocal Fold Paralysis

Paralysis refers to loss of voluntary motor function, whereas **paresis** refers to weakness. Either can arise from damage to the **upper motor neurons**, which are neurons that arise from the brain and end in the spinal column or brain stem; or damage to the **lower motor neurons**, which are neurons that leave the spinal column or brain stem to innervate the muscles involved.

Vocal fold paralysis may take several forms, depending on the nerve damage. If only one side of the recurrent laryngeal nerve (lower motor neuron) is damaged, the result is unilateral vocal fold paralysis. Bilateral vocal fold paralysis results from bilateral lower motor neuron damage.

If the result of damage is **adductor paralysis**, the muscles of adduction are paralyzed and the vocal folds remain in the abducted position. If the damage results in abductor paralysis, the individual is not able to abduct the vocal folds, and respiration is compromised (you may want to read the note "Laryngeal Stridor" in Chapter 5 to get a notion of what happens). If the superior laryngeal nerve is involved, the individual will suffer loss of the ability to alter vocal pitch, because

the cricothyroid is innervated by this branch of the vagus.

In unilateral paralysis, one vocal fold is still capable of motion. Phonation can still occur, but production will be markedly breathy. Bilateral adductor paralysis results in virtually complete loss of phonation.

There are several causes for vocal fold paralysis, but among the leading causes are damage to the nerve during thyroid surgery and blunt trauma, such as from the steering wheel of an automobile. **Cerebrovascular accidents** (CVA), hemorrhage or other condition causing loss of blood supply to the brain, may damage the upper or lower motor neurons, resulting in paralysis; and a host of neurodegenerative diseases can weaken or paralyze the vocal folds. You should also be aware that paralysis may occur as a result of aneurysm of the aortic arch. An aneurysm is a focal ballooning of a blood vessel caused by a weakness in the wall. When the aneurysm balloons out, it compresses the recurrent laryngeal nerve, causing paresis or paralysis. A **phonatory sign** (objective evidence of phonatory deficit) is not to be taken lightly.

raise and lower the larynx, changing the vocal tract length, but the intrinsic laryngeal muscles are responsible for the fine adjustments associated with phonation control.

To say that the musculature works as a unit is clearly an understatement. The simple action of laryngeal elevation must be countered with the controlled antagonistic tone of the laryngeal depressors. Elevation of the tongue tends to elevate the larynx and increase the tension of the cricothyroid, and this must be countered through intrinsic muscle adjustment to keep the articulatory system from driving the phonatory mechanism. In Chapter 5, you will see how these components work together.

Chapter Summary

The larynx consists of the cricoid, thyroid, and epiglottis cartilages, as well as the paired arytenoid, corniculate, and cuneiform cartilages. The thyroid and cricoid cartilages articulate by means of the cricothyroid joint that lets the two cartilages come closer together in front. The arytenoid and cricoid cartilages also articulate with a joint that permits a wide range of arytenoid motion. The epiglottis is attached to the thyroid cartilage and base of the tongue. The corniculate cartilages rest on the upper surface of the arytenoids, while the cuneiform cartilages reside within the aryepiglottic folds.

The cavity of the larynx is a constricted tube with a smooth surface. Sheets and cords of ligaments connect the cartilages, while a smooth mucous membrane covers the medial-most surface of the larynx. The valleculae are found between the tongue and the epiglottis, within folds arising from the lateral and median glossoepiglottic ligaments. The fibroelastic membrane is composed of the upper quadrangular membranes and aryepiglottic folds; the lower conus elasticus; and the vocal ligament, which is actually the upward free extension of the conus elasticus.

The vocal folds are made up of five layers of tissue, the deepest being the muscle of the vocal folds. The aditus is the entryway of the larynx, marking the entry to the vestibule. The ventricular and vocal folds are separated by the laryngeal ventricle. The glottis is the variable space between the vocal folds.

The intrinsic muscles of the larynx include the thyrovocalis, thyromuscularis, cricothyroid, lateral and posterior cricoarytenoid, transverse arytenoid and oblique arytenoid, superior thyroarytenoid, aryepiglotticus, and thyroepiglotticus muscles.

The thyroepiglotticus and aryepiglotticus both serve nonspeech functions. The thyroepiglotticus increases the size of the laryngeal opening for forced inspiration, while the aryepiglotticus protects the airway by narrowing the aditus and vestibule.

Movement of the vocal folds into and out of approximation requires the coordinated effort of the intrinsic muscles of the larynx. The lateral cricoarytenoid muscle rocks the arytenoid cartilage on its axis, tipping the vocal folds in and slightly down. The posterior cricoarytenoid muscle rocks the arytenoid outward. The transverse arytenoid muscle draws the posterior surfaces of the arytenoids closer together. The oblique arytenoid assists the vocal folds in dipping downward when they are adducted. The thyroepiglotticus has no phonatory function but is involved in the swallowing function. Vocal fundamental frequency is increased by increasing tension, a function of the thyrovocalis and cricothyroid.

Extrinsic muscles of the larynx include the infrahyoid and suprahyoid muscles. The digastricus anterior and posterior elevate the hyoid, while the stylohyoid retracts it. The mylohyoid and hyoglossus also elevate the hyoid, and the geniohyoid elevates the hyoid and draws it forward. The thyropharyngeus and cricopharyngeus muscles elevate the larynx, and the sternohyoid, sternothyroid, and omohyoid muscles depress the larynx.

6. Identify the muscles indicated in the following figure.

A. _____

B. _____

C. _____

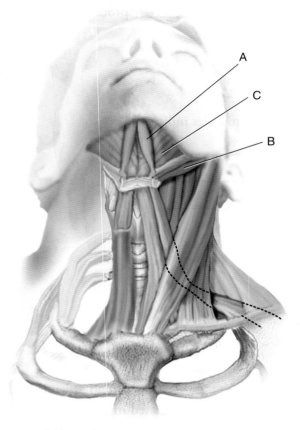

Source: From Seikel/Drumright/King. *Anatomy & Physiology for Speech, Language, and Hearing, 5th Ed.* ©Cengage, Inc. Reproduced by permission.

7. The following figure is a view of the laryngeal opening from above. Identify the structures.

A. _____

B. _____

C. _____

D. _____

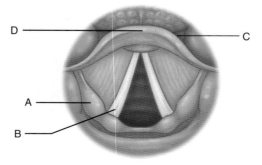

Source: From Seikel/Drumright/King. *Anatomy & Physiology for Speech, Language, and Hearing, 5th Ed.* ©Cengage, Inc. Reproduced by permission.

8. Identify the two muscles indicated in the following figure.

A. _____

B. _____

Source: From Seikel/Drumright/King. *Anatomy & Physiology for Speech, Language, and Hearing, 5th Ed.* ©Cengage, Inc. Reproduced by permission.

9. The _____ muscle is the primary muscle responsible for the change of vocal fundamental frequency.

10. The space between the vocal folds is termed the _____ .

11. Laryngeal cancer sometimes necessitates complete removal of the larynx. Because the respiratory and digestive systems share the pharynx, removal of this protective mechanism poses a problem for accounting for the needs of breathing and swallowing. What surgical changes would permit both processes?

Chapter 4 Study Question Answers

1. The structures are as follows:

    A. **EPIGLOTTIS** cartilage

    B. **THYROID** cartilage

    C. **CRICOID** cartilage

    D. **ARYTENOID** cartilage

    E. **CORNICULATE** cartilage

    F. **HYOID** bone

2. The landmarks are as follows:

    A. **SUPERIOR CORNU**

    B. **INFERIOR CORNU**

    C. **OBLIQUE LINE**

    D. **THYROID NOTCH**

    E. **ANGLE OF THYROID**

    F. **LAMINA**

3. The landmarks are as follows:

    A. **MUSCULAR** process

    B. **VOCAL** process

4. The muscles are as follows:

    A. **TRANSVERSE ARYTENOID**

    B. **OBLIQUE ARYTENOID**

    C. **POSTERIOR CRICOARYTENOID**

5. The muscles are as follows:

    A. **MYLOHYOID**

    B. **DIGASTRICUS ANTERIOR**

    C. **DIGASTRICUS POSTERIOR**

    D. **STYLOHYOID**

6. The muscles are as follows:

    A. **DIGASTRICUS ANTERIOR**

    B. **DIGASTRICUS POSTERIOR**

    C. **MYLOHYOID**

7. The structures are as follows:

   A. **ARYEPIGLOTTIC FOLD**

   B. **TRUE VOCAL FOLDS**

   C. **VALLECULAE**

   D. **EPIGLOTTIS**

8. The two muscles are as follows:

   A. **THYROVOCALIS**

   B. **THYROMUSCULARIS**

9. The **CRICOTHYROID** muscle is the primary muscle responsible for the change of vocal fundamental frequency.

10. The space between the vocal folds is termed the **GLOTTIS**.

11. Removal of the larynx would leave the airway unprotected from intrusion of foreign matter during swallowing. To avoid this danger, the airway is sealed off surgically, and a stoma is surgically opened up through the trachea to permit unhampered respiration.

Bibliography

Aronson, E. A. (1985). *Clinical voice disorders*. New York, NY: Thieme.

Baken, R. J., & Orlikoff, R. F. (1999). *Clinical measurement of speech and voice* (2nd ed.). San Diego, CA: Singular Publishing Group.

Bly, L. (1994). *Motor skills acquisition in the first year*. Tucson, AZ: Therapy Skill Builders.

Broad, D. J. (1973). Phonation. In F. D. Minifie, T. J. Hixon, & F. Williams (Eds.), *Normal aspects of speech, hearing, and language* (pp. 127–168). Englewood Cliffs, NJ: Prentice-Hall.

Chhetri, D. K., Berke, G. S., Lotfizadeh, A., & Goodyer, E. (2009). Control of vocal fold cover stiffness by laryngeal muscles: A preliminary study. *Laryngoscope, 119*(1), 222–227.

Chhetri, D. K., Neubauer, J., & Berry, D. A. (2012). Neuromuscular control of fundamental frequency and glottal pressure at phonation onset. *Journal of the Acoustical Society of America, 13*(2), 1401–1412.

De-Ary-Pires, B., Ary-Pires, R., & Pires-Neto, M. A. (2003). The human digastric muscle: Patterns and variations with clinical and surgical correlations. *Annals of Anatomy-Anatomischer Anzeiger, 185*(5), 471–479.

Dejaeger, E., Pelemans, W., Ponette, E., & Joosten, E. (1997). Mechanisms involved in postdeglutition retention in the elderly. *Dysphagia, 12*(2), 63–67.

Fink, B. R., & Demarest, R. J. (1978). *Laryngeal biomechanics*. Cambridge, MA: Harvard University Press.

Fujiki, R. B., Chapleau, A., Sundarrajan, A., McKenna, V., & Sivasankar, M. P. (2017). The interaction of surface hydration and vocal loading on voice measures. *Journal of Voice, 31*(2), 211–217.

Gaffey, M. M., Sun, R. W., & Richter, G. T. (2018). A novel surgical treatment for posterior glottic stenosis using thyroid ala cartilage: A case report and literature review. *International Journal of Pediatric Otorhinolaryngology, 114*, 129–133.

Gray, H., Bannister, L. H., Berry, M. M., & Williams, P. L. (Eds.). (1995). *Gray's anatomy*. London, UK: Churchill Livingstone.

Gulia, J., Yadav, S., Khaowas, A., Basur, A., & Agrawal, A. (2012). Laryngocele: A case report and review of literature. *Internet Journal of Otorhinolaryngology, 14*(1), 1–4.

Halczy-Kowalik, L., Sulikowski, M., Wysocki, R., Posio, V., Kowalczy, R., & Rzewuska, A. (2012). The role of the epiglottis in the swallow process after a partial or total glossectomy due to neoplasm. *Dysphagia, 27*(1), 20–31.

Hanson, D. G., & Jiang, J. J. (2000). Diagnosis and management of chronic laryngitis associated with reflux. *American Journal of Medicine, 108*(4a), 112S–119S.

Hirano, M., Kiyokawa, K., & Kurita, S. (1988). Laryngeal muscles and glottic shaping. In O. Fujimura (Ed.), *Vocal physiology: Voice production, mechanisms and functions* (pp. 49–65). New York, NY: Raven Press.

Jones-Owens, J. L. (1991). Prespeech assessment and treatment strategies. In M. B. Langley & L. J. Lombardino (Eds.), *Neurodevelopmental strategies for managing communication disorders in children with severe motor dysfunction* (pp. 49–80). Austin, TX: Pro-Ed.

Matteucci, M. L., Rescigno, G., Capestro, F., & Torracca, L. (2012). Aortic arch patch aoroplasty for Ortner's syndrome in the age of endovascular stented grafts. *Texas Heart Institute Journal, 39*(3), 401–404.

McHanwell, S. (2008). Larynx. In S. Standring (Ed.), *Gray's anatomy: The anatomical and clinical basis of practice* (40th ed., pp. 577–594). London, UK: Churchill-Livingstone.

Merati, A. L., & Rieder, A. A. (2003). Normal endoscopic anatomy of the larynx and pharynx. *American Journal of Medicine, 115*, 10S–14S.

Móz, L. E., Domingues, M. A., Castilho, E. C., Branco, A., & Martins, R. H. (2013). Comparative study of the behavior of p53 immunoexpression in smoking associated lesions: Reinke's edema and laryngeal carcinoma. *Inhalation Toxicology, 25*(1), 17–20.

Mu, L., & Sanders, I. (2007). Neuromuscular specializations within human pharyngeal constrictor muscles. *Annals of Otology, Rhinology & Laryngology, 116*(8), 604–617.

Mu, L., & Sanders, I. (2008). Newly revealed cricothyropharyngeus muscle in the human laryngopharynx. *Anatomical Record, 291*(8), 927–938.

Netter, F. H. (1997). *Atlas of human anatomy.* Los Angeles, CA: Icon Learning Systems.

Standring, S. (2008). *Gray's anatomy: The anatomical and clinical basis of practice* (40th ed.). London, UK: Churchill-Livingstone.

Storck, C., Juergens, P., Fischer, C., Wolfensberger, M., Honegger, F., Sorantin, E., . . . Gugatschka, M. (2012). Biomechanics of the cricoarytenoid joint: Three-dimensional imaging and vector analysis. *Journal of Voice, 25*(4), 406–410.

Verdolini, K., Titze, I. R., & Fennell, A. (1994). Dependence of phonatory effort on hydration level. *Journal of Speech and Hearing Research, 37*, 1001–1007.

Weaver, E. M. (2003). Association between gastroesophageal reflux and sinusitis, otitis media, and laryngeal malignancy: A systematic review. *American Journal of Medicine, 115*(3), 81–89.

Wilson, I., Stevens, J., Gnananandan, J., Nabeebaccus, A., Sandison, A., & Hunter, A. (2017). Triticeal cartilage: The forgotten cartilage. *Surgical and Radiologic Anatomy, 39*(10), 1135–1141.

Zhang, Z. (2011). Restraining mechanisms in regulating glottal closure during phonation. *Journal of the Acoustical Society of America, 130*(6), 4010–4019.

CHAPTER 5

Physiology of Phonation

Discussion of the function of the larynx and vocal folds revolves around the movable components and the results of that movement. The nonspeech functions of the larynx are critically important for life because they protect our airway from foreign bodies, so we concentrate on those first (McHanwell, 2008). For the speech-language pathology student, this information will be very useful when you study swallowing and swallowing dysfunction during your graduate studies. Speech function follows naturally from the nonspeech processes. We use these nonspeech functions in our treatment of voice disorders, and this discussion may serve you well.

Nonspeech Laryngeal Function

ANAQUEST LESSON

Protection of the airway is the most important function of the larynx, because failure to prohibit the entry of foreign objects into the lungs is life-threatening. This function is fulfilled through coughing and other associated reflexive actions.

Coughing is a response by the tissues of the respiratory passageway to an irritant or foreign object, mediated by the visceral afferent (sensory) portion of the X vagus nerve innervating the bronchial mucosa. Coughing is a violent and broadly predictable behavior, which includes deep inhalation through widely abducted vocal folds, followed by tensing and tight adduction of the vocal folds and elevation of the larynx (Ludlow, 2015). The axis of movement of the arytenoids guarantees that as they are rocked for adduction, they also are directed somewhat downward, providing more force in opposition to expiration. Significant positive subglottal pressure for the cough comes from tissue recoil and the muscles of expiration. The high pressure of forced expiration blows the vocal folds apart.

The aerodynamic benefit is that the person coughing generates a maximal flow of air through the passageway to expel the irritating object. The negative side of the cough is the force required for its production. Chronic irritation of the respiratory system leads to vocal abuse in the form of repeated coughing.

The near cousin of the cough is throat clearing. It is not as violent as the full cough, but is nonetheless stressful (Dias & Santos, 2016). If you spend a

coughing: forceful evacuation of the respiratory passageway, including deep inhalation through widely abducted vocal folds, tensing and tight adduction of the vocal folds, and elevation of the larynx, followed by forceful expiration

moment clearing your throat and feeling its effects, you can sense increased respiratory effort that is countered by the tightening of the laryngeal musculature. You build pressure in the subglottal region and clamp the vocal folds shut to restrain the pressure. Although this clamping serves a purpose, in that it permits you to clear your respiratory passageway of mucus, it also places the delicate tissues of the vocal folds under a great deal of strain, and the result can be very problematic to a trained voice (D'haeseleer et al., 2017; D'haeseleer, Claeys, Meerschman, & Van Lierde, 2016).

There is a positive clinical side to this action, however. If a client cannot approximate the vocal folds because of muscular weakness, the clinician has a means of achieving this closure. If you can get a client to cough voluntarily, you can very likely get the client to phonate. Both of these actions involve the muscles of adduction: lateral cricoarytenoid, arytenoids, and thyrovocalis. The medial compression generated in the cough is quite large, rivaled only by that required for abdominal fixation.

Abdominal fixation is the process of capturing air within the thorax to provide the muscles with a structure on which to push or pull. The laryngeal movements in this effortful closure are one form of the Valsalva maneuver (O'Connell, Brewer, Man, Weldon, & Hinman, 2016). The preparatory steps for thorax/abdomen fixation are similar to that for the cough: Take in a large inspiratory charge, followed by a tight adduction of the vocal folds. The effect is for the thorax to become a relatively rigid frame, so the forces applied for lifting are translated to the legs. If the thorax is not fixed, those forces will act on the thorax instead, causing the rib cage to be depressed.

You may have wondered why you tend to grunt when lifting heavy objects or pushing your car. All the components required for phonation are present. You are using force that would cause expiration at the same time as your vocal folds are adducted. With sufficient effort, some air escapes through the adducted vocal folds, and you grunt.

So far, we have dealt primarily with laryngeal functions focused on tight adduction of the vocal folds, but abduction has its place as well. Abduction dilates the larynx, an important function for respiration during physical exertion (Røksund, Heimdal, Clemm, Vollsaeter, & Halvorsen, 2017). Recall from Chapter 3 that the physical requirements for oxygen increase significantly during work and exertion. During normal, quiet respiration, the vocal folds are abducted to provide a width of about 8 mm in the adult. During forced respiration, the need for air causes you to **dilate,** or open, the respiratory tract as widely as possible, doubling that width (Figure 5–1).

Reflexes are involuntary, although respiratory reflexes can come under some voluntary control (e.g., you can hold your breath or stifle a yawn). We *must* eventually breathe, which requires reflexively abducting the vocal folds. In cases of drowning and near drowning, the victim may attempt to maintain adducted vocal folds, but must eventually attempt to breathe despite all logic that militates against it (Bierens, Lunetta, Tipton, & Warner, 2016). Similarly, individuals rapidly immersed in cold water reflexively gasp for air; the ability to inhibit this reflex is significantly reduced by alcohol consumption (a fact that explains one of the risks of combining drinking and boating).

abdominal fixation: process of impounding air in thorax to stabilize the torso

Abdominal fixation plays an important role in childbirth, defecation, and vomiting. Review the Clinical Note entitled "Use of Abdominal Muscles for Childbirth and Other Biological Functions" in Chapter 2 to refresh your memory.

dilate: to open or expand an orifice

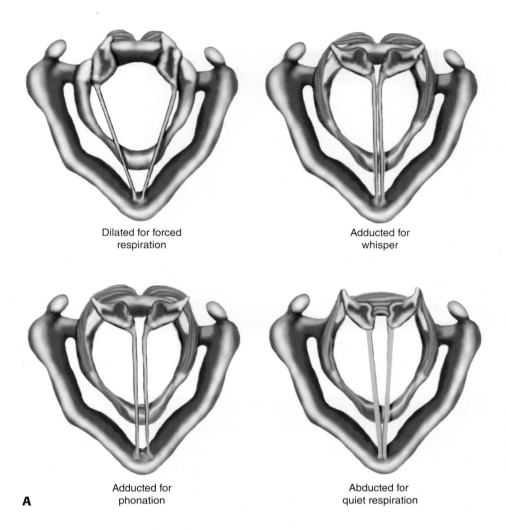

Dilated for forced
respiration

Adducted for
whisper

Adducted for
phonation

Abducted for
quiet respiration

A

Figure 5–1. A. Laryngeal positions for various functions. During adduction for phonation, the vocal folds are approximated. For quiet respiration, the folds are moderately abducted, but for forced respiration, they are widely separated. Adduction for whisper involves bringing the folds close together but retaining a space between the arytenoid cartilages. If one were to use a laryngeal mirror, the image would be reversed. *continues*

We discuss the swallowing reflex more thoroughly in Chapter 8, but it warrants a mention here. During normal deglutition, a **bolus** of food triggers a swallowing reflex as it passes into the region behind the tongue and above the larynx. When the reflex is triggered, the larynx elevates, and the epiglottis (attached to the root of the tongue) drops down to cover the aditus. The aryepiglottic folds tense by the action of the aryepiglottic muscle, and the vocal folds are adducted. Try this: Hold your finger lightly on your thyroid notch and swallow. You may feel your larynx elevate and tense up as you swallow. That finger on the thyroid, by the way, is one component of the clinical swallowing evaluation.

bolus: A mass of chewed food formed into a ball in preparation for swallowing

✓ To summarize:

- We use the larynx and associated structures for many **nonspeech functions**, including coughing, throat clearing, swallowing, and abdominal fixation.

- These functions serve important biological needs and provide us with the background for useful clinical intervention techniques.

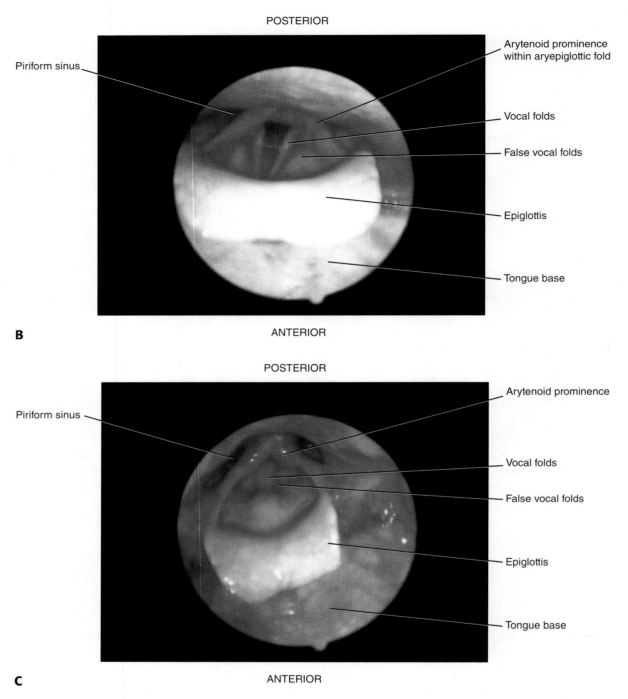

Figure 5–1. *continued* **B.** Fiberendoscopic view of superior larynx with abducted vocal folds. **C.** Fiberendoscopic view of superior larynx with adducted vocal folds. *Source:* From Seikel/Drumright/King. *Anatomy & Physiology for Speech, Language, and Hearing, 5th Ed.* ©Cengage, Inc. Reproduced by permission.

Laryngeal Function for Speech

Before getting into our discussion of phonation, let's review some basic concepts concerning acoustics.

A Brief Discussion of Acoustics

Frequency of Vibration

You are already familiar with the notion that things are capable of vibrating, because you have undoubtedly plucked a guitar string. When a physical body is set into vibration, it tends to continue vibrating (i.e., oscillating), and that vibration tends to continue at the same rate.

Let us examine why a body tends to oscillate. If you have a guitar, pluck one of the strings. As you listen to the twang of the string, you should notice that it continues vibrating for quite a while before finally quieting down. The tone produced remains at about the same **pitch** throughout the audible portion of its vibration.

The actual process of vibration is determined by a lawful interplay of the elastic restoring forces of a material, the stiffness of the material, and the inertia, a quality of its mass (Bless & Abbs, 1995). **Elasticity** is that property of a material that causes it to return to its original shape after being displaced. **Stiffness** refers to the *strength* of the forces within a given material that restore it to its original shape after being distended. **Inertia** is the property of mass dictating that a body in motion tends to stay in motion. If we discuss the vibration of the guitar string in detail, the interaction of these elements may become clearer. Look at Figure 5–2 as we discuss this.

In the first panel of Figure 5–2, the guitar string is at its resting point. At this point, all forces are balanced. Next, the string is being displaced by someone's finger. This displacing force is distending the string. In the next panel, the string has been released and is moving toward its starting point.

pitch: the psychological (perceptual) correlate of frequency of vibration

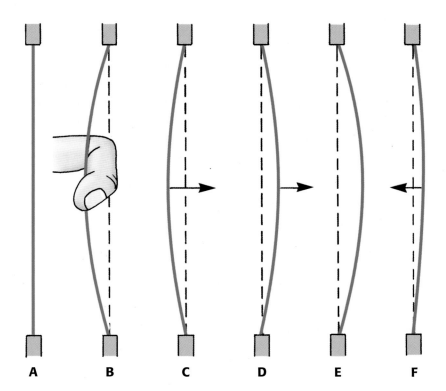

Figure 5–2. A guitar string illustrates oscillation. **A.** The string is at rest. **B.** A finger forces the string into displacement. **C.** The string is released and its elastic elements cause it to return toward the rest position. **D.** The string overshoots the rest position because of its inertia. **E.** The string reaches the extreme point of its excursion past the rest position. **F.** Elastic forces within the string cause the string to return toward the rest position. *Source:* From Seikel/Drumright/King. *Anatomy & Physiology for Speech, Language, and Hearing, 5th Ed.* ©Cengage, Inc. Reproduced by permission.

A   B   C   D   E   F

This is a direct result of the restoring forces of the elastic material. The elastic qualities of the material from which the string is made and the stiffness of that material determine the efficiency with which the string returns.

In Figure 5–2D, when the string reaches the midpoint, it is moving too fast to stop and sails on by that midpoint even though it is the point of equilibrium. This is similar to when you push someone in a swing; the swing does not simply return to the point of rest and stop, but rather overshoots that point. The reason the string travels past the point of rest is that it has mass. It takes energy to move mass and it takes energy to stop it once it has started moving. The string not only returns to its original resting position, due to elastic restoring forces, but flies past that position due to the inertia associated with moving the mass of the object. In Figure 5–2E, the string eventually stops moving because it is now being distended in the opposite direction. The energy you expended in the first distension has now been translated into an opposite distension as a result of inertia. In the final panel (see Figure 5–2F), the string may begin its return trip toward the starting point, but once again overshoots that point because of inertia.

If you had set a pencil into vibration instead of a string and we had moved a sheet of paper in front of it as it vibrated, it might have drawn a picture something like that shown in Figure 5–3, which depicts the periodic motion of a vibrating body. This picture is a graphic representation of the vibration of that object. The drawing represents a waveform, which is the representation of displacement of a body over time, and displays what the pencil or string was doing as it vibrated.

This waveform is **periodic**. When we say that vibration is periodic, we mean that it repeats itself in a predictable fashion. If it took the pencil 1/100 of a second to move from the first point of distension back to that point again, it will take 1/100 of a second to repeat that cycle if it is vibrating periodically.

Moving from one point in the vibratory pattern to the same point again defines one **cycle of vibration**; the time it takes to pass through one cycle of vibration is referred to as the **period**. In our example, the period of vibration was 1/100 second, or 0.01 second. **Frequency** refers to how often something occurs, as in the frequency with which you shop for groceries (e.g., two times

frequency: number of cycles of vibration per second

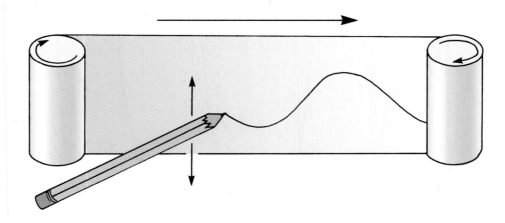

Figure 5–3. Periodic motion of a vibrating body graphically recorded. *Source:* From Seikel/Drumright/King. *Anatomy & Physiology for Speech, Language, and Hearing,* 5th Ed. ©Cengage, Inc. Reproduced by permission.

per month). The frequency of vibration is how often a cycle of vibration repeats itself, which, in our example, is 100 times per second. Frequency and period are the inverse of each other, and that relationship may be stated as $f = 1/T$ or $T = 1/f$. That is, frequency (f) equals 1 divided by period (T for time). For our example, frequency = 1/0.01 second. If you take a moment with your calculator, you can find that this calculation gives a result of 100.

Because frequency refers to the repetition rate of vibration, we speak of it in terms of number of cycles per second. The pencil vibrated with a frequency of 100 cycles per second, but shorthand notation for cycles per second is **hertz** (Hz), after Heinrich Hertz, a brilliant physicist (Mulligan, 2018). When we set the pencil into vibration, it vibrated with a period of 0.01 seconds and a frequency of 100 Hz.

We said that frequency of vibration in a body is governed by the elasticity, stiffness, and mass. If you had added a large weight to the guitar string, it would have vibrated slower. As mass increases, frequency of vibration decreases. (If you are a guitar player, you'll recognize the difference between the high E and low E strings on the guitar: The low E has been wound to add mass to the string.)

If you were to make the string stiffer, it would vibrate more rapidly. Increased stiffness would drive the string to return to its point of equilibrium at a faster rate, increasing the frequency of vibration.

Amplitude and Intensity

There's another aspect of the acoustic signal that we would be quite remiss if we did not mention: intensity. If I were to pluck the string with force, the string would be displaced a lot more than if I had just *lightly* plucked it. The frequency of the vibration is the same whether it is plucked lightly or forcefully, but the amplitude of the vibration is increased. For audible sounds, amplitude corresponds with signal intensity in a lawfully related way. The amplitude of vibration, which translates into the degree to which that waveform deviates from the zero line, correlates well with sound pressure. In fact, if the graph in Figure 5–3 were a microphone output being recorded, the *Y*-axis would be volts, reflecting the degree to which the microphone receiver had moved when we spoke into it. Sound waves consist of oscillations of air molecules, called **compressions** and **rarefactions**. When the vibration is pushing toward the microphone, it is considered to be a compression, and it is a rarefaction when it is moving away from the microphone. These oscillations are direct correlates of the positive and negative movements you see in Figure 5–4, which is a recording of a diphthong from a microphone. These oscillations reflect small changes in pressure. When the waveform goes positive, it translates into a *positive voltage,* and when it goes negative, that is a *negative voltage* change.

Voltage is the correlate of pressure, as in *sound pressure*. There are a couple of things we should say about sound pressure, and then you should seriously consider doing the worksheet on the decibel at the end of the chapter. (As you are probably aware, the decibel is one of those aspects of

compression: the portion of a sound wave in which molecules are closer together than in the quiet state

rarefaction: the portion of a sound wave in which molecules are farther apart, relative to the quiet state

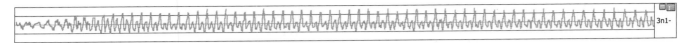

Figure 5–4. Speech waveform of the diphthong /aɪ/, as in "pie," recorded from a microphone. *Source:* From Seikel/ Drumright/King. *Anatomy & Physiology for Speech, Language, and Hearing, 5th Ed.* ©Cengage, Inc. Reproduced by permission.

our field that we tend to shy away from. The activity is designed to walk you through some calculations, without leaving too bad a taste in your mouth!)

As you remember from Chapter 2, pressure is equal to force over a unit area ($P = F/A$). In this case, the area is the surface of the microphone, and the pressure is that which is generated by your voice when you say /a/. In the following sections you will learn that the vocal folds vibrate as a result of physical characteristics of the tissue that interact with airflow, but all you need to know for this discussion is that the vibration results in small changes in air pressure that we (as listeners) translate into sound (*sound* is defined as an audible disturbance in a medium). This air pressure change produces the sound waveform, and you can imagine it looking similar to Figure 5–4. The waveform represents an oscillation that moves from positive pressure (condensation; above the *x*-axis) to negative pressure (rarefaction; below the *x*-axis). Getting back to our original statement, the degree to which the waveform goes beyond the *x*-axis (either negative or positive) is the amplitude of the waveform. The larger the excursion, the louder the sound. Now let us talk about how to measure that.

The ear is one of the true marvels of the universe, although we are admittedly a little biased. It is capable of a range of pressures that is immense, as you should remember from your audiology class. We can measure sound intensity as either power or pressure, which changes our measurement units but not the intensity itself. If we talk of power, we are discussing intensity of a signal as related to the amount of work it is doing (the amount of energy flow per unit area), so the measurement unit is in watts per unit of time. If we are dealing with pressures, we are discussing intensity in terms of force over unit area. These two measures are lawfully related, but we will only work with pressures for this discussion.

You can hear a sound in which the amplitude of air movement is just over the diameter of a molecule of hydrogen atom (20 micropascals = 0 dB SPL), assuming you have young, healthy ears, to a pressure that is a million times larger than that (20,000,000 micropascals= 120 dB SPL). The 120 dB SPL measure would be about the sound pressure your ears would get if you were 200 feet behind a jet engine as the plane is taking off (not recommended). This is an astounding range and is beyond a simple linear description. If you were to have a ruler that represented our range of hearing in micropascals, where 1 mm = 1 micropascal, the ruler's representation of the range of hearing for humans would have to be 1,000 meters long, which would stretch for more than 1/2 mile. Clearly, this is an ungainly way to represent intensity.

To account for our range of hearing, we use a logarithmic scale (von Békésy, & Wever, 1960). The auditory system also functions in a logarithmic way, so the resulting scale comes close to matching our natural perception of loudness. The match is not perfect as we will see in Chapter 10, but it comes much closer than a direct linear measurement of amplitude. Figure 5–5 shows you how logarithms compress a linear scale into a manageable framework. Basically, a logarithm is the power to which the number 10 is raised to reach that given value. (We only talk about base 10 logarithms here, so relax.) The logarithm of 100 is 2; 10^2 is the equivalent of multiplying 10×10, which equals 100. So the exponent (2) is the power to which you raise 10 to get 100. If you have a calculator that will give you logarithms, enter 100 and ask for the log. The answer will be 2.

Now you might start to see the utility of the logarithm. If you have a scale, such as audible sound pressures, that ranges from 20 to 20,000,000, then expressing it using logarithms makes the scale manageable. We talk about the threshold of audibility, which has been defined as 20 micropascals. This is really somewhat arbitrary, because some ears are more sensitive than that; but it gives us the standard for sound pressure level. Sound pressure level (SPL) is defined as 20 micropascals at 1000 Hz. A pascal is the derived measure for pressure that is the equivalent of the force of 1 newton (1 N) exerted on 1 m² (one square meter). (A *newton* is a measure of force defined as the amount of force required to accelerate 1 kilogram of mass 1 meter/second².) A micropascal is 1/1,000,000 of a pascal. The reason we are forced to use such small measures is that we are sensitive to air pressures that represent displacement of molecules by only 1 billionth of a centimeter.

The decibel is actually a ratio of two pressures (or powers). If a sound has a sound pressure level of 40 dB (40 dB SPL), we are talking about the pressure of that sound wave relative to the reference for sound pressure level, 20 micropascals. The calculation is straightforward, and you can get some practice with it by doing the worksheet at the end of the chapter. The formula for the pressure-based decibel is dB = 20 log (input pressure/reference pressure).

As an example, if the input pressure is 20,000,000 micropascals, and we are comparing it to the reference for dB SPL, the formula would be:

$$dB = 20 \log (20{,}000{,}000 \text{ micropascals}/20 \text{ micropascals})$$

First divide 20,000,000 by 20 to get 1,000,000

Then take the logarithm of that (6). This is the power to which you would raise 10 to reach 1,000,000.

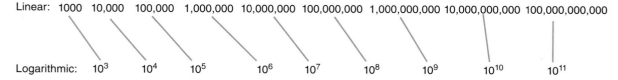

Linear: 1000 10,000 100,000 1,000,000 10,000,000 100,000,000 1,000,000,000 10,000,000,000 100,000,000,000

Logarithmic: 10^3 10^4 10^5 10^6 10^7 10^8 10^9 10^{10} 10^{11}

Figure 5–5. Relationship between linear and logarithmic scales. The top row of numbers reflects linear increases from 1,000 to 100,000,000,000. The bottom row shows what happens if you express the same as the logarithm (base 10). The logarithmic expression makes the ungainly top row much more manageable. *Source:* From Seikel/Drumright/King.. *Anatomy & Physiology for Speech, Language, and Hearing, 5th Ed.* ©Cengage, Inc. Reproduced by permission.

Now multiply that logarithm times 20 (6 × 20 = 120). The answer, then, is that the signal has a sound pressure level of 120 dB.

We can also look at the decibel change from one signal to another, which can be even handier than using the SPL reference. Take a look at the activity at the end of the chapter for some examples of how to do that, and amaze your friends. Knowledge is power!

Frequency and intensity are both critical elements for our discussion in this chapter. As you read this material, don't forget your roots: Frequency is merely looking at how often something happens per unit of time, and intensity is a ratio related to the amount of pressure exerted on a microphone diaphragm (or your ear, for that matter). Both of these concepts will help you as you treat clients with voice disorders.

Instruments for Voicing

Instrumentation for voicing includes tools for processing and analyzing the audio signal (frequency and intensity, mostly) and the physiology of the vocal folds (Baken & Orlikoff, 1999; Behrman, 2007). The standby for intensity is the sound level meter (SLM), which allows you to measure the sound pressure emanating from a source. This is a very useful tool for your work with clients in voice therapy, because inadequate or excessive vocal intensity (intensity of phonation) can arise from both physiological and psychological sources. In voice, the frequency of interest is generally the fundamental frequency (frequency of vibration of the vocal folds), and there are many tools that allow you to measure this in sustained phonation or running speech. A measure of phonatory stability is vocal jitter (or perturbation), which quantifies the cycle-by-cycle differences in vibration. A similar measure of cycle-by-cycle variation in intensity is vocal shimmer. Both of these measures are often bundled with instruments that measure the fundamental frequency. You're going to see that vocal intensity and fundamental frequency can be controlled separately, but also that it is difficult to do so. The phonogram (Pabon & Plomp, 1988) (also known as voice range profile or phonetogram) is a means of showing the interaction between intensity and frequency, revealing the degree of control one can exert on one's physiology and, as importantly, the range of intensity and frequency for an individual (Behrman, 2007).

We know that the respiratory system provides the energy for speech (see Chapter 3), and we can look at the glottal airflow and airway pressures using a number of instruments. Airflow is sensed by means of a pneumotachograph, typically placed within a face mask. Airflow measures allow researchers to examine the relationship between the phonatory and respiratory systems, such as glottal resistance related to phonemes produced, vocal intensity and airflow, and so forth. Measuring subglottal pressure is a little trickier. To get to the region below the vocal folds, you must insert a hypodermic needle through the cricothyroid membrane and read the pressures generated below the level of the vocal folds. Subglottal pressure can be estimated by examining intraoral pressure when the vocal folds are open, such as in production of /p/, which is an indirect measurement.

We can view the upper surface of the vocal folds directly using fiber endoscopy. Nasoendoscopy is a fiber-optic instrument that is inserted transnasally (through the nose and through the velopharyngeal port) so that the fiberoptic bundle can provide an image of the vocal folds and laryngeal structures in real time. While the instrument can certainly be inserted orally and aimed toward the larynx, the view from the velopharyngeal port allows the tongue to move (so it is an excellent tool for swallowing evaluation as well). When a stroboscopic source is used with the endoscope, the examiner can actually stop the action of vibrating vocal folds, a process called videostroboscopy. This process allows close examination of vibratory function of the vocal folds and has provided great insight into the modes of vocal fold vibration, as we will discuss in Chapter 6. Both laryngeal videoendoscopic and videostroboscopic analyses are recommended by the American Speech-Language-Hearing Association (ASHA) in assessment of the vibratory pattern of vocal folds in clinical practice (Patel et al., 2018).

Another excellent tool for examining the vibrating vocal folds is the electroglottograph (EGG; Childers, Hicks, Moore, Eskenazi, & Lalwani, 1990). A pair of electrodes is affixed to the surface of the neck at the thyroid laminae. One electrode emits a very small current, which is read by the other electrode. The EGG trace that is recorded is the impedance (resistance to electrical flow) between the two electrodes (the patient or subject cannot feel the current, by the way). EGG provides a graphic trace that corresponds to the degree of vocal fold contact (see Figure 5–16 later in this chapter).

☑ *To summarize:*

- **Vibration** is governed by the interplay of elastic restoring forces, stiffness, and inertia.

- **Elasticity** is the property of material that causes it to return to its original shape after being displaced.

- **Stiffness** refers to the *strength* of elastic forces.

- **Inertia** is the property of mass that causes it to stay in motion once it is placed into motion.

- **Periodicity** refers to a waveform that is predictable.

- Moving from one point in the vibratory pattern to the same point again defines one **cycle of vibration**.

- The time it takes to pass through one cycle of vibration is referred to as the **period**.

- Frequency refers to how often something occurs. **Frequency of vibration** in sound is measured in cycles per second, abbreviated **Hz**.

- The **intensity of sound** is lawfully related to the amplitude of the waveform.

- **Sound pressure** is the correlate of voltage, so measurement of the output of a microphone can be used to calculate intensity of sound.

- The **decibel (dB)** is a ratio of two sound pressures or powers, which is expressed logarithmically.

- Instrumentation for voicing includes tools for processing and analyzing the audio signal (frequency and intensity, mostly) and the physiology of the vocal folds.

- Intensity is measured using the **sound level meter**, and there are many tools that allow you to measure this in sustained phonation or running speech. **Vocal jitter** (perturbation) quantifies cycle-by-cycle differences in vibration of the vocal folds, and **vocal shimmer** examines cycle-by-cycle differences in intensity.

- The **phonogram** is a means of showing the interaction between intensity and frequency for an individual.

- Airflow is sensed using a **pneumotachograph**, typically placed within a face mask.

- Subglottal pressure may be measured by hypodermic needle through the cricothyroid membrane or estimated by examining intraoral pressure when the vocal folds are open.

- **Nasoendoscopy** involves insertion of a fiber endoscope transnasally to provide an image of the vocal folds and laryngeal structures in real time.

- The **electroglottograph (EGG)** uses a pair of electrodes affixed to the surface of the neck to provide a graphic trace that corresponds to the degree of vocal fold contact.

Now it is time to look at the primary physical principle supporting phonation: the Bernoulli effect.

The Bernoulli Effect

Vocal folds are masses that may be set into vibration. The **larynx** is the cartilaginous structure housing the two bands of tissue we call the vocal folds. The paired vocal folds are situated on both sides of the larynx so that they actually intrude into the airstream, as you can see from the schematic in Figure 5–6. This figure is a view from above and a view from behind. From above, you can see that the vocal folds are bands of tissue that are actually visible from

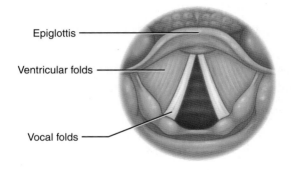

Epiglottis

Ventricular folds

Vocal folds

Figure 5–6. A. Vocal folds from above. *continues*

A   SUPERIOR VIEW

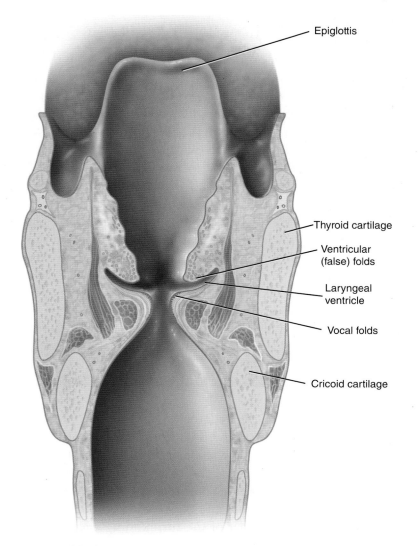

Epiglottis

Thyroid cartilage

Ventricular
(false) folds

Laryngeal
ventricle

Vocal folds

Cricoid cartilage

B   CORONAL SECTION, FROM BEHIND

Figure 5–6. *continued*
B. Coronal section of larynx
looking toward front, showing
constriction in laryngeal
space caused by the vocal
folds. *Source:* From Seikel/
Drumright/King. *Anatomy
& Physiology for Speech,
Language, and Hearing, 5th
Ed.* ©Cengage, Inc. Reproduced by permission.

a point immediately behind your tongue, looking down toward the lungs. From behind, you can see that the vocal folds are also a constriction in the airway, a critical concept for phonation.

Remember from our discussion of respiratory physiology that any constriction in the airway greatly increases airway turbulence. If you are a passenger in a car and put your hand out the window, you can feel the force of the wind dragging against your hand and you can hear the turbulence associated with it. You can rotate your hand so that the turbulence is reduced or increased; as the force on your hand increases, it becomes more difficult to keep your hand in the airstream.

The vocal folds are also a source of turbulence in the vocal tract. Without them, air would pass relatively unimpeded out of the lungs and into the oral cavity. The adduction of the vocal folds results in air having to make a detour around the folds, and the result of that detour invokes a discussion of the Bernoulli effect.

See Chapter 3 for a discussion of respiratory physiology.

The Bernoulli Effect in Everyday Life

The next time you travel in an airplane, feel free to thank Daniel Bernoulli for the flight. While the thrust of the engines has a very large contribution to keeping the plane afloat, the configuration of the wings is critical to keeping you afloat so that you can arrive at your destination. If you viewed a wing in cross section from the end, you would note that the top surface of the wing is fatter, while the bottom is more streamlined. This configuration causes the air on the upper surface of the wing to move a little faster than that of the underbelly of the wing, which corresponds to a reduction in air pressure *above* the wing. This low pressure above sucks up the airplane into the sky as airflow increases, so that the net result is an airplane that rises. (This is why wings are treated for ice in winter: Ice changes the aerodynamics of the wing, destabilizing the difference between upper and lower surfaces, greatly compromising the lift that can be gained.)

For those of you who prefer fly balls to flying, realize that the pitcher in a baseball game is capitalizing on the Bernoulli effect as well. To produce a curve ball, the pitcher ensures that the ball begins its flight with the smooth surface toward the front and that the seam on the ball rotates to the side of the ball sometime during its brief flight. The seam acts as a constriction; the pressure on the seam side is lower than that on the opposite smooth side, and the ball is sucked toward the seam (there are other processes involved, but we will ignore them here). At least one pitcher has demonstrated the ability to weave the ball through a series of fence posts by putting just the right spin on the ball. For an excellent discussion of this effect, see Adair (1995, 2002).

Daniel Bernoulli, an 18th-century Swiss scientist, recognized the effects of constricting a tube during fluid flow. The **Bernoulli effect** states that, given a constant volume flow of air or fluid, at a point of constriction there is a decrease in pressure perpendicular to the flow and an increase in velocity of the flow. If you put a constriction in a tube, air flows faster as it passes through the constriction, and the pressure on the wall at the point of constriction is lower than that of the surrounding area. Let us examine this statement.

Airflow Increase

Figure 5–7 shows a tube with a constriction in it representing the vocal folds. If you have placed your thumb over a garden hose, you know that the rate of water flow increases as a result of that constriction. Likewise, if you have ever been white-water rafting, you will immediately recognize that the rapids arise from constrictions in the flow of the river, in the form of boulders. As the water flows through the constriction, the rate of flow increases, giving you a thrill as you speed uncontrollably toward your fate.

Air Pressure Drop

To get an intuitive feel for the pressure drop, you might think about the flow in terms of molecules of air. Look again at Figure 5–7. We have drawn it so that you can count the number of molecules of air in the tube relative to the

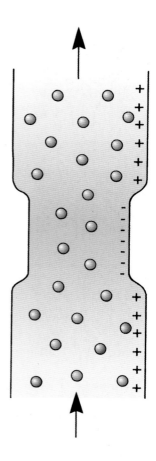

Figure 5–7. Rate of airflow through the tube increases at the point of constriction, and air pressure decreases at that point as well. *Source:* From Seikel/Drumright/King. *Anatomy & Physiology for Speech, Language, and Hearing, 5th Ed.* ©Cengage, Inc. Reproduced by permission.

tube's length. In each unconstricted region, you can count 10 molecules of air. Where the tube becomes narrower, there are fewer air molecules because there is less space for them to occupy and, therefore, you count only five in that area.

When air is forced into a narrower tube, the same total volume of air must squeeze through a smaller space. Because each unit mass of air becomes longer and narrower, it covers a longer stretch of the tube's walls. The pressure exerted by this mass, although the same in an overall sense, is now distributed over more of the wall. The result is that each atom of the wall feels less force from the air molecules, and the narrow part of the tube is more likely to collapse. This effect occurs only when the air is forced to move; air without any forced movement will sooner or later equalize its pressure everywhere. If you remember that pressure is force exerted on an area ($P = F/A$), a drop in pressure makes perfect sense. Less force on the wall translates into lower pressure on the wall. In the case of a constant airflow, airflow will increase in velocity at the constriction as well.

These two elements (pressure drop and velocity increase) are the heart of the Bernoulli effect and help us to understand vocal fold vibration. Return to the notion of vocal folds being a constriction in a tube, as illustrated in Figure 5–8. You will want to refer to this figure as we discuss the Bernoulli principle applied to phonation.

Figure 5–8. One cycle of vocal fold vibration as seen through a frontal section. **A.** Air pressure beneath the vocal folds arises from respiratory flow. **B.** Air pressure causes the vocal folds to separate in the inferior. **C.** The superior aspect of the vocal folds begins to open. **D.** The vocal folds are blown open, the flow between the folds increases, and pressure at the folds decreases. **E.** Decreased pressure and the elastic quality of vocal folds causes folds to move back toward midline. **F.** The vocal folds make contact inferiorly. **G.** The cycle of vibration is completed. *Source:* From Seikel/Drumright/ King. *Anatomy & Physiology for Speech, Language, and Hearing, 5th Ed.* ©Cengage, Inc. Reproduced by permission.

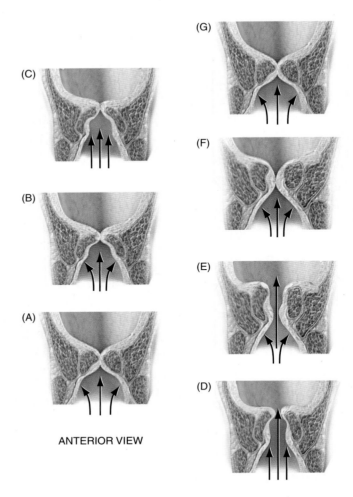

ANTERIOR VIEW

The vocal folds are soft tissue, made up of muscle and epithelial tissue. Because of this characteristic, the folds are also capable of moving when sufficient force is exerted on them, as in the case of your hand extended out of the moving car's window.

By examining Figure 5–8A, you see that the vocal folds are closed. In the next panel (Figure 5–8B), the air pressure generated by the respiratory system is beginning to force the vocal folds open, but there is no transglottal flow because the folds are still making full contact. By panel D (Figure 5–8D), the vocal folds have been blown open. Because the vocal folds are elastic, they tend to return to the point of equilibrium, which is the point of rest. They cannot return to equilibrium, however, as long as the air pressure is so great that they are blown apart. When they are in that position, however, there is a drop in pressure at the point of constriction (the Bernoulli effect), and we already know that if there is a drop in pressure, something is going to move to equalize that pressure.

In the last three panels (Figures 5–8E, F, & G) you can see the result of the negative pressure: The vocal folds are being sucked back toward midline (E) as a result of the negative pressure and aided by tissue elasticity. The final panels (F & G) show the folds again making contact, with airflow being completely halted. When the vocal folds are pulled back toward the midline by their tissue-restoring forces, they completely block the flow of air for an instant as they make contact. At this point, the negative pressure related to flow is gone also. Instead, there is the force of respiratory charge beneath the folds ready to blow them apart once again. Incidentally, the minimum subglottal pressure that will blow the vocal folds apart to sustain phonation is approximately 3 to 5 cm H_2O, although much larger subglottal pressures are required for louder speech (Plant & Younger, 2000).

What you hear as voicing is the product of the repeated opening and closing of the vocal folds. The motion of the tissue and the resultant airflow disturb the molecules of air, causing the phenomenon we call sound.

The act of bringing the vocal folds together for phonation is referred to as **adduction**, and the process of drawing the vocal folds apart to terminate phonation is called **abduction**. As we will see, both of these movements are achieved using specific muscles, but the actual vibration of the vocal folds is the product of airflow interacting with the tissue in the *absence* of repetitive muscular contraction.

If you have followed this introductory discussion of the principles governing vocal fold vibration, you are prepared to examine the structures of the larynx.

⊘ To summarize:

- **Phonation**, or voicing, is the product of vibrating vocal folds within the larynx.
- The **vocal folds** vibrate as air flows past them; the Bernoulli phenomenon and tissue elasticity help maintain phonation.
- The **Bernoulli principle** states that, given a constant volume flow of air or fluid, at a point of **constriction** there will be a **decrease** in **pressure** perpendicular to the flow and an **increase** in **velocity** of the flow.
- The interaction of **subglottal pressure**, **tissue elasticity**, and **constriction** within the airflow caused by the vocal folds produces sustained phonation as long as pressure, flow, and vocal fold approximation are maintained.

Vocal Attack

Phonation is an extremely important component of the speech signal. To accomplish phonation we must achieve three basic laryngeal adjustments. To *start* phonation, we must adduct the vocal folds, moving them into the airstream, a process referred to as **vocal attack** (Orlikoff, Deliyski, Baken, & Watson, 2009; Patel, Forrest, & Hedges, 2017; Watson, Baken, & Roark, 2016). We then hold the vocal folds in a fixed position in the airstream as the aerodynamics of phonation control the actual vibration associated with **sustained phonation**. Finally, we abduct the vocal folds to achieve **termination of phonation**.

sustained phonation: phonation that continues for long durations as a result of tonic contraction of vocal fold adductors

When we are *not* phonating, the vocal folds are sufficiently abducted to prohibit air turbulence in the airway from starting audible vibration of the vocal folds. To initiate voicing, we bring the vocal folds close enough together that the forces of turbulence can cause vocal fold vibration. The process of phonation is considered to consist of two phases: the pre-phonatory adjustment phase and the attack phase. During the pre-phonatory phase, the vocal folds are moved to a position that will support phonation, including adducting the vocal folds and setting the appropriate tensions to balance the subglottal pressure. The **vocal attack** phase is that in which the vocal folds begin to vibrate (Orlikoff et al., 2009).

Vocal attack occurs quite frequently in running speech. If you were to say the sentence "Anatomy is not for the faint of heart," you would have brought the vocal folds together and drawn them apart at least six times in two seconds to produce voiced and voiceless phonemes.

Vocal attack can be characterized in a number of ways that relate to the speed and force of adduction during that attack phase. Vocal attack time (VAT) is a measure of the time between evidence of muscular activation of adduction and the onset of the acoustic result. There are three basic types of attack, and they appear to be well differentiated based upon the VAT measure (Orlikoff et al., 2009). When we initiate phonation using **simultaneous vocal attack**, we coordinate adduction and onset of respiration so that they occur simultaneously. The vocal folds reach the critical degree of adduction at the same time that the respiratory flow is adequate to support phonation, approximately 5 ms after muscular activation. Chances are you are using simultaneous attack when you say the word *zany*, because starting the flow of air before voicing would add the unvoiced /s/ to the beginning of the word, whereas adducting the vocal folds before producing the first sound would add a glottal stop to production. You may want to further explore neuromuscular control of phonation (Chhetri, Neurbauer, & Berry 2012) as it relates to respiration, as well as acoustic phonetics and attack (Watson et al., 2016).

Breathy vocal attack involves starting significant airflow before adducting the vocal folds. This occurs frequently during running speech, because we keep air flowing throughout the production of long strings of words. The vocal attack is much slower, with approximately 26 ms lapsing before onset of phonation. Say the following sentence while attending to the airflow over your tongue and past your lips: "Harry is my friend." If you did this, you felt the constant airflow, which indicates that some of the adductions involved had to be produced with air already flowing.

The third type of attack is **hard** or **glottal attack**. In this attack, adduction of the vocal folds occurs prior to the airflow, much like a cough. Indeed, Orlikoff et al. (2009) found that the VAT for hard attack was approximately −6 ms, revealing that the adduction of the vocal folds occurs during the pre-phonatory adjustment. Try this. Bring your vocal folds together (be gentle!) as if to cough, but instead of opening your vocal folds as you push air through the folds, keep them adducted and say /a/. That was a hard attack. You might have felt a little tension or irritation from doing this exercise, a reminder of the delicacy of the vocal mechanism. We use hard attack when a word begins

vocal attack: movement of vocal folds into the airstream sufficiently to initiate phonation

simultaneous vocal attack: vocal attack in which expiration and vocal fold adduction occur simultaneously

breathy vocal attack: vocal attack in which expiration occurs before the onset of vocal fold adduction

glottal attack: the vocal attack in which expiration occurs after adduction of the vocal folds

with a stressed vowel. Say the following sentence and pay close attention to your vocal folds during the production of the first phoneme of the words: *Okay, I want the car*. If you noticed a buildup of tension and pressure for those words, you were experiencing hard attack.

Vocal Attack Time seems to reliably indicate the mode of attack; and the timing of the attack appears to be relatively unchanged between 24 and 40 years of age, although females have markedly shorter VATs than males (Roark, Watson, Baken, Brown, & Thomas, 2012). All three of these attacks are quite functional in speech and are not at all pathological. Problems occur when an attack is misused. If a hard attack becomes too forceful, the speaker may damage the delicate vocal mechanism tissues. If the speaker inadequately adducts the vocal folds, air may escape between them to produce a **breathy phonation**; a much more common phenomenon is breathy voice caused by a physical tissue change that obstructs adduction.

Termination

We bring the vocal folds together to begin phonation, and termination of phonation requires that we abduct them. We pull the vocal folds out of the airstream far enough to reduce the turbulence, using muscular action. When the turbulence is sufficiently reduced, the vocal folds stop vibrating. As with attack, we terminate phonation many times during running speech to accommodate voiced and voiceless speech sounds.

Both adduction and abduction occur very rapidly. Muscles controlling these functions can complete contraction within about 9 milliseconds (ms) (9/1000 seconds). In running speech, you may see periods of vibration of the vocal folds as brief as three cycles of vibration (approximately 25 ms total) for unstressed vowels, and 9 ms for termination, which would bring the total adduction, phonation, and abduction time to only 43/1000 of a second.

Ventricular Phonation

The false or ventricular vocal folds are technically unable to vibrate for voice, but in some instances, clients may use them for this purpose. Boone, McFarlane, Von Berg, and Zraick (2009) cited instances in which clients used ventricular phonation as an adaptive response to severe vocal fold dysfunction, such as growths on the folds. Apparently, the client forces the lateral superior walls close together during the adductory movement, permitting the folds to make contact and vibrate.

The ventricular folds are thick, and the phonation heard is deep and often raspy. The false folds may **hypertrophy** (increase in size), facilitating ventricular phonation. A study by Young, Wadie, and Sasaki (2012) confirmed that the ventricular folds are innervated by the recurrent laryngeal nerves, and unilateral adductor vocal fold paralysis will result in unilateral paralysis of the ventricular folds.

Fans of old movies may remember the 1930s era "Our Gang" series about rough-and-tumble children set against the world. If you are one of those fans, you may remember Froggy, one of the children who had strong allegiance to Spanky. Take another listen to Froggy's voice and you will hear (and see) an excellent example of ventricular phonation. In Froggy's case, it was a claim to fame that made him a star of the silver screen.

Adduction is a constant in all types of attack. The arytenoid cartilages are capable of moving in three dimensions, involving movement such as **arytenoid rotation**, **rocking**, and **gliding**. It appears that the primary arytenoid movement for adduction is inward rocking. When the arytenoids are pulled medially on the convex arytenoid facet of the cricoid, the arytenoids rock down, with apexes approaching each other. (See Figure 4–11 in Chapter 4 if you wish to review this movement.) Some rotation occurs during the adductory movement of the arytenoid, and this has been demonstrated using cadaver specimens (Storck et al., 2012); but rotatory movement appears to be greatest at the extremes of lateral movement (i.e., nearly abducted; Fink & Demarest, 1978).

Rotation, rocking and gliding of the arytenoid cartilages are the product of the lateral cricoarytenoid muscle and the lateral portion of the thyromuscularis, facilitated by the oblique and transverse arytenoids. The arytenoid

laryngitis: inflammation of the larynx

aphonia: loss of ability to produce voicing for speech

vocal hyperfunction: excessive use of vocal mechanism, for speech or nonspeech function, which has the potential to produce organic pathology

Vocal Fold Nodules

Vocal fold nodules are aggregates of tissue arising from abuse. This condition makes up a large share of the voice disorder cases seen by school clinicians (Aronson & Bless, 2009). Common forms of *vocal abuse* (or phonotrauma) are yelling, screaming, cheerleading, or barking commands (such as by a drill sergeant). The result of this abuse is a sequence of events that can lead to a permanent change in the vocal fold tissue. You are probably familiar with **laryngitis**, which is an inflammation of the larynx. It causes hoarseness, often with loss of voice (**aphonia**). The laryngeal effect is the swelling (**edema**) of the delicate vocal fold tissue, so that it is difficult to make the folds vibrate. In fact, the vocal folds are often bowed so badly that expiratory flow will pass between them, even if you can produce phonation; we refer to this as a **breathy voice** (Sapienza & Stathopoulos, 1994). Laryngitis may easily be caused by **vocal hyperfunction**, which is overadduction of the vocal folds. Laryngitis is a form of vocal abuse, and you may have experienced it after a particularly thrilling football game.

The soreness is a message from your body to stop doing what made the vocal folds sore in the first place. Continued abuse results in the formation of a protective layer of epithelium that is callous-like and is not a very effective oscillator. If the vocal hyperfunction continues, the hardened tissue will increase in size until a nodule forms on one (**unilateral**) or both (**bilateral**) vocal folds. The site of abuse is usually at the juncture of the anterior and middle thirds of the vocal folds, because this is the point of greatest impact during phonation. Although untreated vocal nodules may eventually have to be removed surgically, voice therapy to reverse the vocal behavior driving the phenomenon is always recommended. If the vocal hyperfunction is not eliminated, the vocal nodules will return after surgery; however, surgery may be avoided if therapy is sought in a timely manner (Boone et al., 2009).

cartilages are also capable of limited gliding in the anterior–posterior dimension, which could alter the total vocal fold length (Nishizawa, Sawashima, & Yonemoto, 1988). Adduction does not seem to affect the overall length of the glottis, although it tends to lengthen the membranous portion. The combined forces of the cricothyroid and posterior cricoarytenoid cause the entire glottis to lengthen (Hirano, 1974; Hirano, Kiyokawa, & Kurita, 1988; Hirano, Ohala, & Vennard, 1969).

Sustained Phonation

Sustained phonation is the purpose of adduction and abduction for speech. Let us examine this closely.

Vocal attack requires muscular action, as does termination of phonation. In contrast, sustaining phonation simply requires *maintenance* of a laryngeal posture through **tonic** (sustained) contraction of musculature. This is a very important point. The vibration of the vocal folds is achieved by placing and holding the vocal folds in the airstream in a manner that permits their physical aspects to interact with the airflow, thereby causing vibration. The vocal folds are *held* in place during sustained phonation, and the vibration of the vocal folds is *not* the product of repeated adduction and abduction of the vocal folds. Muscle spindles embedded within the thyrovocalis and thyromuscularis serve an important function in holding the sustained posture. As you will learn in the neurophysiology section (Chapter 12), muscle spindles are responsible for the maintenance of muscle posture. These sensors provide input to the nervous system about the length of muscle in a resting (or in this case, steady-state) posture; and when that muscle moves away from the chosen posture without voluntary contraction, the muscle spindle is responsible for correcting that *accidental* movement. So, during steady-state phonation, the vocal folds are in a steady-state, tonic contraction to control fundamental frequency and to stabilize intensity. The business of vocal fold vibration is purely that of aerodynamic interaction with the elastic characteristics of the vocal folds that have been postured for phonation. The vocal folds need not be touching to vibrate, as you can demonstrate for yourself. Begin the word *hairy* by stretching out the /h/ sound, and then let that breathiness carry forward into the vowel. If you hear a breathy quality, the vocal folds very likely are not touching or are making only very light contact.

Vocal Register

The **mode of vibration** of the vocal folds during sustained phonation refers to the pattern of activity that the vocal folds undergo during a cycle of vibration. Moving from one point in the vibratory pattern to the same point again defines one **cycle** of vibration, and within one cycle the vocal folds undergo some very significant changes. There are actually a number of modes or **vocal registers** that have been differentiated perceptually. Narrowly defined for purposes of phonatory discussion, register refers to differences in the mode of vibration of vocal folds.

*Trained singers refer to combinations of thorax/oral/nasal cavity configurations, laryngeal positions, and muscular **concentrations** to define registers that are perceptually differentiable but about which there are few acoustical or physiological data. See Titze (1994) for a lively discussion of register.*

You can see from the first panel of Figure 5–9 that the vocal folds are approximated at the beginning of a cycle of vibration. In the second panel (Figure 5–9B), air pressure from beneath is forcing the folds apart in the inferior aspect. (This makes sense, because that is where the pressure is located.) In the third panel (C), the bubble of air has moved upward so that the superior portion of the folds is now open, and in panel (E), you can see that they are closing again. Note that they begin closing at the bottom: They open at the bottom first, and they start closing first at the bottom as well. In the final panel (G) the cycle is complete.

There is an observed phase difference in the mucosal wave from inferior to superior, and Titze (1994) demonstrated that this is a result of the mass and elasticity of the vocal folds, and that these conditions support continued oscillation by the vocal folds (i.e., the tissue continues to vibrate after the energy has been removed). You can change the tension and mass per unit length to arrive at a given, relatively constant laryngeal tone.

The vocal folds have one primary frequency of vibration, called the **vocal fundamental frequency**, but they produce an extremely rich set of harmonics as well, which are whole-number multiples of the fundamental frequency. These harmonics provide important acoustical information for identification of voiced phonemes. If the vocal folds were simple tuning forks without these harmonics, we would not be able to tell one vowel from another. The complex vibrational mode of the vocal folds is extremely important.

Can Elephants Purr?

There are two ways for vocal fold tissue to move: active muscle contraction (AMC) (Herbst et al., 2012) or arising from the myoelastic aerodynamic principles we've described here. For many years, speech and hearing scientists fought the battle of determining the mechanism that drives vocal fold vibration, and the theory that is most viable is the myoelastic-aerodynamic theory and its updated version, Titze's mucoviscoelastic-aerodynamic theory (Titze, 1973, 1988, 1994). Before we had a firm notion of the limits of the neuromuscular system, a competing theory, called the neurochronaxic theory, held that each vibratory cycle of the vocal folds was the product of neuromuscular activation. The theory posited that vibration of the vocal folds was a function governed directly by the central nervous system, which activated the X vagus recurrent laryngeal nerve to cause each vibration of the vocal folds. It didn't take the field long to figure out that the motor system could not respond quickly enough to control each vibration (and besides, people with paralyzed vocal folds can still make the fold vibrate if it is within the airflow). The neurochronaxic theory was proven absolutely wrong in humans.

If speech scientists have cats among their ranks, they are not so quick to abandon the neurochronaxic theory. The cat's purr is the product of individual, cyclic contractions of the laryngeal muscles, which is why it is so distinctly different from their *meow*. Herbst et al. (2012) wondered whether the subsonic phonations of elephants might arise from the same mechanism, and he found, using an excised larynx from a deceased elephant, that they could produce the sound *without* muscular contraction. So, cats capitalize on active muscular contraction (neurochronaxic theory) to make their contentment known, but elephants rely on the myoelastic aerodynamic theory to communicate.

The second mode of vibration of the vocal folds is in the anterior–posterior dimension. Whereas the vertical phase difference appears to be consistent in modal vibration, the anterior–posterior mode is less stereotypical. Zemlin (1998) reported that the vocal folds tend to open from posterior to anterior, but that closure at the end of a cycle is made by contact of the medial edge of the vocal fold, with the posterior closing last.

Because the vocal folds offer resistance to air flow, the **minimum driving pressure** of the vocal folds in modal phonation is approximately 3 to 5 cm H_2O subglottal pressure. If pressure is lower than this, the folds are not blown apart. This is clinically important, because a client who cannot generate 3 to 5 cm H_2O and sustain it for 5 seconds will not be able to use the vocal folds for speech. (See the Clinical Note entitled "Clinical Measurement of Subglottal Air Pressure" and Figure 5–10.)

Glottal Fry

The second register is known as **glottal fry** but is also known as **pulse register** and **Strohbass** ("straw bass"). What *fry, pulse,* and *straw bass* all allude to is the crackly, popcorn quality of this voice. Perceptually, this voice is extremely low in pitch and sounds rough, almost like eggs frying in a pan. Some voice scientists jokingly refer to it as the "I'm sick" voice, as it is the weak, low-pitched voice you might use to explain the reason you cannot come to work today.

Glottal fry is the product of a complex glottal configuration, and it occurs in frequencies ranging from as low as 30 Hz, to 80 or 90 Hz. This

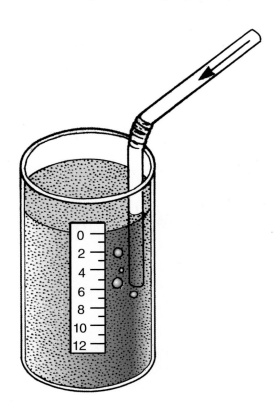

Figure 5–10. A useful clinical tool described by Hixon, Hawley, and Wilson (1982). This portable manometer gives the client feedback concerning respiratory ability and provides the clinician with a measure of function. *Source:* From Seikel/Drumright/King. *Anatomy & Physiology for Speech, Language, and Hearing, 5th Ed.* ©Cengage, Inc. Reproduced by permission.

mode of vibration requires low subglottal pressure to sustain it (on the order of 2 cm H_2O); and tension of the thyrovocalis is significantly reduced relative to modal vibration, so that the vibrating margin is flaccid and thick. The lateral portion of the vocal folds is tensed, so that there is strong medial compression with short, thick vocal folds and low subglottal pressure. If either vocalis tension or subglottal pressure is increased, the popcorn-like perception of this mode of vibration is lost.

In music, syncopation is the change in accent arising from stressing of a weak beat. In the case of glottal fry, this definition is stretched to accommodate the notion of including a weak beat in the rhythm. Glottal fry appears to include both weak and strong beats.

In glottal fry, the vocal folds take on a secondary, syncopated mode of vibration, such that there is a secondary beat for every cycle of the fundamental frequency. In addition to this syncopation, the vocal folds spend up to 90% of the cycle in approximation. Oscillographic waveforms of modal vibration and glottal fry are shown in Figure 5–11, and the presence of the extra beat may be clearly seen. This should reemphasize the notion that the vocal folds are not simply vibrating at a slower rate than in modal phonation, but are vibrating *differently*.

Falsetto

The third and highest register of phonation, the **falsetto**, also is characterized by a vibratory pattern that varies from modal production. In falsetto, the vocal folds lengthen and become extremely thin and reed-like. When set into vibration, they tend to vibrate along the tensed, bowed margins, in contrast to the complex pattern seen in other modes of phonation. The vocal folds make contact only briefly, as compared with modal phonation,

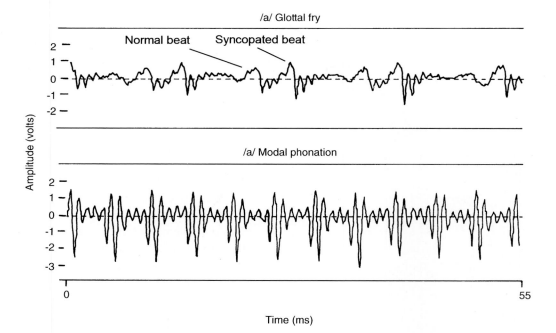

Figure 5–11. Oscillographic comparison of glottal fry (*top*) and modal phonation (*bottom*) for the vowel /a/. *Source: From Seikel/Drumright/King. Anatomy & Physiology for Speech, Language, and Hearing, 5th Ed.* ©Cengage, Inc. Reproduced by permission.

Clinical Measurement of Subglottal Air Pressure

Hixon, Hawley, and Wilson (1982) have provided us with an excellent and simple tool to assess the adequacy of subglottal pressure for speech. In their article, the authors recommend marking a cup of water in cm gradations (see Figure 5–10). Put a paper clip over the straw to hold it to the edge of the glass. Fill the glass up to the top centimeter mark.

As you push the straw deeper into the water, it becomes increasingly difficult to blow bubbles in the water through the straw. At the point where the straw is 3 cm below the water line, you must generate 3 cm H_2O of subglottal pressure to make bubbles.

When assessing a client for adequacy of subglottal pressure, you can have the individual begin blowing as you push the straw into the water. The point at which there are no longer bubbles is the limit of the individual's pressure ability. This is an excellent therapy tool as well, because it provides a practice device with visual feedback of progress toward respiratory support for speech. Realize that this is a measurement of respiratory ability, which is essential for phonation.

and the degree of movement (amplitude of excursion) is reduced. The posterior portion of the vocal folds tends to be damped, so that the length of the vibrating surface is decreased to a narrow opening. Contrast this to elevated pitch in modal phonation, which involves *lengthening* the vocal folds.

The perception of falsetto is one of an extremely thin, high-pitched vocal production. The difference between falsetto and modal vibration is not simply one of the frequency of vibration (in the 300–600 Hz range). Although it is true that falsetto is the highest register, the modal and falsetto registers overlap.

Whistle Register

There is actually a register above falsetto, known as the **whistle register**, but it is not apparently a mode of vibration as much as it is the product of turbulence on the edge of the vocal fold. It occurs at frequencies as high as 2500 Hz, typically in females, and sounds very much like a whistle.

The shift from modal register to glottal fry or falsetto is clearly audible in the untrained voice. If you perform an up-glide of a sung note, reaching up to your highest production, you may hear an audible *break* in the voice as you enter that register. Trained singers learn to smooth that transition so that it is inaudible.

Pressed and Breathy Phonation

There are two variations on modal phonation that we should mention. In **pressed** phonation, medial compression is greatly increased. The product of pressed phonation is an increase in the stridency or harsh quality of the voice, as well as an increase in abuse to the voice. Greater medial compression is translated as stronger, louder phonation, perhaps commanding greater attention. This forceful adduction often results in damage to the vocal fold tissue.

A breathy voice may be the product of the other end of this tension spectrum. If the vocal folds are inadequately approximated, so that the vibrating margins permit excessive airflow between them when in the closed phase, you will hear air escape as a **breathy** phonation. Breathiness is inefficient and causes air wastage, but is not a condition that will damage the phonatory mechanism.

There is a potential danger in the breathy voice, however. The underlying factor keeping the vocal folds from approximating could be any of a number of organic conditions, so that even when the speaker pushes the vocal folds tightly together, air escapes. In this case, a breathy voice may signal the presence of vocal nodules, or even benign or malignant growths such as polyps or laryngeal cancer. In addition, if an individual attempts to overcome the breathy quality caused by nodules or other obstructing pathology, the vocal hyperfunction will result in abuse.

Whispering

Whispering is not really a phonatory mode, because no voicing occurs. This does *not* mean that there are no laryngeal adjustments, but rather that they do not produce vibration in the vocal folds. Prove this to yourself. Exhale forcefully and attend to your larynx, and then on the next forceful exhalation *whisper* the word *Ha!* You probably felt the tension in your larynx increased during whispering. In respiration the vocal folds are abducted, but when whispering they must be partially adducted and tensed to develop turbulence in the airstream, and that turbulence is the noise you use to make speech. The arytenoid cartilages are rotated slightly in but are separated posteriorly, so that there is an enlarged "chink" in the cartilaginous larynx. A whisper is

Puberphonia

During typical development, children undergo a great deal of change during puberty. This occurs between 13 and 15 years of age for boys and between 9 and 16 years of age for girls. Puberty is characterized by rapid muscle development and height and weight gain. The thyroid cartilage and thyroarytenoid are not left out of development. They grow rapidly during this time, although the larynges of boys grow considerably more than those of girls.

The result of this spurt of laryngeal growth is that the child (typically a boy) will have periods of voice change (mutation) in which his voice breaks down in pitch as he is speaking. This is, of course, a normal result of the changing tissue and the young man's attempt to control it for phonation, but it is nonetheless disturbing. **Puberphonia** refers to the maintenance of the childhood pitch despite having passed through the developmental stage of puberty. It surely represents an attempt to hold *something* constant during the roller-coaster ride of puberty, but the result is a significant mismatch between the large body of the developing teenaged boy and the high-pitched voice of the prepubescent child. Typically, the young man is speaking in falsetto but is aware of the lower voice. Therapy performed over the summer to help the individual alter habitual pitch, in the absence of peer pressures associated with the classroom regimen, is quite effective.

not voiced, but is strenuous and can cause vocal fatigue. Whispering is not economical, as you can prove to yourself by sustaining production of an /a/ in modal phonation and again in whispered production. You should see quite a difference in maximum duration.

In Chapter 4 we discussed the notion of frequency of vibration. As mentioned earlier in there as well as in this chapter, the primary frequency of vibration of the vocal folds is called the *fundamental frequency*. This is the number of cycles the vocal folds go through per second, and it is audible. The movement of the vocal folds in air produces an audible disturbance in the medium of air known as **sound**. That sound is transmitted through the air as a wave, with molecules being compressed by movement of the vocal folds.

The interplay of the elasticity and mass of the vocal folds leads them to vibrate in a periodic fashion. However, we have not yet mentioned a final element of phonation, intensity. **Intensity** refers to the relative power or pressure of an acoustic signal, measured in decibels (abbreviated **dB**). In phonation, we may refer to the intensity of voice as **vocal intensity**. Intensity is a direct function of the amount of pressure exerted by the *sound wave* (as opposed to air pressure, as generated by the respiratory system). As molecules vibrate from movement of the vocal folds, the molecular movement exerts an extremely small but measurable force over an area, and that is defined as pressure. The larger the excursion of the vibrating body, the greater the intensity of the signal produced, because air is displaced with greater force. The next two sections deal with frequency and intensity of vocal fold vibration.

intensity: magnitude of sound, expressed as the relationship between two pressures or powers

(✓) *To summarize:*

- We must adduct the vocal folds to **initiate phonation**. This adduction may take several forms, including **breathy, simultaneous**, and **glottal attacks**.

- **Termination** of **phonation** requires abduction of the vocal folds, a process that must occur with the transition of voiced to voiceless speech sounds.

- **Sustained phonation** may take several forms, depending on the laryngeal configuration.

- **Modal phonation** will, by definition, characterize most speech.

- **Falsetto** occupies the upper range of laryngeal function, while **glottal fry** is found in the lower range.

- Vocal fold vibration varies for each of these phonatory modes, and the differences are governed by **laryngeal tension, medial compression**, and **subglottal pressure**.

- **Breathy phonation** occurs when there is inadequate medial compression to approximate the vocal folds. **Whispering** arises from tensing the vocal fold margins while holding the folds in a partially adducted position.

The vocal mechanism is quite flexible and is capable of approximately two octaves of change in fundamental frequency from the lowest possible frequency to the highest. An individual with a low fundamental frequency of 90 Hz will be able to reach a high of about 360 Hz (octave 1 = 90 Hz to 180 Hz; octave 2 = 180 to 360 Hz). This range is often reduced by laryngeal pathology, such as vocal nodules. The normal range can be expanded through voice training. Let us examine how we make changes in vocal fundamental frequency, hence in perceived pitch.

Laryngeal Development

In Chapter 8 we will discuss the development of the larynx in the context of swallowing, but let us discuss some specific laryngeal changes that arise from birth to puberty. At birth, the vocal folds are approximately 4 mm long, as opposed to the adult length of between 12 and 15 mm. If you look at Figure 5–12, you can see the steady progression of vocal fold length as the individual develops. If you look now at the data of Kazarian, Sarkissian, and Isaakian (1978), you can see the life-span development (Figure 5–13). Pay special attention to changes that occur between 11 and 16 years, when puberty begins. The vocal folds of both males and females increase in length, but those of males become much longer. Take a look at Kent's (1976) plot of the vocal fundamental frequency of males and females from birth to adulthood (Figure 5–14), and you can clearly see the effect of this change. The fundamental frequency (denoted as f_0) tends to stabilize in adulthood. As you

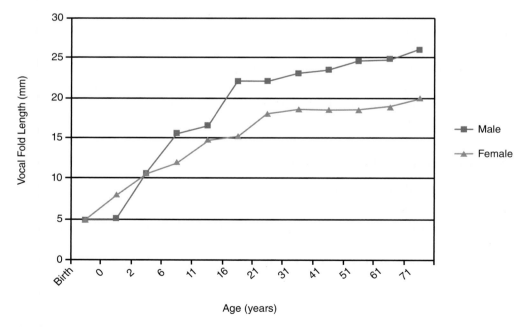

Figure 5–13. Length change of the vocal folds over the lifespan for males and females. *Source:* From Seikel/Drumright/King. *Anatomy & Physiology for Speech, Language, and Hearing, 5th Ed.* ©Cengage, Inc. Reproduced by permission. (Drawn from the data of Kazarian, 1978.)

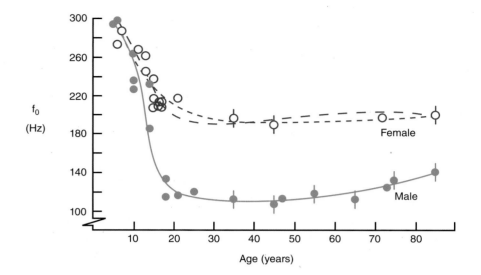

Figure 5–14. Fundamental frequency change over the lifespan for males and females. Note that there are two lines for female because the graph is based on multiple studies. *Source:* From Seikel/Drumright/King. *Anatomy & Physiology for Speech, Language, and Hearing,* 5th Ed. ©Cengage, Inc. Reproduced by permission. (Adapted with permission from Kent, 1994.)

can see from this figure, when you spread out the adult range, males undergo a gradual increase in f_0 after age 50 or so, while females hold quite steady throughout life. You will also see that the average male f_0 is around 130 Hz at 20 years, increasing to about 140 Hz at 80 years of age. Females, on the other hand, hold steady at around 190 Hz throughout adult life.

In Chapter 4 we discussed the importance of a viable respiratory source for phonation. It should not surprise you, then, to know that as our respiratory function matures our ability to sustain phonation increases as well. Kent (1976, 1994) demonstrated that males and females both show a rather steady increase in the ability to sustain phonation. At 3 years of age, a child can sustain a vowel for around 7 seconds, but that ability climbs by about 1.4 seconds per year through young adulthood (until around 17 years of age). By 17, an adolescent should be able to sustain a vowel for 26 seconds or so, although the variability in function is quite large at all ranges.

Pitch-Changing Mechanism

Fundamental frequency increase comes from stretching and tensing the vocal folds using the cricothyroid and thyrovocalis muscles. Here is the mechanism of this change. The changeable elements of the vocal folds are tension, length, and mass. We cannot actually change the mass of the vocal folds, but we can change the mass per unit length by spreading out the muscle, mucosa, and ligament over more distance. We can also change the tension of the vocal folds by stretching them tighter or relaxing them. Both of these changes arise from elongation.

When the cricothyroid muscle is contracted, the thyroid tilts down, lengthening the vocal folds and increasing the fundamental frequency. When the tension on the vocal folds is increased, the **natural frequency of vibration** increases.

The thyrovocalis is a tensor of the vocal folds as well, because contraction of this muscle pulls both cricoid and thyroid closer together, an action

The natural frequency of vibration: the frequency at which a body vibrates given the mass, tension, and elastic properties of the body.

opposed by the simultaneously contracted cricothyroid. This tensing process must be opposed by contraction of the posterior cricoarytenoid, although this muscle is not classified as a tensor of the vocal folds. The posterior cricoarytenoid is invested with **muscle spindles**, structures responsible for monitoring and maintaining tonic muscle length. As the length of this muscle changes, its length may be reflexively controlled to compensate for the stretching force on the vocal folds. See Chapter 12 for a discussion of the muscle spindle.

These tensors tend to operate together, but for slightly different functions. It is currently believed that the cricothyroid contracts to approximate the degree of tension required for a given frequency of vibration. The thyrovocalis appears to fine-tune this adjustment. That is, the cricothyroid makes the gross adjustment, and the thyrovocalis causes the fine movement.

We have still not dealt with mass changes. As the mass of a vibrating body decreases, frequency of vibration increases. The mass of the vocal folds is constant, because to actually increase or decrease mass would require growth of tissue or atrophy, neither of which occurs quickly. Instead, the mass is rearranged by lengthening. When the vocal folds are stretched by contraction of the tensors, the mass of the folds is distributed over a greater distance, thus reducing mass per unit length.

The effect of the lengthening and tensing actions is to make vocal folds longer and thinner in appearance. Interestingly, there is evidence that the vocal folds do not lengthen continuously as fundamental frequency increases, but rather that, at some point near or in the falsetto range, the vocal folds again begin to shorten as frequency increases (Nishizawa et al., 1988). Others have found that increased medial compression may effectively shorten the vibrating surface, increasing frequency (Van den Berg, 1958, 1968; Van den Berg & Tan, 1959).

Lowering fundamental frequency requires the opposite manipulation. As mass per unit length increases and tension decreases, fundamental frequency decreases. We relax the vocal folds by shortening them, moving the cricoid and thyroid closer together in front. This process is achieved by contraction of the thyromuscularis. When it contracts, the vocal folds are relaxed and shortened so that they become more massive and less tense. It appears that there is help from some of the suprahyoid musculature that indirectly pulls up on the thyroid cartilage, shortening the vocal folds by distancing the thyroid from the cricoid.

Subglottal Pressure and Fundamental Frequency

There are also changes in subglottal pressure that must be reckoned with. Increasing pitch requires increasing the tension of the system, thereby increasing the glottal resistance to airflow. If airflow is to remain constant through the glottis, pressure must increase. It appears, however, that the increases in subglottal pressure are a *response* to the increased tension required for frequency change rather than its *cause*. Subglottal pressure does increase, but the primary influence on fundamental frequency change is muscular tension (Titze, 1994). It is a delicate balancing act that we perform. It appears that the cricothyroid and posterior cricoarytenoid tense the vocal folds, while the thyroarytenoid (thyromuscularis and thyrovocalis) increase medial contact of the vocal folds (Chhetri et al., 2012).

✅ *To summarize:*

- **Pitch** is the psychological correlate of frequency of vibration, although the term has come into common usage when referring to perception of the physical vibration of the vocal folds.

- **Optimal pitch** refers to the frequency of vibration that is most efficient for a given pair of vocal folds, and **habitual pitch** is the frequency of vibration habitually used by an individual.

- The **pitch range** of an individual spans approximately two octaves, although the range will be reduced by pathology and may be increased through vocal training.

- Changes in **vocal fundamental frequency** are governed by the tension of the vocal folds and their mass per unit length.

- Increasing the length of the vocal folds increases vocal fold tension as well as decreases the mass per unit area, thus increasing the fundamental frequency.

- The **respiratory system** responds to increased vocal fold tension with **increased subglottal pressure**, so that pitch and subglottal pressure tend to covary.

- Increased subglottal pressure is a response to increased vocal fold tension.

Intensity and Intensity Change

Just as pitch is the psychological correlate of frequency, **loudness** is the psychological correlate of intensity. **Intensity** (or its correlate, sound pressure level) is a ratio of the physical measure of power (or pressure), but loudness is how we perceive power or pressure differences. As with pitch, there is a close relationship between loudness and intensity.

> **vocal intensity:** sound pressure level associated with a given speech production

To increase vocal intensity of the vibrating vocal folds, one must somehow increase the vigor with which the vocal folds open and close. In sustained phonation, the vocal folds move only as a result of the air pressure beneath them and the flow between them. Subglottal pressure and flow provide the energy for this vocal engine, so to increase the intensity or strength of the phonatory product we have to increase the energy that drives it. We increase subglottal pressure to increase vocal intensity. To prove this to yourself, do the following. You need to feel what you do to produce loud speech. You may be in a quiet setting right now and you really may not want to yell, but that is fine. Pay attention to your lungs and larynx as you *prepare to yell as loudly as you can* to someone across the room. Without even yelling, you should have been able to feel your lungs take in a large charge of air, and you should have also felt your vocal folds tighten up. These are the two steps of significance for increasing vocal intensity: increased subglottal pressure and medial compression.

Subglottal pressure and increased medial compression vary together, but the causal relationship is better established for vocal intensity than for the tension–pressure relationship for pitch. For intensity to increase, the energy source must also increase, so subglottal pressure must rise. To explain the effect that medial compression has on vocal intensity requires a return to the discussion of a cycle of vocal fold vibration.

We can break a cycle of vibration into stages, such as an **opening stage**, in which the vocal folds are opening up; a **closing stage**, in which the vocal folds are returning to the point of approximation; and a **closed stage**, in which there is no air escaping between the vocal folds (Figures 5–15 and 5–16). In modal phonation at conversational intensities, it has been found

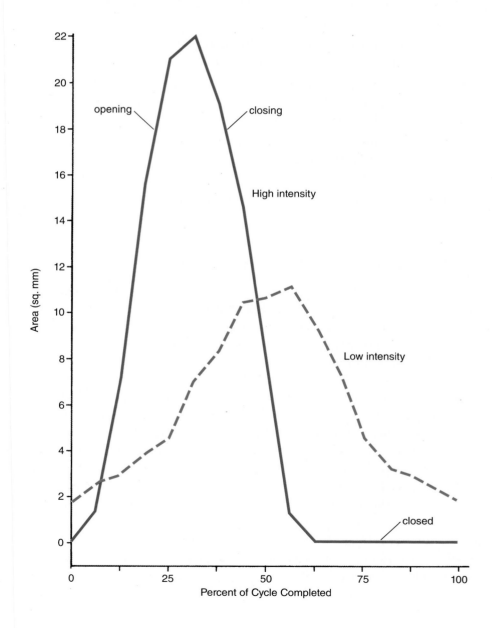

Figure 5–15. Effect of vocal intensity on vocal fold vibration. During low-intensity speech the opening and closing phases occupy most of the vibratory cycle, as revealed in the area of the glottis. During high-intensity speech the opening phase is greatly compressed, as is the closing phase, while the time spent in the closed phase is greatly increased. *Source:* From Seikel/Drumright/King. *Anatomy & Physiology for Speech, Language, and Hearing, 5th Ed.* ©Cengage, Inc. Reproduced by permission. (Data from Fletcher, 1950.)

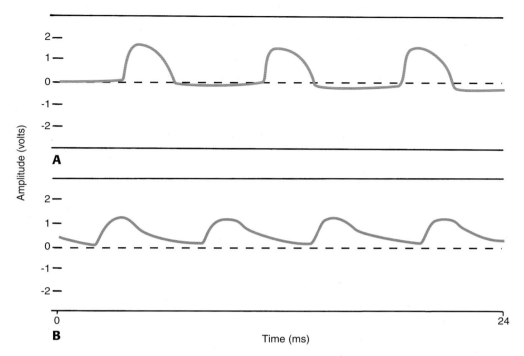

Figure 5–16. Effect of vocal intensity, as shown through electroglottographic trace. The electroglottograph measures impedance across the vocal folds, and the peak represents the closed phase of the glottal cycle. **A.** Conversational-level sustained vowel. **B.** High-level sustained vowel. *Source:* From Seikel/Drumright/King. *Anatomy & Physiology for Speech, Language, and Hearing, 5th Ed.* ©Cengage, Inc. Reproduced by permission.

that the vocal folds spend about 50% of their time in the opening phase, 37% of the time in the closing phase, and 13% of the cycle completely closed. When the vocal folds are tightly adducted for increased vocal intensity, they tend to return to the closed position more quickly and to stay closed for a longer period of time. The opening phase reduces to approximately 33%, while the closed phase increases to more than 30%, depending on the intensity increase.

Electroglottography

The electroglottograph (EGG) is a useful and nonintrusive instrument for the examination of vocal function. A pair of surface electrodes is placed on the thyroid lamina, typically held in place by an elastic band. An extremely small and imperceptible current is introduced through one electrode, and the impedance (resistance to current flow) is measured at the other electrode. When the vocal folds are approximated during phonation, there is less resistance to flow. The less contact the vocal folds make, the greater the impedance.

This nice arrangement permits researchers to examine at least some aspects of vocal fold function with ease. As you can see from the EGG trace of Figure 5–16, there are marked differences in the duration of vocal fold contact for quiet (A) versus loud (B) speech. For further reading, you may want to review Childers et al. (1990).

The concept you should retain is this: To increase vocal intensity, the vocal folds are tightly compressed, it takes more force to blow them open, they close more rapidly, and they tend to stay closed because they are tightly compressed. This is the *cause* side of the equation. The *effect* portion is that, because so much energy is required to hold the folds in compression, the release of the folds from this condition is markedly stronger. Each time the folds open, they do so with vigor, producing an explosive compression of the air medium. The harder that eruption of the vocal folds is, the greater is the amplitude of the cycle of vibration. Remembering that as the amplitude of the signal increases, so does the intensity, you should recognize the increase in intensity between the two panels of Figure 5–17.

The two waveforms in Figure 5–17 are different in intensity, but not in frequency. The time between the cycles is exactly the same, so the frequency must be the same. From this comes a very important point: Intensity and frequency are controlled independently, and you can increase intensity without increasing frequency. Here is the paradox. Increases in intensity and fundamental frequency depend on the same basic mechanism (tension/compression and subglottal pressure), so it is difficult to increase intensity without increasing pitch; but trained or well-controlled speakers can do this. The tendency is for frequency and intensity to increase together, which is a natural process that you can demonstrate to yourself. Find a place where

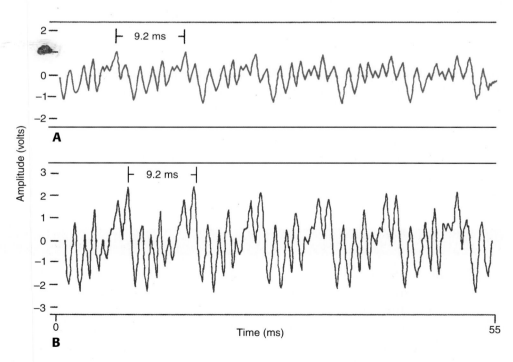

Figure 5–17. Oscillogram of sustained vowel at two vocal intensities. **A.** Sustained vowel at conversational level. **B.** Sustained vowel at increased vocal intensity. Although the vocal intensity increases, the period of each cycle of vibration remains constant at 9.2 milliseconds. *Source:* From Seikel/Drumright/King. *Anatomy & Physiology for Speech, Language, and Hearing, 5th Ed.* ©Cengage, Inc. Reproduced by permission.

you can shout, and then say a word before shouting it. Your pitch will most certainly go up when you shout, unless you try very hard to avoid it.

The relationship between subglottal pressure and the actual sound pressure level output of the vocal folds depends on the speaker. However, it appears that for a 1 cm H_2O increase in subglottal pressure there is a 5 dB increase in vocal intensity, so that for each doubling of subglottal pressure, there is an increase of about 10 decibels in vocal intensity (Björklund & Sundberg, 2016). Plant and Younger (2000) found that this relationship breaks down for some individuals, with marked changes in intensity without corresponding subglottal pressure changes, dependent on the fundamental frequency. It would appear that we, as humans, are capable of solving physical problems in multiple ways. Don't despair for lack of simple answers to complex questions: This complexity represents what many refer to as the "degree of freedom" problem. Given multiple degrees of flexibility in a system (in this case, the ability to simultaneously manipulate subglottal pressure, muscular tension, and adductory force), the problem of intensity control can be solved through various combinations of the tools at hand.

☑ To summarize:

- **Vocal intensity** refers to the increase in sound pressure of the speech signal.
- To increase vocal intensity of phonation, a speaker must increase **medial compression** through the muscles of adduction.
- This increased adductory force requires greater **subglottal pressure** to produce phonation and forces the vocal folds to remain in the closed portion of the phonatory cycle for a longer period of time.
- The increased **laryngeal tension** required for increasing intensity can also increase the vocal fundamental frequency, although the trained voice is quite capable of controlling fundamental frequency and vocal intensity independently.

Clinical Considerations

The phonatory mechanism is extraordinarily sensitive to the physical well-being of a speaker. When individuals are ill, their voices often get weak and, in the case of upper respiratory problems, "rough." Diseases that weaken individuals also tend to compromise phonatory effort, so that the voice weakens in intensity, and pitch range is reduced. Increasing muscle tension for pitch and intensity variation requires work, and illness tends to reduce the ability to exert such forces. A number of neuromuscular diseases have been shown to affect phonation, and many methods of measuring phonatory stability and ability have gained clinical acceptance.

Frequency perturbation is a measure of cycle-by-cycle variability in phonation. Perturbation, or **vocal jitter**, provides an exquisite index of muscle tone and stability but requires instrumentation for measurement. The

vocal jitter: cycle-by-cycle variation in fundamental frequency of vibration

client is asked to sustain a vowel as steadily as possible while it is recorded. Following this, a computer program measures each cycle of vibration and calculates how closely each cycle corresponds to the next in duration. The program measures the duration of the first cycle (e.g., 10.2 ms), subtracts it from that of the next cycle (e.g., 10.4 ms), and stores that number. It performs this for all succeeding cycles of vibration and calculates the average of the differences, treating all amplitudes as positive. It then compares this average with the average period of vibration. The resulting percent of perturbation (or percent jitter) is an indication of how perfectly this imperfect system is oscillating. The broad rule of thumb is that variation in excess of 1% to 2% will be perceived as hoarse. This is a good measure of client change over time and a less effective means of comparison among clients.

This measure has been shown to be sensitive to a number of characteristics. Individuals who are more physically fit have lower perturbation values than those who are not. Individuals with **neuromotor dysfunction** (neurological conditions that affect motor function) have higher perturbation than healthy individuals. Finally, increased mass on the vocal folds (such as vocal nodules and laryngeal polyps) increases perturbation (Jiang, Zhang, MacCallum, Sprecher, & Zhou, 2009), while therapy to reduce the mass results in a decrease in the jitter.

More prosaic measures do not require this degree of instrumentation, but nonetheless provide insight into the phonatory function. The process of assessment often requires us to stress the system under examination so that its weakness can be seen with relation to normal abilities. Kent et al. (1987) provided an excellent overview of methods of stressing the phonatory system.) As mentioned earlier, **maximum phonation time** refers to the duration an individual is capable of sustaining a phonation. Sustained phonation provides an index of phonatory-plus-respiratory efficiency. You can examine the respiratory system by itself, to determine the ability of your client to sustain expiration in the absence of voicing, and you can have some confidence that length and steadiness of a sustained vowel are an indicator of laryngeal function (Kurtz & Cielo, 2010).

Another time-honored measure is the diadochokinetic rate. **Oral diadochokinesis** refers to the alternation of articulators (you may hear it referred to as *alternating motor rate* as well). Specifically, it is the number of productions of a single or multiple syllables an individual produces per second. This is an excellent tool for assessing the articulators (the topic of Chapters 6 and 7), but also helps the assessment of the coordination of phonatory and articulatory systems.

As mentioned earlier, pathological conditions often have an impact on vocal range and vocal intensity. For instance, the presence of vocal nodules may reduce an individual's vocal range from two octaves to one-half octave or less, and the breathy component will have a real impact on vocal intensity. Similarly, physical weakness may limit a client's ability to exert effort for either pitch or vocal intensity change.

The exquisitely sensitive vocal mechanism is an excellent window to the health and well-being of a client, as you will find in your advanced studies of voice.

Linguistic Aspects of Pitch and Intensity

Pitch and intensity play significant roles in the suprasegmental aspects of communication. **Suprasegmental** elements are the parameters of speech that are above the segment (phonetic) level. This term generally refers to elements of **prosody**, the system of stress used to vary meaning in speech. The prosodic elements include pitch, intonation, loudness, stress, duration, and rhythm; these elements not only convey a great deal of information concerning emotion and intent but also provide information that can disambiguate meaning. Even though it is not the purpose of an anatomy text to delve into these suprasegmental elements, pitch and intensity play such a heavy role that we should at least glance at them.

Intonation refers to the changes in pitch during speech, whereas **stress** refers to syllable or word emphasis relative to an entire utterance. For example, say the following sentence out loud: "That's a cat." You end it with a falling *intonation* and put more *stress* on "that's" than on "a" or "cat." To a large extent, both these elements arise out of variation in vocal intensity and fundamental frequency. Intonation may be considered the melodic envelope that contains the sentence and may serve to mark the sentence type. Generally, statements tend to have falling intonation at the end; questions tend to have rising intonation. Figure 5–18 shows traces of the fundamental frequency for the productions of "Bev bombed Bob." and "Bev bombed Bob?" If you say these two sentences, you can hear for yourself the changes that are so strong in the second sentence. Hirano et al. (1969) used this sentence contrast to show that the lateral cricoarytenoid, thyrovocalis, and cricothyroid are all quite active in making these rapid laryngeal adjustments.

Stress helps punctuate speech, providing emphasis to syllables or words through both intensity and frequency changes. To increase stress, we increase the fundamental frequency and intensity by increasing subglottal pressure, medial compression, and laryngeal tension. Remember from our earlier discussion in this chapter that changes in both frequency and intensity

suprasegmental: parameters of speech that include prosody, pitch, and loudness changes for meaning

prosody: the system of stress used to vary the meaning in speech

intonation: the melody of speech, provided by variation of the fundamental frequency during speech

stress: the product of relative increase in fundamental frequency, vocal intensity, and duration

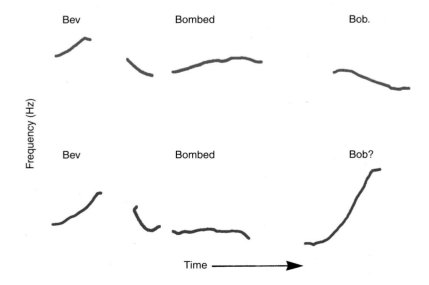

Figure 5–18. Fundamental frequency fluctuation for declarative statement and question form. Note the difference in falling and rising intonation between these two sentence forms. *Source:* From Seikel/Drumright/King. *Anatomy & Physiology for Speech, Language, and Hearing, 5th Ed.* ©Cengage, Inc. Reproduced by permission.

Prosody and Neuromuscular Disorder

The prosodic element of speech can be a window to speech physiology in neuropathology. *Prosody* is the combination of changes in fundamental frequency, vocal intensity, and duration that produce linguistically relevant intonation and stress characteristics. When the neuromuscular system is compromised, prosody may be affected. When muscle tone increases (hypertonus) due to spasticity, the individual may demonstrate prosody characterized by even and equal stress with inappropriately high vocal intensity on each syllable or word, in combination with a harsh phonatory quality.

When an individual has ataxic signs from cerebellar damage, that person will have disrupted prosody from the discoordination of respiratory, phonatory, and articulatory systems. Speech syllable timing will be defective, and the control of phonatory elements will be seriously deficient.

In many of the hyperkinetic dysarthrias, the element of speech control is overridden by movements of speech structures that are involuntary and uncontrollable. In these cases, prosody will be seriously affected.

involve adjustments of these variables. We capitalize on the fact that both intensity and fundamental frequency vary together, so stressed syllables or words will show changes in both. If you look at the frequency and intensity traces of Figure 5–19, you can see how they vary together.

The musculature involved in stress is not unlike that of intonation, although we must factor in the increase in subglottal pressure. The changes in fundamental frequency are to the order of 50 Hz (Netsell & Hixon, 1978), governed by the lateral cricoarytenoid, the thyrovocalis, and the cricothyroid. The changes in subglottal pressure are small but rapid, or pulsatile (Hixon, 1973). Because changes in fundamental frequency and subglottal pressure require bursts of increased expiratory force, they will be driven by expiratory muscles.

Although stress and intonation are not *essential* for communication, they *are* essential for naturalness. Clearly you can speak in a **monopitch** (unvarying vocal pitch) or **monoloud** voice (unvarying vocal loudness), but the effect is so distracting that it certainly interferes with communication. You may find individuals with neurological impairments who show both of

Figure 5–19. Fundamental frequency and intensity changes during production of a question form. *Source:* From Seikel/Drumright/ King. *Anatomy & Physiology for Speech, Language, and Hearing, 5th Ed.* ©Cengage, Inc. Reproduced by permission.

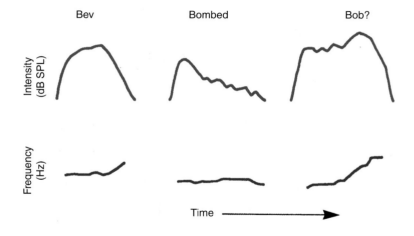

Laryngeal Stridor

Laryngeal stridor refers to a harsh sound produced during respiration. The sound is associated with some obstruction in the respiratory passageway and is always a sign of dysfunction. Stridor may arise from a growth in the larynx or trachea causing turbulence during respiration, or it may arise from the vocal folds. If the vocal folds are paralyzed in the adducted position (**abductor paralysis**), they will not only obstruct the airway but will also vibrate as the air of inspiration passes by them. In this case, the harsh sound is referred to as **inhalatory stridor**. You may want to imitate this sound in yourself so that you will come to recognize this sign of obstruction. Phonate while breathing out, and then, without abducting your vocal folds, force your inspiration through the closed vocal folds. You should notice not only a harsh sound but also the extreme difficulty of inhaling through an obstruction.

these characteristics. Treatment directed toward increasing muscular effort at points requiring stress will greatly enhance the naturalness of speech, because increasing vocal effort at these points will inevitably increase both fundamental frequency and vocal intensity (Connaghan & Patel, 2017).

Theories of Phonation

The history of theories of vocal fold vibration is long and colorful, leading certainly from Helmholtz of the 1800s to the present. Although it has long been known that the vocal folds are the source of voicing, only recently did we develop an understanding of the mechanism of phonation, and refinements continue. Certainly, the underlying principles discussed in this chapter are broadly accepted, although it has not always been so.

An early battle arose within the field of speech science when some researchers questioned whether the vocal folds vibrated as a result of direct stimulation of the intrinsic laryngeal muscles (active muscle contraction). The theory that proposed this view (the neurochronaxic theory of vocal fold vibration) was abandoned when it was understood that the neuromuscular system was not capable of producing a fundamental frequency greater than about 200 Hz through this means (Herbst et al., 2012). It became clear that some version of the myoelastic-aerodynamic theory would explain vocal fold dynamics. As discussed earlier in this chapter, the myoelastic-aerodynamic theory of phonation states that vibration of the vocal folds depends on the elements embodied in the name of the theory. The myoelastic element is the elastic component of muscle (*myo* = muscle) and the associated soft tissues of the larynx, and the aerodynamic component is that of the airflow and pressure through this constricted tube. Van den Berg (1958) recognized that the combination of tissue elasticity, which causes the vocal folds to return to their original position after being distended, and the Bernoulli effect, which helps promote this return by dropping the pressure at the constriction, could account for the sustained vibration shown in even a cadaverous specimen provided with an artificial source of expiratory charge.

Work by Hirano and Kakita (1985) and expanded by Titze (1994) has sought to explain how complex acoustic output can come from a simple oscillator such as the vocal folds. We have long recognized that the vocal folds are not simple oscillators, but rather undulate in the modes discussed earlier. Titze recognized that this complex vibration arises from the loosely bound masses associated with the membranous **cover** of the vocal folds (the epithelium and superficial layer of the lamina propria) and the **body** of the vocal folds (the intermediate and deep layers of lamina propria and thyro-vocalis muscle). The loosely bound elastic tissue supports oscillation, and viewing the soft tissue as an infinite (or at least uncountable) number of masses reveals that a very large number of modes of vibration are possible. This discussion in no way does justice to the elegance of this theory, and we recommend that you take time for the exceptionally readable work of Titze (1973, 1988, 1994).

The phonatory mechanism is an important component of the speaking mechanism, providing the voiced source for speech. It is time for us to see what happens to the voice source after it leaves the larynx. See Chapter 6 for a continuation of this story.

Pathologies That May Affect Phonation

Pathologies affecting phonation are broadly those that affect the larynx and its related structures. Phonation is extremely sensitive to pathology, such that a small mass difference between vocal folds, for instance, can cause a marked phonatory effect. The vocal mechanism is sensitive to muscular weakness, vascular disturbance, neurological problems, tumors, and even emotional stress. Because phonation provides the voicing source for speech, anything that affects phonatory function is likely to affect speech. Furthermore, the larynx is intrinsically involved in swallowing, a topic we'll cover in Chapter 8. In the sections that follow, we describe a small sample of pathologies that can affect phonation.

Before moving forward, however, let's define a few terms:

- Aphonia: complete loss of voice
- Diplophonia: perception of two pitches in voicing
- Dysphonia: reduction in any vocal function, including appropriate vibration, pitch change, or intensity change
- Edema: swelling
- Frequency of vibration: number of vibrations per second of a vibrating body (hertz, Hz)
- Glottis: the space between the vocal folds
- Intensity: the level of sound, measured in decibels (dB)
- Larynx: the cartilaginous structure at the superior end of the trachea designed for protection of the airway from foreign objects

- Loudness: the psychological correlate of intensity
- Metastasis: spreading of cancerous cells
- Metastasize: verb implying spread of cancerous cells
- Paralysis: complete loss of function due to neurological lesion
- Paresis: partial loss of muscle function due to neurological lesion
- Phonation: voicing for speech arising from vibration of the vocal folds
- Pitch: the psychological correlate of frequency
- Subglottal: the region below the vocal folds
- Supraglottal: the region above the vocal folds

In the following section, we'll talk about two major classes of etiologies of voice disorder: structural and neurological. Structural etiologies include those conditions that alter the physical structure of the vocal mechanism. Neurological lesions reflect damage to the nervous system arising from disease or trauma that cause vocal folds or laryngeal mechanisms to no longer perform protective phonatory function properly.

Structural Etiologies

Laryngeal Trauma

Laryngeal trauma can arise from a number of causes, most related to motor vehicle accidents (MVA). Laryngeal trauma from MVA is seen in 12 of 3000 emergency room visits within the population. Sports is a close second etiology to MVA, followed by gunshot wounds. Eighty-five percent of these injuries are of the blunt force variety, but obviously gunshot wounds are penetrating.

Trauma from MVAs includes those involving snowmobiles, jet skis, and other recreational vehicles. Often, neck extension on impact causes blunt injury from the steering wheel, but the larynx can also be injured by contact with the dashboard. Seat belts and airbags have decreased laryngeal injuries markedly.

Children are not immune to laryngeal injuries from trauma, although they are not as common in children because the larynx is higher in the pharynx than in adults. For children, laryngeal trauma can arise from bicycle accidents, other play accidents (e.g., bumping into furniture in play), clothesline injury (e.g., blunt contact with an object such as a clothesline, rope suspended between posts, fence wire). Laryngeal trauma is also seen as a result of physical child abuse.

Common childhood injuries arise from contact sports. Again, children have fewer injuries than adults because of the laryngeal location in the pharynx. Soccer (including football) and rugby cause most injuries through player and ball contact. Ice hockey, martial arts, gymnastics, and cheerleading are also listed as etiologies for trauma. Baseball players can have blunt impact from a baseball, resulting in laryngeal collapse.

Signs and symptoms of laryngeal trauma are dysphonia (phonatory dysfunction), stridor (harsh voice), and respiratory distress (remembering that the larynx is a significant component of the respiratory system). There may be dysphagia (swallowing disorder), as well as odynophagia (pain during swallowing). There will be neck pain and a change in voicing. Treatment always involves first ensuring an open airway, perhaps through emergency tracheotomy. Reconstruction of the laryngeal anatomy may be required.

Gastroesophageal reflux disease (GERD), also known as acid reflux, involves refluxing of gastric contents into the pharynx. The trauma arising from GERD involves tissue change of the esophagus, pharynx, vocal mechanism, arising from recurring contact with the acidic contents of the stomach. Reflux causes laryngeal irritation, ulceration, and may lead to laryngeal cancer, so it's a serious condition. The signs and symptoms of GERD are heartburn, chest pain, an acid taste in the mouth, bad breath, vomiting, and damage to dental enamel. Phonation may be hoarse. There are several potential causes of GERD, including esophagitis (inflammation of the esophagus), esophageal stricture, or relaxed upper esophageal sphincter.

Neoplasm

Neoplasms (literally "new tissue") are either benign or cancerous (metastatic) growths. There are several benign growths that affect the larynx and vocal folds. We'll talk about nodules, contact ulcers (granulomas), hemangiomas, hyperkeratosis, papilloma, and polyps.

Vocal nodules and polyps are tissue aggregates arising from vocal abuse, including yelling, throat clearing, loud speech, or other activities that cause hard contact between the vocal folds. Vocal nodules are a thickening of the vocal folds at the contact site, usually on the anterior two thirds of vocal folds. They typically results from excessive force during phonation, and can be either unilateral or bilateral. Signs and symptoms of vocal nodules include hoarseness, breathiness, and harsh phonation. The individual may also experience pain in the throat region, loss of the ability to alter the vocal fundamental frequency, and very often reduced phrase length in speech due to phonatory inefficiency.

Contact ulcers are also known as granulomas, consisting of granulated tissue sacs that arise from vocal abuse, GERD, or as a tissue response to surgery. Just like vocal nodules, contact ulcers can be created by excessive force coupled with a hard glottal attack. They are typically found in the posterior vocal folds as the arytenoids. They are also associated with GERD. Contact ulcers produce severe dysphonia, including breathiness, hoarseness, and the continual feeling that the throat needs to be cleared. They need to be surgically removed, but the individual also needs voice therapy to keep them from returning.

Hemangiomas are similar to granulomas but are vascularized. They are soft, pliable, blood-filled sacs, found typically on the posterior vocal folds. They also arise from vocal hyperfunction (abuse), GERD, or intubation during surgery. They must be surgically removed, and then the patient needs to have a vocal hygiene program to keep them from re-developing

Hyperkeratosis is a nonmalignant growth that may be a precursor of malignant tissue change. Hyperkeratosis is a reactive lesions from tissue irritation, occurring typically under the tongue, and on the anterior and posterior vocal folds. These growths typically arise from either tobacco smoking or from being in an environment of smoke. They may have mild or severe voice effects, including hoarseness and dysphonia.

Laryngeal webbing can occur either as a congenital condition, or can be acquired through physical trauma. When it is from a congenital etiology, laryngeal webbing is detected at birth because of the respiratory distress it causes. The infant will have stridor, shortness of breath, and a high-pitched cry. The webbing must be immediately surgically removed. Acquired webs often come from bilateral trauma of the vocal folds, often from intubation during surgery. Any irritant of mucosal surface can cause webbing, which is a tissue response in itself. The healing vocal folds grow together, forming the laryngeal web on the inner margins. The webs must be surgically separated and kept apart during the healing process.

Papillomas are wart-like growths that are viral in origin. They often occur in children, and because they can grow quite rapidly they pose a threat to the airway of the child. The result of papillomas is hoarseness and shortness of breath. They are removed surgically, but typically do not recur after puberty.

Polyps are masses that appear to arise from vocal hyperfunction (vocal abuse), and can be either pedunculated (on a stalk) or sessile (attached directly to the vocal folds), typically on the inner margin of the anterior two thirds of the folds. Polyps are soft, fluid-filled sacs that often form from a single irritating event. The voice is hoarse, breathy, and often diplophonic due to the added mass to one vocal fold.

Leukoplakia are whitish patches on the surface membranes of the larynx that typically extend beneath the surface. These are precursors to cancer, similar to hyperkeratosis. They often lead to squamous cell carcinoma. The phonatory result of leukoplakia may be lowering of the vocal fundamental frequency and hoarseness. Leukoplakia may cause diplophonia if only one vocal fold is involved.

Laryngeal cancer (carcinoma) is a life-threatening growth, typically caused by tobacco smoking. It makes up 2 to 5% of malignancies annually in the United States. Tumor locations are classified as glottal, supraglottal, or subglottal. Glottal cancers involve only the vocal folds, while supraglottal cancers involve the area above the vocal folds, including the aryepiglottic folds, epiglottis, and walls of the hypopharynx (laryngopharynx). Subglottal cancers involve the cricoid cartilage and trachea. Treatment for cancer often includes partial or radical laryngectomy, which is removal of part or all of the larynx. Radiation therapy and chemotherapy may be employed either separately or in conjunction with laryngectomy. The signs and symptoms of laryngeal cancer include persistent hoarseness without other cause, pain to the ear, neck swelling, inspiratory stridor, and difficulty breathing. The patient often has unremitting and nonproductive cough, fullness in the laryngeal area, sometimes breathiness, and unexpected weight loss.

The most common type of laryngeal cancer is squamous cell carcinoma. The connective tissue covering of the vocal folds and oral cavity is made up of squamous cells, and the carcinoma begins as a thickening of this lining. Treatment is surgical removal of the cancer and surrounding tissue to reduce the risk of metastasis (spreading) of the cancer. Irradiation (radiation therapy) is used to kill any remaining cells.

Speech is obviously affected if the person undergoes a laryngectomy. The individual may learn esophageal speech (introduction of air into the pharynx from the esophagus), or use of an external electrolarynx. Removal of the larynx necessitates closing off the trachea from the pharynx, and a stoma (literally "mouth") is surgically opened in the anterior trachea to permit breathing. The stoma must be protected from foreign bodies, water, and other intrusive elements (including pet hair). Tracheoesophageal puncture (TEP) may be employed, in which a one-way valve is placed between the trachea and the esophagus. The TEP allows the individual to occlude the stoma during exhalation, forcing air into the esophagus as a means of causing the esophageal sphincter to vibrate and thus providing a phonatory source for speech.

There are typically significant iatrogenic results of surgical procedures. Radiation therapy causes tissue to swell, muscle to weaken, and mucous glands to stop functioning. Sensation is reduced, and if the vocal folds are not surgically affected one can still have dysphonia due to poor muscle contraction, loss of lubrication, and edema.

Degenerative Neurological Diseases

We'll be talking about neurogenic etiologies in Chapter 12, but realize that most degenerative neurological diseases result in speech problems, with many of them affecting phonation. As an example, Parkinson's disease results in reduced vocal intensity and reduced adductory force. Amyotrophic lateral sclerosis (ALS), caused by a degeneration of upper and lower motor neurons, results in a flaccid-spastic dysarthria. Phonation in ALS is characterized as low in vocal intensity, monopitch, and strain-strangle phonation. Multiple sclerosis arises from degeneration of the myelin sheath of axons, and the effect on phonation varies. The phonation can have spastic harshness, as well as irregularities arising from degeneration of the cerebellar pathways. Cerebrovascular accident (CVA) can cause phonatory deficits, with manifestations depending on the site of lesion.

Vocal fold paralysis arises from lower motor neuron lesion to the recurrent laryngeal nerve of X vagus. It can be either unilateral or bilateral, and can occur as a result of physical insult (e.g., trauma from MVA), CVA, trauma during surgery, or as an idiopathic disorder (i.e., no known cause). The signs of vocal fold paralysis are breathiness, hoarseness, low vocal intensity, and ineffective coughing.

Chapter Summary

Frequency of vibration of sound is measured in cycles per second, abbreviated Hz. The intensity of sound is measured in decibels, which represent a ratio of pressures or powers, expressed logarithmically. Instrumentation for phonation includes the sound level meter for intensity, various instruments for measurement of fundamental frequency, as well as vocal jitter and vocal shimmer. The phonetogram shows the interaction of intensity and frequency in an individual's speech. The electroglottograph is a useful tool for estimating vocal fold contact during phonation, while the nasoendoscope and videostroboscope allow viewing the vocal folds during phonation.

Phonation is the product of vibrating vocal folds within the larynx. The vocal folds vibrate as air flows past them, capitalizing on the Bernoulli phenomenon and tissue elasticity to maintain phonation. The interaction of subglottal pressure, tissue elasticity, and constriction within the airflow caused by the vocal folds produces sustained phonation as long as pressure, flow, and vocal fold approximation are maintained.

The larynx is an important structure for a number of nonspeech functions as well, including coughing, throat clearing, and abdominal fixation. The degree of muscle control during phonation is greatly increased, however, because the successful use of voice requires careful attention to vocal fold tension and length.

Adduction takes several forms, including breathy, simultaneous, and hard attacks, and termination of phonation requires abduction of the vocal folds. The attacks are reflected in consistent vocal attack times that are stable during midlife but vary between males and females. Sustained phonation depends on the laryngeal configuration. The modal pattern of phonation is most efficient, capitalizing on the optimal combination of muscular tension and respiratory support for the vocal folds.

The falsetto requires increased vocal fold tension, and glottal fry demands a unique glottal and respiratory configuration. Each of these modes of vocal fold vibration is different, and the variations are governed by laryngeal tension, medial compression, and subglottal pressure. Breathy phonation occurs when there is inadequate medial compression to approximate the vocal folds, and whispering results from tensing the vocal fold margins while holding the folds partially adducted.

Pitch is the psychological correlate of the frequency of vibration, and loudness is the correlate of intensity, although both the terms *pitch* and *intensity* have been used to represent physical phenomena. Optimal pitch is the most efficient frequency of vibration for a given pair of vocal folds, and habitual pitch is the frequency of vibration used habitually by an individual. The pitch range of an individual spans approximately 2 octaves but can be reduced by pathology or increased through vocal training.

Vocal fundamental frequency changes are governed by vocal fold tension and mass per unit length. To increase the fundamental frequency, we increase the length of the vocal folds, which increases the tension of the vocal folds and decreases the mass per unit length. To compensate for increased tension, subglottal pressure increases.

Medial compression is increased to produce an increase in vocal intensity of phonation, and this is performed largely through the muscles of adduction. Increased adductory force requires greater subglottal pressure to produce phonation, and that forces the vocal folds to remain in the closed portion of the phonatory cycle for a longer time. The increased laryngeal tension increases the vocal fundamental frequency as well, although the fundamental frequency and vocal intensity may be controlled independently.

Decibel Practice Activity

The Decibel Practice Activity was produced through a grant funded by the Fund for Improvement of Postsecondary Education (FIPSE), No. P116B90965–90. Seikel, J. A. (1990–1992). Project to Enhance Graduate and Undergraduate Education in Speech and Hearing Sciences. Department of Education: Fund for the Improvement of Postsecondary Education (FIPSE; $93,234).

The decibel practice activity involves practice working with exponents, logarithms, and finally figuring the decibel.

I. EXPONENTS AND LOGARITHMS

If you are comfortable with exponents and logarithms, go directly to the next page and do the problems marked "FIGURING EXPONENTS AND LOGARITHMS." Otherwise, continue reading.

An exponent is the power to which a number is raised. For instance, 2 is the exponent in 4^2 (4 squared, which is 4×4, which = 16)

What are the exponents and answers below?

	Exponent	Answer		Exponent	Answer
$4^2 =$	_____	_____	$10^3 =$	_____	_____
$2^3 =$	_____	_____	$10^2 =$	_____	_____
$3^3 =$	_____	_____	$10^5 =$	_____	_____
$4^6 =$	_____	_____	$10^1 =$	_____	_____

The exponent tells the number of times you will multiply an item times itself:

$3^2 = 3 \times 3 = 9$

$4^2 = 4 \times 4 = 16$

$3^3 = 3 \times 3 \times 3 = 27$

$5^3 = 5 \times 5 \times 5 = 125$

Logarithms (LOGS) are exponents (in our work we will only talk about logarithms to the base 10, so relax. A logarithm will be presented as log10, which means to take the base 10 logarithm of a number).

I know that $10^3 = 10 \times 10 \times 10 = 1000$

So, the $\log_{10}$ of 1000 = 3: That is, the "exponent for 10" to give me 1000 is 3. Or I could say, the "power to which I must raise 10 to get 1000 is 3."

Figure the logarithms$_{10}$ ($\log_{10}$) for the following:

$\log_{10} (1000) =$ _____ $\log_{10} (10,000) =$ _____

$\log_{10} (100) =$ _____ $\log_{10} (100,000) =$ _____

$\log_{10} (100,000) =$ _____ $\log_{10} (1,000,000) =$ _____

So, by now you should see that if the exponent is a whole number, the $\log_{10}$ will be the number of zeros after the 1.

Figure a few more:

$\log_{10}(10{,}000{,}000) = $ _____

$\log_{10}(100{,}000{,}000) = $ _____

$\log_{10}(10) = $ _____

If you have a logarithm key on your calculator, you are all set. If not, you may count zeros.

FIGURING EXPONENTS AND LOGARITHMS

What are the exponents in the following?

$2^2 = $ _____ $\qquad$ $9^4 = $ _____

$3^4 = $ _____ $\qquad$ $6^3 = $ _____

$6^{10} = $ _____ $\qquad$ $10^1 = $ _____

$7^5 = $ _____ $\qquad$ $41^2 = $ _____

$8^1 = $ _____ $\qquad$ $15^6 = $ _____

Determine the logarithms ($\log_{10}$) in the following statements:

$\log_{10}(1000) = $ _____ $\qquad$ $\log_{10}(10) = $ _____

$\log_{10}(100) = $ _____ $\qquad$ $\log_{10}(1{,}000{,}000) = $ _____

$\log_{10}(100{,}000) = $ _____ $\qquad$ $\log_{10}(10{,}000) = $ _____

II. dB SPL PROBLEMS

A. Figure dB SPL in the following examples. If you have a calculator that will figure logarithms, this could be fun. If you do not have a calculator, do those that are marked "no calculator."

Note: If your calculator calculates only natural logarithms (ln), then simply multiply the result times .4343: that is, log10 = ln × .4343

Example for figuring dB SPL

dB SPL = 20 log10 (Pressure$_{out}$/Pressure$_{ref}$)

Given a pressure output = 2,000,000 micropascals

dB SPL = 20 log10 (2,000,000 micropascals / 20 micropascals)

$\qquad$ = 20 log10 (100,000)

$\qquad\qquad$ (*Note:* Count zeros to get log10)

$\qquad$ = 20(5)

$\qquad$ = 100 dB SPL

1. No calculator: Given pressure output = 200 micropascals. Figure dB SPL. (Answer: 20 dB SPL)

2. No Calculator: Given pressure output = 2,000 micropascals. Figure dB SPL. (Answer: 40 dB SPL)

3. No Calculator: Given pressure output = 20,000 micropascals. Figure dB SPL. (Answer: 60 dB SPL)

4. No Calculator: Given pressure output = 200,000,000 micropascals. Figure dB SPL. (Answer: 140 dB SPL)

III. SPL: MORE COMPLEX EXAMPLES

Given 12,000,000 micropascals as output. Figure dB SPL.

x dB SPL = 20 log10 ($PRESSURE_{out}/PRESSURE_{ref}$)

= 20 log10 (12,000,000 micropascals / 20 micropascals)

= 20 log10 (600,000)

= 20 × 5.778

= 115.56 db SPL

1. Calculator: Figure dB SPL with $Pressure_{out}$ = 346,000 micropascals (Answer = 84.7 dB SPL)

2. No Calculator: Figure dB SPL with $Pressure_{out}$ = 200,000 micropascals (Answer = 80 dB SPL)

3. Calculator: Figure dB SPL with $Pressure_{out}$ = 25,000 micropascals (Answer = 61.9 dB SPL)

4. No Calculator: Figure dB SPL with $Pressure_{out}$ = 20,000 micropascals (Answer = 60 dB SPL)

5. Calculator: Figure dB SPL with $Pressure_{out}$ = 486,000 micropascals (Answer = 87.71 dB SPL)

6. No Calculator: Figure dB SPL with $Pressure_{out}$ = 2,000,000 micropascals (Answer = 100 dB SPL)

7. Calculator: output = 17,022 micropascals. Figure dB SPL. (Answer = 58.59 dB SPL)

8. No Calculator: output = 2,000 micropascals. Figure dB SPL. (Answer = 40 dB SPL)

IV. dB INCREASE AND DECREASE (a really useful thing to learn! e.g., reading from an oscilloscope trace)

A. Example: You measure a sine wave = 3 volts, zero-to-peak.

B. After raising the volume control (or lowering attenuation), you measure the output voltage to be 96 V.

C. What is the change in dB?

x dB = 20 log10 ($volts_{output}/volts_{reference}$) = 20 log10(96 volts/3 volts)

= 20 log10 (32 volts)

= 20 (1.505)

= 30.1 dB re: 3 volt reference (or dB increase)

So if your original signal was 10 dB SPL, this new output signal is 40 dB SPL (assuming a perfect world).

1. Given an initial reading of 11.3 V (your reference), you raise the sound output and get a reading of 431 V. What is dB change?
(Answer: 31.62 dB re: 11.3 V)

2. Given an initial reading of 640 V, you turn the loudness control down and get an output of 21 V. How many dB did you drop?
(Answer: –29.68 dB re: 640 V) (note that "re:" means "with reference to," which is inserted so that you always know your referent. If we were calculating dB SPL we could insert re: 20 micropascals, but that is implied in the "SPL" notation)

3. You measure a sine wave from an audiometer. The dial says 20 dB (which you know is HL), and you read a voltage on your oscilloscope of 46 V at 20 dB. What is the voltage if you turn up the audiometer 6 dB? Hint: remember that voltage is the correlate of pressure. What happens to dB when you double pressure?).
(Answer: 92 V)

4. Given an initial voltage of 3 volts. You increase the volume control and now read 300 V. What is the dB difference?
(Answer: 40 dB re: 3 V)

5. You turn on the radio and measure .006 volts. After cranking it up until it parts your hair, you measure output as 600 volts. How many dB have you increased the signal?
(Answer: 100 dB re: .006 V)

6. Your upstairs neighbor has his stereo set to a mind-boggling level. After verbally assaulting him, you slap an oscilloscope on the speaker leads and get a reading of 43 volts. After he turns it down, under protest, it reads .00043 volts. How many dB did you drop the intensity? (Hint: 43 volts is your reference.)
(Answer: –100 dB re: 43 V)

FINISHED!

Baken, R. J., & Orlikoff, R. F. (1999). *Clinical measurement of speech and voice* (2nd ed.). San Diego, CA: Singular Publishing Group.

Behrman, A. (2007). *Speech and voice science*. San Diego, CA: Plural Publishing.

Bierens, J. J., Lunetta, P., Tipton, M., & Warner, D. S. (2016). Physiology of drowning: A review. *Physiology, 31*(2), 147–166.

Björklund, S., & Sundberg, J. (2016). Relationship between subglottal pressure and sound pressure level in untrained voices. *Journal of Voice, 30*(1), 15–20.

Bless, D. M., & Abbs, J. H. (1995). *Vocal fold physiology* (2nd ed.). San Diego, CA: Singular Publishing Group.

Boone, D. R., McFarlane, S. C., Von Berg, S. L., & Zraick, R. I. (2009). *The voice and voice therapy* (8th ed.). Upper Saddle River, NJ: Pearson.

Chhetri, D. K., Neurbauer, J., & Berry, D. A. (2012). Neuromuscular control of fundamental frequency at phonation onset. *Journal of the Acoustical Society of America, 131*(2), 1401–1412.

Childers, D. G., Hicks, D. M., Moore, G. P., Eskenazi, L., & Lalwani, A. L. (1990). Electroglottography and vocal fold physiology. *Journal of Speech and Hearing Research, 33*, 245–254.

Connaghan, K. P., & Patel, R. (2017). The impact of contrastive stress on vowel acoustics and intelligibility in dysarthria. *Journal of Speech, Language, and Hearing Research, 60*(1), 38–50.

D'haeseleer, E., Claeys, S., Meerschman, I., Bettens, K., Degeest, S., Dijckmans, C., . . . Van Lierde, K. (2017). Vocal characteristics and laryngoscopic findings in future musical theater performers. *Journal of Voice, 31*(4), 462–469.

D'haeseleer, E., Claeys, S., Meerschman, I., & Van Lierde, K. (2016, January). *The impact of a theater performance on the vocal quality of actors*. Presentation at the 45th Annual Symposium of the Voice Foundation, Philadelphia, PA.

Dias, M. D. R., & Santos, I. S. (2016). Laryngopharyngeal reflux and vocal quality in senior population: "Mr./Ms. Gluttony." *International Journal of Development Research, 6*, 10048–10053.

Fink, B. R., & Demarest, R. J. (1978). *Laryngeal biomechanics*. Cambridge, MA: Harvard University Press.

Fletcher, W. W. (1950). *A study of internal laryngeal activity in relation to vocal intensity* (Doctoral dissertation). Northwestern University, Evanston, IL.

Herbst, C. T., Stoeger, A. S., Frey, R., Lohscheller, J., Titze, I. R., Gumpenberger, M., & Fitch, W. T. (2012). How low can you go? Physical production mechanisms of elephant infrasonic vocalization. *Science, 337*, 595–598.

Hirano, M. (1974). Morphological structure of the vocal cord as a vibrator and its variations. *Folia Phoniatrica, 26*, 89–94.

Hirano, M., & Kakika, Y. (1985). Cover-body theory of vocal fold vibration. In R. Daniloff (Ed.), *Speech science* (pp. 1–46). San Diego, CA: Singular Publishing Group.

Hirano, M., Kiyokawa, K., & Kurita, S. (1988). Laryngeal muscles and glottic shaping. In O. Fujimura (Ed.), *Vocal physiology: Voice production, mechanisms, and functions* (pp. 49–65). New York, NY: Raven Press.

Hirano, M., Ohala, J., & Vennard, W. (1969). The function of laryngeal muscles in regulation of fundamental frequency and intensity of phonation. *Journal of Speech and Hearing Research, 12*, 616–628.

Hixon, T. J. (1973). Respiratory function in speech. In F. D. Minifie, T. J. Hixon, & F. Williams (Eds.), *Normal aspects of speech, hearing, and language* (pp. 73–125). Englewood Cliffs, N.J., Prentice-Hall.

Hixon, T. J., Hawley, J. L., & Wilson, K. J. (1982). An around-the-house device for the clinical determination of respiratory driving pressure: A note on making simple even simpler. *Journal of Speech and Hearing Disorders, 47*, 413–415.

Jiang, J. J., Zhang, Y., MacCallum, J., Sprecher, A., & Zhou, L (2009). Objective analysis of pathological voices with vocal nodules and polyps. *Folia Phoniatrica et Logopedica, 61*, 342–349.

Kaplan, H. M. (1971). *Anatomy and physiology of speech*. New York, NY: McGraw-Hill.

Kazarian, A. G., Sarkissian, L. S., & Isaakian, D. G. (1978). Length of human vocal cords by age. (Article in Russian). *Zhurnal Eksperimentalnoi I Klinicheskoi Meditsiny, 18*, 105–109.

Kent, R. (1976). Anatomical and neuromuscular maturation of the speech mechanism: Evidence from acoustic studies. *Journal of Speech and Hearing Research, 19*, 421–447.

Kent, R. (1994). *Reference manual for communication sciences & disorders*. Austin, TX: Pro-Ed.

Kent, R. D., Kent, J. F., & Rosenbek, J. C. (1987). Maximum performance tests of speech production. *Journal of Speech and Hearing Disorders, 52*, 367–387.

Kurtz, L. O., & Cielo, C. A. (2010). Maximum phonation time of vowels in adult women with vocal nodules. *Pro Fono, 22*(4), 451–454.

Ludlow, C. L. (2015). Laryngeal reflexes: Physiology, technique and clinical use. *Journal of Clinical Neurophysiology, 32*(4), 284–293.

McHanwell, S. (2008). Larynx. In S. Standring (Ed.), *Gray's anatomy: The anatomical and clinical basis of practice* (40th ed., 577–594). London, UK: Churchill Livingstone.

Mulligan, J. F. (Ed.). (2018). *Heinrich Rudolf Hertz (1857–1894): A collection of articles and addresses*. London, UK: Routledge.

Netsell, R., & Hixon, T. J. (1978). A noninvasive method for clinically estimating subglottal air pressure. *Journal of Speech and Hearing Disorders, 43*, 326–330.

Nishizawa, N., Sawashima, M., & Yonemoto, K. (1988). Vocal fold length in vocal pitch change. In O. Fujimua (Ed.), *Vocal physiology: Voice production, mechanisms and functions* (pp. 49–65). New York, NY: Raven Press.

O'Connell, D. G., Brewer, J. F., Man, T. H., Weldon, J. S., & Hinman, M. R. (2016). The effects of forced exhalation and inhalation, grunting, and Valsalva maneuver on forehand force in collegiate tennis players. *Journal of Strength & Conditioning Research, 30*(2), 430–437.

Orlikoff, R. F., Deliyski, D. D., Baken, R. J., & Watson, B. C. (2009). Validation of a glottographic measure of vocal attack. *Journal of Voice, 23*(2), 164–168.

Pabon, J. P. H., & Plomp, R. (1988). Automatic phonetogram recording supplemented with acoustical voice-quality parameters. *Journal of Speech, Language, and Hearing Research, 31*(4), 710–722.

Patel, R. R., Awan, S. N., Barkmeier-Kraemer, J., Courey, M., Deliyski, D., Eadie, T., . . . Hillman, R. (2018). Recommended protocols for instrumental assessment of voice: American Speech-Language-Hearing Association expert panel to develop a protocol for instrumental assessment of vocal function. *American Journal of Speech-Language Pathology, 27*(3), 887–905.

Patel, R. R., Forrest, K., & Hedges, D. (2017). Relationship between acoustic voice onset and offset and selected instances of oscillatory onset and offset in young healthy men and women. *Journal of Voice, 31*(3), 389.e9–389e17.

Plant, R. L., & Younger, R. M. (2000). The interrelationship of subglottal pressure, fundamental frequency, and vocal intensity during speech. *Journal of Voice, 14*(2), 170–177.

Ptacek, P. H., & Sander, E. K. (1963). Maximum duration of phonation. *Journal of Speech and Hearing Disorders, 28*(2), 171–182.

Rastatter, M. P., & Hyman, M. (1982). Maximum phoneme duration of /s/ and /z/ by children with vocal nodules. *Language, Speech, and Hearing Services in Schools, 13*, 197–199.

Roark, R. M., Watson, B. C., Baken, R. J., Brown, D. J., & Thomas, J. M. (2012). Measures of vocal attack time for healthy young adults. *Journal of Voice, 26*(1), 12–17.

Røksund, O. D., Heimdal, J. H., Clemm, H., Vollsaeter, M., & Halvorsen, T. (2017). Exercise inducible laryngeal obstruction: Diagnostics and management. *Paediatric Respiratory Reviews, 21*, 86–94.

Sapienza, C. M., & Stathopoulos, E. T. (1994). Respiratory and laryngeal measures of children and women with bilateral vocal fold nodules. *Journal of Speech and Hearing Research, 37*, 1229–1243.

Sorensen, D. N., & Parker, P. A. (1992). The voiced/voiceless phonation time in children with and without laryngeal pathology. *Language, Speech, and Hearing Services in Schools, 23*, 163–168.

Storck, C., Juergens, P., Fischer, C., Wolfensberger, M., Honegger, F., Sorantin, E., . . . Gugatschka, M. (2012). Biomechanics of the cricoarytenoid joint: Three-dimensional imaging and vector analysis. *Journal of Voice, 25*(4), 406–410.

Tait, N. A., Michel, J. F., & Carpenter, M. A. (1980). Maximum duration of sustained /s/ and /z/ in children. *Journal of Speech and Hearing Disorders, 15*, 239–246.

Titze, I. R. (1973). The human vocal cords: A mathematical model, Part I. *Phonetica, 28*, 129–170.

Titze, I. R. (1988). The physics of small amplitude oscillation of the vocal folds. *Journal of the Acoustical Society of America, 83*(4), 1536–1552.

Titze, I. R. (1994). *Principles of voice production*. Englewood Cliffs, NJ: Prentice-Hall.

Van den Berg, J. W. (1958). Myoelastic-aerodynamic theory of voice production. *Journal of Speech and Hearing Research, 1*, 227–244.

Van den Berg, J. W. (1968). Sound production in isolated human larynges. *Annals of the New York Academy of Sciences, 155*, 18–27.

Van den Berg, J. W., & Tan, T. S. (1959). Results of experiments with human larynxes. *Practica Oto-Rhino-Laryngologica, 21*, 425–450.

von Békésy, G., & Wever, E. G. (1960). *Experiments in hearing* (Vol. 8). New York, NY: McGraw-Hill.

Watson, B. C., Baken, R. J., & Roark, R. M. (2016). Effect of voice onset type on vocal attack time. *Journal of Voice, 30*(1), 11–14.

Young, N., Wadie, M., & Sasaki, C. T. (2012). Neuromuscular basis for ventricular fold function. *Annals of Otology, Rhinology and Laryngology, 121*(5), 317–321.

Zemlin, W. (1998). *Speech and hearing science: Anatomy and physiology* (4th ed.). Needham Heights, MS: Allyn & Bacon.

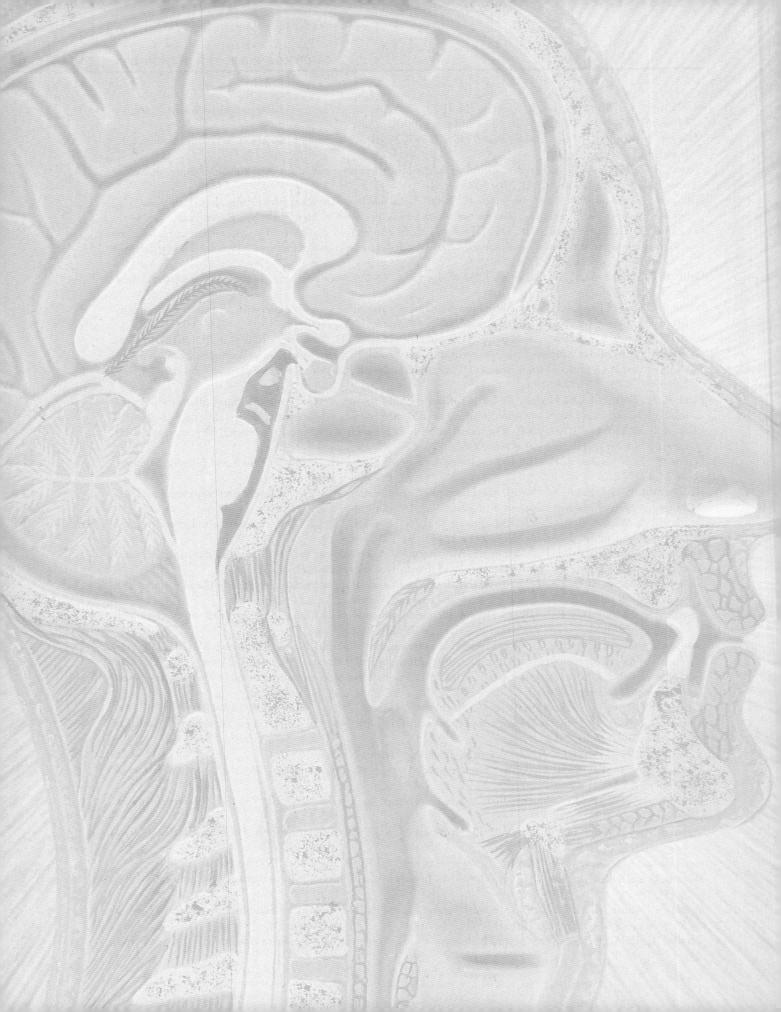

CHAPTER 6

Anatomy of Articulation and Resonation

When laypeople think of the process of speaking, they are more than likely actually thinking about articulation. You, of course, now know that there is much more to speech than moving the lips, tongue, mandible, and so forth. Nonetheless, the articulatory system is an extremely important element in our communication system.

Articulation is the process of joining two elements, and the **articulatory system** is the system of mobile and immobile articulators brought into contact for the purpose of shaping the sounds of speech. Remember from Chapters 4 and 5 that laryngeal vibration produces the sound required for voicing in speech. We are capable of rapidly starting and stopping phonation, depending on whether we want voiced or voiceless production. This chapter focuses on what happens after that sound reaches the oral cavity. In this cavity, the undifferentiated buzz produced by the vocal folds is shaped into the sounds we call *phonemes*. Let us present an overview of how the oral cavity is capable of creating phonemes.

articulation: the process of joining two elements

ANAQUEST LESSON ▶

Source-Filter Theory of Vowel Production

A widely accepted description of how the oral cavity shapes speech sounds is the **source-filter theory** of vowel production. In general terms, the theory states that a voicing source is generated by the vocal folds and routed through the vocal tract where it is shaped into the sounds of speech. Changes in the shape and configuration of the tongue, mandible, soft palate, and other articulators govern the resonance characteristics of the vocal tract, and the resonances of the tract determine the sound of a given vowel. Here is how that works.

The **vocal tract** consists of the mouth (oral cavity), the region behind the mouth (pharynx), and the nasal cavity. It may be thought of as a series of linked tubes (Figure 6–1A). From your experience, you know that if you blow carefully across the top of a water bottle, you will hear a tone. If you decrease the volume of the air in the bottle by adding water to it, the frequency of vibration of the tone increases. Likewise, if you blow across the top of a bottle with larger volume, the tone decreases in frequency. *As the volume of the air in the bottle increases, the frequency of the tone decreases. As*

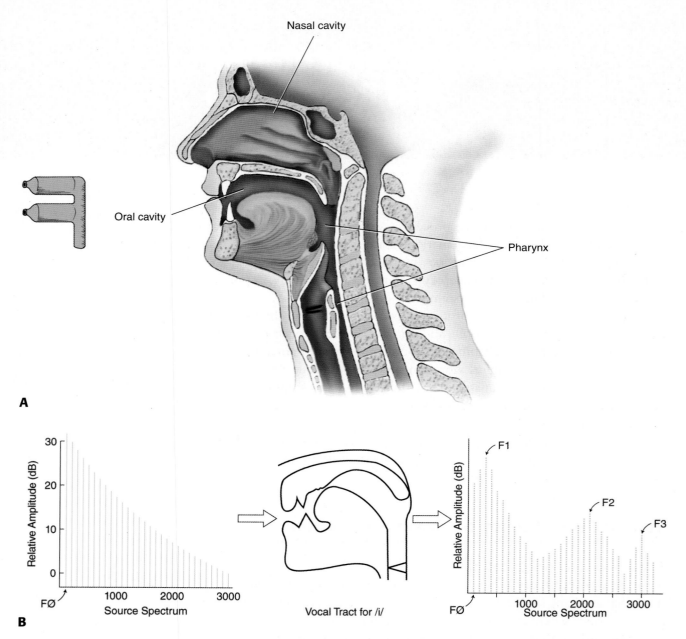

Figure 6–1. A. Visualization of the oral, nasal, and pharyngeal cavities as a series of linked tubes. This linkage provides the variable resonating cavity that produces speech. **B.** Relationship among source (spectrum of output from vocal folds), filter (vocal tract transfer function), and filtered output of the vocal tract (formants). *Source:* From Seikel/Drumright/King. *Anatomy & Physiology for Speech, Language, and Hearing, 5th Ed.* ©Cengage, Inc. Reproduced by permission.

resonant frequency: frequency of stimulation to which a resonant system responds most vigorously

the volume decreases, the frequency increases. This exercise is an experiment with the **resonant frequency** of a cavity, which is the frequency of sound to which the cavity most effectively responds. You might think of the bottle as a filter that lets only one frequency of sound through and rejects the other frequencies, much as a coffee filter lets the liquid through but traps the grounds. The airstream blowing across the top of the bottle is actually producing a very broad-spectrum signal, but the bottle selects the frequency components that are at its resonant frequency. The resonant frequency of a cavity is largely governed by its volume and length. Now, if you were somehow able to blow across two bottles (one low-resonant frequency and one high-resonant frequency), the two tones would combine.

When you move your tongue around in your mouth, you are changing the shape of your oral cavity, making it smaller or larger, lengthening or shortening it. It is as if you had a series of bottles that you could manipulate in your mouth, changing their shape at will. When you change the shape of the oral cavity, you are changing the resonant frequencies, and therefore you are changing the sound that comes out of the mouth. This, then, is the source-filter theory view of speech production. The vocal folds produce a quasi-periodic tone (see Chapters 4 and 5), which is passed through the filter of your vocal tract. The vocal tract filter is manipulable, so that you can change its shape and therefore change the sound.

The resonant frequencies govern our perception of vowels. To prove that vocal folds do not govern the nature of a vowel, whisper the words *he* and *who*. Could you tell the difference? The vocal folds were not vibrating, but you excited the oral cavity filter through the turbulence of your whispered production, and the vowels were quite intelligible.

The source-filter theory can be easily expanded to other phonemes as well. The source of the sound may vary. With vowels, the source always is phonation in normal speech. With consonants, other sources include the turbulence of frication or combinations of voicing and turbulence. In all cases, you produce a noise source and pass it through the filter of the oral cavity that has been configured to meet your acoustic needs. Now look at Figure 6–1B. On the left is the spectrum output of the vocal folds before the sound has filtered through the vocal tract. Notice that the spectrum is made up of a fundamental frequency (lowest bar in the graph) and whole-number multiples, known as harmonics. These harmonics are evenly spaced and diminish in intensity by about 12 dB per octave. In the middle of that figure is the filter itself: the vocal tract through which the sound source is being fed. We have drawn this so the shape of the articulators is making the /i/ vowel. The /i/ vowel is a high-front vowel, which means its constriction is forward in the mouth, near the alveolar ridge, behind the upper teeth. This means that the space in front of the constriction is very small. Now look at the right-most part of that figure. The spectrum that entered the vocal tract filter on the left has been shaped into the output spectrum on the right, which is the spectrum for the vowel /i/. We identify that vowel by the second formant (F2), which is produced by the space anterior to the constriction. That F2 frequency, by the way, is approximately 2500 Hz, while the F1 frequency is about 300 Hz.

Look at Figure 6–2 and notice the difference between production of the /s/ and /ʃ/ phonemes. Sustain an /s/ and realize that when you produce it, your tongue is high, forward, and tense. You pass a compact stream of air over

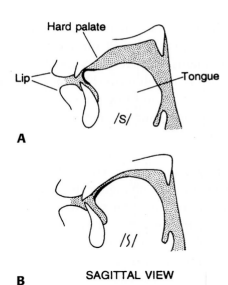

Figure 6–2. Comparison of the articulatory posture used for production of /s/ and /ʃ/. (After the data and view of Shriberg & Kent, 2002.)

the surface of the tongue, and then between the tongue tip and the upper front teeth. Now produce the /ʃ/ and recognize that the tongue is farther back in your mouth, much as in the figure. The source in both cases is the turbulence associated with the airstream escaping from its course between your tongue and an immobile structure of your mouth (front teeth or roof of your mouth). The turbulence excites the cavity in front of the constriction, and you have a recognizable sound. Which of the two phonemes has the larger cavity distal to the constriction? The /ʃ/ has a larger resonant cavity than the /s/, so its resonant frequency is lower, following our discussion of bottles. Now make the /s/ again, but without stopping, slide your tongue back in your mouth until you reach the /ʃ/ position. As you do this, you should hear the noise drop in frequency because the cavity is increasing in size. The source-filter theory dictates this change.

✓ To summarize:

- The source-filter theory states that speech is the product of sending an acoustic source, such as the sound produced by the vibrating vocal folds, through the filter of the vocal tract that shapes the output.

- The ever-changing speech signal is the product of moving articulators.

- Sources may be voicing, as in the case of vowels, or the product of turbulence, as in fricatives. Articulators may be moveable (such as the tongue, lips, pharynx, and mandible) or immobile (such as the teeth and hard palate).

Let us now examine the structures of the articulatory system. As with the phonatory system, we must examine the support structures (the skull and bones of the face) and the muscles that move the articulators. Before we begin discussion of the structures, we define the articulators used in speech production.

The Articulators

As noted, articulators may be either mobile or immobile. In speech, we often move one articulator to make contact with another, thus positioning a mobile articulator in relation to an immobile articulator.

The largest mobile articulator is the *tongue*, with the lower jaw (*mandible*) a close second (Figure 6–3). The *velum* or *soft palate* is another mobile articulator, used to differentiate nasal sounds such as /m/ or /n/ from nonnasal sounds. The *lips* are moved to produce different speech sounds, and the *cheeks* play a role in changes of resonance of the cavity. The region behind the oral cavity (the **fauces** and the *pharynx*) may be moved through muscular action, and the *larynx* and *hyoid bone* both change to accommodate different articulatory postures.

There are three immobile articulators. The *alveolar ridge* of the upper jaw (*maxilla*) and the *hard palate* are both significant articulatory surfaces. The *teeth* are used in the production of a variety of speech sounds.

The process of **articulation for speech** is quite automatic. To get a feel for changes in speech that occur when you alter the function of an articulator, try this. Place a small stack of tongue depressors between your molars on one side of your mouth and bite lightly (this creates a *bite block*). Now say, "You wish to know all about my grandfather." Now say the same sentence after placing your tongue between your front teeth and biting lightly. Finally, say the sentence while pulling your cheeks out with your fingers. There are two important points to this demonstration. First, your speech changed when you altered the articulatory and resonatory characteristics of the vocal tract. You restrained the articulators, and they had to work harder to make yourself understood. Second, you were able to overcome most of these difficulties. Despite having a bite block or clamped tongue tip, you were able to make yourself understood. In fact, you automatically adjusted your articulation to match the new physical constraints. As a student in speech-language pathology, you should be quite heartened by the extraordinary flexibility of motor planning exhibited in this demonstration, because you can use this feature to your advantage in treatment.

Of these mobile and immobile articulators, the tongue, mandible, teeth, hard palate, and velum are the major players, although all surfaces and cavities within the articulatory/resonatory system are contributors to the production of speech.

You may wish to refer to Figures 6–4 through 6–9 as we begin our discussion of the bones of the facial and cranial skeleton. In addition, Table 6–1 may help you to organize this body of material.

fauces: the pillars at the posterior margin of the oral cavity

Maxilla is the singular of maxillae.

articulation for speech: the process of bringing two or more moveable speech structures together to form the sounds of speech

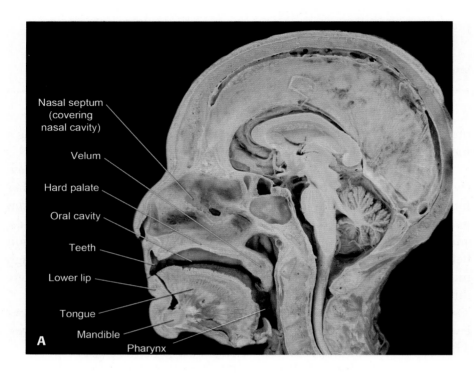

Nasal septum
(covering
nasal cavity)

Velum

Hard palate

Oral cavity

Teeth

Lower lip

Tongue

Mandible

A

Pharynx

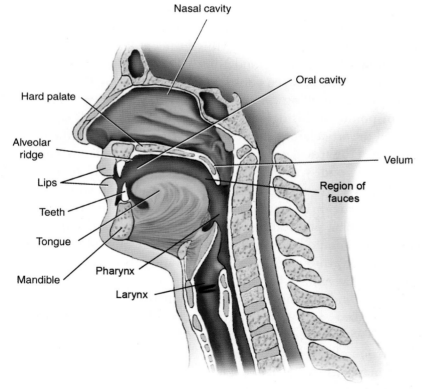

Nasal cavity

Oral cavity

Hard palate

Alveolar
ridge

Velum

Lips

Region of
fauces

Teeth

Tongue

Pharynx

Mandible

Larynx

B   SAGITTAL VIEW

Figure 6–3. A. Photograph of articulators seen through sagittal section. **B.** Relationships among the articulators. *Source:* From Seikel/ Drumright/King. *Anatomy & Physiology for Speech, Language, and Hearing, 5th Ed.* ©Cengage, Inc. Reproduced by permission.

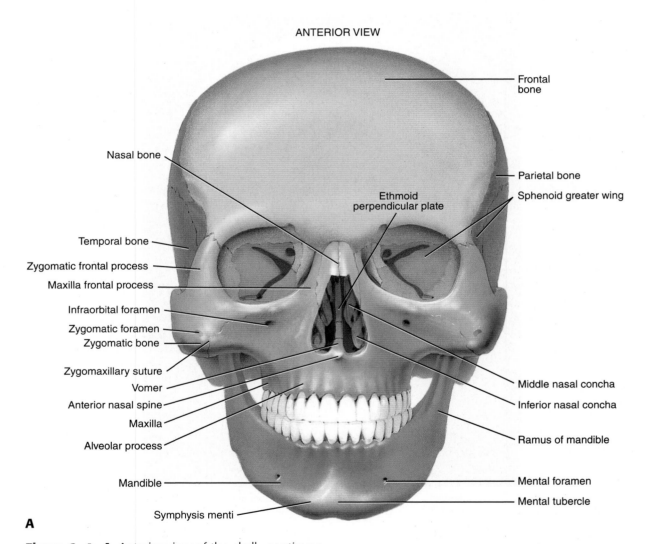

ANTERIOR VIEW

Figure 6–4. A. Anterior view of the skull. *continues*

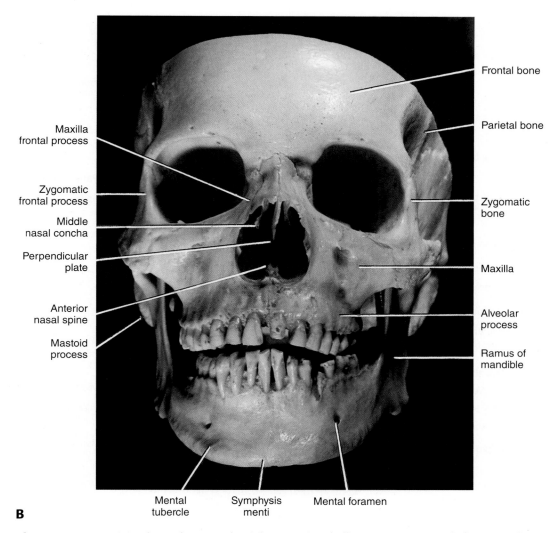

B

Figure 6–4. *continued* **B.** Photograph of the anterior skull. *Source:* From Seikel/Drumright/King. *Anatomy & Physiology for Speech, Language, and Hearing, 5th Ed.* ©Cengage, Inc. Reproduced by permission.

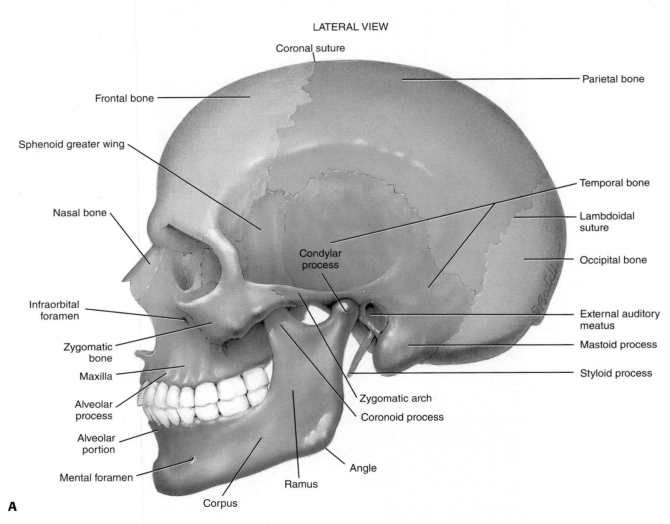

Figure 6–5. A. Lateral view of the skull. *continues*

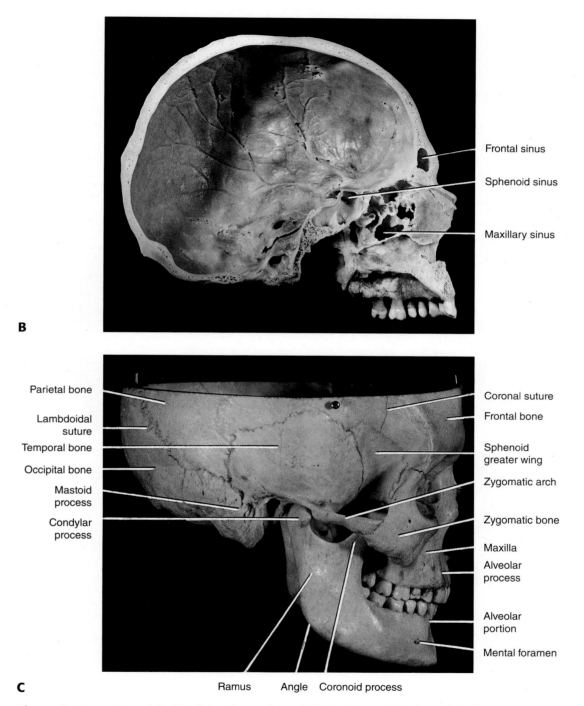

Figure 6–5. *continued* **B.** Medial surface of the skull. **C.** Photo of the lateral skull. *Source:* From Seikel/Drumright/King. *Anatomy & Physiology for Speech, Language, and Hearing, 5th Ed.* ©Cengage, Inc. Reproduced by permission.

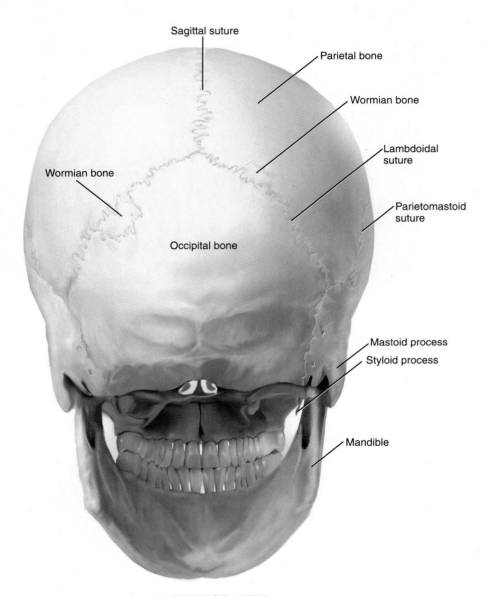

POSTERIOR VIEW

Figure 6–6. Posterior view of the skull. *Source:* From Seikel/Drumright/King. *Anatomy & Physiology for Speech, Language, and Hearing, 5th Ed.* ©Cengage, Inc. Reproduced by permission.

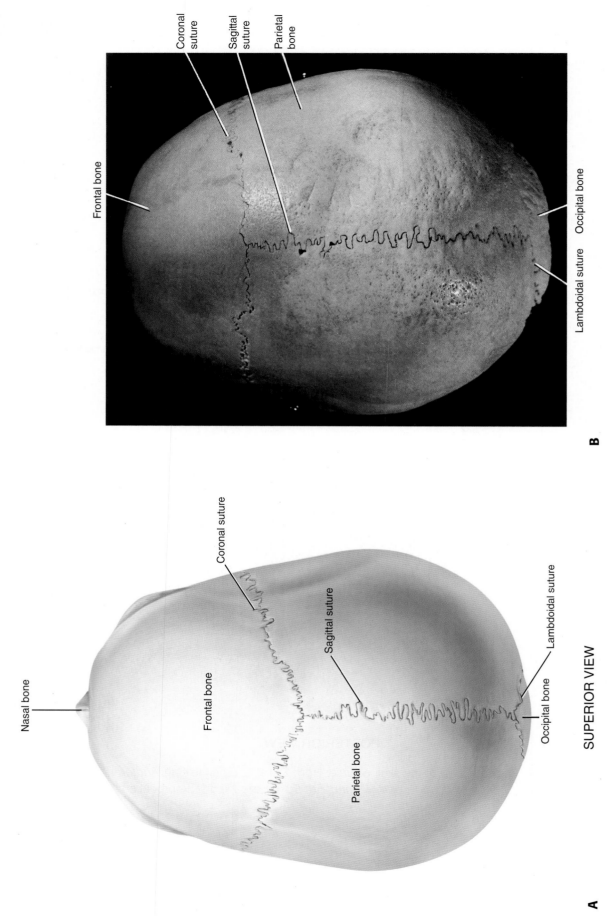

Figure 6–7. A. Superior view of the skull. **B.** Superior view photo of the skull. *Source:* From Seikel/Drumright/King. *Anatomy & Physiology for Speech, Language, and Hearing, 5th Ed.* ©Cengage, Inc. Reproduced by permission.

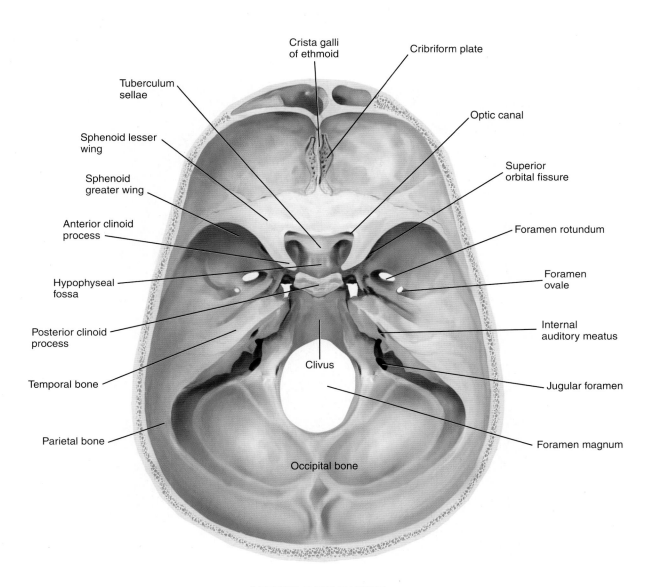

A

INTERNAL BASE OF SKULL

Figure 6–8. A. Internal view of base of the skull. *continues*

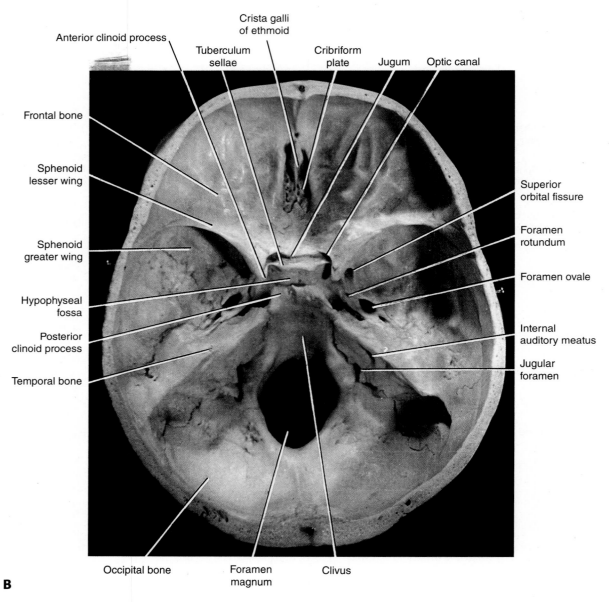

B

Figure 6–8. *continued* **B.** Photo of the internal skull. *Source:* From Seikel/Drumright/King. *Anatomy & Physiology for Speech, Language, and Hearing, 5th Ed.* ©Cengage, Inc. Reproduced by permission.

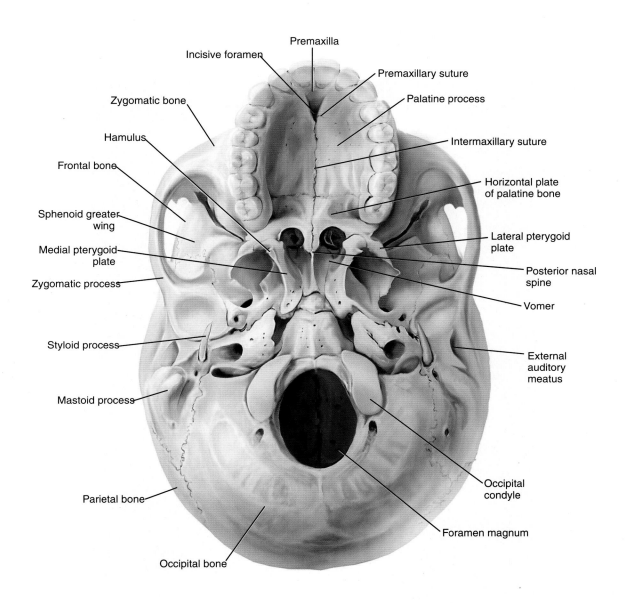

A   INFERIOR VIEW

Figure 6–9. A. Inferior view of the skull. *Source:* From Seikel/Drumright/King. *Anatomy & Physiology for Speech, Language, and Hearing, 5th Ed.* ©Cengage, Inc. Reproduced by permission. *continues*

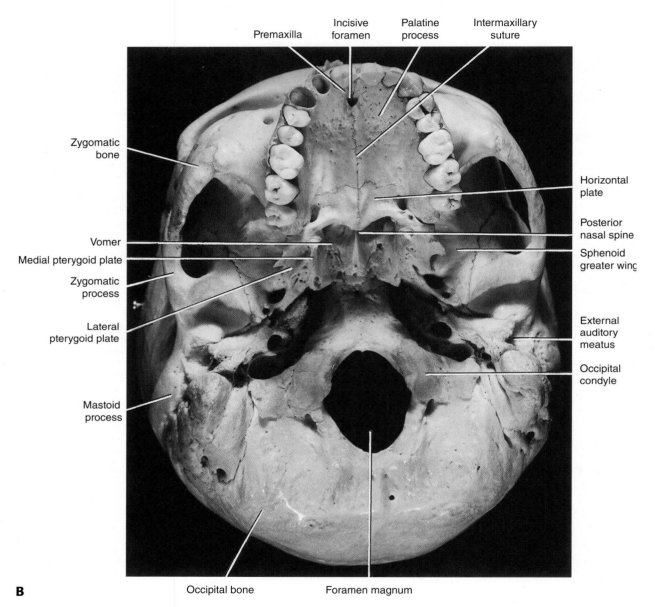

B

Figure 6–9. *continued* **B.** Photo of inferior view of the skull. *Source:* From Seikel/Drumright/King. *Anatomy & Physiology for Speech, Language, and Hearing, 5th Ed.* ©Cengage, Inc. Reproduced by permission.

Table 6–1

Bones of the Face and Cranial Skeleton	
Bones of the Face	**Bones of the Cranial Skeleton**
Mandible	Ethmoid bone
Maxillae	Sphenoid bone
Nasal bones	Frontal bone
Palatine bones and nasal conchae	Parietal bone
Vomer	Occipital bone
Zygomatic bone	Temporal bone
Lacrimal bones	
Hyoid bone	

Bones of the Face and Cranial Skeleton

ANAQUEST LESSON

Bones of the Face

There are numerous bones of the face with which you should become familiar. As with the respiratory and phonatory systems, learning the landmarks will serve you well as you identify the course and function of the muscles of articulation.

- Mandible
- Maxillae
- Nasal bones
- Palatine bones and nasal conchae
- Vomer
- Zygomatic bone
- Lacrimal bones
- Hyoid bone

Mandible

The mandible is the massive unpaired bone making up the lower jaw of the face. It begins as a paired bone but fuses at the midline by the child's first birthday. As you can see from Figure 6–10, there are several landmarks of interest on both outer and inner surfaces. The point of fusion of the two halves of the mandible is the **symphysis menti** or **mental symphysis**, marking the midline mental **protuberance** (or **prominences**) and separating the paired mental **tubercles**. Lateral to the tubercles on either side is the

mental: L., mentum, chin

symphysis: Gr., growing together

protuberance: Gr., pro, before; tuber, bulge

tubercles: little swelling

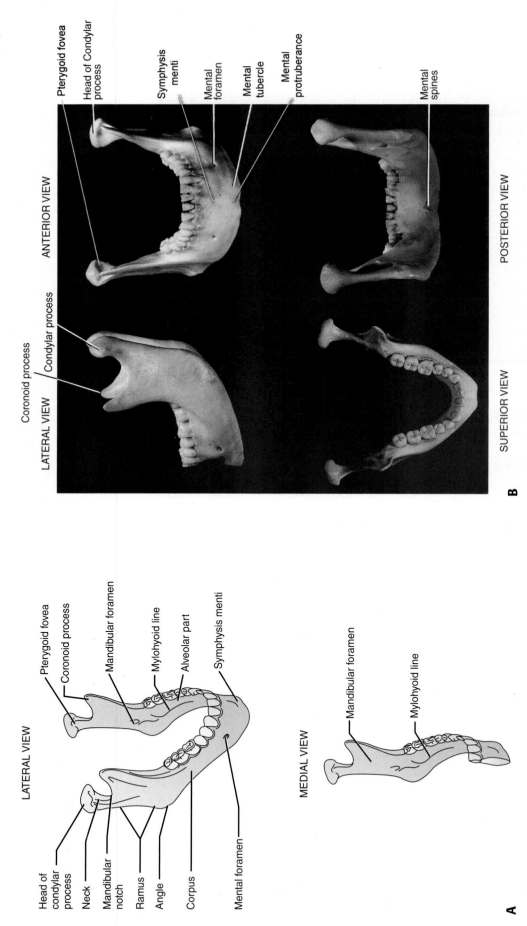

Figure 6-10. A. Lateral and medial views of the mandible. **B.** Photo of the mandible from lateral, anterior, superior, and posterior aspects. *Source:* From Seikel/Drumright/King. *Anatomy & Physiology for Speech, Language, and Hearing, 5th Ed.* ©Cengage, Inc. Reproduced by permission.

On Use of the Bite Block

A *bite block* is a device used to stabilize the mandible so that other articulators can be evaluated or exercised. Bite blocks come in many shapes, sizes, and textures, ranging from acrylic blocks about 1 cm square to bite blocks that are created from dental impression material. The softer, more pliable dental impression bite block provides a better surface for sustained use and is particularly good for clients who have limited motor control.

A bite block is used when you cannot differentiate the contribution of the mandible from that of the lips or tongue during articulation. For instance, if you say /ta ta ta ta/ repeatedly while lightly holding your mandible, you feel the mandible move, even though the dominant articulator is the tongue. If you want to strengthen the tongue, such as having it push toward the roof of the mouth against a resistance, you could place a bite block between the molars and have your client push up against a tongue depressor.

Having your client perform oral motor activities such as the one mentioned here requires that you have a firm understanding of the anatomy and physiology of articulation, as well as a deep knowledge of motor development. Oral motor therapy focuses on remediating muscle imbalance, and inappropriate application of oral motor activities can create even greater problems. For an excellent discussion, see Langley and Lombardino (1991).

---

mental foramen, the hole through which the mental nerve of V trigeminal passes in life. The lateral mass of bone is the **corpus** or body, and the point at which the mandible angles upward is the **angle**. The rhomboidal plate rising up from the mandible is the **ramus**. The **condylar** and **coronoid** processes are important landmarks and are separated by the **mandibular notch**. The prominent **head** of the condylar process articulates with the skull, permitting the rotation of the mandible. The **pterygoid fovea** on the anterior surface of the condylar process marks the point of attachment of the lateral pterygoid muscle, which is discussed later. In the healthy mandible, teeth are found within small **dental alveoli** (sacs) on the upper surface of the **alveolar part** of the mandible (Standring, 2008; Zhang, 2008).

On the inner surface of the mandible are prominent midline **superior** and inferior **mental spines** and the laterally placed **mylohyoid line**, landmarks that will figure prominently as we attach muscles to this structure. The **mandibular foramen** is the conduit for the inferior alveolar nerve of V trigeminal, providing sensory innervation for the teeth and gums (Black, 2008).

Maxillae

The paired maxillae (singular, **maxilla**) are the bones making up the upper jaw. These bones deserve careful study, for they make up most of the roof of the mouth (**hard palate**), nose, and upper dental ridge and are involved in clefting of the lip and hard palate. As you study the landmarks of this complex bone, it might help you to realize that the various processes are logically named. For example, the *frontal* process of maxilla articulates with the *frontal* bone. Thus, learning the names of the larger structures early on will facilitate learning the processes and attachments later.

foramen: L., a passage, opening, orifice

corpus: body

ramus: L., branch

pterygoid: Gr., pterygodes, wing; referring to one of two prominent processes arising from the base of the sphenoid bone

fovea: L., a pit

orbital: L., orbita, orbit

In Figure 6–11 you can see the significant landmarks of the maxillae. As you can see, the **frontal process** is the superior-most point of this bone. You can palpate this process on yourself by placing your finger on your nose at the nasal side of your eye. You could run your finger down the **infra-orbital margin** from there to the lower midpoint of your eye. The **orbital** process projects into the eye socket, providing support for the eyeball. Just below your finger is the **infraorbital foramen**, the conduit for the infraor-bital nerve arising from the maxillary nerve of the V trigeminal, providing sensory innervation of the lower eyelid, upper lip, and nasal alae (Kandel, Schwartz, Jessell, Siegelbaum, & Hudspeth, 2013). Lateral to your finger is the **zygomatic process** of the maxilla bone, which articulates with the zygomatic bone.

At the midline you can see the **anterior nasal spine (nasal crest)**, and lateral to this is the **nasal notch**. The lower tooth-bearing ridge, the **alveolar process**, contains alveoli that hold teeth in the intact adult maxilla. The

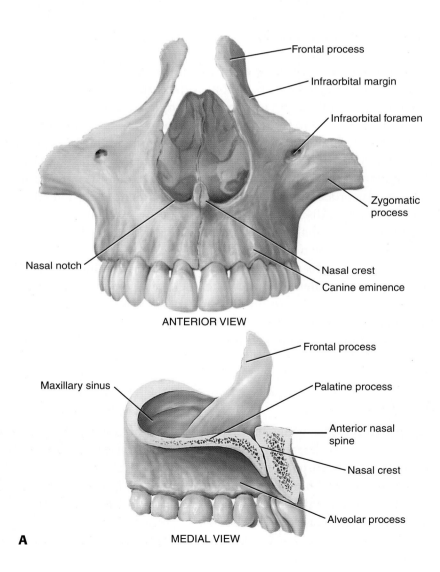

Figure 6–11. A. Anterior and medial views of the maxilla. *continues*

A

ANTERIOR VIEW

MEDIAL VIEW

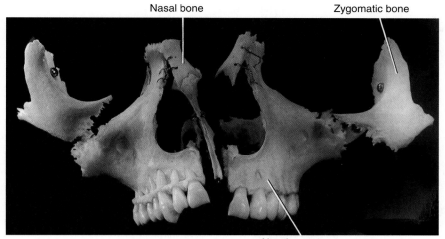

Nasal bone   Zygomatic bone

Alveolar process

ANTERIOR VIEW

B

Figure 6–11. *continued* **B.** Anterior view of maxillae, showing the relationship with nasal and zygomatic bones. *Source:* From Seikel/Drumright/King. *Anatomy & Physiology for Speech, Language, and Hearing, 5th Ed.* ©Cengage, Inc. Reproduced by permission.

region between the **canine eminence** and the **incisive foramen** (not shown) will become important as we discuss cleft lip.

A medial view requires disarticulation of left and right maxillae. This view reveals the **maxillary sinus**, the **palatine process**, and the important inner margin of the alveolar process.

Figure 6–12 shows an inferior view of the maxilla. As you can see from this view, the two palatine processes of the maxilla articulate at the **intermaxillary suture** (also known as the **median palatine suture**). When a cleft of the hard palate occurs, it is on this **suture**. The palatine process makes up three fourths of the hard palate, with the other one fourth being the horizontal plate of the palatine bone.

The incisive foramen in the anterior aspect of the hard palate is the conduit for the nasopalatine nerve serving the nasal mucosa. Trace the **premaxillary suture** forward from the incisive foramen to the alveolar process to identify the borders of the **premaxilla**. The premaxilla is difficult

suture: L., sutura, seam; the fibrous union of skull bones

Mandibular Hypoplasia and Micrognathia

Congenital mandibular hypoplasia is a condition in which there is inadequate development of the mandible. Although some specific genetic syndromes have this as a trait (e.g., Robin syndrome), **micrognathia** (small jaw) may occur without any known mediating condition. The misalignment of the mandibular and maxillary arches may be corrected through surgery to extend the mandible. It is hypothesized that, during development, micrognathia may lead to cleft palate: the mandible may not develop adequately to accommodate the tongue, which, in turn, blocks the extension of the palatine processes of the maxillae.

micrognathia: Gr., micro, small; gnathos, jaw

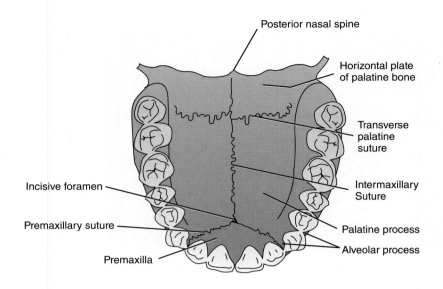

INFERIOR VIEW

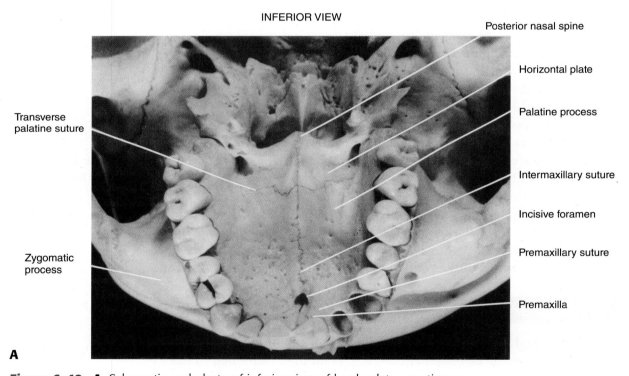

A

Figure 6–12. A. Schematic and photo of inferior view of hard palate. *continues*

to see on the adult skull, but it is an important topic of discussion. Note that the premaxillary suture separates the lateral incisors from the cuspids. If there is a cleft of the lip, it will occur at this location, and it may include the lip, alveolar bone, and the region of the premaxillary suture. A cleft lip may be either unilateral or bilateral, but in virtually all cases, it occurs at this suture (there is very rarely a midline cleft lip).

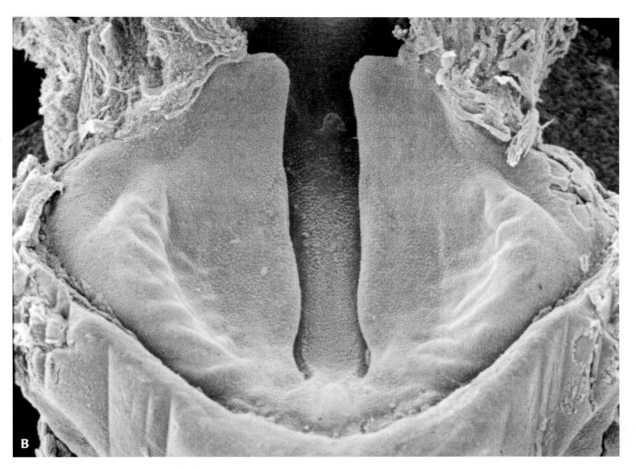

Figure 6–12. *continued* **B.** Experimentally induced cleft palate in mouse. Photograph courtesy of Marilyn Russell, Ph.D. *Source:* From Seikel/Drumright/King. *Anatomy & Physiology for Speech, Language, and Hearing, 5th Ed.* ©Cengage, Inc. Reproduced by permission.

Nasal Bones

The nasal bones are small, making up the superior nasal surface. As you can see from Figure 6–4 (shown earlier), the nasal bones articulate with the frontal bones superiorly, the maxillae laterally, and the perpendicular plate of the ethmoid bone and the nasal septal cartilage.

Palatine Bones and Nasal Conchae

Recall that the posterior one fourth of the hard palate is made up of the horizontal plate of the palatine bones. Let us now examine this small, but complex bone (Figure 6–13).

When viewed from the front, you can see that the articulated palatine bones echo the nasal cavity defined by the maxillae. The **posterior nasal spine** and **nasal crest** provide midline correlates to the anterior nasal spine and nasal crest of the maxillae, while the **horizontal plate** parallels the palatine

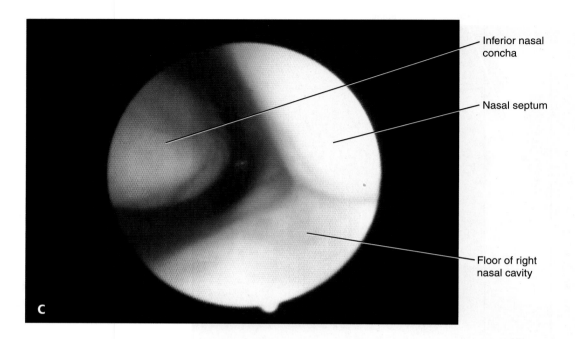

Inferior nasal concha

Nasal septum

Floor of right nasal cavity

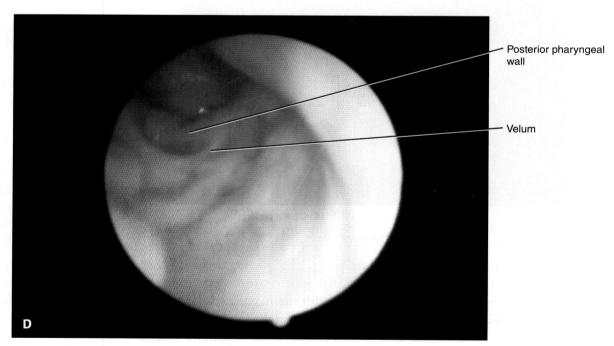

Posterior pharyngeal wall

Velum

Figure 6–13. *continued* **C.** Nasoendoscopic view of entry to right naris. Note the prominent inferior nasal concha arising from the left side (medial wall of nasal cavity). **D.** Nasoendoscopic view of nasopharynx as seen from the right naris, showing superior surface of velum and posterior pharyngeal wall. *continues*

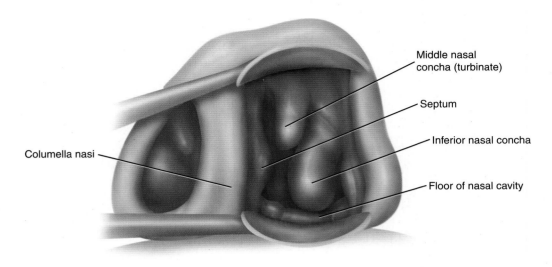

Middle nasal
concha (turbinate)

Septum

Inferior nasal concha

Columella nasi

Floor of nasal cavity

E   SPECULUM VIEW

Figure 6–13. *continued* **E.** View of left nares opened using speculum for visualization, showing inferior and middle conchae. *Source:* From Seikel/Drumright/King. *Anatomy & Physiology for Speech, Language, and Hearing, 5th Ed.* ©Cengage, Inc. Reproduced by permission.

Vomer

The vomer (Figure 6–14) is an unpaired, midline bone making up the inferior and posterior **nasal septum**, the dividing plate between the two nasal cavities (Figure 6–15). The vomer has the appearance of a knife blade or a plowshare, with its point aimed toward the front. It articulates with the sphenoid **rostrum** and perpendicular plate of the ethmoid bone in the posterior–superior margin, and with the maxillae and palatine bones on the inferior margin. The posterior **ala** of the vomer marks the midline terminus of the nasal cavities. As you examine Figure 6–15, attend to the fact that the bony nasal **septum** is made up of two elements: the vomer and the perpendicular plate of the ethmoid bone. With the addition of the midline **septal cartilage**, the nasal septum is complete.

rostrum: L., beak or beaklike

ala: L., wing

septum: L., partition

Zygomatic Bone

The **zygomatic** bone makes up the prominent structures we identify as cheekbones. As you can see from Figure 6–16, the zygomatic bone articulates with the maxillae, frontal bone, and temporal bone, as well as with the sphenoid bone (not shown), and makes up the lateral orbit.

Fortunately, the landmarks of the zygomatic bone make intuitive sense. At the base of the **orbital margin** is the **maxillary process**, the point of articulation of the zygomatic bone and maxilla. The **temporal process** seen in the lateral aspect projects back, forming half of the **zygomatic arch**.

zygomatic: zygoma, yoke

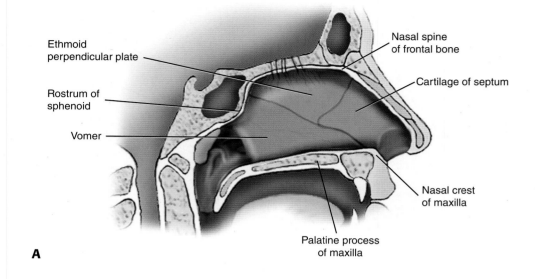

Ethmoid
perpendicular plate

Rostrum of
sphenoid

Vomer

Nasal spine
of frontal bone

Cartilage of septum

Nasal crest
of maxilla

Palatine process
of maxilla

A

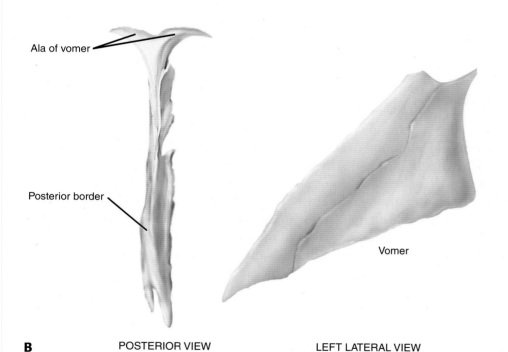

Ala of vomer

Posterior border

Vomer

B   POSTERIOR VIEW   LEFT LATERAL VIEW

Figure 6–14. Lateral view of the vomer. **A.** Vomer *in situ* as part of the nasal septum. **B.** Posterior and lateral views of vomer. *Source:* From Seikel/Drumright/King. *Anatomy & Physiology for Speech, Language, and Hearing, 5th Ed.* ©Cengage, Inc. Reproduced by permission.

(The zygomatic arch consists of the temporal process of the zygomatic bone and the zygomatic process of the temporal bone.) The **frontal process** forms the articulation with the frontal and sphenoid bones.

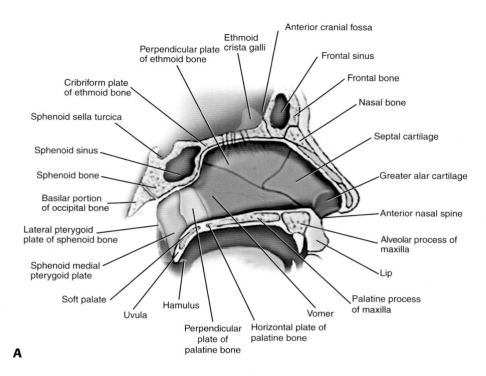

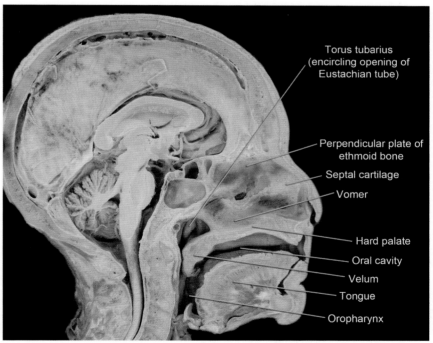

Figure 6–15. A. Medial view of the nasal septum. Note that the septum is composed of the perpendicular plate of the ethmoid, the vomer, and the septal cartilage. **B.** Photograph of specimen with intact nasal septum. *continues*

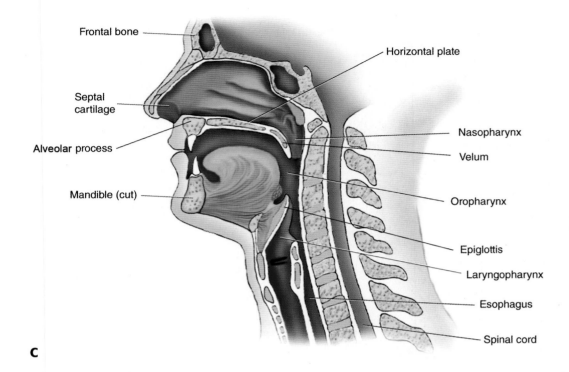

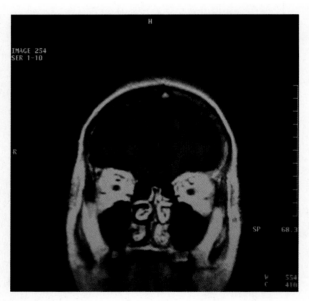

Figure 6–15. *continued* **C.** Drawing of the sagittal section through the nasal septum. **D.** Frontal magnetic resonance image showing deviated nasal septum and hypertrophied nasal mucosa and turbinates. *continues*

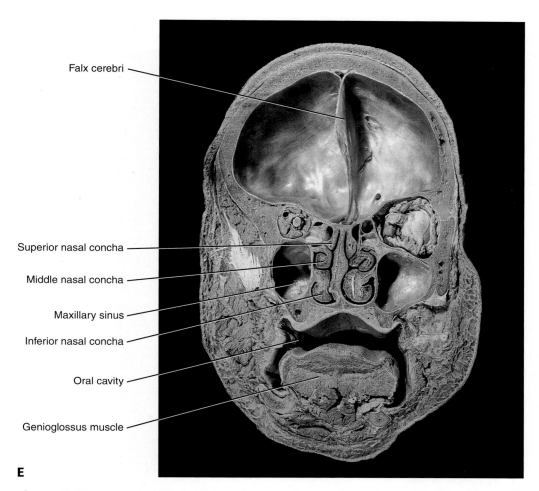

Falx cerebri

Superior nasal concha

Middle nasal concha

Maxillary sinus

Inferior nasal concha

Oral cavity

Genioglossus muscle

E

Figure 6–15. *continued* **E.** Frontal section revealing maxillary sinuses, nasal cavities, and the relationship of oral articulators. *continues*

Cleft Lip and Cleft Palate

Cleft lip and cleft palate arise during early development. Cleft lip may be either unilateral or bilateral, occurring along the premaxillary suture. Cleft lip is almost never midline, but may involve soft tissue alone or include a cleft of the maxilla up to the incisive foramen. Cleft palate may involve both hard and soft palates. Cleft lip appears to result from a failure of embryonic facial and labial tissue to fuse during development (Moore, Persaud, & Torchia, 2019).

With cleft lip, it looks as though tissues migrate and develop normally but, for some reason, either fail to fuse or the fusion of the migrating medial nasal, maxillary, and lateral nasal processes breaks down. Cleft palate apparently arises from some mechanical intervention in development. Prior to the seventh embryonic week, the palatine processes of the maxillae have been resting alongside the tongue so that the tongue separates the processes. As the oral cavity and mandible grow, the tongue drops away from the processes, and the processes can extend, make midline contact, and fuse. If something (such as micrognathia) blocks the movement of the tongue, the palatine processes will not move in time to make contact. The head grows rapidly, and the plates will have missed their chance to become an intact palate.

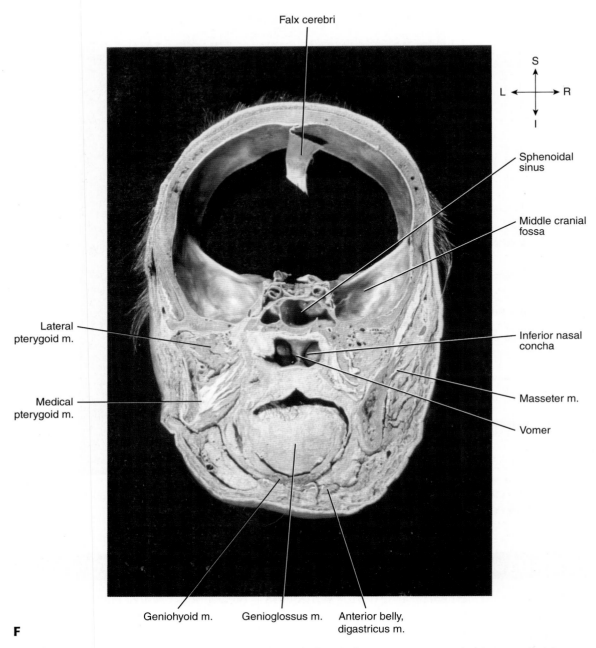

F

Figure 6–15. *continued* **F.** Coronal section through the skull. *Source:* From Seikel/Drumright/King. *Anatomy & Physiology for Speech, Language, and Hearing, 5th Ed.* ©Cengage, Inc. Reproduced by permission.

Lacrimal Bones

lacrimal: L., lacrima, tear

The small **lacrimal** bones are almost completely hidden in the intact skull. They articulate with the maxillae, frontal bone, nasal bone, and inferior conchae. They constitute a small portion of the lateral nasal wall and form a small portion of the medial orbit as well.

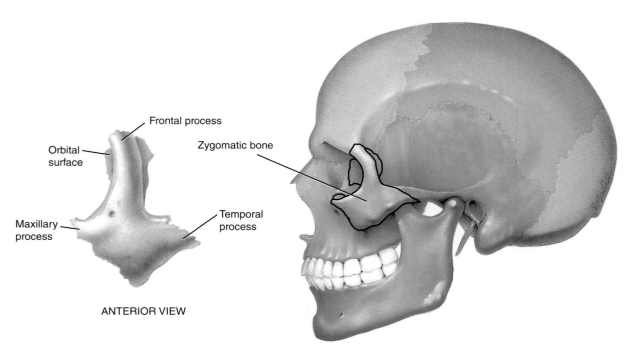

ANTERIOR VIEW

Figure 6–16. Anterior view of the zygomatic bone. *Source:* From Seikel/Drumright/King. *Anatomy & Physiology for Speech, Language, and Hearing, 5th Ed.* ©Cengage, Inc. Reproduced by permission.

Hyoid Bone

The hyoid bone was discussed in Chapters 4 and 5, but rightfully belongs in this chapter as well. Its presence in this listing should remind you of the interconnectedness of the phonatory and articulatory systems.

Bones of the Cranial Skeleton

ANAQUEST LESSON

The bones of the cranium include those involved in the creation of the cranial cavity.

- Ethmoid bone
- Sphenoid bone
- Frontal bone
- Parietal bone
- Occipital bone
- Temporal bone

Ethmoid Bone

The **ethmoid** bone is a complex, delicate structure with a presence in the cranial, nasal, and orbital spaces. If the cranium and facial skeleton were an apple, the ethmoid would be the core (Figure 6–17).

ethmoid: Gr., ethmos, sieve

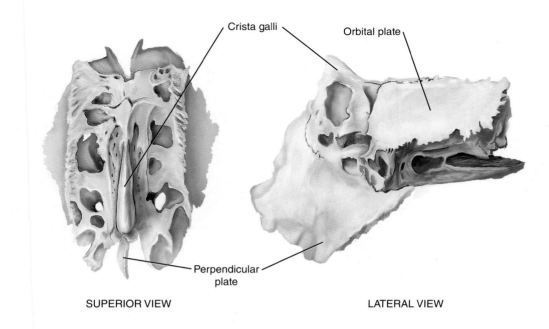

SUPERIOR VIEW   LATERAL VIEW

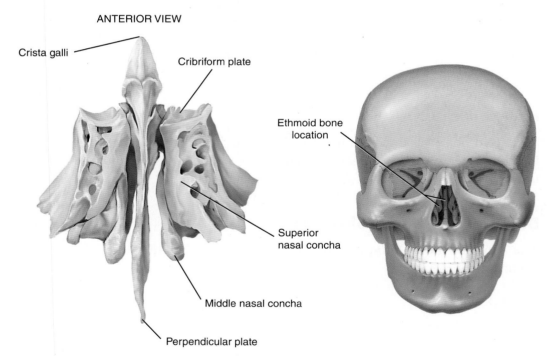

ANTERIOR VIEW

Figure 6–17. Views of the ethmoid bone. *Source:* From Seikel/Drumright/King. *Anatomy & Physiology for Speech, Language, and Hearing, 5th Ed.* ©Cengage, Inc. Reproduced by permission.

When viewed from the front, the superior surface is dominated by the **crista galli**, which protrudes into the cranial space. The perpendicular plate projects down, making up the superior nasal septum. Lateral to this plate are the middle and superior nasal conchae. On both sides of the perpendicular plate and perpendicular to it are the **cribriform plates**. The **cribriform** plates separate the nasal and cranial cavities and provide the conduit for the olfactory nerves as they enter the cranial space. The lateral **orbital plates** articulate with the frontal bone, lacrimal bone, and maxilla to form the medial orbit.

cribriform: L., cribum, sieve; forma, the porous component of the ethmoid bone

Sphenoid Bone

The **sphenoid** bone is much more complex than the ethmoid bone and is a significant contributor to the cranial structure (Figure 6–18). The sphenoid consists of a corpus and three pairs of processes, the greater wings, lesser wings, and pterygoid processes. The sphenoid also contains numerous foramina through which nerves and blood vessels pass.

sphenoid: Gr., spheno, wedge

When viewed from above, you can see that the medially placed **corpus** is dominated by the **hypophyseal fossa** (also known as the **sella turcica** or **pituitary fossa**), the indentation holding the pituitary gland (hypophysis) in life. This gland projects down from the hypothalamus and is placed at the point where the optic nerve decussates, the **chiasma**. The anterior portion of the **fossa** is the **tuberculum sellae**, and the posterior aspect is the **dorsum sellae**. The **anterior clinoid processes** project from the lesser wing of the sphenoid, lateral to the **tuberculum** sellae. The optic nerve passes under these

sella turcica: L., Turkish saddle

chiasma: Gr., khiasma, cross; an X-shaped crossing

fossa: L., furrow or depression

tuberculum: L., little swelling

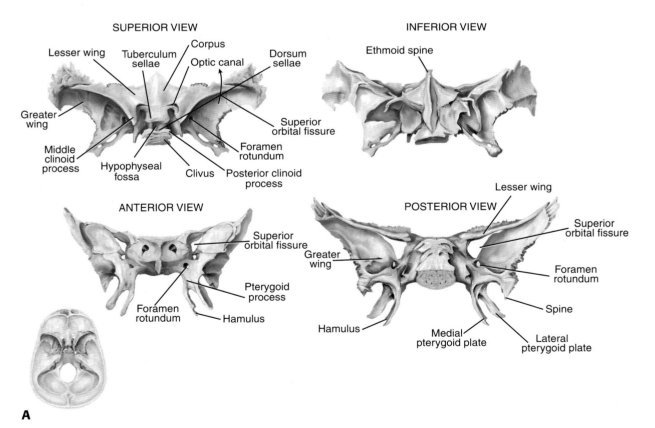

SUPERIOR VIEW

Lesser wing — Tuberculum sellae — Corpus — Optic canal — Dorsum sellae

Greater wing

Superior orbital fissure

Middle clinoid process — Hypophyseal fossa — Clivus — Posterior clinoid process — Foramen rotundum

INFERIOR VIEW

Ethmoid spine

ANTERIOR VIEW

Superior orbital fissure

Foramen rotundum — Hamulus — Pterygoid process

POSTERIOR VIEW

Lesser wing

Superior orbital fissure

Greater wing

Foramen rotundum

Spine

Hamulus — Medial pterygoid plate — Lateral pterygoid plate

A

Figure 6–18. A. Schematic sphenoid bone, including superior, inferior, anterior, and posterior views. *continues*

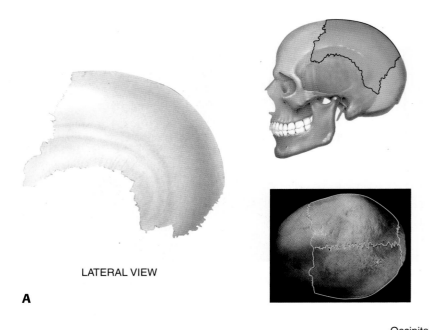

LATERAL VIEW

A

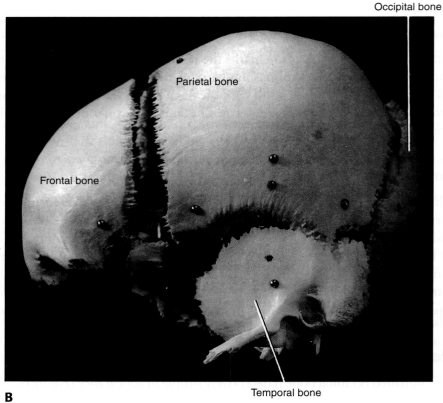

Occipital bone

Parietal bone

Frontal bone

Temporal bone

B

Figure 6–20. A. Lateral view of the parietal bone. **B.** Photo of disarticulated parietal, frontal, temporal, and occipital bones. *Source:* From Seikel/Drumright/King. *Anatomy & Physiology for Speech, Language, and Hearing, 5th Ed.* ©Cengage, Inc. Reproduced by permission.

the skull, wrapping beneath the brain. The **foramen magnum** provides the opening for the spinal cord and beginning of the medulla oblongata, and the **condyles** mark the resting point for the first cervical vertebra. The **basilar part** articulates with the corpus of the sphenoid.

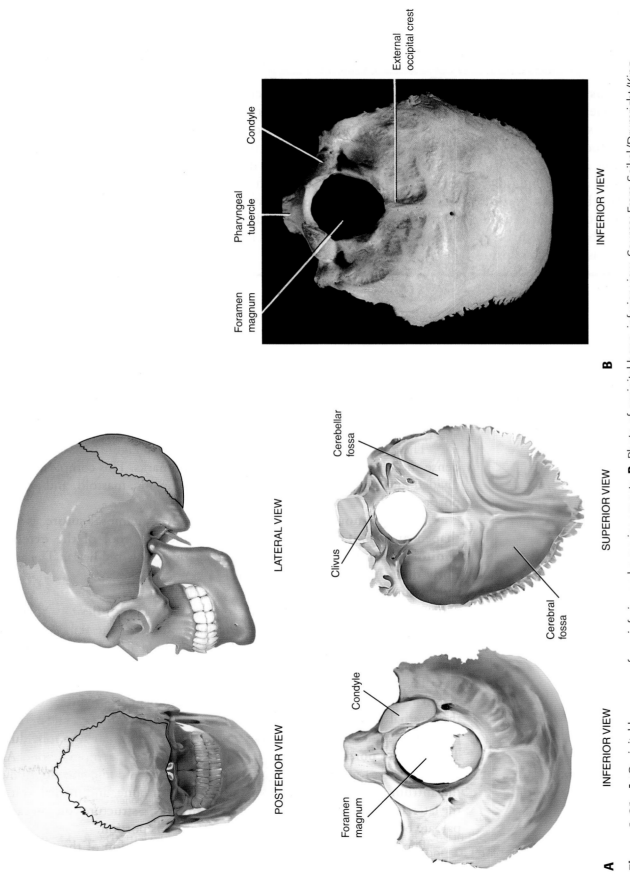

Figure 6–21. A. Occipital bone seen from inferior and superior aspects. **B.** Photo of occipital bone, inferior view. *Source:* From Seikel/Drumright/King. *Anatomy & Physiology for Speech, Language, and Hearing, 5th Ed.* ©Cengage, Inc. Reproduced by permission.

reveals the **internal auditory meatus** through which the VIII cranial nerve will pass on its way to the brain stem.

✔ *To summarize:*

- The bones of the **face** and **skull** work together in a complex fashion to produce the structures of **articulation**.
- The **mandible** provides the lower **dental arch** (lower set of teeth), **alveolar region**, and resting location for the tongue.
- The **maxillae** provide the **hard palate**, point of attachment for the **soft palate**, **alveolar ridge**, upper **dental arch**, and dominant structures of the **nasal cavities**.
- The midline **vomer** articulates with the perpendicular plate of the **ethmoid** and the **cartilaginous septum** to form the **nasal septum**.
- The **zygomatic bone** articulates with the **frontal bone** and **maxillae** to form the cheekbone. The small **nasal bones** provide the upper margin of the nasal cavity.
- The **ethmoid bone** serves as the core of the skull and face, with the prominent **crista galli** protruding into the **cranium** and the **perpendicular plate** dividing the nasal cavities.
- The **frontal, parietal, temporal**, and **occipital** bones of the skull overlie the lobes of the brain of the same names.
- The **sphenoid bone** has a marked presence within the braincase, with the prominent **greater** and **lesser wings** of the sphenoid being found lateral to the **corpus**. The **hypophyseal fossa** houses the pituitary gland. The **clivus** joins the **occipital** bone near the **foramen magnum**.
- The **squamous portion of the temporal bone** includes the roof of the **external auditory meatus**. The zygomatic process articulates with the temporal process of the zygomatic bone to form the **zygomatic arch**. The **mandibular fossa** is the temporal bone component of the temporomandibular joint.
- The **styloid process** of the temporal bone is medial to the mastoid process. The **petrous portion** includes the cochlea and semicircular canals in a living person. The **mastoid portion** makes up the posterior part of the temporal bone. The **mastoid process** is found in the posterior temporal bone.

 ANAQUEST LESSON ▶

Dentition

The teeth are vital components of the speech mechanism. Housed within the alveoli of the maxillae and mandible, teeth provide the mechanism for mastication, as well as articulatory surfaces for several speech sounds.

Before we discuss the specific teeth, let us begin with an orientation to the dental arch itself. The upper and lower dental arches contain equal numbers of teeth of four types: incisors, cuspids, bicuspids, and molars. It is convenient to think of half-arches, knowing that left and right sides will have equal distribution of teeth (Figure 6–23).

Generally, teeth in the upper arch are larger than those in the lower arch, and the upper arch typically overlaps the lower arch in front. Each tooth has a **root**, hidden beneath the protective **gingiva** or gum line (Figure 6–24). The **crown** is the visible one third of the tooth, and the juncture of the crown and root is termed the **neck**. The surface of the crown is composed of dental **enamel**, an extremely hard surface that overlies the **dentin**, or ivory, of the tooth. At the heart of the tooth is the **pulp**, in which the nerve supplying the tooth resides. The tooth is held in its socket by **cementum**, which is

gingival: L., gingiva, gum

dentin: L., dens, tooth

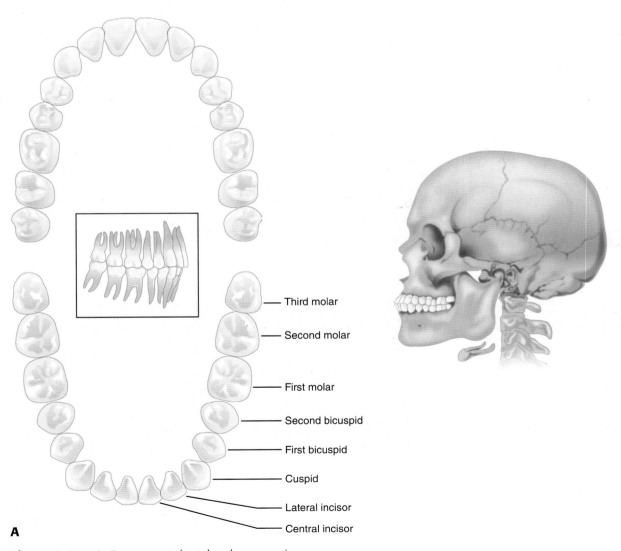

- Third molar
- Second molar
- First molar
- Second bicuspid
- First bicuspid
- Cuspid
- Lateral incisor
- Central incisor

A

Figure 6–23. A. Permanent dental arches. *continues*

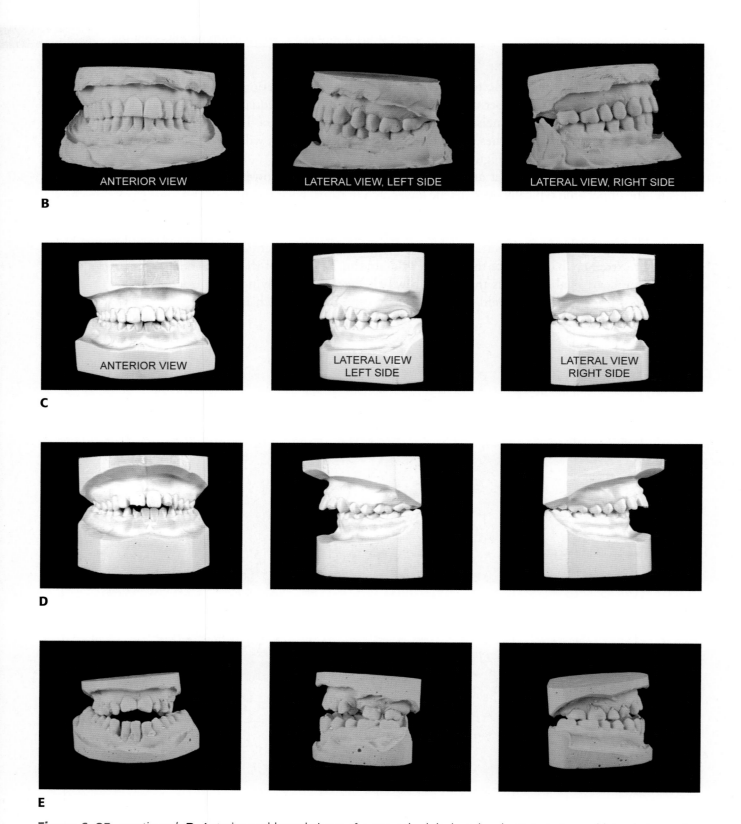

Figure 6–23. *continued* **B.** Anterior and lateral views of a normal adult dental arch. **C.** Anterior and lateral views of the deciduous dental arch. **D.** The dental arch of a child with significant oromyofunctional disorder. Note the marked labioversion of the incisors. **E.** The deciduous dental arch of a child with significant oromyofunctional disorder. Note significant cross-bite, open bite, and malocclusion. *Source:* From Seikel/Drumright/King. *Anatomy & Physiology for Speech, Language, and Hearing, 5th Ed.* ©Cengage, Inc. Reproduced by permission.

a thin layer of bone. Teeth shift as a result of pressures (such as the forces accompanying tongue thrust), and the cementum develops as a result of those pressures to ensure that the tooth remains firmly in its socket.

Five surfaces are important when discussing teeth. To understand the terminology, you need to alter your thinking about the dental arch a bit. Examine Figure 6–25 and you can see that the center of the dental arch is considered the point between the two central incisors, in front. Follow the

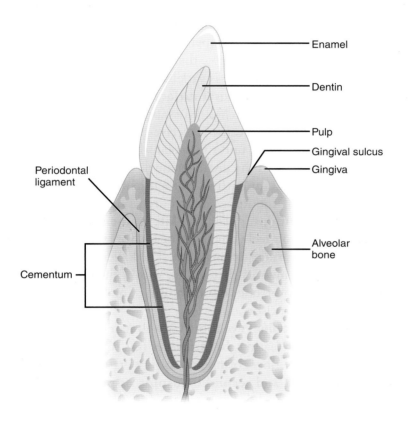

Figure 6–24. Components of a tooth. *Source:* From Seikel/Drumright/King. *Anatomy & Physiology for Speech, Language, and Hearing, 5th Ed.* ©Cengage, Inc. Reproduced by permission.

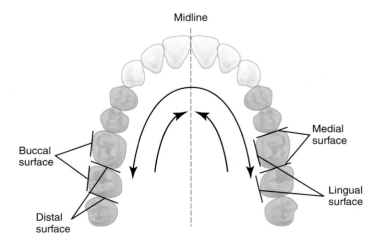

Figure 6–25. Surface referents of teeth and the dental arch. *Source:* From Seikel/Drumright/King. *Anatomy & Physiology for Speech, Language, and Hearing, 5th Ed.* ©Cengage, Inc. Reproduced by permission.

arch around toward the molars in back, and you have traced a path distal to those incisors. That is, *medial* refers to movement along the arch toward the midline between the central incisors, whereas *distal* refers to movement along the arch away from that midpoint. So the **medial surface** (or **mesial**) of any tooth is the surface looking along the arch toward the midpoint between the central incisors. The **distal surface** is the surface of any tooth that is farthest from that midline point. Every tooth has a medial and a distal surface. Table 6–2 provides descriptions of terms related to dentition.

The **buccal surface** of a tooth is that which could come in contact with the **buccal** wall (cheek), and the **lingual surface** is the surface facing the tongue. The **labial surface** is the superficial surface of the incisors, as they would be in contact with the lips (note that buccal and labial have a great deal of overlap, since the buccal surface is variable based upon the opening of the mouth at any moment). The **occlusal surface** is the contact surface between teeth of the upper and lower arches. Not surprisingly, the thickest enamel overlies the occlusal surface, because it receives the most abrasion. However, the habit of chewing ice can undo this plan of nature causing premature **attrition** or wearing away of the dental enamel.

Incisors are designed for cutting, as their name implies (Figure 6–26). The **central incisors** of the upper dental arch present a large, spade-like surface with a thin cutting surface. The **lateral incisors** present a smaller but similar surface. If you feel your superior incisors with your tongue, you should feel a prominent ridge or **cingulum**. The lower incisors are markedly smaller than the upper incisors that resting within the upper arch, and you must slightly open and protrude your mandible to make contact between the occlusal surfaces of the incisors.

The **cuspid** (also **canine**, **eye tooth**) is well named. It has a single cusp or point that is used for tearing. In carnivores this tooth is particularly well suited for separating the fibers of muscle to support meat eating. Lateral to the cuspids are the **first** and **second bicuspids** or **premolars**. These teeth have two cusps on the occlusal surface that are absent in the deciduous dental arch.

Molars are large teeth with great occlusal surfaces designed to grind material, and their placement in the posterior arch capitalizes on the significant force available in the muscles of mastication. This mix of cutting teeth (incisors, cuspids, and bicuspids) and grinding teeth (molars) is just right for omnivorous humans: We can eat virtually anything.

There are three molars in each half of the adult dental arch. The medialmost **first molar** is the largest of the group, with the **second** and **third molars** descending in size. The first molar has four cusps, the second molar may have three or four, and the third molar has three. The third molar is sometimes known as the **wisdom tooth**, often erupting well into adulthood. The third molar is very likely a safeguard against losing teeth. In days before dental hygiene, it was not uncommon to lose many teeth to **caries**. A late-emerging set of molars, useful for grinding grain and pulverizing fibers, would have been an ideal item to extend the life of our ancestors. Now those wisdom teeth seem less "wise," as they tend to crowd the other teeth and

buccal: L., bucca, cheek

labial surface: the surface of a tooth that could readily come in contact with the lips

incisor: L., cutter; referring to either lateral or central incisors of the upper or lower dental arch

cingulum: L., girdle

cuspid: L., cuspis, point

canine: L., caninus, related to dog

molars: L., molaris, grinding; referring to the posterior six teeth in either upper or lower dental arch

Table 6–2

Terms Related to Dentition	
Surfaces	
Medial/mesial	Surface of an individual tooth closest to midline point on arch between central incisors
Distal	Surface of an individual tooth farthest from midline point on arch between central incisors
Buccal	Surface of a tooth that could come in contact with the buccal wall
Lingual	Surface of a tooth that could come in contact with the tongue
Occlusal	The contact surface between teeth of the upper and lower arches
Development	
Deciduous tooth eruption	Eruption of deciduous (temporary) dentition
Permanent tooth eruption	Eruption of permanent dentition
Intraosseous eruption	Eruption of teeth through the alveolar process
Clinical eruption	Eruption of teeth into the oral cavity
Successional teeth	Teeth that replace deciduous teeth
Superadded teeth	Teeth in the adult arch not present within the deciduous arch
Supernumerary	Teeth in excess of the normal number for an arch
Dental Occlusion	
Overjet	Normal projection of upper incisors beyond lower incisors in transverse plane
Overbite	Normal overlap of upper incisors relative to lower incisors
Class I occlusal relationship	Relationship between upper and lower teeth in which the first molar of the mandibular arch is one-half tooth advanced of the maxillary molar
Class I malocclusion	Occlusal relationship in which there is normal orientation of the molars, but an abnormal orientation of the incisors
Class II malocclusion	Relationship of upper and lower arches in which the first mandibular molars are retracted at least one tooth from the first maxillary molars
Class III malocclusion	Relationship of upper and lower arches in which the first mandibular molar is advanced more than one tooth beyond the first maxillary molar
Relative micrognathia	Condition in which mandible is small in relation to the maxillae
Axial Orientation	
Torsiversion	Condition in which an individual tooth is rotated or twisted on its long axis
Labioversion	Condition in which an individual tooth tilts toward the lips
Linguaversion	Condition in which an individual tooth tilts toward the tongue
Buccoversion	Condition in which an individual tooth tilts toward the cheek
Distoversion	Condition in which an individual tooth tilts away from midline of dental arch
Mesioversion	Condition in which an individual tooth tilts toward the midline of the dental arch
Infraversion	Condition in which a tooth is inadequately erupted
Supraversion	Condition in which a tooth protrudes excessively into the oral cavity, causing inadequate occlusion of other dentition
Persistent open bite	Condition in which the front teeth do not occlude because of excessive eruption of posterior teeth
Persistent closed bite	Condition in which the posterior teeth do not occlude because of excessive eruption of anterior dentition

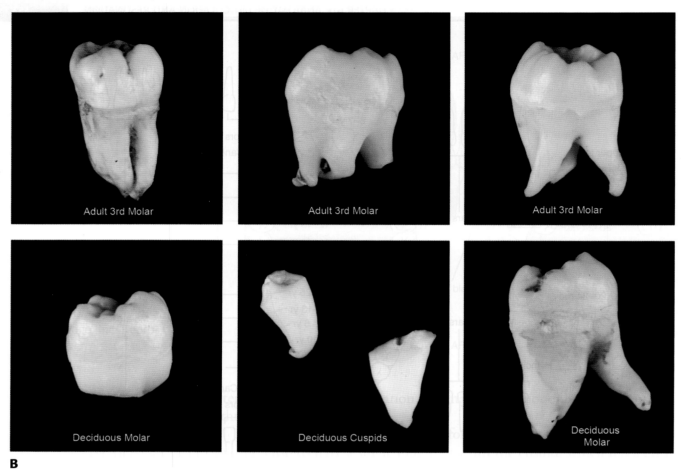

Adult 3rd Molar   Adult 3rd Molar   Adult 3rd Molar

Deciduous Molar   Deciduous Cuspids   Deciduous Molar

B

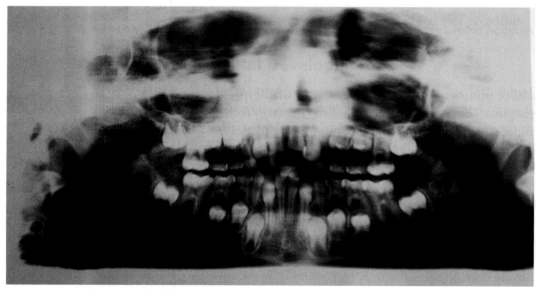

C

Figure 6–27. *continued* **B.** Individual deciduous and permanent teeth: *Top row:* adults 3rd molars; *Bottom, left to right:* deciduous molar, deciduous cuspids, deciduous molar. **C.** Pantomagraph of mixed dentition. Note the presence of unerupted permanent teeth within the maxilla and mandible. Photograph courtesy of Dr. P. Chad Ellis, D.D.S. *Source:* From Seikel/Drumright/King. *Anatomy & Physiology for Speech, Language, and Hearing, 5th Ed.* ©Cengage, Inc. Reproduced by permission.

Table 6–3

Timeline for Eruption of Mandibular and Maxillary Dentition			
Earliest Age of Expected Eruption	Type of Dentition	Mandibular Dentition	Maxillary Dentition
5 mo.	Deciduous	Central incisors	
6 mo.	Deciduous		Central incisors
7 mo.	Deciduous	Lateral incisors	
8 mo.	Deciduous		Lateral incisors
10 mo.	Deciduous	First molars	
16 mo.	Deciduous	Cuspids	Cuspids
20 mo.	Deciduous	Second molars	
36 mo.			Second molars
6 yrs.	Permanent	Central incisors First molars	First molars
7 yrs.	Permanent	Lateral incisors	Central incisors
8 yrs.	Permanent		Lateral incisors
9 yrs.	Permanent	Cuspids	
10 yrs.	Permanent	First bicuspids	First bicuspids Second bicuspids
11 yrs.	Permanent	Second bicuspids	Cuspids
12 yrs.	Permanent	Second molars	Second molars
17 yrs.	Permanent	Third molars	Third molars

Source: Based on data of Behrman and Vaughan (1987).

Dental Occlusion

The primary purpose of dentition is mastication, and this fact makes the orientation of teeth of the utmost importance. **Occlusion** is the process of bringing the upper and lower teeth into contact, and proper occlusion is essential for successful mastication. Clearly, if the upper molars do not make contact with the lower molars, no grinding will occur. We discuss the orientation of the upper and lower dental arches, as well as orientation that the individual teeth can take within the arches, later in this chapter. These terms of orientation will serve you well as you prepare for your clinical work, because they are central to the oral-peripheral examination of teeth.

To discuss this orientation, first examine your own dental arch relationship. Lightly tap your molars, and then bite down lightly and leave them occluded. This sets the orientation of the arches. With your teeth making contact in this manner, open your lips so that you can see the front teeth while looking in a mirror. If you have a **Class I occlusal relationship** between your upper and lower teeth, the first molar of the mandibular arch is one-half tooth advanced of the maxillary molar. Your upper incisors project beyond the lower incisors vertically by a few millimeters (termed **overjet**), and the upper incisors naturally hide the lower incisors (termed **overbite**) so that only a little of the lower teeth show. This Class I occlusion (also known as **neutroclusion**) (Figure 6–28) is considered the normal relationship between the molars of the dental arches.

In **Class II malocclusion**, the first mandibular molars are retracted at least one tooth from the first maxillary molars. This is sometimes the product of **relative micrognathia**, a condition in which the mandible is small in relation to the maxillae (Figure 6–29).

A **Class III malocclusion** is identified if the first mandibular molar is advanced farther than one tooth beyond the first maxillary molar. Thus, in Class II malocclusion the mandible is retracted, whereas in Class III the mandible is protruded. There is a **Class I malocclusion** as well. This is

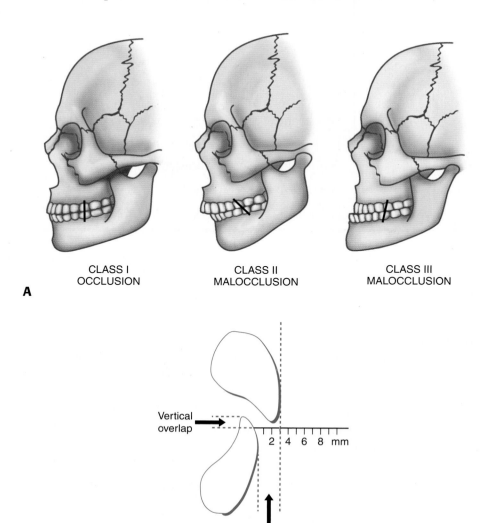

CLASS I
OCCLUSION

CLASS II
MALOCCLUSION

CLASS III
MALOCCLUSION

A

Vertical overlap

2 4 6 8 mm

Horizontal overlap

B

Figure 6–28. A. Types of malocclusion. **B.** Normal occlusal relationship between upper and lower central incisors. *Source:* From Seikel/Drumright/King. *Anatomy & Physiology for Speech, Language, and Hearing, 5th Ed.* ©Cengage, Inc. Reproduced by permission.

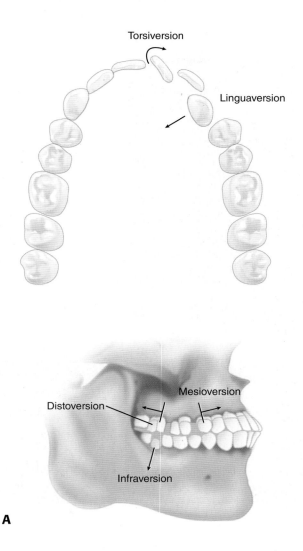

Figure 6–29. A. Graphic representation of torsiversion, linguaversion, infraversion, distoversion, and mesioversion. *continues*

Dental Anomalies

There are numerous developmental dental anomalies. Children may be born with **supernumerary teeth** (teeth in addition to the normal number), or teeth may be smaller than appropriate for the dental arch (**microdontia**). Teeth may **fuse** together at the root or crown. In addition to this, enamel may be extremely thin or even missing from the surface of the tooth (**amelogenesis imperfecta**), or the enamel may be stained by use of the antibiotic tetracycline or fluoride.

---

defined as an occlusion in which there is normal orientation of the molars, but an abnormal orientation of the incisors.

Individual teeth may be misaligned as well. If a tooth is rotated or twisted on its long axis, it has undergone **torsiversion**. If it tilts toward the lips, it is referred to as **labioverted** whereas tilting toward the tongue is **linguaverted** (see Figure 6–29A). When molars tilt toward the cheeks, it is called **buccoversion**. A tooth that tilts away from the midline along the arch is said to be **distoverted**, whereas one tilting toward that midline between

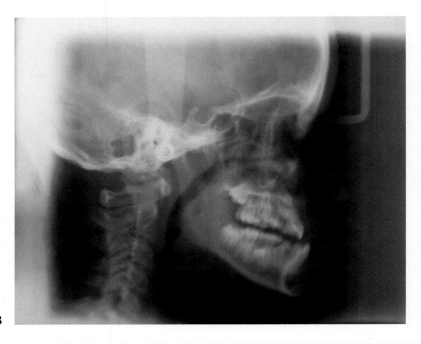

B

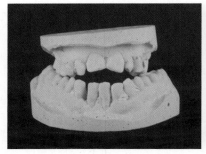 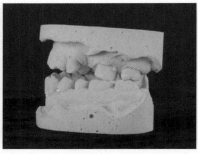 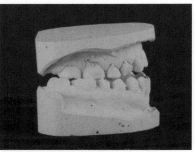

C

Figure 6–29. *continued* **B.** Radiograph of prognathic mandible that was later surgically corrected. **C.** Dental impression of young adult with significant oromyofunctional disorder, revealing extreme palatal arch, distoversion, torsiversion, linguaversion, and labioversion secondary to tongue thrust. Note the evidence of gingival lesion (gum recession) secondary to retained tongue thrust. Photography courtesy of Tanis Trenka. *Source:* From Seikel/Drumright/King. *Anatomy & Physiology for Speech, Language, and Hearing, 5th Ed.* ©Cengage, Inc. Reproduced by permission.

the two central incisors is **mesioverted**. When a tooth does not erupt sufficiently to make occlusal contact with its pair in the opposite arch, it is said to be **infraverted**; the tooth that erupts too far is said to be **supraverted**. In some cases, the front teeth may not demonstrate the proper occlusion because teeth in the posterior arch prohibit anterior contact, a condition that is termed **persistent open bite**. If supraversion prohibits the posterior teeth from occlusion, it is called **persistent closed bite**. As you examine the dental orientation of the photographs in Figure 6–29B and 6–29C, attend closely to the variety of misalignments in this dentition. The cast in Figure 6–29C was made from the teeth of a young person who had low muscle tone as well as marked and uncorrected tongue thrust.

Supernumerary Teeth

Supernumerary teeth arise from a developmental anomaly in which the embryonic dental lamina produces excessive numbers of tooth buds. When this occurs, the individual is born with more teeth than predicted, often resulting in "twinning" of incisors. Following is a report from J. M. Harris, DDS, of a child he saw in his dental practice in Idaho Falls, Idaho.

An eight-year-old girl was brought to Dr. Harris's clinic with the complaint that one of her deciduous teeth needed to be extracted due to her age. Dr. Harris performed panelipse radiography to verify that the permanent teeth were present prior to the extraction, but the radiograph revealed supernumerary teeth in the left mandibular arch in the bicuspid region.

Extraction of the decayed deciduous tooth revealed a pocket of 15 supernumerary teeth: Some were simply tooth buds, but some had developed small roots and looked like fully formed molars. In an arch built ultimately for 16 teeth, that would be a significant addition!

The cluster was removed, Gelfoam® was placed in the cavity, and sutures closed the space. There were no further complications.

✓ *To summarize:*

- The **teeth** are housed within the **alveoli** of the **maxillae** and **mandible** and consist of **incisors, cuspids, bicuspids**, and **molars**.

- Each tooth has a **root** and **crown**, with the surface of the crown composed of **enamel** overlying **dentin**.

- Each tooth has a **medial, distal, lingual, buccal** (or labial), and **occlusal** surface; the occlusal surface reflects the function of the teeth in the omnivorous human dental arch.

- **Clinical eruption** of the **deciduous** arch begins between 5 and 9 months of age, while the **permanent arch** emerges between 6 and 9 years.

- **Class I occlusion** refers to normal orientation of mandible and maxillae, while **Class II malocclusion** refers to a relatively retracted mandible. **Class III malocclusion** refers to a relatively protruded mandible.

- Individual teeth may have aberrant orientation within the alveolus, including buccoversion, **torsiversion, labioversion, linguaversion, distoversion**, and **mesioversion**.

- Inadequately erupted or hypererupted teeth are referred to as **infraverted** and **supraverted**.

Cavities of the Articulatory System

ANAQUEST LESSON ▶

We mentioned that the source-filter theory depends on cavities to shape the acoustic output. Before we show you the muscles associated with articulation, let us discuss how the cavities are shaped by the movements of those muscles.

These are the oral, buccal, pharyngeal(including oropharyngeal, nasopharyngeal, and laryngopharyngeal cavities), and nasal cavities (Figure 6–30).

The **oral cavity** is the most significant cavity of the speech mechanism, as it undergoes the most change during the speech act. Its shape can be altered by the movement of the tongue or mandible.

The oral cavity extends from the oral opening, or mouth, in front to the faucial pillars in back. The oral opening is strongly involved in articulation, being the point of exit of sound for all orally emitted phonemes (i.e., all sounds except those emitted nasally). The lips of the mouth are quite important for the articulation of many consonants and vowels.

This is a good opportunity to take a guided tour of your own mouth (Figure 6–31). Palpate the roof of your mouth (you can use your tongue to feel this if you wish). The hard roof of your mouth is the **hard palate**. The prominent ridges running laterally are the **rugae**, potentially useful structures in the formation of the bolus of food during deglutition and serving as a landmark in articulation. The **median raphe** divides the hard palate into two equal halves.

As you run your tongue back along the roof of your mouth, you can feel the point at which the hard palate suddenly becomes soft. This is the juncture of the hard and soft palates, and the soft portion is the **soft palate** or **velum**,

rugae: Gr., creases

velum: L., veil

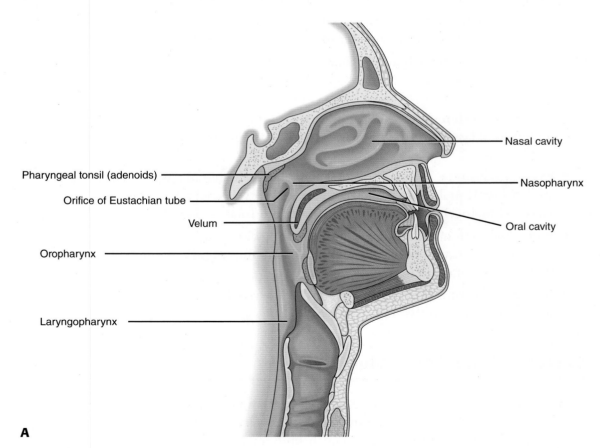

Nasal cavity

Pharyngeal tonsil (adenoids)

Orifice of Eustachian tube

Nasopharynx

Velum

Oral cavity

Oropharynx

Laryngopharynx

A

Figure 6–30. A. Oral, nasal, and pharyngeal cavities. *continues*

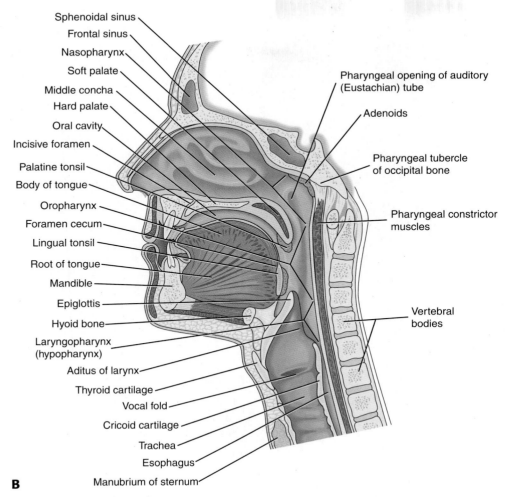

Sphenoidal sinus
Frontal sinus
Nasopharynx
Soft palate
Middle concha
Hard palate
Oral cavity
Incisive foramen
Palatine tonsil
Body of tongue
Oropharynx
Foramen cecum
Lingual tonsil
Root of tongue
Mandible
Epiglottis
Hyoid bone
Laryngopharynx
(hypopharynx)
Aditus of larynx
Thyroid cartilage
Vocal fold
Cricoid cartilage
Trachea
Esophagus
Manubrium of sternum

Pharyngeal opening of auditory
(Eustachian) tube
Adenoids
Pharyngeal tubercle
of occipital bone
Pharyngeal constrictor
muscles
Vertebral
bodies

B

Figure 6–30. *continued* **B.** Detail of structures and cavities. *Source:* From Seikel/ Drumright/King. *Anatomy & Physiology for Speech, Language, and Hearing, 5th Ed.* ©Cengage, Inc. Reproduced by permission.

with the **uvula** marking the terminus of the velum. The velum is the movable muscle mass separating the oral and nasal cavities (or more technically, the oropharynx and nasopharynx, as you will soon see). The velum is attached in front to the palatine bone (not shown) and is thus a muscular extension of the hard palate.

On either side of the soft palate and continuous with it are two prominent bands of tissue. These are the **anterior** and **posterior faucial pillars**, and they mark the posterior margin of the oral cavity. The teeth and alveolar ridge of the maxillae make up the lateral margins of the oral cavity. The tongue occupies most of the lower mouth.

Between the anterior and posterior faucial pillars you may see the **palatine tonsils**. These masses of lymphoid tissue are situated between the pillars on either side and even invade the lateral undersurface of the soft palate. Medial to these tonsils, on the surface of the tongue, are the lingual tonsils (not shown).

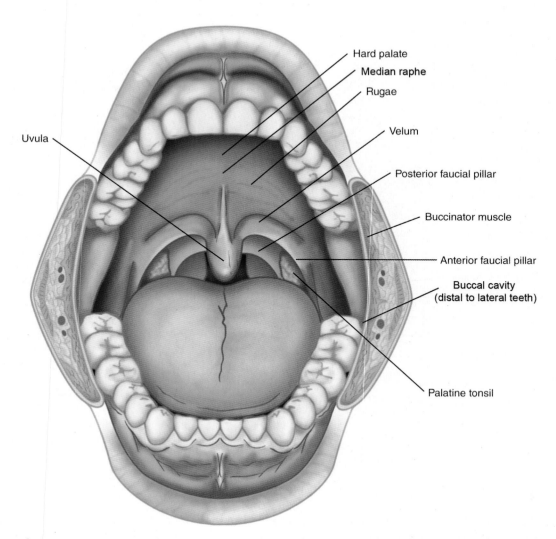

Figure 6–31. Anterior view of the oral cavity. *Source:* From Seikel/Drumright/King. *Anatomy & Physiology for Speech, Language, and Hearing, 5th Ed.* ©Cengage, Inc. Reproduced by permission.

The **buccal cavity** lies lateral to the oral cavity, composed of the space between the posterior teeth and the cheeks of the face. It is bounded by the cheeks laterally, the lips in front, and the teeth medially. The posterior margin is at the third molar. The buccal cavity plays a role in oral resonance when the mandible is depressed to expose it, is involved in high-pressure consonant production, and is the source of the distortion heard in the misarticulation known as the lateral /s/.

The **pharyngeal cavity**, or **pharynx** (Figure 6–30A), is broken into three logically named regions. You can envision the pharynx as a tube approximately 12 cm in length, extending from the vocal folds below to the region behind the nasal cavities above. This tube is lined with muscle capable of constricting the size of the tube to facilitate deglutition, and this musculature plays an important role in effecting the closure of the **velopharyngeal port**, the opening between the oropharynx and the nasopharynx.

The **oropharynx** is the portion of the pharynx immediately posterior to the fauces, bounded above by the velum. The lower boundary of the oropharynx is the hyoid bone, which marks the upper boundary of the laryngopharynx. The **laryngopharynx** (or **hypopharynx**) is bounded anteriorly by the epiglottis and inferiorly by the esophagus.

The third pharyngeal space is the **nasopharynx**, the space above the soft palate, bounded posteriorly by the pharyngeal protuberance of the occipital bone and by the nasal **choanae** in front. The lateral nasopharyngeal wall contains the **orifice** of the **auditory tube** (also known as the **Eustachian tube**, named after Bortolomeo Eustachi, a 16th-century anatomist; see Figures 6–30 and 6–32).

choanae: Gr., funnel; posterior entry of the nasal cavities

Although minute, the auditory tube serves an extremely important function in that it provides a means of aerating the middle ear cavity. The nasopharynx is level with the ears, so that the tube connecting the nasopharynx with the middle ear space must course slightly up, back, and out to reach that cavity. The auditory tube is actively opened through contraction of the tensor veli palatini muscle. The bulge of tissue partially encircling the orifice of the auditory tube is the **torus tubarius**, and the ridge of tissue coursing down from the orifice is the **salpingopharyngeal fold**—the salpingopharyngeus muscle covered with mucous membrane.

Also within the nasopharynx are the **pharyngeal tonsils** (also known as **adenoids**). This mass of lymphoid tissue is typically found to arise from the base of the posterior nasopharynx. By virtue of its proximity to the velopharyngeal port, the tissue of the pharyngeal tonsil may provide support for velar

Palpation of the Oral Cavity

This palpation exercise is best performed with one of your friends and requires aseptic procedures. You will want to perform it under the guidance of your instructor, as this will be a procedure that will carry into the oral peripheral examination in your clinical practice. A flashlight will help you identify structures.

Look inside your friend's open mouth. Ensure that your nondominant hand (e.g., left hand if you are right-handed) is the only hand that holds the flashlight, as the other hand is gloved and must not touch anything but your friend. Ask your friend to say *ah* and watch the velum in back elevate. Look for presence or absence of the palatine tonsils between the faucial pillars. Shine the light on the hard palate and note the median **raphe** and rugae. Now palpate both these structures, running your finger back along both sides of the median raphe of

the hard palate. Palpate the margin of the hard and soft palate, being sensitive to the fact that this may elicit a gag reflex in some people. As you palpate the hard palate, be sensitive to the potential presence of occult (hidden, submucous) clefts of the hard palate.

Have your friend bite lightly on the molars and hold the teeth closed but lips open for an /i/ vowel. With the gloved finger, palpate the lateral margins of the teeth and gums. With a tongue depressor, move the cheeks away from the teeth and examine the relationship between the upper and lower teeth for occlusion.

Gently pull down the lower lip and examine the labial frenulum. Ask your friend to open the mouth and elevate the tongue so you can examine the lingual frenulum.

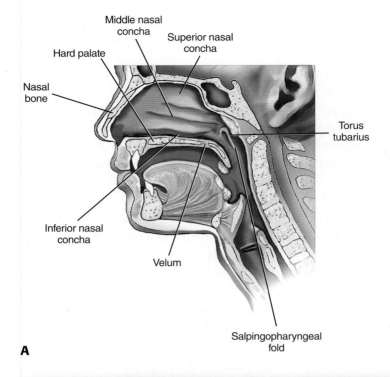

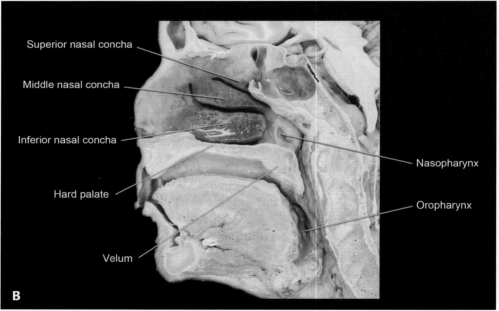

Figure 6–32. A. Drawing of nasal cavity and nasopharynx. **B.** Photograph of sagittal section through nasal cavity and nasopharynx. *Source:* From Seikel/Drumright/King. *Anatomy & Physiology for Speech, Language, and Hearing, 5th Ed.* ©Cengage, Inc. Reproduced by permission.

function. Removal of the adenoids from children with short or hypotrophied soft palates may result in persistent hypernasality.

The final cavities of concern to articulation are the **nasal cavities** (see Figure 6–32). The nasal cavities are produced by the paired maxillae, palatine, and nasal bones, and are divided by the nasal septum, made up of the singular vomer bone, perpendicular plate of the ethmoid, and the cartilaginous septum. The superior border is made up of the nasal bones, while the lateral boundaries are the frontal process of the maxillae. The inferior border is made up of the paired palatine processes of the maxillae, while the anterior border are the nares. The posterior border is the nasal choanae (Table 6–4). The nasal cavities and turbinates are covered with mucous membrane endowed with beating and secreting epithelia, as well as a rich vascular supply. The moisture inherent in the nasal mucosa, combined with the vascular supply of the nasal tissue, humidifies and warms the air as it enters the passageway. Beating epithelia propel encapsulated pollutants toward the nasopharynx,

Table 6–4

Cavities of the Articulatory System

Cavity	Superior Boundary	Inferior Boundary	Anterior Boundary	Posterior Boundary
Oral cavity	Hard palate	Floor of mouth	Lips	Faucial pillars and depressed velum
Buccal cavity	Cheeks	Floor of mouth	Lips	Third molars and pterygomandibular raphe
Pharyngeal cavity	Pharyngeal protruberance of occipital bone	Esophagus	Nasal choanae in nasopharynx Fauces in oropharynx Epiglottis in laryngopharynx	Posterior pharyngeal wall
Oropharynx	Velum	Hyoid bone	Fauces	Posterior pharyngeal wall
Laryngopharynx	Hyoid bone	Esophagus	Epiglottis	Posterior pharyngeal wall
Nasopharynx	Pharyngeal protuberance of occipital bone	Velum	Nasal choanae	Posterior pharyngeal wall
Nasal cavities	Nasal bones	Palatine processes of maxillae; horizontal processes of palatine bones	Nares	nasal choanae

Auditory Tube Development

The Eustachian tube is the communicative port between the nasopharynx and middle ear cavity. It is opened during deglutition and yawning and provides a means of aeration of the middle ear cavity. In the adult, the auditory tube courses down at an angle of about 45°. In the infant, the tube is more horizontal, with the shift in the angle of descent brought about by head growth. It is felt that this horizontal course in the infant contributes to middle ear disease, with the assumption being that liquids and bacteria have a low-resistance path to the middle ear from the nasopharynx of an infant being bottle-fed in the supine position.

from whence they slowly work their way toward the esophagus, to be swallowed (a much better fate than being deposited in the lungs).

The **nares** or nostrils mark the anterior boundaries of the nasal cavities, while the **nasal choanae** are the posterior portals connecting the nasopharynx and nasal cavities. The floor of the nasal cavity is the hard palate of the oral cavity, specifically the palatine processes of the maxillae and horizontal plates of the palatine bones.

✓ To summarize:

- The **cavities** of the articulatory system can be likened to a series of linked tubes.
- The most posterior of the tubes is the vertically directed **pharynx**, made up of the **laryngopharynx**, **oropharynx**, and **nasopharynx**.
- The horizontally coursing tube representing the nasal cavities arises from the nasopharynx, with the nasal and nasopharyngeal regions entirely separated from the oral cavity by elevation of the **soft palate**.
- The large tube representing the **oral cavity** is flanked by the small **buccal cavities**.
- The shape and size of the oral cavity is altered through movements of the tongue and mandible, and the nasal cavity may be coupled with the oral/pharyngeal cavities by means of the **velum**.

Let us examine the muscles involved in the articulatory system. Appendix E may assist you in your study of these muscles.

ANAQUEST LESSON

Muscles of the Face and Mouth

The articulatory system is dominated by three significant structures: the lips, the tongue, and the velum. Movement of the lips for speech is a product of the muscles of the face, while the tongue capitalizes on its own musculature and that of the mandible and hyoid for its movement. The muscles of the velum elevate that structure to completely separate the oral and nasal regions. Table 6–5 may assist you in organizing the muscles of the face and mouth, while Figure 6–33 will help you recognize their functions.

Table 6–5

Muscles of Articulation	
Muscles of the Face	
Orbicularis oris	Levator anguli oris
Risorius	Zygomatic major
Buccinator	Depressor labii inferioris
Levator labii superioris	Depressor anguli oris
Zygomatic minor	Mentalis
Levator labii superioris alaeque nasi	Platysma
Intrinsic Tongue Muscles	
Superior longitudinal	
Inferior longitudinal	
Transverse	
Vertical	
Extrinsic Tongue Muscles	
Genioglossus	
Hyoglossus	
Styloglossus	
Chondroglossus	
Palatoglossus	
Mandibular Elevators and Depressors	
Masseter	Digastricus muscle
Temporalis muscle	Mylohyoid muscle
Medial pterygoid muscle	Geniohyoid muscle
Lateral pterygoid muscle	Platysma
Muscles of the Velum	
Levator veli palatini	
Musculus uvulae	
Tensor veli palatini	
Palatoglossus	
Palatopharyngeus	
Pharyngeal Musculature	
Superior pharyngeal constrictor	Thyropharyngeus muscle
Middle pharyngeal constrictor	Salpingopharyngeus muscle
Inferior pharyngeal constrictor	Stylopharyngeus muscle
Cricopharyngeal muscle	

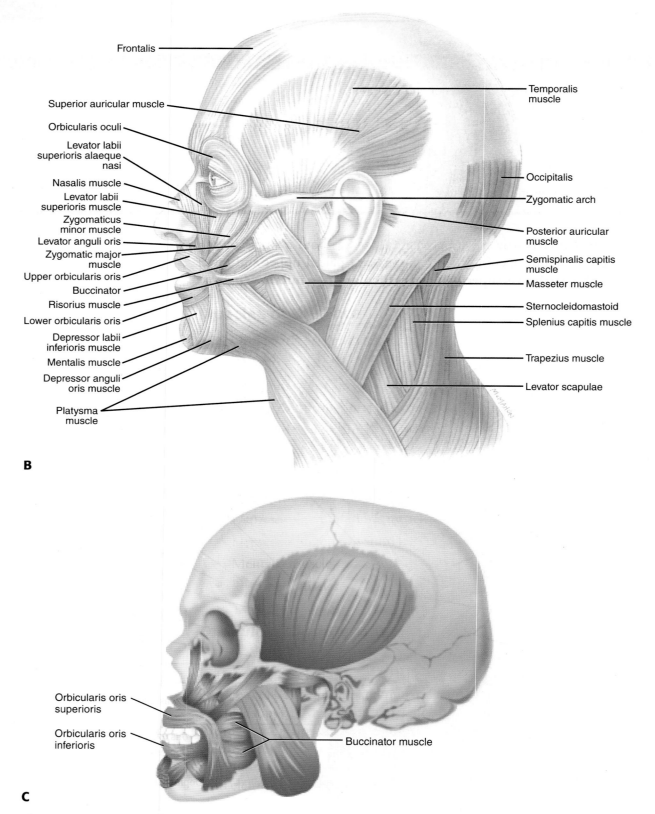

B

Frontalis

Temporalis muscle

Superior auricular muscle

Orbicularis oculi

Levator labii superioris alaeque nasi

Nasalis muscle

Levator labii superioris muscle

Zygomaticus minor muscle

Levator anguli oris

Zygomatic major muscle

Upper orbicularis oris

Buccinator

Risorius muscle

Lower orbicularis oris

Depressor labii inferioris muscle

Mentalis muscle

Depressor anguli oris muscle

Platysma muscle

Occipitalis

Zygomatic arch

Posterior auricular muscle

Semispinalis capitis muscle

Masseter muscle

Sternocleidomastoid

Splenius capitis muscle

Trapezius muscle

Levator scapulae

C

Orbicularis oris superioris

Orbicularis oris inferioris

Buccinator muscle

Figure 6–34. *continued* **B.** The lateral view of facial muscles. **C.** The relationship among facial muscles and pharyngeal constrictor muscles. Note that the orbicularis oris are continuous with the buccinator muscle, and ultimately with the superior pharyngeal constrictor. *Source:* From Seikel/Drumright/King. *Anatomy & Physiology for Speech, Language, and Hearing, 5th Ed.* ©Cengage, Inc. Reproduced by permission.

will see in Chapter 7, there is ample evidence for *functional* differentiation of the upper and lower orbicularis oris. The upper and lower orbicularis oris act much like a drawstring to pull the lips closer together and effect a labial seal. The orbicularis oris is innervated by the mandibular marginal and lower buccal branches of the VII facial nerve.

The orbicularis oris serves as the point of insertion for many other muscles and interacts with the muscles of the face to produce the wide variety of facial gestures of which we are capable. The muscles inserting into the orbicularis oris have different effects, based on their course and point of insertion into the lips. The **risorius** and buccinator muscles insert into the corners of the mouth and retract the lips. The depressor labii inferioris depresses the lower lip, and the **levator** labii superioris, zygomaticus minor, and levator labii superioris alaeque nasi muscles elevate the upper lip. The zygomatic major muscle elevates and retracts the lips, whereas the depressor anguli oris depresses the corner of the mouth. The levator anguli oris pulls the corner of the mouth up and medially.

risorius: L., laughing; most superficial of the buccal muscles

levator: L., lifter

Risorius Muscle

It is evident from the course of the buccinator and risorius that they retract the corners of the mouth (see Figure 6–34). The buccinator is the dominant muscle of the cheeks. The **risorius muscle** is the most superficial of the pair, originating from the posterior region of the face along the fascia of the masseter muscle. The risorius is considerably smaller than the buccinator, coursing forward to insert into the corners of the mouth. The function of the risorius muscles is to retract the lips at the corners, facilitating smiling and grinning. Innervation of the risorius is by means of the buccal branch of the VII facial nerve.

Buccinator Muscle

The **buccinator muscle** ("bugler's muscle") lies deep to the risorius, following a parallel course. It originates at the pterygomandibular ligament, a tendinous slip running from the hamulus of the internal pterygoid plate of the sphenoid to the posterior mylohyoid line of the inner mandible. Fibers of the buccinator also arise from the posterior alveolar portion of the mandible and maxillae, while the posterior fibers appear to be continuous with those

Muscle:	Risorius
Origin:	Posterior region of the face along the fascia of the masseter
Course:	Forward
Insertion:	Orbicularis oris at the corners of mouth
Innervation:	Buccal branch of the VII facial nerve
Function:	Retracts lips at the corners

of the superior pharyngeal constrictor. The buccinator courses forward to insert into the upper and lower orbicularis oris.

The buccinator, like the risorius, is primarily involved in mastication. The buccinator is used to move food onto the grinding surfaces of the molars, and contraction of this muscle tends to constrict the oropharynx. The buccinator is innervated by the buccal branch of the VII facial nerve.

Levator Labii Superioris, Zygomatic Minor, and Levator Labii Superioris Alaeque Nasi Muscles

The levator labii superioris, zygomatic minor, and levator labii superioris alaeque nasi share a common insertion into the mid-lateral region of the upper lip, such that some anatomists refer to them as heads of the same muscle. The three hold the major responsibility for the elevation of the upper lip.

The medial-most **levator labii superioris alaeque nasi** courses nearly vertically along the lateral margin of the nose, arising from the frontal process of the maxilla. The intermediate **levator labii superioris** originates from the infraorbital margin of the maxilla, coursing down and in to the upper lip. The **zygomatic minor** begins its downward course from the facial surface of the zygomatic bone.

Muscle:	Buccinator
Origin:	Pterygomandibular ligament
Course:	Forward
Insertion:	Orbicularis oris at the corners of mouth
Innervation:	Buccal branch of the VII facial nerve
Function:	Moves food onto the grinding surfaces of the molars; constricts oropharynx

Muscle:	Levator labii superioris
Origin:	Infraorbital margin of the maxilla
Course:	Down and in to the upper lip
Insertion:	Mid-lateral region of the upper lip
Innervation:	Buccal branches of the VII facial nerve
Function:	Elevates the upper lip

Muscle:	Levator labii superioris alaequae nasi
Origin:	Frontal process of maxilla
Course:	Vertically along the lateral margin of the nose
Insertion:	Mid-lateral region of the upper lip
Innervation:	Buccal branches of the VII facial nerve
Function:	Elevates the upper lip

Together, these three muscles are the dominant forces in lip elevation. Working in conjunction, these muscles readily dilate the oral opening, and fibers from the levator labii superioris alaeque nasi that insert into the wing (ala) of the nostril flare the nasal opening. The levator labii superioris, zygomatic minor, and levator labii superioris alaeque nasi are innervated by the buccal branches of the VII facial nerve.

Levator Anguli Oris Muscle

The **levator anguli oris** arises from the canine fossa of the maxilla, coursing to insert into the upper and lower lips. This muscle is obscured by the levator labii superioris. The levator anguli oris draws the corner of the mouth up and medially. The levator anguli oris is innervated by the superior buccal branch of the VII facial nerve.

Zygomatic Major Muscle

The **zygomatic major muscle** (zygomaticus) arises lateral to the zygomatic minor on the zygomatic bone. It takes a more oblique course than the minor, inserting into the corner of the orbicularis oris. The zygomatic major elevates and retracts the angle of the mouth, as in the gesture of smiling.

Muscle:	Levator anguli oris
Origin:	Canine fossa of maxilla
Course:	Down
Insertion:	Corners of upper and lower lips
Innervation:	Superior buccal branches of VII facial nerve
Function:	Draws corner of mouth up and medially
Muscle:	Zygomatic major (zygomaticus)
Origin:	Lateral to the zygomatic minor on zygomatic bone
Course:	Obliquely down
Insertion:	Corner of the orbicularis oris
Innervation:	Buccal branches of the VII facial nerve
Function:	Elevates and retracts the angle of mouth
Muscle:	Zygomatic minor
Origin:	Facial surface of the zygomatic bone
Course:	Downward
Insertion:	Mid-lateral region of upper lip
Innervation:	Buccal branches of the VII facial nerve
Function:	Elevates the upper lip

The zygomatic major muscle is innervated by the buccal branches of the VII facial nerve.

Depressor Labii Inferioris Muscle

The **depressor labii inferioris** is the counterpart to the levator triad listed previously. It originates from the mandible at the oblique line, coursing up and in to insert into the lower lip. Contraction of the depressor labii inferioris dilates the orifice of the mouth by pulling the lips down and out. The depressor labii inferioris is innervated by the mandibular marginal branches of the VII facial nerve.

Depressor Anguli Oris Muscle

The **depressor anguli oris** (triangularis) originates along the lateral margins of the mandible on the oblique line. Its fanlike fibers converge on the orbicularis oris and upper lip at the corner. Contraction of the depressor anguli oris will depresses the corners of the mouth and, by virtue of attachment to upper lip, help compress the upper lip against the lower lip, as well as help produce a frown. The depressor anguli oris is innervated by the mandibular marginal branch of the VII facial nerve.

Mentalis Muscle

The **mentalis muscle** arises from the region of the incisive fossa of the mandible, coursing down to insert into the skin of the chin below. Contraction of the mentalis elevates and wrinkles the chin and pulls the lower lip out, as in pouting. The mentalis receives its innervation via the mandibular marginal branch of the VII facial nerve.

Muscle:	Depressor labii inferioris
Origin:	Mandible at the oblique line
Course:	Up and in to the lower lip
Insertion:	Lower lip
Innervation:	Mandibular marginal branch of the VII facial nerve
Function:	Dilates the orifice by pulling the lips down and out
Muscle:	Depressor anguli oris (triangularis)
Origin:	Lateral margins of the mandible on the oblique line
Course:	Fanlike upward
Insertion:	Orbicularis oris and upper lip corner
Innervation:	Mandibular branch of the VII facial nerve
Function:	Depresses corners of mouth and helps compress the upper lip against the lower lip

Muscle:	Mentalis
Origin:	Region of the incisive fossa of mandible
Course:	Down
Insertion:	Skin of the chin below
Innervation:	Mandibular marginal branch of the VII facial nerve
Function:	Elevates and wrinkles the chin and pulls the lower lip out

Muscle:	Platysma
Origin:	Fascia overlaying pectoralis major and deltoid
Course:	Up
Insertion:	Corner of the mouth, region below symphysis menti, lower margin of mandible, and skin near masseter
Innervation:	Cervical branch of the VII facial nerve
Function:	Depresses the mandible

Platysma Muscle

The **platysma** is more typically considered a muscle of the neck, but it is discussed here because of its function as a mandibular depressor. The platysma arises from the fascia overlying the pectoralis major and deltoid, coursing up to insert into the corner of the mouth, the region below the symphysis menti, and the lower margin of the mandible, fanning as well to insert into the skin near the masseter. The platysma is highly variable but assists in the depression of the mandible. The platysma is innervated by the cervical branch of the VII facial nerve.

platysma: Gr., plate

✓ To summarize:

- The muscles of **facial expression** are important for articulation involving the lips.

- Numerous muscles insert into the **orbicularis oris** inferior and superior muscles, providing a flexible system for lip **protrusion, closure, retraction, elevation,** and **depression**.

- The **risorius** and **buccinator** muscles assist in the retraction of the lips, as well as support entrapment of air within the oral cavity.

- The contraction of the **levator labii superioris, zygomatic minor,** and **levator labii superioris alaeque nasi** elevates the upper lip, and the contraction of the **depressor labii inferioris** depresses the lower lip.

- The contraction of the **zygomatic major** muscle elevates and retracts the angle of the mouth, while the **depressor labii inferioris** pulls the lips down and out.

- The **depressor anguli oris** muscle depresses the corner of the mouth, the **mentalis** muscle elevates and wrinkles the chin and pulls the lower lip out, and the **platysma** depresses the mandible.

ANAQUEST LESSON

Muscles of the Mouth

Musculature of the mouth is dominated by intrinsic and extrinsic muscles of the tongue, as well as those responsible for the elevation of the soft palate. The movement of the tongue is an interesting engineering feat, as you will see.

The Tongue

The tongue is a massive structure occupying the floor of the mouth. If you take a moment to examine Figure 6–35, you can get some notion of the magnitude of this organ. When people use the tongue as an expressive instrument, they protrude only a small portion of it, leaving the bulk of the tongue within the mouth. We divide the muscles of the tongue into intrinsic and extrinsic musculature, a division that proves to be both anatomical and functional. The extrinsic muscles tend to move the tongue into the general region desired, while the intrinsic muscles tend to provide the fine, graded control of the articulatory gesture. The tongue is primarily involved in mastication and deglutition, being responsible for the movement of food within the oral cavity to position it for chewing and to propel it backward for swallowing.

The tongue is divided longitudinally by the **median fibrous septum**, a dividing wall between right and left halves that serves as the point of origin for the transversus muscle of the tongue. The septum originates at the body of the hyoid bone via the hyoglossal membrane, forming the tongue attachment with the hyoid. The septum courses the length of the tongue.

It is useful to divide the tongue into regions as we discuss its characteristics. The superior surface is referred to as the **dorsum**, and the anterior-most portion is the **tip** or **apex**. The ventral surface of the tongue would be that underside of the tongue seen if you elevated your tongue to the roof of your mouth. On Figure 6–35 it is represented as the region beneath the tip. The

Figure 6–35. Demarcation of the regions of the tongue. *Source:* From Seikel/ Drumright/King. *Anatomy & Physiology for Speech, Language, and Hearing, 5th Ed.* ©Cengage, Inc. Reproduced by permission.

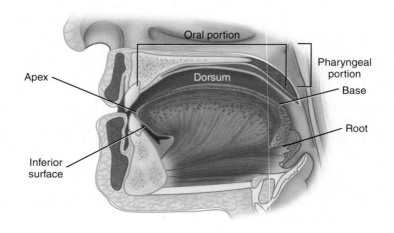

base of the tongue is the portion of the tongue that resides in the oropharynx (also known as the **pharyngeal portion**). The portion of the tongue surface within the oral cavity, referred to as the **oral** or **palatine surface**, makes up about two-thirds of the surface of the tongue. The other third of the tongue surface lies within the oropharynx and is referred to as the **pharyngeal surface**. The **root** has variable definition by anatomists. Some refer to the pharyngeal portion as the root and call the palatine surface the body, while others view the base of the tongue as the root, as we have indicated in Figure 6–35. Phoneticians use the palatine definition, such that "advancement of the root" results in "fronting" of a sound (D. Cooper, personal communication, January 22, 2013; Edmonson & Esling, 2006).

The mucous membrane covering the tongue dorsum has numerous landmarks (Figures 6–36 and 6–37). The prominent central or **median sulcus** divides the tongue into left and right sides. The dorsum of the posterior of the tongue is invested with **circumvallate (or vallate) papillae**, small, irregular prominences on the surface of the tongue. The **terminal sulcus** marks the posterior palatine surface, and the center of this groove is the **foramen cecum**, a deep recess in the tongue. **Foliate papillae** are found on the lateral posterior tongue, while **fungiform papillae** are predominantly on the anterior tip of the tongue.

Beneath the membranous lining of the pharyngeal surface of the tongue are **lingual tonsils**, groups of lymphoid tissue. Working in conjunction with the pharyngeal and palatine tonsils, the lingual tonsils form the final portion

papillae: L., nipple; small prominences on the tongue that hold taste sensors

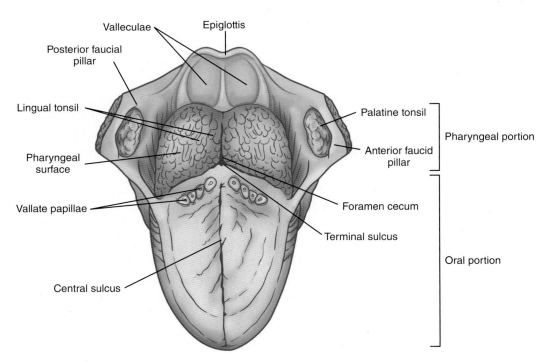

Figure 6–36. Landmarks of the tongue. *Source:* From Seikel/Drumright/King. *Anatomy & Physiology for Speech, Language, and Hearing, 5th Ed.* ©Cengage, Inc. Reproduced by permission.

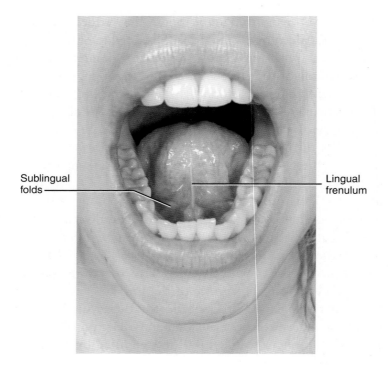

Sublingual folds

Lingual frenulum

Figure 6–37. Inferior surface of the tongue. *Source:* From Seikel/Drumright/King. *Anatomy & Physiology for Speech, Language, and Hearing, 5th Ed.* ©Cengage, Inc. Reproduced by permission.

of the ring of lymphatic tissue in the oral and pharyngeal cavities. Tonsils tend to atrophy over time. Although the pharyngeal and palatine tonsils may be quite prominent during childhood, they are markedly diminished in size by puberty.

The tongue is invested with taste buds to convey the gustatory sense. Sensors for all types of tastes are found throughout the oral cavity (Roper & Chaudhari, 2017), although there are regions of concentration of receptor types (e.g., Bushman, Ye, & Liman, 2015; Kochem, 2017). The anterior tongue has a higher propensity for sensation of sweetness, starchiness, and a savory (meaty) perception, while the posterior tongue has a propensity for bitter taste (Choi et al., 2016; Colvin, Pullicin, & Lim, 2018). Bitter tastes are generally sensed near the terminal sulcus in circumvallate papillae (Choi et al., 2016).

If you examine the inferior surface of your tongue in a mirror, you can see three important landmarks (see Figure 6–37). Notice the rich **vascular supply** on that undersurface: Medications administered under the tongue are very quickly absorbed into the bloodstream. You can see a prominent band of tissue running from the inner mandibular mucosa to the underside of the tongue. The **lingual frenulum** (or **lingual frenum**) joins the inferior tongue and the mandible, perhaps stabilizing the tongue during the movement. Also notice the transverse band of tissue on either side of the tongue (the **sublingual folds**). At this point are the ducts for the sublingual salivary glands. Lateral to the lingual frenulum are the ducts for the submandibular salivary glands that are hidden under the mucosa on the inner surface of the mandible. These salivary glands and their functions are discussed in detail in Chapter 8.

Intrinsic Tongue Muscles

The intrinsic muscles of the tongue include two pairs of muscles running longitudinally, as well as muscles coursing transversely and vertically. At the outset we should note that the intrinsic muscles interact in a complex fashion to produce the rapid, delicate articulations needed for speech and nonspeech activities. As we discuss each muscle, we provide you with the basic function but will deal thoroughly with the integration of these muscles in Chapter 7. Figure 6–38 can assist you in our discussion of these very important lingual muscles.

- Superior longitudinal muscle
- Inferior longitudinal muscle

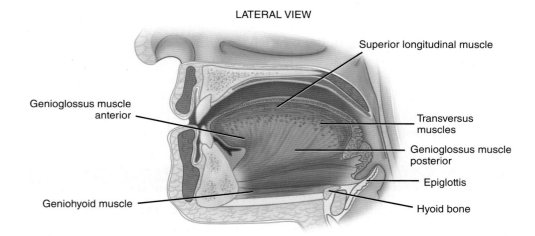

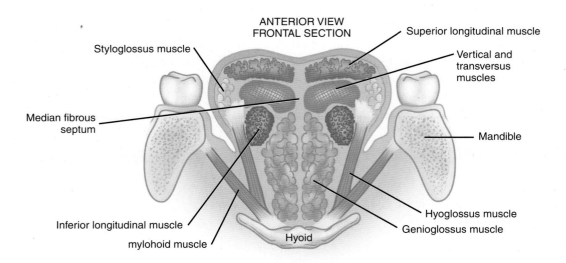

Figure 6–38. Intrinsic muscles of the tongue. *Source:* From Seikel/Drumright/King. *Anatomy & Physiology for Speech, Language, and Hearing, 5th Ed.* ©Cengage, Inc. Reproduced by permission. (From the data of Netter, 1997).

- Transversus muscles
- Vertical muscles

Superior Longitudinal Muscle of the Tongue

The **superior longitudinal muscle** courses along the length of the tongue, comprising the upper layer of the tongue. This muscle originates from the fibrous submucous layer near the epiglottis, from the hyoid, and from the median fibrous septum. Its fibers fan forward and outward to insert into the lateral margins of the tongue and region of the apex. By virtue of their course and insertions, fibers of the superior longitudinal muscle tend to elevate the tip of the tongue. If one superior longitudinal muscle is contracted without the other, the tongue tends to be pulled toward the side of contraction. Innervation of all intrinsic muscles of the tongue is by means of the XII hypoglossal nerve.

Inferior Longitudinal Muscle of the Tongue

The **inferior longitudinal muscle** originates at the root of the tongue and corpus hyoid, with fibers coursing to the apex of the tongue. This muscle occupies the lower sides of the tongue but is absent in the medial tongue base, which is occupied by the extrinsic genioglossus muscle. The inferior longitudinal muscle pulls the tip of the tongue downward and assists in the retraction of the tongue if co-contracted with the superior longitudinal. As

Ankyloglossia (Tongue Tie)

The *lingual frenulum* is a band of tissue connecting the tongue to the floor of the mouth. It appears to assist in stabilizing the tongue during movement but occasionally may be too short for proper lingual function. This condition, known as ankyloglossia ("ankyl" = stiffness or immobility, "glossia" = tongue) and colloquially referred to as **tongue tie**, will result in difficulty elevating the tongue for phonemes requiring palatal or alveolar contact. The tongue may appear heart-shaped when protruded, resulting from the excessive tension on the midline by the short frenulum. A surgical procedure to correct the condition may be useful, although such surgery is not minor. Recent evidence indicates that retention of uncorrected ankyloglossia may predict later-life oropharyngeal dysphagia (Moulton, Seikel, Loftin, & Devine, in press).

Muscle:	Superior longitudinal
Origin:	Fibrous submucous layer near the epiglottis, the hyoid, and the median fibrous septum
Course:	Fans forward and outward
Insertion:	Lateral margins of the tongue and region of apex
Innervation:	XII hypoglossal nerve
Function:	Elevates, assists in retraction, or deviates the tip of the tongue

with the superior longitudinal, unilateral contraction of the inferior longitudinal causes the tongue to turn toward the contracted side and downward. Innervation of all intrinsic muscles of the tongue is by means of the contralateral XII hypoglossal nerve.

Transversus Muscles of the Tongue

The **transversus muscles of the tongue** provide a mechanism for narrowing the tongue. Fibers of these muscles originate at the median fibrous septum and course laterally to insert into the side of the tongue in the submucous tissue. Some fibers of the transversus muscle continue as the palatopharyngeus muscle. The transversus muscle of the tongue pulls the edges of the tongue toward the midline, effectively narrowing the tongue. Innervation of all intrinsic muscles of the tongue is by means of the XII hypoglossal nerve.

Vertical Muscles of the Tongue

The **vertical muscles of the tongue** run at right angles to the transversus muscles and flatten the tongue. Fibers of the vertical muscle course from the base of the tongue and insert into the membranous cover. The fibers of the transversus and vertical muscles interweave. Contraction of the vertical muscles pulls the tongue down into the floor of the mouth. Innervation of all intrinsic muscles of the tongue is by means of the XII hypoglossal nerve.

Muscle:	Inferior longitudinal
Origin:	Root of the tongue and corpus hyoid
Course:	Forward
Insertion:	Apex of the tongue
Innervation:	XII hypoglossal nerve
Function:	Pulls tip of the tongue downward, assists in retraction, and deviates the tongue
Muscle:	Transversus muscles of the tongue
Origin:	Median fibrous septum
Course:	Laterally
Insertion:	Side of the tongue in the submucous tissue
Innervation:	XII hypoglossal nerve
Function:	Provides a mechanism for narrowing the tongue
Muscle:	Vertical muscles of the tongue
Origin:	Base of the tongue
Course:	Vertically
Insertion:	Membranous cover
Innervation:	XII hypoglossal nerve
Function:	Pulls the tongue down into the floor of the mouth

Extrinsic Tongue Muscles

The intrinsic muscles of the tongue are responsible for precise articulatory performance, and the extrinsic muscles of the tongue tend to move the tongue as a unit. It appears that extrinsic tongue muscles set the general posture for articulation, with the intrinsic muscles performing the refined perfection of that action.

- Genioglossus muscle
- Hyoglossus muscle
- Styloglossus muscle
- Chondroglossus muscle
- Palatoglossus muscle

Genioglossus Muscle

The **genioglossus** is the prime mover of the tongue, making up most of its deeper bulk. As you can see from Figure 6–39, the genioglossus arises from the inner mandibular surface at the symphysis and fans to insert into the tip and dorsum of the tongue, as well as to the corpus of the hyoid bone.

The genioglossus muscle occupies a medial position in the tongue, with the inferior longitudinal muscle, hyoglossus, and styloglossus being lateral to it. Fibers of the genioglossus insert into the entire surface of the tongue but are sparse to absent in the tip. Contraction of the anterior fibers of the genioglossus muscle results in the retraction of the tongue, whereas contraction of the posterior fibers draws the tongue forward to aid protrusion of the apex. If both anterior and posterior portions are contracted, the middle

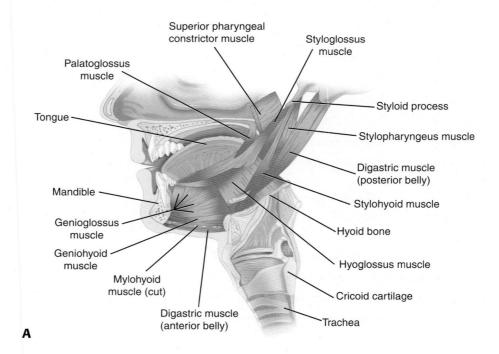

Figure 6–39. A. Genioglossus and related muscles. *continues*   **A**

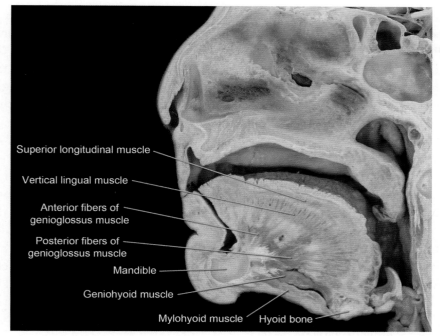

B

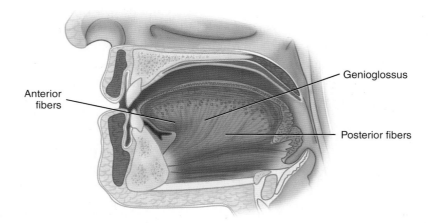

C

Figure 6–39. *continued*
B. Photograph showing genioglossus muscle. **C.** Schematic of genioglossus. *A and C Source:* From Seikel/ Drumright/King. *Anatomy & Physiology for Speech, Language, and Hearing, 5th Ed.* ©Cengage, Inc. Reproduced by permission.

portion of the tongue is drawn down into the floor of the mouth, functionally cupping the tongue along its length. The genioglossus is innervated by the XII hypoglossal nerve.

Muscle:	Genioglossus
Origin:	Inner mandibular surface at the symphysis
Course:	Fans up, back, and forward
Insertion:	Tip and dorsum of tongue and corpus hyoid
Innervation:	XII hypoglossal nerve
Function:	Anterior fibers retract the tongue; posterior fibers protrude the tongue; together, anterior and posterior fibers depress the tongue

Hyoglossus Muscle

As the name implies, the **hyoglossus** arises from the length of the greater cornu and lateral body of the hyoid bone, coursing upward to insert into the sides of the tongue between the styloglossus (to be discussed shortly) and the inferior longitudinal muscles. The hyoglossus pulls the sides of the tongue down, in direct antagonism to the palatoglossus (to be discussed shortly). The hyoglossus is innervated by the XII hypoglossal nerve.

Styloglossus Muscle

If you examine Figure 6–39 again, you will see that the **styloglossus** originates from the anterolateral margin of the styloid process of the temporal bone, coursing forward and down to insert into the inferior sides of the tongue. It divides into two portions: One interdigitates with the inferior longitudinal muscle, and the other with the fibers of the hyoglossus. As you can guess from the examination of the course and insertion of this muscle, contraction of the paired styloglossi draws the tongue back and up. The styloglossus is innervated by the XII hypoglossal nerve.

Chondroglossus Muscle

chondroglossus: Gr., chondros, cartilage; glossus, tongue

The **chondroglossus** muscle is often considered to be part of the hyoglossus muscle. As with the hyoglossus, the chondroglossus arises from the hyoid (lesser cornu), coursing up to interdigitate with the intrinsic muscles of the tongue medial to the point of insertion of the hyoglossus. The chondroglossus is a depressor of the tongue. The chondroglossus is innervated by the XII hypoglossal nerve.

ANAQUEST LESSON ▶

Palatoglossus Muscle (Glossopalatine Muscle)

The **palatoglossus** may be functionally defined as a muscle of the tongue or of the velum, although it is more closely allied with palatal architecture and

Muscle:	Hyoglossus
Origin:	Length of greater cornu and lateral body of hyoid
Course:	Upward
Insertion:	Sides of the tongue between styloglossus and inferior longitudinal muscles
Innervation:	XII hypoglossal nerve
Function:	Pulls sides of the tongue down

Muscle:	Styloglossus
Origin:	Anterolateral margin of styloid process
Course:	Forward and down
Insertion:	Inferior sides of the tongue
Innervation:	XII hypoglossal nerve
Function:	Draws the tongue back and up

Muscle:	Chondroglossus
Origin:	Lesser cornu hyoid
Course:	Up
Insertion:	Interdigitates with intrinsic muscles of the tongue medial to the point of insertion of hyoglossus
Innervation:	XII hypoglossal nerve
Function:	Depresses the tongue

Muscle:	Palatoglossus (Glossopalatine)
Origin:	Anterolateral palatal aponeurosis
Course:	Down
Insertion:	Sides of posterior tongue
Innervation:	Pharyngeal plexus from the XI accessory and X vagus nerves
Function:	Elevates the tongue or depresses the soft palate

origin. We've added the alternate name here to emphasize this dual function. It will be described in a later section, but you should realize that it serves the dual purpose of depressing the soft palate or elevating the back of the tongue. The palatoglossus makes up the anterior faucial pillar. The palatoglossus is endowed with muscle spindles (Kuehn, Templeton, & Maynard, 1990; Liss, 1990), which underscores the need to sustain an elevated velum for nonnasalized phonemes.

⊘ *To summarize:*

- The **tongue** is a massive structure occupying the floor of the mouth. It is divided by a **median fibrous septum** from where the transversus intrinsic muscle of the tongue originates.

- The tongue is divided into **dorsum**, **apex** (tip), and **base**.

- Fine movements of the tongue are produced by the contraction of the intrinsic musculature (**transversus**, **vertical**, **inferior longitudinal**, and **superior longitudinal** muscles of the tongue).

- Larger adjustments of lingual movement are completed through the use of **extrinsic muscles**. The **genioglossus** retracts, protrudes, or depresses the tongue. The **hyoglossus** and **chondroglossus** depress the tongue, while the **styloglossus** and **palatoglossus** (**glossopalatine**) elevate the posterior tongue.

Muscles of Mastication: Mandibular Elevators and Depressors

The process of chewing food, or **mastication**, requires the movement of the mandible so that the molars can make a solid, grinding contact. The muscles of mastication are among the strongest of the body, and the coordinated

mastication: L., masticare, chewing

contraction of these muscles is required for proper food preparation. The muscles of mastication include the mandibular elevators (masseter, temporalis, and medial pterygoid), muscle of protrusion (lateral pterygoid), and depressors (digastricus, mylohyoid, geniohyoid, and platysma).

- Masseter muscle
- Temporalis muscle
- Medial pterygoid muscle
- Lateral pterygoid muscle
- Digastricus muscle
- Mylohyoid muscle
- Geniohyoid muscle
- Platysma muscle

Masseter Muscle

As you may see from Figure 6–40, the **masseter** is the most superficial of the muscles of mastication. This massive quadrilateral muscle originates on the lateral, inferior, and medial surfaces of the zygomatic arch, coursing down to insert primarily into the ramus of the mandible, but with some of the deeper fibers terminating on the coronoid process. The course and attachments of the masseter make it ideally suited for placing maximum force on the molars. Contraction of this muscle elevates the mandible, and when the teeth are clenched, the prominent muscular belly is clearly visible. The masseter is innervated by the anterior trunk of the mandibular nerve arising from the V trigeminal.

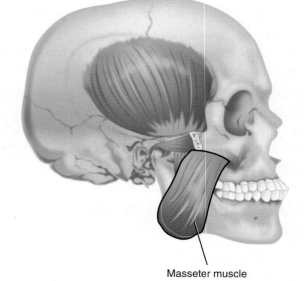

Figure 6–40. Graphic representation of masseter. *Source: From Seikel/Drumright/ King. Anatomy & Physiology for Speech, Language, and Hearing, 5th Ed.* ©Cengage, Inc. Reproduced by permission.

Masseter muscle

Temporalis Muscle

The **temporalis muscle** is deep to the masseter, arising from a region of the temporal and parietal bones known as the **temporal fossa**. As you can see in Figure 6–41, it arises from a broad region of the lateral skull, converging as it courses down and forward. The terminal tendon of the temporalis passes deep to the zygomatic arch and inserts into the coronoid process and ramus of the mandible. The temporalis elevates the mandible and draws it back if protruded. The temporalis muscle appears to be capable of more rapid contraction than the masseter. The temporalis is innervated by the temporal branches arising from the mandibular nerve of V trigeminal.

Medial Pterygoid Muscle

The **medial pterygoid muscle** (also known as the **internal pterygoid muscle**) originates from the medial pterygoid plate and fossa lateral to it (Figure 6–42). Fibers from the muscle course down and back to insert into the mandibular ramus. The medial pterygoid muscle elevates the mandible, acting in conjunction with the masseter. The medial pterygoid muscle is innervated by the mandibular division of the V trigeminal nerve.

Muscle:	Masseter
Origin:	Zygomatic arch
Course:	Down
Insertion:	Ramus of the mandible and coronoid process
Innervation:	Anterior trunk of mandibular nerve arising from the V trigeminal
Function:	Elevates the mandible
Muscle:	Temporalis
Origin:	Temporal fossa of temporal and parietal bones
Course:	Converging downward and forward, through the zygomatic arch
Insertion:	Coronoid process and ramus
Innervation:	Temporal branches arising from the mandibular nerve of V trigeminal
Function:	Elevates the mandible and draws it back if protruded
Muscle:	Medial pterygoid
Origin:	Medial pterygoid plate and fossa
Course:	Down and back
Insertion:	Mandibular ramus
Innervation:	Mandibular division of the V trigeminal nerve
Function:	Elevates the mandible

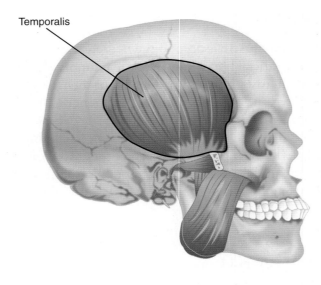

Figure 6–41. Graphic representation of the temporalis. *Source:* From Seikel/ Drumright/King. *Anatomy & Physiology for Speech, Language, and Hearing, 5th Ed.* ©Cengage, Inc. Reproduced by permission.

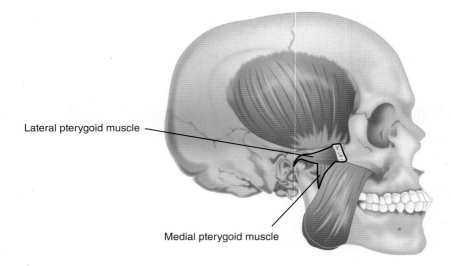

Figure 6–42. Lateral and medial pterygoid muscles. *Source:* From Seikel/ Drumright/King. *Anatomy & Physiology for Speech, Language, and Hearing, 5th Ed.* ©Cengage, Inc. Reproduced by permission.

Lateral Pterygoid Muscle

The **lateral** (or external) **pterygoid muscle** arises from the sphenoid bone. One head of the lateral pterygoid arises from the lateral pterygoid plate (hence the name of the muscle); another head attaches to the greater wing

Muscle:	Lateral pterygoid (external pterygoid)
Origin:	Lateral pterygoid plate and the greater wing of sphenoid
Course:	Back
Insertion:	Pterygoid fovea of the mandible
Innervation:	Mandibular branch of the V trigeminal nerve
Function:	Protrudes the mandible

Tongue Thrust

As with other motor functions, swallowing develops from immature to mature forms. The immature swallow capitalizes on the needs of the moment: An infant needs to compress the nipple to stimulate release of milk, so the tongue moves forward naturally during this process. As the infant develops teeth, anterior movement of the tongue is blocked even as the need for it diminishes. The child begins eating semisolid and solid food, and chewing becomes more important than sucking. The mature swallow propels a bolus back toward the oropharynx, a maneuver requiring posterior direction of the tongue.

If the child fails to develop the mature swallow, we call this condition **tongue thrust**. The anterior force of the tongue in its rest posture will cause labioversion of the incisors. This child may have flaccid oral musculature, weak masseter action during swallow, and a disorganized approach to generation of the bolus. Considering that we swallow between 400 and 600 times per day, the immature swallow is difficult (but far from impossible) to reorganize into a mature swallow. Many speech-language pathologists specialize in **orofacial myofunctional therapy** directed toward remediation of such problems, a rich and rewarding practice that results in (literally) smiling clients (see Zickefoose, 1989). There is recent evidence that uncorrected tongue thrust may place a person at risk for later-life oropharyngeal dysphagia (Seikel et al., 2016). Chapter 8 discusses issues related to tongue thrust.

of the sphenoid. Fibers course back to insert into the pterygoid fovea of the mandible, the lower inner margin of the condyloid process of the mandible (see Figure 6–42). Contraction of the lateral pterygoid muscle protrudes the mandible, and this muscle works in concert with the mandibular elevators for grinding action at the molars. The lateral pterygoid muscle is innervated by the mandibular branch of the V trigeminal nerve.

Digastricus Muscle

The dual-bellied digastricus was described in Chapter 4, so it is only briefly discussed here. The **digastricus anterior** originates at the inner surface of the mandible at the digastricus fossa, near the symphysis, while the **digastricus posterior** originates at the mastoid process of the temporal bone. The anterior fibers course medially and down to the hyoid, where they join with the posterior digastricus by means of an intermediate tendon that inserts into the hyoid at the juncture of the hyoid corpus and greater cornu. If the hyoid bone is fixed by infrahyoid musculature, contraction of the anterior

Muscle:	Digastricus anterior
Origin:	Inner surface of the mandible at digastricus fossa, near the symphysis
Course:	Medially and down
Insertion:	Intermediate tendon to juncture of hyoid corpus and greater cornu
Innervation:	Mandibular branch of V trigeminal nerve via the mylohyoid branch of the inferior alveolar nerve
Function:	Pulls the hyoid forward; depresses the mandible if in conjunction with digastricus posterior

Muscle:	Digastricus posterior
Origin:	Mastoid process of temporal bone
Course:	Medially and down
Insertion:	Intermediate tendon to juncture of hyoid corpus and greater cornu
Innervation:	Digastric branch of the VII facial nerve
Function:	Pulls the hyoid back; depresses mandible if in conjunction with anterior digastricus

component results in the depression of the mandible. The anterior belly is innervated by the mandibular branch of the V trigeminal nerve via the mylohyoid branch of the inferior alveolar nerve. The posterior belly is supplied by the **digastric** branch of the VII facial nerve.

digastric: L., two belly; refers to the two-bellied muscle, digastricus

Mylohyoid Muscle

This muscle was described in Chapter 4. The **mylohyoid** originates at the underside of the mandible and courses to the corpus hyoid. This fanlike muscle courses from the **mylohyoid line** of the mandible to the median fibrous raphe and inferiorly to the hyoid, forming the floor of the mouth. With the hyoid fixed in position, the mylohyoid depresses the mandible. The mylohyoid is innervated by the alveolar nerve, arising from the V trigeminal nerve, mandibular branch.

Geniohyoid Muscle

Also described in Chapter 4, the **geniohyoid muscle** originates at the mental spines of the mandible and projects parallel to the anterior digastricus from

Muscle:	Mylohyoid
Origin:	Mylohyoid line, inner mandible
Course:	Back and down
Insertion:	Median fibrous raphe and inferiorly to hyoid
Innervation:	Alveolar nerve, arising from the V trigeminal nerve, mandibular branch
Function:	Depresses the mandible

Muscle:	Geniohyoid
Origin:	Mental spines of the mandible
Course:	Medially
Insertion:	Corpus hyoid
Innervation:	XII hypoglossal nerve and spinal C1 nerve
Function:	Depresses the mandible

the inner mandibular surface to insert into the corpus hyoid. Contraction of the geniohyoid depresses the mandible if the hyoid is fixed. Innervation of the geniohyoid is by means of the XII hypoglossal nerve.

Platysma Muscle

The platysma was discussed in the "Muscles of the Face" section of this chapter.

✓ To summarize:

- The muscles of **mastication** include mandibular **elevators** and **depressors**, as well as muscles to **protrude** the mandible.

- Mandibular elevators include the **masseter, temporalis**, and **medial pterygoid** muscles, while the **lateral pterygoid** protrudes the mandible.

- Depression of the mandible is performed by the **mylohyoid, geniohyoid**, and **platysma** muscles. The grinding action of the molars requires coordinated and synchronized contraction of the muscles of mastication.

Muscles of the Velum

Only three speech sounds in English require that the soft palate be depressed (/m/, /ŋ/, and /n/). During most speaking time and swallowing, the soft palate is actively elevated. We discuss the general configuration of the soft palate here and then talk about how we go about elevating and depressing this important structure.

The **soft palate** or **velum** is a combination of muscle, aponeurosis, nerves, and blood supply covered by the mucous membrane lining. The **palatal aponeurosis** makes up the mid-front portion of the soft palate, being an extension of an aponeurosis arising from the tensor veli palatini. The palatal aponeurosis divides around the musculus uvulae but serves as the point of insertion for other muscles of the soft palate. The mucous membrane lining is invested with lymph and mucous glands, and the oral side of the lining also has taste buds.

Muscles of the soft palate include elevators (levator veli palatini and musculus uvulae), an auditory tube dilator (tensor veli palatini), and depressors (palatoglossus and palatopharyngeus). Although the superior constrictor muscle is a pharyngeal muscle, we should note that it is also an important muscle for the function of the soft palate. We discuss the muscles of the pharynx following the discussion of the muscles of the soft palate. Figure 6–43 can assist you in the following discussion.

- Levator veli palatini muscle
- Musculus uvulae muscle
- Tensor veli palatini muscle

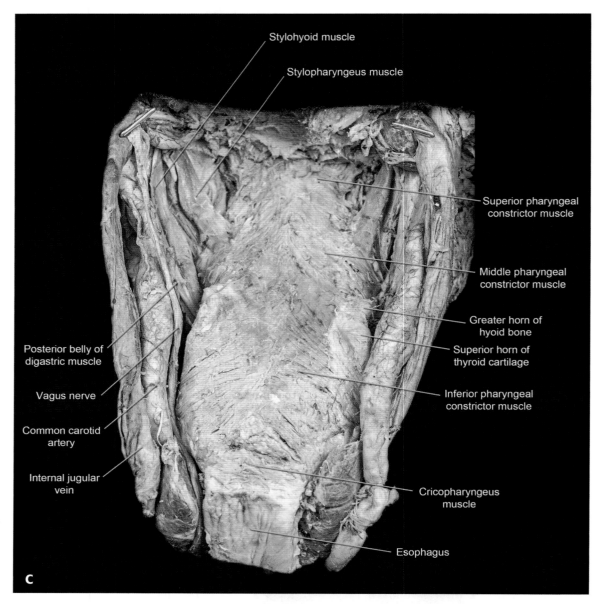

Figure 6–44. *continued* **C.** Photograph of posterior larynx, showing pharyngeal constrictors. Note cricopharyngeus muscle.

other fibers arise from the sides of the tongue. Contraction of the superior pharyngeal constrictor muscle pulls the pharyngeal wall forward and constricts the pharyngeal diameter, an especially prominent movement during swallowing. This contraction assists in effecting the velopharyngeal seal and thereby prevents the bolus from entering the nasopharynx.

Middle Pharyngeal Constrictor Muscle

The **middle pharyngeal constrictor** arises from the horns of the hyoid bone, as well as from the **stylohyoid ligament** that runs from the styloid process to the lesser horn of the hyoid. The middle constrictor courses up and back, inserting into the median pharyngeal raphe. The middle constrictor narrows the diameter of the pharynx. The middle pharyngeal constrictor is innervated by the X vagus and IX glossopharyngeal nerves.

Inferior Pharyngeal Constrictor Muscle

The **inferior pharyngeal constrictor** makes up the inferior pharynx. The portion arising from the sides of the cricoid cartilage forms the cricopharyngeal portion, frequently referred to as a separate muscle, the **cricopharyngeus muscle (upper esophageal sphincter**). This portion, which courses back to form the muscular orifice of the esophagus, is an important muscle for swallowing and is the structure set into vibration during esophageal speech, as will discussed in Chapter 8. The upper thyropharyngeal portion (or **thyropharyngeus muscle**) arises from the oblique line of the thyroid lamina, coursing up and back to insert into the median pharyngeal raphe. Contraction of the inferior constrictor reduces the diameter of the lower pharynx.

Salpingopharyngeus Muscle

The **salpingopharyngeus muscle** arises from the lower margin of the auditory tube, descending the lateral pharynx to join the palatopharyngeus muscle (Figure 6–45). The **salpingopharyngeal fold** is a prominence in the lateral

Muscle:	Middle pharyngeal constrictor
Origin:	Horns of the hyoid and stylohyoid ligament
Course:	Up and back
Insertion:	Median pharyngeal raphe
Innervation:	X vagus, pharyngeal branch and IX glossopharyngeal nerve, pharyngeal branch
Function:	Narrows diameter of the pharynx

Muscle:	Cricopharyngeus muscle (upper esophageal sphincter)
Origin:	Cricoid cartilage
Course:	Back
Insertion:	Orifice of the esophagus
Innervation:	X vagus, pharyngeal branch and IX glossopharyngeal nerve, pharyngeal branch
Function:	Constricts superior orifice of esophagus

Muscle:	Inferior pharyngeal constrictor; thyropharyngeus
Origin:	Oblique line of thyroid lamina
Course:	Up and back
Insertion:	Median pharyngeal raphe
Innervation:	X vagus nerve, pharyngeal branch and IX glossopharyngeal nerve, pharyngeal branch
Function:	Reduces the diameter of the lower pharynx

4. In the figure below, identify the bones and landmarks indicated.

A. _____ bone   J. _____

B. _____ bone   K. _____ process

C. _____ (bone)   L. _____ process

D. _____ (bone)   M. _____ process

E. _____ bone   N. _____

F. _____ bone   O. _____ process

G. _____ bone   P. _____ process

H. _____ bone   Q. _____

I. _____

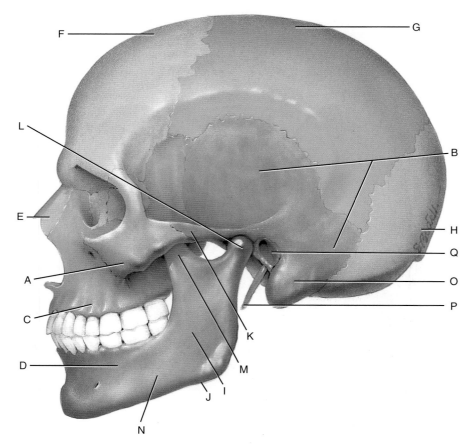

Source: From Seikel/Drumright/King. *Anatomy & Physiology for Speech, Language, and Hearing*, 5th Ed. ©Cengage, Inc. Reproduced by permission.

5. In the figure below, identify the structures indicated.

A. _____ process

B. _____ (bone)

C. _____ bone

D. _____

E. _____ foramen

F. _____ suture

G. _____ process

H. _____ plate

I. _____ plate

J. _____ process

K. _____

L. _____

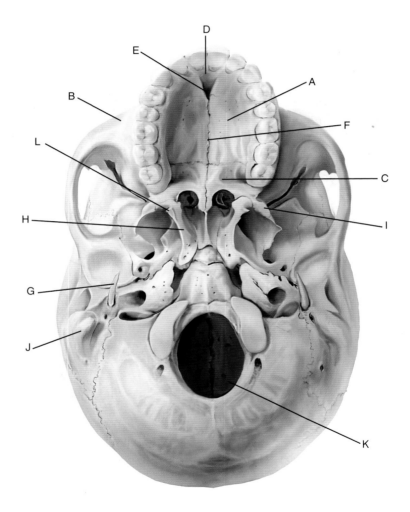

INFERIOR VIEW

Source: From Seikel/Drumright/King. *Anatomy & Physiology for Speech, Language,
and Hearing, 5th Ed.* ©Cengage, Inc. Reproduced by permission.

The lips are deceptive in another sense as well. At first glance, one might assume that the upper and lower lips have very similar qualities. In reality, however, the lower lip achieves a greater velocity and force than the upper lip and seems to do most of the work in lip closure (Barlow & Netsell, 1986; Barlow & Rath, 1985; Folkins & Canty, 1986). The extra force is a function of the mentalis muscle, for which there is no parallel in the upper lip, and the doubled velocity is facilitated by the variable movement and placement of the mandible. The lower lip is attached to a movable articulator (the mandible), and it must quickly adapt to being closer or farther from the maxillary upper lip. That is, for sound to be accurately perceived as a chosen phoneme, the lips must make contact within closely timed tolerances. The lower lip is capable of rapidly altering its rate of closure to accommodate a variety of jaw positions, unflinchingly.

The notion of variable mandible position reinforces another fine point of labial function. The lips (as with the other articulators) are amazingly resistant to interference. We can easily adjust to perturbations of our articulators, or to even gross malformation (e.g., see Folkins & Abbs, 1975). As an example, you could ask someone to recite a poem with eyes closed. At an unpredictable point, if you briefly pulled down on the lower lip, the person would quickly adjust to the distorted articulatory position and continue talking with the new configuration (within limits, of course).

Similarly, you are able to adapt to other restrictions on supportive articulators. Try this. Repeat the syllable *puh* as rapidly as you can, counting the number of syllables you can produce in 5 seconds. Note that your mandible was helping, and it moved when you closed your lips. Now bite lightly on a pencil using your incisors and perform the same task. Your rate of repetition was probably very similar, despite the fact that your mandible was no longer able to help your lips close.

We are amazingly resistant to interference with the articulatory mechanism. This resistance, by the way, is evidence that the plan for an articulatory movement (e.g., see Ostry, Vatikiotis-Bateson, & Gribble, 1997; Steeve & Moore, 2009) is not micromanaged by central cortical control, but rather that the details of motor execution are left to be worked out by some type of coordinative structures, as will be discussed shortly. If the neural command, for instance, said simply to elevate the lower lip by 1.3 cm, either of the distortions mentioned previously would have resulted in a faulty articulation.

proprioceptive: L. proprio, own; captive, sense; sensation of one's body, particularly of movement

This does not mean that we do not use the **proprioceptive** information provided by sensors in our facial muscles to help us note muscle tone and position. As we mentioned in our introduction to neuroanatomy and neurophysiology in Chapter 1, muscle spindles are a powerful means of maintaining a specific articulatory posture, particularly when faced with the forces of gravity that are attempting to passively move elements of the anatomy. For instance, the mandible would tend to hang open as a result of the pull of gravity, but when gravity pulls on the mandible, the muscle spindles tell the muscles that elevate the mandible (especially the masseter and temporalis) to contract, thereby counteracting the forces of gravity.

Although we do not have spindles in facial muscles to assist in maintaining a specific articulatory posture (Blair & Muller, 1987; Folkins & Larson, 1978; Seibel & Barlow, 2007), we do have other sensors (e.g., those for pressure and touch) that provide feedback on the condition of facial muscles (Møller, 2003). Reflexive contraction of the orbicularis oris occurs with increased intraoral pressure, such as that produced during production of a bilabial stop or plosive. The oral mucosa and lips have sensors for light mechanical stimulation, such as would occur during linguadental articulation. There are mechanoreceptors in the lips, and the perioral reflex can be elicited through the mechanical deformation of the angles of the mouth (Weber & Smith, 1987; Wohlert, 1996; Wohler & Goffman, 1994).

Evidence that you *do* use this type of information to control muscles may be found in the recollection of your last trip to the dentist. You may remember accidentally biting your lip while chewing or talking after the dentist's anesthetic deadened it. Your unconscious perception of its position generally keeps that from happening. Mechanical stimulation of the lips affects other articulators as well. When the lower lip is stimulated, reflexive excitation in both the masseter and genioglossus can be recorded. The *degree* to which this information is *required* for speech accuracy is still a lively topic of debate. That having been said, Abbs (1973) provided solid evidence that the muscle spindle system involved in mandibular movement is also used in control of the lips and mandible for speech, and the velum is well endowed with muscle spindles to support its tonic contraction against gravity (Kuehn, Templeton, & Maynard, 1990; Liss, 1990).

Mandible

The mandible is something of an unsung hero among articulators. It quietly and unceremoniously does its business, assisting the lips, changing its position for tongue movement, and tightly closing when necessary. It *does* move, however, and you can remind yourself of that movement by placing one finger of your right hand on your upper lip, and another finger on your chin. Close your eyes and count to 20 quickly, paying attention to the degree of movement you feel. You probably felt very little movement, but the mandible *did* move. Now clamp your mandible and count to 20. Were you still intelligible? (Yes.) Now do the opposite: Let your mouth hang absolutely slack-jaw open, and count to 20.

If you really relaxed your jaw and refused to elevate it for your speech, you probably noticed that you were largely unintelligible. The mandible is an extremely important articulator (e.g., see Tasko & Greilik, 2010) in its supportive role of carrying the lips, tongue, and teeth to their targets in the maxilla (i.e., lips, teeth, alveolar ridge, and hard palate), but its adjustments are rather minute in normal speech. For this reason, paralysis of the muscles of mastication can be devastating to speech intelligibility.

The muscles of mandibular elevation (temporalis, masseter, and medial pterygoid) are endowed with muscle spindles, although those of mandibular depression (digastricus, mylohyoid, geniohyoid, and lateral pterygoid) are not. You can easily see the effects of muscle spindles on yourself. Relax your jaw while looking into a mirror. Now apply a firm rubbing pressure on the masseter in a downward-pulling direction. You should see your mandible elevate slightly as you trigger the mandibular reflex. There are also sensors of joint position within the temporomandibular joint that permit extremely accurate positioning of the jaw (within 1 mm). If these sensors are anesthetized, the speaker's accuracy diminishes markedly.

The mandible is, of course, quite important for mastication, and the function of the muscles of mastication is distinctly different for speech and for chewing. It appears that there is a central pattern generator within the brain stem that produces the rhythmic muscular contraction needed for chewing (Ostry et al., 1997; Wilson, Green, & Weismer, 2012). The mandible must elevate, grind laterally, and depress, requiring coordinated activation of the elevators and depressors in a synergistic, rhythmic fashion. We will discuss this pattern further in Chapter 8.

For speech, in contrast, the mandibular elevators and depressors stay in dynamic balance, so that a slight modification in muscle activation (and inhibition by antagonists) permits a quick adjustment of the mandible (Moore, 1993). Indeed, depression of the mandible seems to be not only a function of the classically defined mandibular depressors (digastricus, mylohyoid, geniohyoid, and lateral pterygoid), but, to a significant extent, of the infrahyoid musculature as well (Westbury, 1988). The hyoid undergoes a great deal of movement during depression of the mandible.

Tongue

Arguably, the tongue is the most important of the articulators. It is involved in the production of the majority of phonemes in English. Let us look at how we achieve the individual movements of the tongue.

Although the tongue is capable of generating a great deal of force through contraction, we typically use only about 20% of its potential force for speech activities. The tongue is endowed with muscle spindles, Golgi tendon organs, and tactile sensors. Muscle spindles have been found in the tongue muscles, and Golgi tendon organs have been found in the transverse intrinsic muscles. Passive movement of the tongue (pulling outward) results in a reflexive retraction of the tongue, and mechanical stimulation of the tongue dorsum causes excitation of the genioglossus muscle. Stimulation of the tongue dorsum has an effect on other articulators as well, causing excitation of the masseter and lower orbicularis oris.

The tongue is also remarkably sensitive to touch. We can differentiate two points on the tongue tip separated by only about 1.5 mm. Another extremely sensitive region of the mouth is the periodontal ligament of the dental arch, which can sense movement of particles as slight as 10 microns (if you have ever had a strawberry seed wedged between your teeth, you can verify this sensitivity). It is likely that this sensitivity is used to monitor production of dental consonants.

As a first approximation, you can think of the tongue as a group of highly organized (intrinsic) muscles being carried on the "shoulders" of the extrinsic muscles. Much as the muscles of the legs and trunk move your upper body to a position where your arms and head can interact with the environment, the extrinsic muscles set the basic posture of the tongue, whereas the intrinsic muscles have a great deal of responsibility for the microstructure of articulation. The two groups of muscles work closely together to achieve the target articulatory motion. Let us examine each of the basic actions required for speech (Table 7–1).

Tongue Tip Elevation

Elevation of the tongue is the primary responsibility of the superior longitudinal muscles of the tongue. When these fibers are shortened, the tip and lateral margins of the tongue are pulled up.

Table 7–1

Muscles of Tongue Movement	
Movement	**Muscle**
Elevate tongue tip	Superior longitudinal muscles
Depress tongue tip	Inferior longitudinal muscles
Deviate tongue tip	Left and right superior and inferior longitudinal muscles for left and right deviation, respectively
Relax lateral margin	Posterior genioglossus for protrusion; superior longitudinal for tip elevation; transverse intrinsic for pulling sides medially
Narrow tongue	Transverse intrinsic
Deep central groove	Genioglossus for depression of the tongue body; vertical intrinsic for depression of central dorsum
Broad central groove	Moderate genioglossus for depression of the tongue body; vertical intrinsic for depression of dorsum; superior longitudinal for elevation of margins
Protrude tongue	Posterior genioglossus for advancement of the tongue body; vertical muscles to narrow tongue; superior and inferior longitudinal to balance and point tongue
Retract tongue	Anterior genioglossus for retraction of tongue into the oral cavity; superior and inferior longitudinal for shortening of tongue; styloglossus for retraction of tongue into the pharyngeal cavity
Elevate posterior tongue	Palatoglossus for elevation of sides of tongue; transverse intrinsic to bunch tongue
Depress tongue body	Genioglossus for depression of medial tongue; hyoglossus and chondroglossus for depression of sides of tongue if hyoid is fixed by infrahyoid muscles

Hypernasality refers to excessive, linguistically inappropriate nasal resonance arising from failure to adequately close the velopharyngeal port during nonnasal speech sound production. In contrast, hyponasality refers to the absence of appropriately nasalized speech sounds, such that the velopharyngeal port is inadequately opened for the /n/, /m/, and /ŋ/ phonemes.

with such a complex structure in so simple a fashion. The velum is capable of a range of motion and rate of movement that, in the normally endowed individual, matches the needs of rapid speech and nonspeech functions.

The velum generally is closed for nonnasal speech, and this is the result of contraction of the levator veli palatini, a direct antagonist to the palatoglossus muscle. In speech, the opening and closing of the velar port must occur precisely and rapidly, or the result is hyper- or hyponasality. Failure to open the port turns a 70 ms nasal phoneme into a voiced stop consonant, an unacceptable result. The soft palate opens and closes in coordination with the other articulators, thus avoiding the effect of nasal resonance on other phonemes, which is called nasal **assimilation**. In reality, some nasal assimilation is inevitable, acceptable; and in some geographic regions, dialectically appropriate.

Production of high-pressure consonants (such as fricatives and stops) requires greater velopharyngeal effort. To accomplish this seal, additional help is needed from the superior pharyngeal constrictor and uvular muscles. Even then, the pressures for speech are far less than those for, say, playing a wind instrument. Individuals may have difficulty avoiding nasal air escape when playing in the brass section but otherwise have perfectly normal speech.

The hard and soft palates are richly endowed with receptors that provide feedback concerning pressure, and it appears that these sensors facilitate or inhibit motor lingual activity. Indeed, the tensor veli palatini, palatoglossus, and levator veli palatini muscles have been found to have muscle spindles, and the input from these sensors may be important to the initiation of the pharyngeal swallowing reflex (Kuehn et al., 1990; Liss, 1990). In cats, when the soft palate is stimulated electrically, extrinsic tongue movement is inhibited. In contrast, when the hard palate is stimulated (as it would be by food crushed during oral preparation), the extrinsic lingual muscles are excited, producing a rhythmic movement of the tongue. Stretching the faucial pillars by pulling on the tongue or the pillars themselves also inhibits the activity of the extrinsic tongue muscles.[1] It appears that the interaction of the soft palate, fauces, and tongue is a well-organized and integrated system. Palatal, laryngeal, and pharyngeal stimulation activates protrusion of the tongue, whereas stimulation of the anterior oral region appears to stimulate retraction of the tongue.

✔ *To summarize:*

- Each of the articulators has both speech and nonspeech functions that do not necessarily share the same patterns.

- The lower lip is much faster and stronger than the upper lip and responds reflexively to increases of pressure. This added

---

[1]It's worth note that this level of electrical stimulation is low and not painful, as it is lower than the level you would feel if you had muscle stimulation in physical therapy. The whole issue of medical research on non-humans, however, is large and controversial, and strongly deserves our attention as humans.

responsiveness makes it quite effective at overcoming incidental **perturbations** while performing its assigned tasks.

- Movement of the **mandible** for speech is slight when compared with its movement for chewing. In addition, the mandibular posture for speech is one of sustained dynamic tension between antagonists.

- The **tongue** is an extremely versatile organ, with the **extrinsic muscles** providing the major movement of the tongue, and the **intrinsic muscles** providing the shaping of the tongue.

- The **velum** must be maintained in a reasonably elevated position for most speech sounds, although it is capable of a range of movements.

Development of Articulatory Ability

Infants are faced with an enormous task during development. They begin life with no knowledge of the universe and with a motor system in which movement is governed by reflexes that are out of their control. They spend the next several years (perhaps the rest of their lives!) making sense of the world around them and learning to manipulate their environment. Fortunately, they are born with an innate desire to acquire information and learn about their environment, and it appears that this desire drives the often-painful process of development.

The primitive human motor system is actually an extremely complex network of protective reflexes. **Reflexes** provide the means for an immature infant to respond to the environment in a stereotyped manner, without volition. This is not to argue that infants have no will, but rather to point out that they cannot express it voluntarily. If a breast touches the lips of an infant, the infant orients to the breast and starts sucking reflexively (you can stimulate this reflex with a stroke of your fingers). The infant does not need to think, "Gee, I'm hungry. I wonder whether there is anything to eat around here?" Rather, nature has hardwired the infant to meet its needs.

This reflexive condition results in what Langley and Lombardino (1991) referred to as "primitive mass patterns of movement." Movements are gross responses to environmental stimuli that help the infant meet its basic needs. Development is a process of gaining cortical control of the motor patterns for volitional purposes, and the development of the articulatory system has its roots in learning to walk.

The most pervasive postnatal experience an infant has is gravity (Bly, 1983, 1994). Always present, gravity provides the ultimate challenge to an infant who wants to experience a universe that is out of reach. Reflexive movement against gravity provides the child with information about the effects of movement. Infants can see their hands as they move them and learn that there is a relationship between the sensation and the hands they see. These are the essential elements of motor development: reflexive response to environmental stimuli, providing *feedback* to an intact neuromotor system.

reflexes: neural responses that are involuntary and unconscious

conditions. If you pay attention to your tongue as you say the words *beat* and *toot*, you will note that the tongue is in two very different locations as it moves up for the final /t/, yet you are perfectly able to achieve both goals. Central control theories are forced to establish individual articulatory patterns to represent each allophone to accommodate this need—a very weighty proposition. Although the notions of central control remain robust and promising (e.g., see MacKay, 1982), clearly there is a need to explain how we are able to articulate with such precision in the face of continuous variability.

Dynamic or Action Theory Models

As theorists worked to explain accurate and variable articulatory ability, the notion of **articulatory goals** evolved. The end product of muscle activity (and central control) was viewed as being a major determinant in execution. Saltzman (1986) viewed goal-related movement as composed of an **effector system**, a portion of which is the **terminal device**. The effector system would include the entire group of articulators involved in a given action, and the terminal device, or **end-effector** (e.g., the dorsum of the tongue for the articulation of the phoneme /i/), is that portion of the effector system directly related to the articulatory goal. By differentiating these components, one can account for the problem of having to coordinate large numbers of muscle fibers in concert. From this point, one can view the articulatory effector system in a dynamic fashion. The components of the effector system are assigned the goal of articulation but are free to work within the degrees of freedom inherent in the system to accomplish the task. That is, no two acts are ever produced the same way twice, and yet there are definitely commonalities among motor acts. The dynamic models state that the commonality is that the motor act is accurately achieved within the bounds of variability.

The functional units of activation are groups of **coordinative structures**. Coordinative structures are functionally defined muscle groups that, when activated, contribute to achieving the goal at the terminal effector. An important element of achieving the terminal goal is the concept of motor equivalence. If the goal is, for instance, production of the vowel /i/, there might be many different articulatory solutions to the problem of getting an acoustic production that would be judged as correct. The mandible could be clamped and immobile, which would require a different gesture than that of someone with a slack jaw. Motor equivalence states that a goal can be achieved through various means and systems.

Trajectories, or movement paths, can be seen as targets of movement, and the structures involved in achieving a target are grouped as coordinative structures. If the movement is disturbed during execution, the coordinative structures are capable of altering their degree of activation to compensate for this perturbation without an altered central command. As an example, if you were to pick up a glass of milk, your target would be the accurate movement of the glass rim to your lips. Unknown to you, the glass has a very heavy base. When you lift the glass, you expect it to be lighter than it is, so your muscular

effector system: those components involved in completing an action

terminal device: structure involved in the final component of a movement

trajectories: movement paths

effort is less than if you had expected a heavier glass. If you depended on a central program to correct your movement, the glass might not reach your lips, and you would probably pour the milk down your shirt. As it is, your effector system adapts its activities to match the trajectory (table to lips), you add extra force, your thirst is quenched, and your shirt stays dry. This ability to compensate is essential for speech production.

The **dynamic models** take into account the physical properties of the systems involved in articulation. Muscles and connective tissue have elastic properties that result in recoil, and dynamic models account for these variables in the equation. These models have more quickly accommodated the role of afferent information concerning the state of the musculature. According to Kelso & Ding (1993), there are many solutions to achieving any trajectory, and the relationship of the coordinative structures simply defines the solution from a given point of trajectory initiation to the point of termination.

Models of speech production must also somehow account for the fact that speech occurs at an extraordinarily rapid rate and that, somehow, the articulatory system is very resistant to perturbation. We can accommodate a wide range of surprises in speech with no trouble at all. Dynamic models account for the dynamic aspects of the physical system required to achieve a

dynamic models: those models that take into account the changing physical properties of the system

Apraxia

Apraxia refers to a deficit in programming of musculature for voluntary movement that is not attributable to muscular weakness or paralysis. There appear to be many types and subtypes of apraxia. **Limb apraxia** is identified as the inability to perform volitional gestures using the limbs. A patient with limb apraxia might reveal deficits in voluntarily using multiple objects to perform a sequence of acts upon request, such as making a sandwich. The act may be fluent, but the objects are used inappropriately. The patient's ability to perform the act through imitation would be much less impaired.

Patients with oral apraxia might reveal difficulty using the facial and lingual muscles of nonspeech acts. When they are asked to blow out a candle, they may experience a great deal of effortful groping in an attempt to find the right configuration of their lips in coordination with the outward flow of air. Often the individual with oral apraxia also has a verbal apraxia.

Verbal apraxia refers to a deficit in planning the motor act and programming the articulators for speech sound production. The individual with verbal apraxia makes errors in correct articulation of the sounds of speech, although the errors vary widely from one attempt to another. The individual is aware of the error and makes frequent attempts at production, so that the flow of speech is greatly impeded. This patient will have more difficulty with multisyllabic than monosyllabic words, and semiautomatic speech (such as greetings) may be quite fluent.

By definition, apraxias occur without muscular weakness, although muscular weakness or paralysis may co-occur with the apraxia. Apraxias may arise from lesions to a variety of brain structures. Damage to the left hemisphere premotor region of the cerebral cortex appears to have the greatest probability of producing apraxia. The specific premotor region involved with speech is known as Broca's area, and the insular cortex, which is deep to Broca's area, was identified by Dronkers (1996) and Dronkers, Pinker, and Damasio (2000) as a site involved with verbal apraxia, although others disagree (Hillis et al., 2004).

removed, the individual may benefit from a lingual prosthesis. In this case, the prosthesis is elevated to the hard palate by elevation of the mandible.

Another cause of tongue trauma is partial amputation. Traumatic amputation can occur, for instance, when an individual is stricken in the face with tongue protruded beyond the teeth, sometimes seen in motor vehicle accidents. Self-inflicted gunshot wounds to the head may also penetrate and sever the tongue and dentition.

Oral Disease

Disease states affecting tongue function include those that cause sufficient pain to limit lingual movement. Tongue ulcers (canker sores) can impede movement, as can burning tongue syndrome (also known as burning mouth syndrome), in which the tongue feels like it is burning. Lichen planus is seen as white patches on the tongue, and results in a great deal of pain, also limiting movement. Moeller's glossitis (also known as bald tongue) is a condition causing the tongue surface to become smooth and damaging the taste buds. Immune dysfunction can cause Moeller's glossitis, as well as Sjogren's syndrome, which results in dry mouth.

Developmental Tongue Problems

A number of developmental conditions affect tongue function. Ankyloglossia (tongue tie) is a congenital shortness of the lingual frenulum, reducing superior, anterior, and posterior mobility of the tongue. As a result, articulation of palatal and alveolar sounds may be affected, and swallowing is compromised. Macroglossia is a condition in which the tongue is excessively large for the oral cavity. Frequently, the condition is one of relative macroglossia, in which the tongue is appropriately sized for the head but large relative to a small mandible. In either case, the tongue has limited movement within the oral cavity when the mandible is elevated, reducing articulatory precision and resulting in protruding tongue.

Mandibular and Maxillary Problems

Retruded and Prognathic Mandible

Retruded mandible, also known as retrognathia, is a condition in which the mandible is short relative to the maxilla (Class II malocclusion). When this happens, there is typically malocclusion of the upper and lower dentition. This condition can be remediated through surgical advancement of the mandible. A prognathic mandible is one in which the mandible is advanced relative to the maxilla, which is a Class I malocclusion. Both Class I and II malocclusions can cause articulatory problems, but as likely the individual will have normal speech production. The malocclusions can have detrimental effects on mastication and deglutition.

Trauma

Gunshot wounds to the face often affect the mandible and maxilla, because these areas make up the bulk of the face. In these cases, surgery will stabilize the injury and injury site, and often prostheses will be created to accommodate the defect.

Problems Affecting Lips and Palate

Lip Trauma

Lip trauma can arise from many sources. Physical assault and motor vehicle accidents are frequent causes of labial trauma, but sports injuries are another significant contributor. Surgical repair and tissue grafting may be required if the injury is significant. Labial sounds are affected by labial trauma, although mandibular compensation often serves to overcome the speech problems.

Congenital Lip and Palatal Problems

A significant developmental issue with relation to speech is seen in craniofacial malformations. Craniofacial malformations are conditions present at birth that alter the structure and function of hard palate, soft palate, and lip, arising from some congenital condition. A cleft of the palate involves incomplete closure of the left and right palates, in various configurations, including incomplete or complete cleft of the hard palate and soft palate. When the cleft includes the alveolar ridge and soft tissue of the lip, it is classified as a cleft lip. A cleft palate occurs along the intermaxillary suture, while a cleft lip involves the premaxillary suture on one or both sides. In cleft palate, problems with the velum can take many forms, ranging from hypotrophy (inadequate muscular tissue), muscular weakness, and clefting. When the velum is involved in the cleft palate, the oral resonance is affected, because the normal decoupling of the oral and nasal cavities may no longer be possible due to tissue insufficiency or immobility. A cleft that extends into the bone but which is hidden by the oral mucosal layer is termed an occult or submucous cleft. If a child has a seemingly normal palate, but a bifid (split) uvula is seen during oral examination, there is a good chance that the child has a submucous cleft. Even though the oral and nasal cavities aren't actually open to each other, with submucous cleft there is still an acoustic manifestation of the defect.

Speech is significantly affected in individuals with cleft palate. Because speech is a process of manipulating resonances to achieve communication, anything that alters our ability to do this will cause speech problems. In this case, the inability to decouple the oral and nasal cavities results in hypernasality. Acoustically, coupling the nasal cavity has the effect of significantly attenuating the intensity of the signal at frequencies above about 500 Hz. Because place of articulation is largely a product of the second formant

Bibliography

Abbs, J. H. (1973). The influence of the gamma motor system on jaw movements during speech: A theoretical framework and some preliminary observations. *Journal of Speech and Hearing Research, 16*, 175–200.

Bailey, E. F., Rice, A. D., & Fuglevand, A. J. (2007). Firing pattern of human genioglossus motor units during voluntary tongue movement. *Journal of Neurophysiology, 97*, 933–936.

Baken, R. J., & Orlikoff, R. F. (1999). *Clinical measurement of speech and voice* (2nd ed.). San Diego, CA: Singular Publishing Group.

Ballard, K. J., Halaki, M., Sowman, P. F., Kha, A., Daliri, A., Robin, D., . . . & Guenther, F. (2018). An investigation of compensation and adaptation to auditory perturbations in individuals with acquired apraxia of speech. *Frontiers in Human Neuroscience, 12*. (Article ID 510)

Barlow, S. M., & Netsell, R. (1986). Differential fine force control of the upper and lower lips. *Journal of Speech and Hearing Research, 29*, 163–169.

Barlow, S. M., & Rath, E. M. (1985). Maximum voluntary closing forces in the upper and lower lips of humans. *Journal of Speech and Hearing Research, 28*, 373–376.

Blair, C., & Muller, E. (1987). Functional identification of the perioral neuromuscular system: A signal flow diagram. *Journal of Speech, Language, and Hearing Research, 30*(1), 60-70.

Bly, L. (1983). *The components of normal movement during the first year of life and abnormal motor movement.* Chicago, IL: Neuro-Developmental Treatment Association.

Bly, L. (1994). *Motor skills acquisition in the first year.* Tucson, AZ: Therapy Skill Builders.

Brumberg, J. S., Nieto-Castanon, A., Kennedy, P. R., & Guenther, F. H. (2010). Brain–computer interface for speech production. *Speech Communication, 52*, 367–379.

Callan, D. E., Kent, R. D., Guenther, F. H., & Vorperian, H. K. (2000). An auditory-feedback-based neural network model of speech production that is robust to developmental changes in the size and shape of the articulatory system. *Journal of Speech, Language, and Hearing Research, 43*, 721–736.

Dronkers, N. F. (1996). A new brain region for coordinating speech articulation. *Nature, 384*(6605), 159.

Dronkers, N. F., Pinker, S., & Damasio, A. (2000). Language and the aphasias. *Principles of Neural Science, 4*, 1169–1187.

Fairbanks, G. (1954). Systematic research in experimental phonetics: A theory of the speech mechanism as a servosystem. *Journal of Speech and Hearing Disorders, 19*(2), 133–139.

Folkins, J. W., & Abbs, J. H. (1975). Lip and jaw motor control during speech: Responses to resistive loading of the jaw. *Journal of Speech and Hearing Research, 18*, 207–220.

Folkins, J. W., & Canty, J. L. (1986). Movements of the upper and lower lip during speech: Interactions of the lips with the jaw fixed at different positions. *Journal of Speech and Hearing Research, 29*, 348–356.

Folkins, J. W., & Larson, C. R. (1978). In search of a tonic vibration reflex in the human lip. *Brain Research, 151*, 409–412.

Guenther, F. H., Ghosh, S. S., & Tourville, J. A. (2006). Neural modeling and imaging of cortical interactions underlying syllable production. *Brain and Language, 96*(3), 280–301.

Guenther, F. H., Hampson, M., & Johnson, D. (1998). A theoretical investigation of reference frames for the planning of speech movements. *Psychological Review, 105*, 611–633.

Guenther, F. H., Satrajit, S. G., Nieto-Castanon, A., & Tourville, J. A. (2006) A neural model of speech production. In J. Harrington & M. Tabain (Eds.), *Speech production: Models, phonetic processes, and techniques* (pp. 27–39). New York, NY: Psychology Press.

Guenther, F. H., & Vladusich, T. (2012). A neural theory of speech acquisition and production. *Journal of Neurolinguistics, 25*, 408–422.

Hall, P. K., Hardy, J. C., & LaVelle, W. E. (1990). A child with signs of developmental apraxia of speech with whom a palatal lift prosthesis was used to manage palatal dysfunction. *Journal of Speech and Hearing Disorders, 55*, 454–460.

Hillis, A. E., Work, M., Barker, P. B., Jacobs, M. A., Breese, E. L., & Maurer, K. (2004). Re-examining the brain regions crucial for orchestrating speech articulation. *Brain, 127*(7), 1479–1487.

Katz, W. F., Kripke, C., & Tallal, P. (1991). Anticipatory coarticulation in the speech of adults and young children: Acoustic, perceptual, and video data. *Journal of Speech and Hearing Research, 34*, 1222–1249.

Kelso, J. A. S., & Ding, M. (1993). Fluctuations, intermittency, and controllable chaos in biological coordination. *Variability and Motor Control*, 291–316.

Kelso, J. A. S., Tuller, B., Vatikiotis-Bateson, E., & Fowler, C. A. (1984). Functionally specific articulatory cooperation following jaw perturbations during speech: Evidence for coordinative structures. *Journal of Experimental Psychology: Perception and Performance, 19*, 812–832.

Kent, R. D., & Vorperian, H. K. (1995). *Development of the craniofacial-oral-laryngeal anatomy: A review.* San Diego, CA: Singular.

Kuehn, D. P., Templeton, P. J., & Maynard, J. A. (1990). Muscle spindles in the velopharyngeal musculature of humans. *Journal of Speech and Hearing Research, 33*, 488–493.

Langley, M. B., & Lombardino, L. J. (1991). *Neurodevelopmental strategies for managing communication disorders in children with severe motor dysfunction.* Austin, TX: Pro-Ed.

Lashley, K. S. (1951). *The problem of serial order in behavior* (Vol. 21). Bobbs-Merrill.

Liss, J. M. (1990). Muscle spindles in the human levator veli palatini and palatoglossus muscles. *Journal of Speech and Hearing Research, 33*, 736–746.

MacKay, D. G. (1982). The problem of flexibility, fluency, and speed-accuracy trade-off in skilled behavior. *Psychological Review, 89*, 483–506.

Mithen, S. (2008). The diva within. *New Scientist, 197* (2644), 38–39.

Møller, A. R. (2003). *Sensory systems: Anatomy and physiology.* New York, NY: Academic Press.Moore, C. A. (1993). Symmetry of mandibular muscle activity as an index of coordinative strategy. *Journal of Speech and Hearing Research, 36*, 1145–1157.

Moore, C. A. (1993). Symmetry of mandibular muscle activity as an index of coordinative strategy. *Journal of Speech, Language, and Hearing Research, 36*(6), 1145–1157.

Ostry, D. J., Vatikiotis-Bateson, E., & Gribble, P. L. (1997). An examination of the degrees of freedom of human jaw motion in speech and mastication. *Journal of Speech, Language, and Hearing Research, 40*(6), 1341–1351.

Peeva, M. G., Guenther, F. H., Tourville, J. A., Nieto-Castanon, A., Anton, J., Nazarian, B., & Alario, F. (2010). Distinct representations of phonemes, syllables, and supra-syllabic sequences in the speech production network. *Neuroimage, 50*, 626–638.

Prather, J. F., Peters, S., Nowicki, S., & Mooney, R. (2008). Precise auditory-vocal mirroring in neurons for learned vocal communication. *Nature, 451*, 305–310.

Saltzman, E. (1986). Task dynamic coordination of the speech articulators: A preliminary model. *Experimental brain research* (pp. 129–144). Berlin-Heidelberg, Germany: Springer-Verlag.

Seibel, L. M., & Barlow, S. M. (2007). Automatic measurement of nonparticipatory stiffness in the perioral complex. *Journal of Speech, Language, and Hearing Research, 50*, 1272–1279.

Steeve, R. W., & Moore, C. A. (2009). Mandibular motor control during the early development of speech and nonspeech behaviors. *Journal of Speech, Language, and Hearing Research.*

Tasko, S. M., & Greilik, K. (2010). Acoustic and articulatory features of diphthong production: A speech clarity study. *Journal of Speech, Language, and Hearing Research, 53*, 84–99.

Vorperian, H. K., Kent, R. D., Lindstrom, M. J. Kalina, C. M., Gentry, L. R., & Yandell, B. S. (2005). Development of vocal tract length during early childhood: A magnetic resonance imaging study. *Journal of the Acoustical Society of America, 117*(1), 338–350.

Vorperian, H. K., Wang, S., Chung, M. K., Schimek, E. M., Durtschi, R. B., Kent, R. D., . . . Gentry, L. R. (2009). Anatomic development of the oral and pharyngeal portions of the vocal tract: An imaging study. *Journal of the Acoustical Society of America, 125*(3), 1666–1678.

Vorperian, H. K., Wang, S., Schimek, E. M., Durtschi, R. B., Kent, R. D., Gentry, L. R., & Chung, M. K. (2011). Developmental sexual dimorphism of the oral and pharyngeal portions of the vocal tract: An imaging study. *Journal of Speech, Language, and Hearing Research, 54*(4), 995–1010.

Weber, C. M., & Smith, A. (1987). Reflex responses in human jaw, lip, and tongue muscles elicited by mechanical stimulation. *Journal of Speech and Hearing Research, 30*, 70–79.

Westbury, J. R. (1988). Mandible and hyoid bone movements during speech. *Journal of Speech and Hearing Research, 31*, 405–416.

Wilson, E. M., Green, J. R., & Weismer, G. (2012). A kinematic description of the temporal characteristics of jaw motion for early chewing: Preliminary findings. *Journal of Speech, Language and Hearing Research, 55*, 626–638.

Wohlert, A. B. (1996). Reflex responses in lip muscles in younger and older women. *Journal of Speech and Hearing Research, 39*, 578–589.

Wohlert, A. B., & Goffman, L. (1994). Human perioral muscle activation patterns. *Journal of Speech and Hearing Research, 37*, 1032–1040.

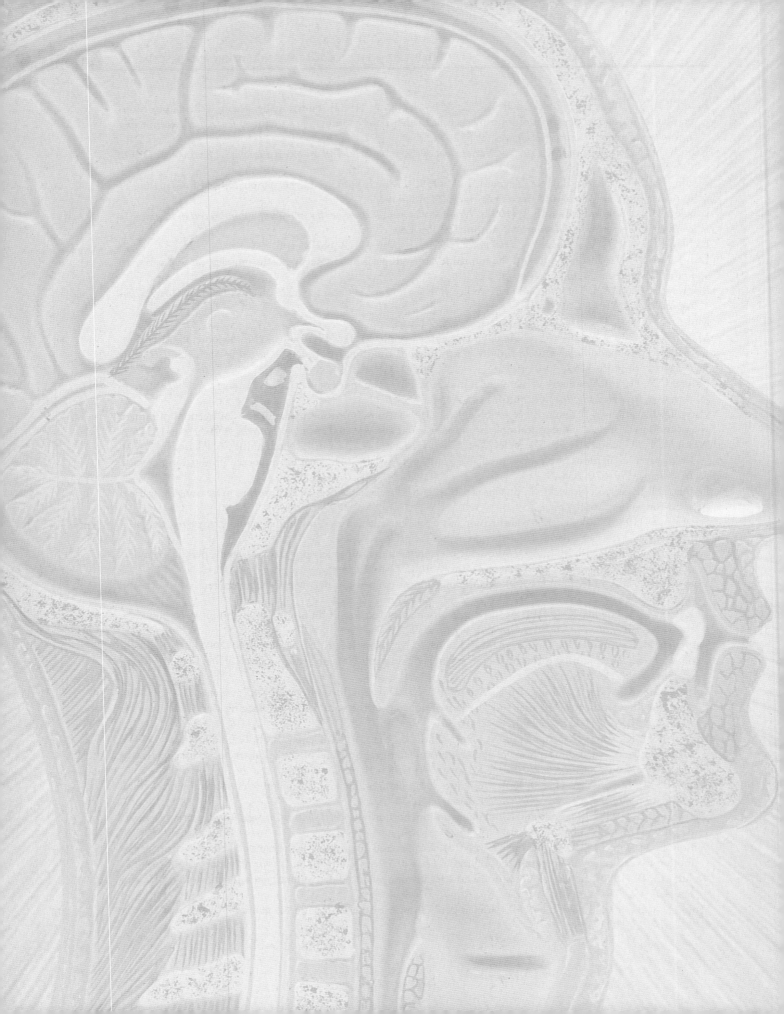

CHAPTER 8

Physiology of Mastication and Deglutition

I n Chapter 1, we introduced you to the concept of the relationship between the biological and speech function in anatomy and physiology. Humans have done a marvelous job of taking the anatomical structures and their physiology and capitalizing on those functions for speech. In many ways, the physiology of **mastication** (the process of preparing food for swallowing, also known as chewing) and **deglutition** (the processes of swallowing) provides an exquisite view of those integrated systems we use so effortlessly in speech. As we discuss these very basic and fundamental processes, you will see how we invoke the respiratory, phonatory, articulatory, and nervous systems. Furthermore, keep an eye on the Clinical Notes we provide in boxes to see just how problematic it can be when the anatomy and physiology of *any one of these systems* is disrupted. As practicing speech-language pathologists, you may very likely be deeply involved in these processes, so we hope you take this information to heart.

mastication: the process of preparing food for swallowing

deglutition: the process of swallowing

Mastication and Deglutition

ANAQUEST LESSON

Mastication refers to the processes associated with grinding and crushing food in preparation for swallowing. *Deglutition* refers to swallowing, which is a complex process of moving the bolus into the pharynx and propelling it into the esophagus. These two biological processes require the integration of lingual, velar, pharyngeal, and facial muscle movement (see Chapter 7) with laryngeal adjustments (see Chapter 5) and respiratory control (see Chapter 2). Consider this: During the adult's mastication and deglutition process, all muscles inserting into the orbicularis oris may be called into action to open, close, purse, and retract the lips as food is received into the oral cavity. All intrinsic and extrinsic muscles of the tongue are called into action to move the food into position for chewing and preparation of the **bolus** (either liquid or a mass of food) for swallowing. (The term *bolus* comes from the Greek word for "lump." It's that "lump" of food in your mouth that is being prepared for swallowing.) The velar elevators seal off the nasal cavity to prevent regurgitation, and the pharyngeal constrictors must contract in a highly predictable fashion to move the bolus down the pharynx and into the esophagus. With the addition of tongue movement and laryngeal elevation, we have just invoked more than 55 pairs of muscles whose timing and

bolus: ball of food or liquid to be swallowed

movement of the mandible during speech in normal development. Tongue protrusion distal to the mouth during suckling evolves into a sucking gesture that does not require tongue protrusion.

Early postnatal development is a time for organization. The infant must develop the coordination of sucking, swallowing, and breathing. Early on, infants may take up to three sucks before swallowing and have an apneic period between suck–swallow runs (Arvedson & Brodsky, 2002). As the infant develops, the ratio of sucks to swallows moves from 3:1 to 1:1, with respiration occurring after between 10 and 30 suck–swallow sequences (Arvedson & Brodsky, 2002; Lau, Smith, & Schanler, 2003).

Figures 8–1 and 8–2 compare the adult and infant oral-pharyngeal structures. If you look closely at these figures, you should realize that there are marked differences between these two systems. The infant's oral cavity is necessarily smaller; but notice also the location of the laryngeal structures and the size of the velum relative to the pharynx. The larynx is markedly elevated at birth but descends over the course of the first 4 years. The hyoid is elevated and relatively forward as compared with the adult, and there is no dentition in the neonate. The relatively larger velum and elevated larynx play a vital role in respiration and deglutition, as we will see.

The suckling response is critically important because it is the means by which the infant gets nutrition. An absent or weak suckling reflex requires intervention by a feeding specialist who can help to stimulate it, and alternative forms of nutrient intake may be required until the reflex is established. This reflex is elicited by the tactile stimulation of the lips and perioral space, as well as through the visual presentation of a food source in older infants (Miller, 2002), and involves protrusion of the tongue with sufficient force to initiate the flow of milk from the breast. Repeated forward pumping of the tongue-mandible unit results in milk entering the oral cavity. After a few thrusts of the tongue, a swallow is triggered, with the tongue base lowered to permit the milk bolus to enter the oropharynx during the next forward pumping action of the tongue. This suckling response evolves into a more mature sucking response that includes tongue elevation and greater lip seal.

This swallow pattern of the neonate is precisely supported by the anatomy of the infant. Take a look at Figure 8–2 again. You can see that the larynx is high in the pharynx, and the soft palate (velum) of the infant "locks" into the space between the epiglottis and tongue at the location of the valleculae, partially protecting the infant's airway from the liquid bolus.

With typical development, this relationship changes as the oral cavity increases in size and as the hyoid and larynx drop relative to the oropharynx, to their adult positions. The adult pharynx serves as a passageway for both the respiratory and gastrointestinal systems, a clear incompatibility. The adult human swallow pattern compensates for this vulnerability by reflexively closing and protecting the airway.

Around the 6th month, dentition begins erupting, and the infant is introduced to relatively solid food. The dentition blocks the anterior protrusion of the tongue and supports retraction of the tongue during the swallow. Furthermore, dentition supports chewing and grinding movements, which

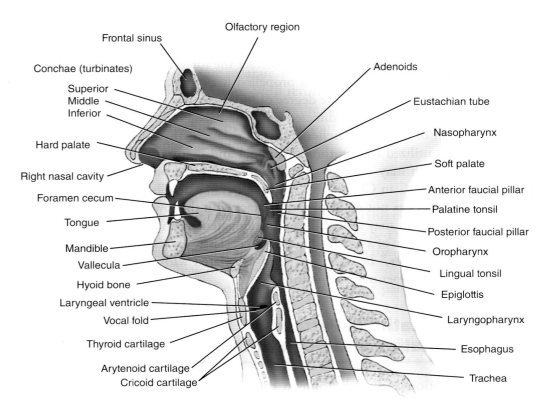

Figure 8–1. Oral, pharyngeal, and laryngeal structure of an adult. *Source:* From Seikel/ Drumright/King. *Anatomy & Physiology for Speech, Language, and Hearing, 5th Ed.* ©Cengage, Inc. Reproduced by permission.

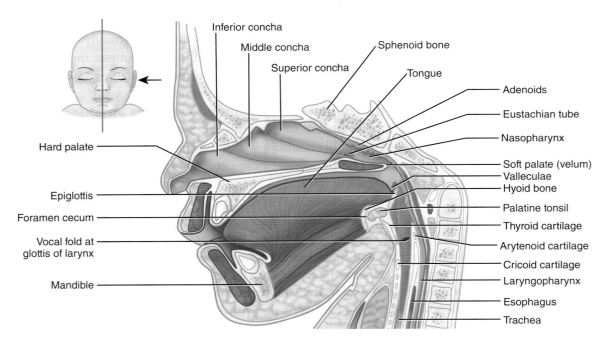

Figure 8–2. The relationship between oral and velar structures in the neonate. *Source:* From Seikel/ Drumright/King. *Anatomy & Physiology for Speech, Language, and Hearing, 5th Ed.* ©Cengage, Inc. Reproduced by permission.

Table 8–1

Muscles of the Oral Preparation Stage

Muscle	Function	Innervation (cranial nerve)
Facial muscles		
Orbicularis oris	Maintains oral seal	VII
Mentalis	Elevates lower lip	VII
Buccinator	Flattens cheeks	VII
Risorius	Flattens cheeks	VII
Mandibular muscles		
Masseter	Elevates mandible	V
Temporalis	Elevates mandible; retracts and protrudes mandible	V
Medial pterygoid	Elevates mandible; moves mandible, grinds mandible laterally	V
Lateral pterygoid	Protrudes and grinds mandible	V
Tongue muscles		
Mylohyoid	Elevates floor of mouth	V
Geniohyoid	Elevates hyoid; depresses mandible	XII
Digastric	Elevates hyoid; depresses mandible	V, VII
Superior longitudinal	Elevates tip; deviates tip	XII
Inferior longitudinal	Depresses tip; deviates tip	XII
Vertical	Cups and grooves tongue	XII
Genioglossus	Moves tongue body; cups tongue	XII
Styloglossus	Elevates posterior tongue	XII
Palatoglossus	Elevates posterior tongue	X, XI
Soft palate muscles		
Palatoglossus	Depresses velum	X, XI
Palatopharyngeus	Depresses velum	X, XI

bunches up in the back and the soft palate is pulled down to keep the food in the oral cavity.

The tongue cups in preparation for the input food. A food bolus must be ground up (the reduction phase) so that it can easily pass through the esophagus for digestion, and this is performed by the coordinated activity of the muscles of mastication as well as the lingual muscles. The tongue is in charge of keeping the food in the oral cavity, and it does so by creating a seal along the alveolar ridge. As it holds the food in place, the tongue may compress it against the hard palate, partially crushing it in preparation for the teeth. The tongue then begins moving the food onto the grinding surfaces of the teeth, pulling the food back into the oral cavity to be mixed with saliva, and then moving it back to the teeth for more of a workup. The salivary glands (parotid, submandibular, and sublingual glands) secrete saliva into the oral cavity to help form the mass of food into a bolus for swallowing. The facial muscles of the buccal wall (risorius and buccinator) contract to keep the food from entering the lateral sulcus (between the gums and cheek wall). The cheeks are critical players in mastication: When they are experimentally inhibited from functioning, the bolus is poorly mixed and poorly formed (Mazari, Heath, & Prinz, 2007).

This oral preparation is quite a feat of coordination. To prove this to yourself, take a bite of a cracker and attend to the process. If you count the number of times you chew on the cracker, you should realize that you grind it between 15 and 30 times before you swallow any of it. As you introduce the cracker into your mouth, your tongue may push it up against the anterior hard palate to begin breaking it down. Your tongue then performs the dance of mastication, flicking in between the molars as your mandible lowers, then quickly moving out of the way before the jaw closes forcefully to continue grinding. Your tongue organizes the ground food onto its dorsum, mixes the food with saliva, and moves it back out to the teeth if the bolus does not meet your specification for "ready to swallow." We are quite adept at creating the ideal bolus for swallowing, which is amazingly similar in consistency among individuals (Hoebler et al., 1998; Mishellany, Woda, Labas, & Peyron, 2006; Peyron, Mishellany, & Woda, 2004; Printz & Lucas, 1995). That is, humans have a common perception of how dense, large, masticated and moist a bolus should be, and unconsciously strive to create such a bolus before swallowing. This person-to-person consistency of bolus may reflect an important organizing principle: We do not have to worry about *how* we create the bolus (i.e., how many times we chew, or how often we have to mix saliva with the particles), but we are very aware of the outcome (Mishellany et al., 2006). For a healthy individual, bolus creation is relatively stable over the life span (Peyron, Woda, Bourdiol, & Hennequin, 2017), although we do adapt our mastication as musculature weakens with age. Illness in the aged is cause for concern, as weakened musculature or cognitive decline can significantly alter mastication efficiency and safety (Lamster, Asadourian, Del Carmen, & Friedman, 2016; Suma, Furuta, Yamashita, & Matsushita, 2019). To create the ideal bolus may require a degree of grinding and manipulation, but the product is the same: When we achieve the physical qualities of the ideal bolus, the swallow is initiated.

The sensory receptors in your oral cavity monitor the bolus continually as it is being prepared (Ertekin & Aydogdu, 2003). Mechanoreceptors in the tongue and hard and soft palates provide input to the nervous system concerning the physical characteristics of the bolus, including the particle size, texture, ductility (ability to be pulled apart) and malleability (ability to be compressed), and degree of cohesion. Chemoreceptors (receptors that differentially respond to chemical composition) play an important role in the

Deficits of the Oral Preparatory Stage

Numerous problems arise when the neuromuscular control of mastication is compromised. Loss of sensation and awareness, coupled with weak buccal musculature, can lead to pocketing of food in the lateral or anterior sulci. Weak muscles of mastication can cause inadequately chewed food; weak lingual muscles may result in poor mixing of saliva with the food, inadequate bolus production, poor lip seal and posterior tongue elevation to impound the bolus, and difficulty compressing the bolus onto the hard palate. If the muscles of the soft palate are compromised, the velum may not be fully elevated and the tongue may not be elevated in the back, permitting food to escape into the pharynx before initiation of the pharyngeal reflexes. This condition is life-threatening because food entering the pharynx in the absence of the reflexive response may well reach the open airway. Aspiration pneumonia (pneumonia secondary to aspirated matter) is a constant concern for individuals with dysphagia (a disorder of swallowing).

component of foods, but also have an important place in stimulation of the pharyngeal swallow, as we will discuss later in this chapter. Thermoreceptors provide sensation concerning the temperature of the bolus, which is also important for both taste and stimulation of the pharyngeal swallow.

If you still question the grace of this process, try to remember the last time you bit your tongue, lip, or cheek. A snack of 10 crackers may invoke at least 600 oscillations of the mastication musculature, and a full meal clearly requires thousands of grinding gestures. Despite this, you can scarcely remember the last painful time your tongue and mandible failed the coordination test.

Oral Stage: Transport

oral transport stage: the stage of swallow in which the bolus is transmitted to the pharynx

When the bolus of food is finally ready to swallow, the **oral transport stage** of swallowing begins (Table 8–2). Interestingly, oral transport can be either voluntary or involuntary (automatic might be a better term). We can voluntarily and willfully move the bolus into the oropharynx as part of the oral preparatory stage, or it may arise as part of the involuntary, automatic sequence that leads to the pharyngeal and esophageal stages of swallowing. In either case, the motor sequence is the same.

In the oral transport stage, several processes must occur sequentially. The tongue base is elevated at the posterior during mastication, but now it drops down and pulls posteriorly. Mastication stops, and the anterior tongue elevates to the hard palate as the vocal folds close to terminate respiration at about 0.1 seconds after initiation. The tongue tip and dorsum move to squeeze the bolus back toward the faucial pillars. Importantly, the tongue movement is characterized as a front-to-back squeezing motion. Tongue tip function shows a lot of variability among people (Dodds et al., 1990), referred to "tippers" and "dippers" as individuals who elevate the tip or depress the tip during swallow, but the dorsum and posterior tongue are easier to characterize. X-ray microbeam studies of swallowing using water verify the anterior-to-posterior movement of the tongue during swallowing

Table 8–2

Muscles of the Oral Stage Required to Propel the Bolus Into the Oropharynx		
Muscle	**Function**	**Innervation (cranial nerve)**
Mandibular muscles		
Masseter	Elevates mandible	V
Temporalis	Elevates mandible	V
Internal pterygoid	Elevates mandible	V
Tongue muscles		
Mylohyoid	Elevates tongue and floor of mouth	V
Superior longitudinal	Elevates tongue tip	XII
Vertical	Cups and grooves tongue	XII
Genioglossus	Moves tongue body; cups tongue	XII
Styloglossus	Elevates posterior tongue	XII
Palatoglossus	Elevates posterior tongue	X, XI

Deficits of the Oral Transit Stage

Deficits of the oral stage center around sensory and motor dysfunction. Weakened movements cause reduced **oral transit time** of the bolus toward the pharynx. With greater motor involvement, food may remain on the tongue or hard palate following transit.

In patients with oral-phase involvement, there is a tendency for the epiglottis to fail to invert over the laryngeal opening and to have limited elevation of the hyoid. Perlman, Grayhack, and Booth (1992) found that individuals with such a deficit showed increased pooling of food or liquid within the valleculae.

Difficulty initiating a reflexive swallow may be the result of sensory deficit. Application of a cold stimulus to the anterior faucial pillars coupled with instructions to attempt to swallow is a time-honored method to assist these individuals in initiating a swallow, although ongoing clinical research is needed to determine its efficacy (Rosenbek, Robbins, Fishback, & Levine, 1991).

oral transit time: time required to move the bolus through the oral cavity to the point of initiation of the pharyngeal stage of swallowing

of liquid (Tasko, Kent & Westbury, 2002). Notably, the mandible elevates to counteract the pressure of the tongue on the roof of the mouth, although the extent and degree of movement are quite variable as well.

Contact with the faucial pillars, soft palate, or posterior tongue base has been proposed as the stimulus that triggers the reflexes of the pharyngeal stage (Ertekin et al., 2011), but Lang (2009) stated that the physical presence of adequate bolus in the oropharynx is the prerequisite for the patterned pharyngeal swallow to occur. Indeed, the pharyngeal swallow does not occur with every completed transport event that occurs, but only after there is adequate mass of bolus in the oropharynx.

Pharyngeal Stage

pharyngeal stage: the stage of swallow in which the bolus moves from the oral cavity, through the pharynx, and to the entryway to the esophagus; involves numerous physiological protective responses.

The **pharyngeal stage** consists of a complex sequence of reflexively controlled events (Table 8–3 and Figure 8–4). As the bolus reaches the region of the faucial pillars (or, alternatively, farther back at the posterior base of the tongue near the valleculae in older individuals), the pharyngeal swallow stage begins. (For examinations of the effects of age on pharyngeal stage initiation, see Martin-Harris, Brodsky, Michel, Lee, and Walters [2007] and Stephens, Taves, Smith, & Martin [2005]. For age effects on transit time, see Mendell & Logemann, [2007].) Events happen fast during the pharyngeal stage, which is a highly coordinated and well-orchestrated sequence of patterned motor operations. It's important to realize that, although the pharyngeal stage is classically referred to as "reflexive" in nature, it is considerably more complex than that. The pharyngeal stage is a programmed stage of transit, such that the sequence of events that we conveniently label as the pharyngeal stage really reflects a component of oropharyngeal transit. Assemblies of neurons called central pattern generator (CPG) circuits create the control mechanism for highly organized and yet involuntary movements, such as those that control swallowing from tongue tip to lower esophageal sphincter. (We should mention here that we are talking only about single swallows: If a person takes multiple swallows or if the bolus is large, the pharyngeal stage may not be initiated until the bolus is in the valleculae [Stephens et al., 2005].)

CPGs are neural circuits that, when initiated, produce the same sequence of events unless modified by influences from the cerebral cortex. They are similar to reflexes (which are simple patterned responses to an environmental stimulus), but consist of a complex sequence of motor responses. Here is a way to contrast between reflexes and central pattern generators. If you hold your mandible in a relaxed state and pull rapidly down on your chin with your thumb, your mouth may snap closed. The stretch receptors in the masseter and temporalis are stimulated by your movement of the mandible and cause the muscles to contract. That's the bite reflex. On the other hand, when you take a bite of cookie, you automatically start chewing it (unless you consciously decide not to), and the movement is a complex interaction among the masseter, temporalis, internal and external pterygoid muscles, and muscles of the tongue. To grind a hard bolus, we must alternate contraction of the muscles of mastication side-to-side, all the while controlling where our tongue is. This complex movement is the product of a central pattern generator. If you think of the very complex process of the pharyngeal stage of swallowing, which uses many muscles in a highly orchestrated manner to protect the airway and transfer the bolus from the mouth to the esophagus, you should quickly recognize how elegant this CPG is.

Table 8–3

Muscles of the Pharyngeal Stage Required to Propel the Bolus Toward the Esophagus, Elevate the Larynx, and Close the Airway		
Muscle	**Function**	**Innervation (cranial nerve)**
Tongue muscles		
Mylohyoid	Elevates hyoid and tongue	V
Geniohyoid	Elevates hyoid and larynx; depresses mandible	XII
Digastricus	Elevates hyoid and larynx	V, VII
Genioglossus	Retracts tongue	XII
Styloglossus	Elevates posterior tongue	XII
Palatoglossus	Narrows fauces; elevates posterior tongue	X, XI
Stylohyoid	Elevates hyoid and larynx	VII
Hyoglossus	Elevates hyoid	XII
Thyrohyoid	Elevates hyoid	XII
Superior longitudinal	Elevates tongue	XII
Inferior longitudinal	Depresses tongue	XII
Transverse	Narrows tongue	XII
Vertical	Flattens tongue	XII
Soft palate muscles		
Levator veli palatini	Elevates soft palate	X, XI
Tensor veli palatini	Dilates auditory tube	V
Musculus uvulae	Shortens soft palate	X, XI
Pharyngeal muscles		
Palatopharyngeus	Constricts oropharynx to channel bolus	X, XI
Salpingopharyngeus	Elevates pharynx	XI
Stylopharyngeus	Raises larynx	IX
Cricopharyngeus	Relaxes esophageal orifice	X, XI
Middle constrictor	Narrows pharynx	X, XI
Inferior constrictor	Narrows pharynx	X, XI
Laryngeal muscles		
Lateral cricoarytenoid	Adducts vocal folds	X
Transverse arytenoid	Adducts vocal folds	X
Oblique arytenoid	Adducts vocal folds	X
Aryepiglotticus	Retracts epiglottis; constricts aditus	X
Thyroepiglotticus	Dilates airway following swallow	X

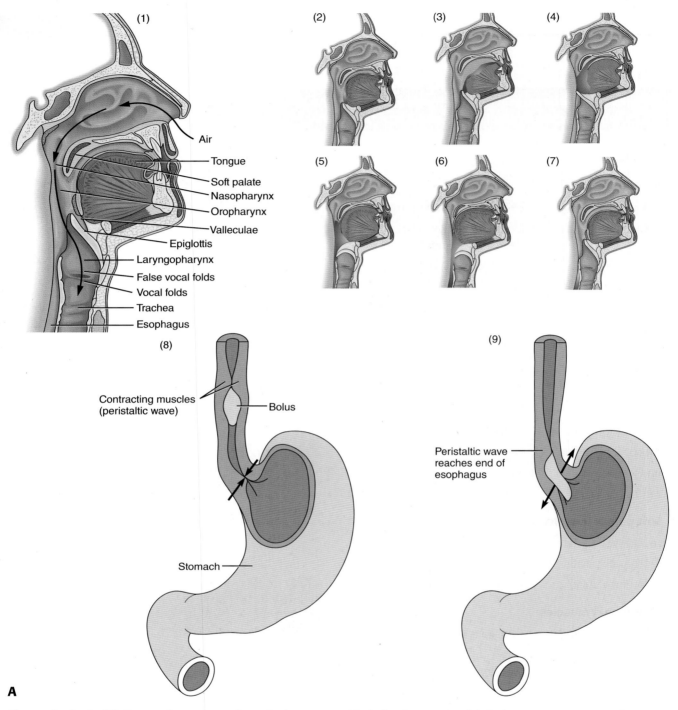

A

Figure 8–4. A. (1) Tongue is at rest and respiration occurs. No bolus is present. (2) Bolus rests on tongue after having been prepared for swallowing. (3) Anterior tongue elevates to hard palate, and hyoid elevates. (4) Posterior tongue elevates, which propels the bolus into the oropharynx. At the same time, the larynx moves up and forward, and the velum elevates. The upper esophageal sphincter opens as the larynx elevates. Vocal folds adduct. (5) The epiglottis inverts, closing off the vestibule. The bolus passes over inverted epiglottis, divides into two portions, and enters the pyriform sinuses of the hypopharynx. (6) Tongue moves posteriorly to contact posterior pharyngeal wall, increasing pharyngeal pressure. The divided boluses recombine at the esophageal opening, and bolus passes through upper esophageal sphincter into esophagus. (7) Bolus has cleared the hypopharynx, epiglottis elevates, hyoid and larynx descend, velum depresses, and respiration (typically expiration) is initiated. (8) Bolus is swept along esophagus by peristaltic contractions; lower esophageal sphincter (*arrows*) is closed. (9) Lower esophageal sphincter (*arrows*) opens; bolus moves into stomach. (Modified from Campbell, 1990.) *Source:* From Seikel/Drumright/King. *Anatomy & Physiology for Speech, Language, and Hearing, 5th Ed.* ©Cengage, Inc. Reproduced by permission. *continues*

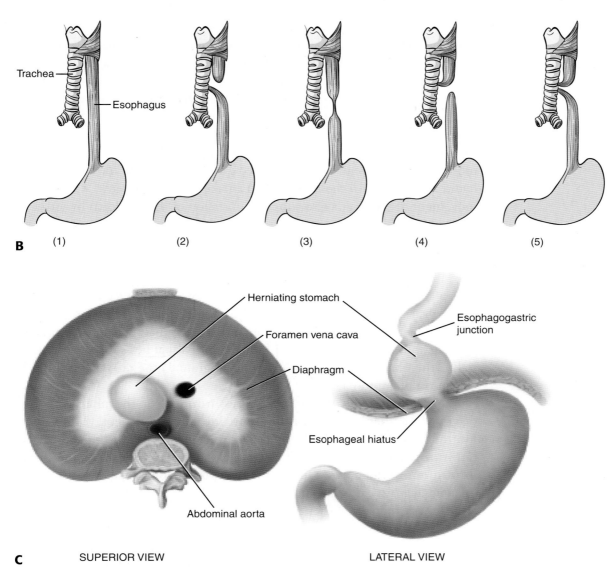

Figure 8–4. *continued* **B.** Developmental malformations of the esophagus. (B–1) Normal esophagus. (B–2) Esophagus anastomosing with trachea. (B–3) Esophageal stenosis. (B–4) Esophageal discontinuity with tracheal porting. (B–5) Esophageal fusing with trachea, resulting in esophageal porting. (Adapted from Newman and Randolph, 1990.) *Source:* From Seikel/Drumright/King. *Anatomy & Physiology for Speech, Language, and Hearing, 5th Ed.* ©Cengage, Inc. Reproduced by permission. **C.** Herniation of stomach through esophageal hiatus of diaphragm. *Left*: View from above the diaphragm, showing herniation of stomach. *Right*: Lateral view. Note the position of the lower esophageal sphincter (esophagogastric junction). (Modified from Healey & Seybold, 1969; Payne & Ellis, 1984.) *Source:* From Seikel/Drumright/King. *Anatomy & Physiology for Speech, Language, and Hearing, 5th Ed.* ©Cengage, Inc. Reproduced by permission.

Because of the complexity of the pharyngeal stage (see Figure 8–3), we will characterize the activities as separate functional operations, including hyolaryngeal elevation, pharyngeal pressurization, airway protection, pharyngeal timing, and upper esophageal sphincter (UES) action. (Remember discussion of the cricopharyngeus muscle in Chapter 7: It makes up the bulk of the upper esophageal sphincter, which is responsible for keeping the esophagus closed until a bolus is ready to enter the esophagus.) Realize this sequence is simply a way to organize discussion of the movements, but these are not isolated events during the pharyngeal stage of the swallow.

Hyolaryngeal elevation: Movement of the hyolaryngeal complex (hyoid and larynx) begins with anterior movement of the tongue base and tongue tip at the initiation of the swallow. Nearly simultaneously, the hyoid and larynx elevate as a result of contraction of the suprahyoid muscles (Pearson, Langmore, Uy, & Zumwalt, 2012), followed quickly by anterior movement of the hyoid and larynx. All these movements make mechanical sense. The upward movement of the larynx also supports inversion of the epiglottis by virtue of its mechanical attachment to the larynx and proximity to the tongue. As we will discuss shortly, elevation of the larynx is a key player in relaxation of the upper esophageal sphincter and protection of the airway.

Laryngeal elevation is extremely important. If the larynx fails to elevate, the epiglottis may not invert to cover the laryngeal entrance and the upper esophageal sphincter may not open. The bolus could enter the pharynx with an unprotected airway and fail to pass into the esophagus, resulting in bolus pooling above the level of the UES. If the individual lies supine with material in the pharynx, that material could migrate to the airway, resulting in aspiration pneumonia.

Pressurization of the pharynx: Pressurization of the pharynx is the driving force behind bolus propulsion into the esophagus (McCulloch, Hoffman, & Ciucci, 2010). You can think of the swallowing process in terms of manipulation of oral, pharyngeal, and esophageal pressures that, in turn, move the bolus. During the oral preparatory stage, because of the open nasal airway, the oral and pharyngeal cavity pressures are equalized with atmospheric pressure. When entering the transit stage of the swallow, the soft palate tightly closes, separating the oropharynx and nasopharynx, and the tongue begins squeezing the bolus posteriorly. The positive pressure created by the movements of the tongue propels the bolus toward the oropharynx. The tongue makes contact with the posterior oropharynx, transferring the bolus into the pharynx with an additional pressure gradient. The pharyngeal walls compress the bolus, increasing the pressure to prompt it toward the esophagus. Elevation of the larynx creates a relatively lower pressure at the esophageal entryway, and relaxation of the cricopharyngeus muscle further increases the superior-inferior pressure gradient. The laryngeal entryway is tightly clamped to avoid confounding the pressures of deglutition with those of respiration so that the bolus is naturally drawn to the area of lower pressure, the esophageal entrance. The cricopharyngeus muscle contracts most forcefully during inspiration, thereby prohibiting inflation of the esophagus. Peristaltic contraction of the superior, middle, and inferior constrictor muscles helps to clear the pharynx of residue to protect the airway, but the pressures generated are the primary means of propelling the bolus into the esophagus (Gumbley, Huckabee, Doeltgen, Witte, & Moran, 2008).

Airway protection: The airway must be protected. To accomplish the protective function, the vocal folds tightly adduct at the initial stage of the swallow, as part of what Dodds et al. (1990) referred to as the "leading complex" of actions (see Figure 8–3). As the larynx elevates, the false folds close (in most people), and the epiglottis inverts to cover the laryngeal aditus. If you reflect on Figure 8–3, you'll see that vestibular closure (closing of the laryngeal vestibule, which is the entryway to the larynx) is completely sealed off as long as the bolus is in the pharynx.

Pharyngeal timing: Doty and Bosma (1956) performed the seminal research that defined the muscular sequence of the pharyngeal swallow, and since that time researchers have acknowledged that the highly complex neuromuscular activity arises from a centrally generated neuromuscular pattern. Thexton, Crompton, and German (2007) elaborated the sequence of events in the pharyngeal swallow, as you can see from Figure 8–5. Although this study was performed on nonhumans, it should be noted that the swallow across mammals is extraordinarily similar in both sequence and timing (Jean, 2001). In Figure 8–5, the term *leading complex* refers to the first set of muscles that are activated in the patterned response. Those muscles are the hyoglossus, stylohyoid, mylohyoid, middle pharyngeal constrictor, and styloglossus, and they contract about 300 ms (about one-third second) after the liquid bolus is introduced orally. This contraction coincides with the timeline identified by Dodds et al. (1990; see Figure 8–3), with three of these muscles causing hyoid elevation and one (styloglossus) involved in tongue retraction (the Dodds et al. timeline is relative to the first muscle activation rather than introduction of the bolus, which is how we have drawn Figure 8–5). An

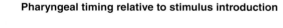

Pharyngeal timing relative to stimulus introduction

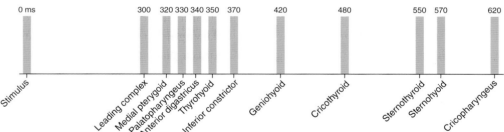

Figure 8–5. Pharyngeal swallow data as described by Thexton, Crompton, and German (2007). Timing of muscle contraction during pharyngeal stage of swallow. Stimulus presentation was a milk bolus delivered orally to decerebrate pigs. EMG recordings were verified through videoradiograph recordings. Note that the leading complex included the hyoglossus, stylohyoid, mylohyoid, middle pharyngeal constrictor, and styloglossus muscles. The following are implied muscular functions and timings: 300 ms leading complex, including hyoglossus (hyoid elevation), stylohyoid (hyoid elevation), mylohyoid (hyoid elevation), Middle pharyngeal constrictor (pharyngeal constriction), and styloglossus (tongue retraction); 320 ms medial pterygoid (mandible elevation); 330 ms palatopharyngeus (pharyngeal elevation and constriction), omohyoid (hyoid depression or fixation); 340 ms anterior digastricus (forward hyoid movement); 350 ms thyrohyoid (elevation of larynx); 370 ms inferior constrictor (narrowing of hypopharynx); 420 ms geniohyoid (hyoid elevation); 480 ms cricothyroid (anterior rocking of thyroid); 550 ms sternothyroid (fixation of larynx); 570 ms sternohyoid (fixation of hyoid); 620 ms cricopharyngeus (UES activation). (From data of Thexton, Crompton, & German, 2007.) *Source:* From Seikel/Drumright/King. *Anatomy & Physiology for Speech, Language, and Hearing, 5th Ed.* ©Cengage, Inc. Reproduced by permission.

Deficits of the Esophageal Stage

Although the disorders of the esophageal stage are not directly treated by a speech-language pathologist (SLP), a working knowledge of problems associated with this stage is certainly important to the SLP. Gastroesophageal reflux disease (GERD) is significant and potentially life-threatening. You may have experienced heartburn at one time or another, but that burning feeling actually may have been the acids from your stomach (i.e., gastric region) being refluxed into your esophagus or pharynx. In some individuals the lower esophageal sphincter relaxes, allowing gastric juices to enter the esophagus. If the upper sphincter is likewise weakened or flaccid, these acids may reflow (reflux) into the pyriform sinus, assaulting the delicate pharyngeal tissue. If this occurs during the night when you are supine, the acid may flow into the airway, resulting in aspira-

tion. (We know of one client with oral, pharyngeal, and esophageal dysphagia secondary to irradiation for cancer. Her pharyngeal dysphagia was being well controlled through treatment directed toward improving pharyngeal responses, and her esophageal reflux had been controlled surgically. The surgical procedure to prevent reflux failed, and she was hospitalized with aspiration pneumonia.)

The stomach can herniate through the esophageal hiatus (see Figure 8–4C), a condition termed a *hiatal hernia*. When this occurs, the lower esophageal sphincter may malfunction, allowing reflux into the esophagus. More rarely, a congenital malformation of the esophagus, such as stenosis (see Figure 8–4B), may cause a severe, life-threatening loss of nutrition in a newborn. Rare maldevelopment of the esophagus may even result in the esophageal contents directly entering the trachea.

without the bolus being retained in the oropharynx. In this manner, the classical oral preparation stage of swallowing is revised to include ingestion and Stage I and Stage II transport. The pharyngeal phase is equivalent to the hyolaryngeal transport phase, and the esophageal stage is the same as the classical esophageal stage.

✓ To summarize:

- Mastication and deglutition involve a complex set of motor acts that are strongly governed by the sensory environment.

- The oral stage can be subdivided into the oral preparatory and transport stages. In the **oral preparatory stage**, food is introduced into the oral cavity, moved onto the molars for chewing, and mixed with saliva to form a concise bolus between the tongue and the hard palate. In the **oral transport stage**, the bolus is moved back toward the oropharynx by the tongue.

- The **pharyngeal stage** begins when the bolus reaches the faucial pillars. The soft palate and larynx have begun elevation during the transport stage, and contact of the tongue with the posterior pharyngeal wall pressurizes the pharynx, propelling the bolus to the upper esophageal sphincter, which has relaxed to receive the material. The epiglottis has dropped to partially cover the laryngeal opening, whereas the intrinsic musculature of the larynx has effected a tight seal to protect the airway. Food passes over the epiglottis and through the pyriform sinuses to the esophagus.

- The final, **esophageal stage** involves the peristaltic movement of the bolus through the esophagus.

- **Central pattern generators (CPGs)** govern the complex, hierarchical movement of muscles in oral, pharyngeal and esophageal stages. Although each stage is independently controlled, the control systems are linked, providing efficiently controlled deglutition. The oral preparatory stage is considered to be a voluntary stage.

Neurophysiological Underpinnings of Mastication and Deglutition

ANAQUEST LESSON ⊙

It is critically important for the experience of eating to be pleasant and behaviorally reinforcing. Natural drives related to hunger bring you to the process of acquiring nutrition, but the food must be palatable for it to be consumed in sufficient quantities to properly nourish you. Furthermore, there must be an adequate neuroanatomical substrate that supports the stages of swallowing. Let us discuss these substrates in turn, and then see how they integrate into the acts of mastication and deglutition.

There are three primary brain stem elements that govern swallowing: the sensory (afferent) component, the cranial motor nuclei, and the network that organizes these two elements into "the program" for swallowing, or the swallowing CPG (Broussard & Altschuler, 2000; Ertekin & Aydogdu, 2003; Jean, 2001). Let us look at each of these elements.

Sensation Associated with Mastication and Deglutition

Numerous types of stimulus receptors are critical for completion of the chewing, sucking, and swallowing (CSS) elements associated with mastication and deglutition. (For a thorough review of sensory systems, see Møller, 2003, and Kandel, Schwartz, Jessell, Siegelbaum, & Hudspeth, 2013). Among these are the gustatory (taste), tactile (touch), temperature (thermal), and pressure senses, as well as pain sensation (nociception) (Møller, 2003). Each plays a critical role in successful completion of the CSS routines. We will go into considerable detail in our discussion of these senses, but some of the material may become clear to you only upon studying the underlying neuroanatomy in Chapters 11 and 12.

Gustation

Gustation (taste) is a complex and critical component of CSS. Taste drives the desire to continue eating, which fulfills the nutritional requirements of the body. Taste receptors (**taste buds** or **taste cells**) consist of a class of sensors known as **chemoreceptors**, in that they respond when specific chemicals come in contact with them. Taste receptors are found interspersed in the epithelia of the tongue within **papillae**, or prominences (Figure 8–6). The

chemoreceptors: neural receptors that respond to specific chemical compositions

papillae: prominences

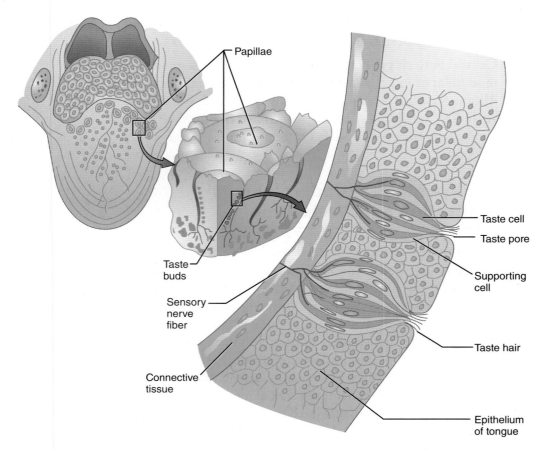

Figure 8–6. Taste sensor. Note that taste receptors are found in papillae of the epithelium of the tongue, within taste pores. (Adapted from Buck, 2000.) *Source:* From Seikel/ Drumright/King. *Anatomy & Physiology for Speech, Language, and Hearing, 5th Ed.* ©Cengage, Inc. Reproduced by permission.

taste pore: opening in the lingual epithelium that houses taste cells

microvilli: small, hair-like fibers projecting from the taste cell into the taste pore

tongue is invested with taste buds to convey the gustatory sense. Sensors for all types of tastes are found throughout the oral cavity (Roper & Chaudhari, 2017), although there are regions of concentration of receptor types (e.g., Bushman, Ye, & Liman, 2015; Kochem, 2017). The anterior tongue has a higher propensity for sensation of sweetness, starchiness, and a savory (meaty) perception, while the posterior tongue has a propensity for bitter taste (Choi, Lee, et al., 2016; Colvin, Pullicin, & Lim, 2018). Bitter tastes are generally sensed near the terminal sulcus in circumvallate papillae (Choi, Lee, et al., 2016). An opening in the epithelium called the **taste pore** permits the isolation of a sample of the tasted substance, which is held in place by **microvilli** (small hair-like fibers projecting from the taste cell into the taste pore). There are five basic tastes: sweet, salty, sour, bitter, and umami. We are familiar with the first four terms, but you may have never run across *umami*, though you most certainly have tasted it. Umami is the taste of monosodium glutamate, which tastes meaty or protein-like. For more than a century, we believed that taste receptors were restricted to zones of the tongue, with sweet tastes being sensed at the tip, salty at the sides in front, and sour at the sides in back. Bitterness was thought to be sensed on the posterior tongue. The reality is that all the tastes can be sensed all over the tongue.

If you examine Figure 8–6 (also see Figure 6–36 in Chapter 6), you can see that the tongue is richly invested with papillae of various forms. The filiform papillae are the dominant papillary formation of the tongue. They appear as small threads on the surface of the tongue, are pink or gray in color, and make the dorsum of the tongue look rough. They include not only taste sensors but also mechanoreceptors to provide a fine tactile sensory ability to the tongue, permitting fine discrimination of the bolus characteristics (Table 8–4). Fungiform papillae are bright red and are found interspersed with filiform papillae on the tip and sides of the tongue. Vallate papillae are

What Did They Do with the Tongue Map?

Hanig (1901 as cited in Collings, 1974) T was the first to hypothesize that the basic tastes of sweet, sour, salty, and bitter were represented in zones of the tongue, so that sweet taste was mediated by the tongue tip, bitter taste was sensed by the posterior tongue, and so on. His work was based on that of Hoffmann in 1875 (as cited in Collings, 1974) arose from both the observation that there was differential anatomy among taste receptors (circumvallate papillae are found in the posterior middle of the tongue, and foliate papillae are in the posterior lateral aspect; fungiform papillae are found on the anterior and lateral surfaces of the tongue) and that humans tended to taste the four basic tastants in different locations. The work of many perceptual scientists who followed Hoffmann and Hanig defined the tongue tip as sensitive to sweet taste, the anterior and anterolateral surface as responsive to salty, with sour taste being sensed at the mid-lateral regions. Bitter taste was reserved for the posterior dorsum of the tongue, just above the junction of the hard and soft palates. This view began to blur, however, as knowledge of taste receptors improved. Hoon et al. (1999) showed that taste receptors were actually a subset of what is termed G protein coupled receptor signal pathways (GPCR). Two specific GPCRs were identified: T1R1 (found predominantly in the circumvallate papillae) and T1R2 (found in abundance in the foliate papillae). What the authors also found was that the receptors were mixed, rather than isolated: T1R2 dominated the foliate papillae, but there were T1R1 receptors there as well. Eventually, two more receptors were found (T1R3 and T12Rs) and added to the mix. Perception studies revealed that, in humans, the sense of sweetness is mediated by the combined activation of T1R2 and T1R3 receptors (Nelson et al., 2001), and bitter sense is activated by the T2Rs receptors. The taste of amino acids (such as umami, the taste of monosodium glutamate) is mediated by a combination of T1R1 and T1R3 sensors. A receptor for sour taste (PK2DL1; Huang et al., 2006) left salt as the only outlier without a receptor. Salty taste evidently is mediated by direct sodium migration into the cell (Oka, Butnaru, von Buchholtz, Ryba, & Zuker, 2013). The taste bud itself, which is not neural tissue, can be genetically altered in lab animals so that, for instance, a bitter TRC feeds a sweet neural fiber. When this is done, a lab animal is likely to develop an affinity for the bitter taste, ostensibly because the animal perceives sweet when bitter taste is presented (Mueller, Hoon, Erlenbach, Zuker, & Ryba, 2005).

Where did that leave our historical taste map? Although it is appealing to think that specific regions of the tongue are sensitive to specific tastes, this view gets blurred quite a bit by the reality of the receptor distribution. Each taste bud has many TRCs, and there is a great deal of overlap of TRC fields. As Hoon et al. (1999) stated, there is a correlation between perception of taste and receptors, but there is no room for a rigidly demarcated tongue map in current physiology.

Table 8–4

Taste Mediation in the Mouth

Taste	Papillae and Location on Tongue	Numbers of Receptors Per Papillae	Stimulus	Receptors	Function in Humans
Sweet	Foliate papillae: mostly posterior edge of tongue Circumvallate papillae: mostly posterior tongue fungiform (Kochem, 2017; Witt & Miller, 1992; Yee et al., 2011); mostly anterior tongue	Type I taste receptors: hundreds	Sugars, saccharin, carbohydrates, aspartame, monellin, thaumatin, D-amino acids, starches	G-coupled receptors: T1R2 and T1R3 In foliate and circumvallate papillae	Attractant for humans
Sour	NA	NA	Acidic food and drink	Perhaps specific ion channels	Repellant for humans (perhaps avoiding spoiled foods)
Salty	NA	NA	NaCl	Specific ion channels	Attractant for humans
Bitter	Circumvallate papillae: posterior central tongue (Choi, Cho, et al., 2016) Fungiform papillae: mostly anterior two-thirds of tongue (Buck & Bargman, 2013; Lipchock et al., 2017)	Type II receptors: 5 per pore	Caffeine, nicotine, alkaloids, denatonium, quinine	G-coupled receptors: T2Rs	Repellant for humans (perhaps avoiding poisons)
Umami	Fungiform papillae: mostly anterior two-thirds of tongue	5 taste buds per pore	Monosodium glutamate, purine nucleo-tides (inosine 5+'-monophos-phate [IMP])	T1R1 & T1R3 receptors in fungiform papillae	Attractant for humans (promotes protein consumption)
Spiciness (pungency)	NA	NA	Capsaicin; chili peppers, pepper, ginger, horseradish	TRPV1 & TRPA1 receptors	Burning sensation (chemesthesis)
Coolness	NA	NA	Peppermint, spearmint, menthol	TRPM8 receptors	

Note that taste sensors are widely distributed throughout the papillae. There is a preponderance of Type I sensors in the anterior fungiform papillae and a preponderance of Type II bitter sensors in the circumvallate papillae on the posterior dorsum. That said, it is the combination of sensor types that give the broad and diverse perceptions that humans experience, and there are Type II sensors in anterior papillae and Type I sensors in posterior papillae.

Source From data of Buck and Bargmann (2013); Choi, Cho, Chung, and Kim (2016); Kochem (2017); Linden (1993); Lipchock, Spielman, Mennella, Mansfield, Hwang, Douglas, and Reed, (2017); Roper and Chaudhari (2017); Takeda, Shishido, Kitao, and Suzuki (1982); Witt and Miller (1992); Yee, Sukumaran, Kotha, Gilbertson, and Margolskee (2011).

the large V-shaped formation of circles seen in the posterior dorsum of the tongue. There are typically a dozen or so on a tongue, and each has a "moat" surrounding it. Foliate papillae are sparsely present on the lateral margins of the tongue.

Taste is mediated by means of four cranial nerves. The VII facial nerve mediates the sense of taste from the anterior two thirds of the tongue, predominantly involving sweet, salty, and sour sensations (Segerstad & Helle-kant, 1989; Figure 8–7), whereas the IX glossopharyngeal nerve transmits information from the posterior one third of the tongue (Geran & Travers, 2011; Ninomaya, Imoto, & Sugimura, 1999). Taste receptors of the palate are innervated by the VII facial nerve. Although not shown in Figure 8–7, taste receptors of the epiglottis and esophagus are innervated by the X vagus nerve. The V trigeminal is responsible for the mediation of chemesthetic sense, as we will discuss shortly.

Taste stimulus to the VII facial nerve is relayed through the genicu-late ganglion to the solitary tract within the medulla, to terminate at the rostral and lateral aspects of the solitary tract nucleus in the gustatory region of the brain stem. Taste sensation from the IX glossopharyngeal nerve is mediated via the petrosal ganglion, and fibers also terminate in the solitary tract nucleus. Epiglottal and esophageal taste senses are transmitted via the

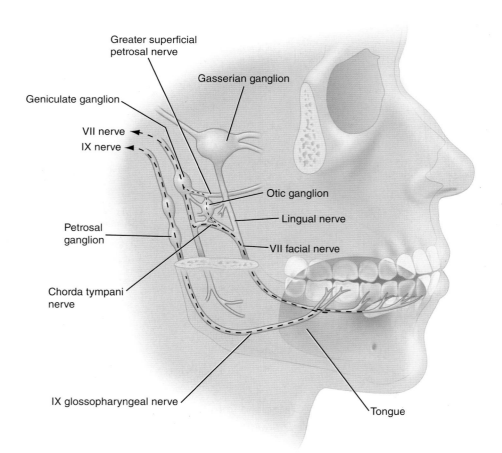

Figure 8–7. Innervation schematic for anterior and posterior tongue. *Source:* From Seikel/Drumright/ King. *Anatomy & Physiology for Speech, Language, and Hearing, 5th Ed.* ©Cengage, Inc. Reproduced by permission. (Adapted from Mountcastle, 1974.)

X vagus nerve through the nodose ganglion, likewise to the solitary tract nucleus. This taste information is then relayed to the ventral posterior medial nucleus (VPMN) of the thalamus, which subsequently relays this information ipsilaterally to the anterior portion of the insula of the cerebral cortex. Figure 8–8 illustrates the taste pathways in humans.

Now examine Figure 8–9, which illustrates the relative contribution of each nerve to taste perception. First, notice the relative magnitude of tastes mediated by each of the nerves (VII, IX, and X) in relation to their locations and distribution. This information converges on the rostral nucleus of the solitary tract (rNST) and is then sent to the ventral posterior nucleus (VPN) of the thalamus. The sensation is subsequently transmitted to the primary sensory cortex (located in the postcentral gyrus of the cerebrum) and to the

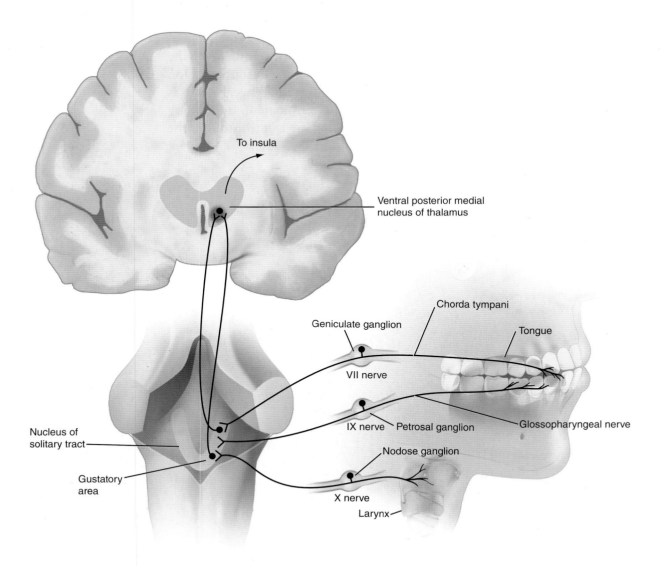

Figure 8–8. Pathways mediating the sensations of taste. (Modified from Buck, 2000.) *Source:* From Seikel/Drumright/King. *Anatomy & Physiology for Speech, Language, and Hearing, 5th Ed.* ©Cengage, Inc. Reproduced by permission.

insular cortex of the frontal lobe (located in a fold of the cerebral cortex underlying the operculum), as well as the operculum overlying the insula. Taste and smell are probably integrated at the insula (Møller, 2003). Fibers from the insula project into the limbic system and the motor regions of the brain stem.

The nucleus of the solitary tract (NST) also projects into the motor cortex, specifically the region serving the tongue. This is important. Our nutritional needs govern our selection of sweet and umami tastes, as these indicate the presence of carbohydrates (sweet) and protein (umami). Salt is also a necessary mineral, so we crave that taste as well. These tastes may elicit salivation, as well as ingestive responses, including tongue protrusion to receive the food, release of insulin, mastication, and deglutition. In contrast, bitter and sour tastes typify poisons, and they often elicit protective responses

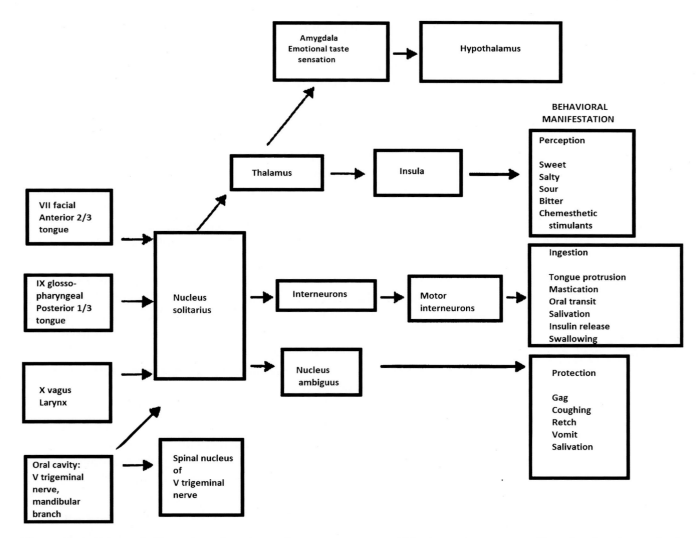

Figure 8–9. Schematic illustration of routing and response to taste within the nervous system. Note that the chemesthetic sense is mediated by the V trigeminal nerve. (Modified from Simon & Roper, 1993.) *Source:* From Seikel/Drumright/King. *Anatomy & Physiology for Speech, Language, and Hearing, 5th Ed.* ©Cengage, Inc. Reproduced by permission.

that include gagging, coughing, apnea, and salivation (Huang et al., 2006) (salivation in this case encapsulates the material and protects the oral cavity). The receptors sensitive to bitter taste are even found in the cilia of the airway, and presence of bitter materials increases the beating of those cilia, apparently as a means of eliminating a potentially toxic material from the airway (Shah, Ben-Shahar, Moninger, Kline, & Welsh, 2009). Admittedly, we *do* eat sour and bitter foods (think coffee), but notice next time you encounter a particularly bitter taste how you find it difficult to swallow, or at least become wary of it. This reaction underscores a critically important point. Tastes can elicit motor responses that may or may not be under volitional (or even conscious) control. The gag response is a complex motor act involving elevation of the larynx and clamping of the vocal folds, elevation of the velum, and protrusion of the tongue. Coughing entails tightly closing the vocal folds, compressing the abdomen and thorax, and forcefully blowing the vocal folds apart. Now recognize that each of these responses has components of the swallow embedded within it, and you can see that deglutition is made up of a complex set of motor responses dictated by stimuli in the oral and pharyngeal spaces.

Some foods are capable of activating nontaste sensors, which can have both positive and negative effects on swallowing. Oral chemesthesis is the process of detection of chemical stimuli by thermal and pain receptors within the mouth (Green, 2012). Obviously, pain is an aversive stimulus that typically causes a person to stop whatever activity induced the pain (think of the last time you burned your finger). In contrast, thermal stimuli (heat and cold) mediate qualities of the bolus that are important, although there are extremes there as well. A warm drink is very satisfying in winter, but if it is too hot, the sense of pain takes over. We will talk about pain and thermal sense shortly, but first let us consider the interaction of these protective senses in gustation.

The study of oral chemesthesis has provided insight into swallowing behavior. Some chemesthetic stimuli enhance swallowing function by lowering the threshold of the swallow, although others signal the body that a foreign and potentially dangerous material has been introduced. Oral chemesthesis can tell your body that it has been invaded by bacteria that have caused chemical changes in the oral mucosa, for instance, causing sneezing or nasal rhinorrhea (Green, 2012).

These chemosensor components are only one side of chemesthesis, however. We regularly indulge in foods that trigger responses from pain and thermal sensors. Chili powder, for instance, contains capsaicin that triggers pain and thermal receptors in the mouth, giving the burning sensation and, some would say, sense of pain from the chili (Cometto-Muñiz, Cain, & Abraham, 2004). (There are at least two words for "hot" in Spanish: *picante* and *caliente*, with *picante* referring to the heat associated with capsaicin and *caliente* referring to the heat associated with cooking.) Researchers are examining the possibility that clinicians can utilize oral chemesthesis to their advantage in therapy. There are several examples of the cross-modality function of chemesthesis. For example, carbonation triggers a painful sensation, and gingerol in very strong ginger ale stimulates thermal receptors. The conversion of CO_2 to carbonic acid in carbonated water, a reaction catalyzed by the salivary enzyme carbonic anhydrase, activates lingual nociceptors, which causes trigeminal neurons to signal oral irritation to higher centers (Cowart, 1998; Dessirier, Simons, Carstens, O'Mahony, & Carstens, 2000). Carbonated water, with and without the addition of the thermal irritant ginger (in strong ginger ale) (Krival & Bates, 2012), as well as high concentrations of sucrose, salt, and citric acid (Pelletier & Dhanaraj, 2006) all have increased linguapalatal pressure in people with normal swallow function. In adults with dysphagia, high levels of citric acid and carbonation have each been shown to reduce the latency of swallow initiation as well as to reduce the occurrence of aspiration in experimental MBSS studies (Bülow, Olsson, & Ekberg, 2003; Logemann, 1995; Pelletier & Lawless, 2003; Sdravou, Walshe, & Dagdilelis, 2012). Although to date no studies have examined the effectiveness of these chemesthetic stimuli on swallowing over time, the fact that immediate changes in swallowing occur suggests that capitalizing on the oral chemesthetic sense has promise for increasing lingual force and pharyngeal swallowing in people with dysphagia. A caution: In many of these studies, the effect on swallowing was achieved only when the bolus was so strongly irritating that it was deemed unpalatable by the research participants (Logemann, 1995; Pelletier & Dhanaraj, 2006).

Olfaction

Olfaction (the sense of smell) plays a vital role in appetite and taste. Molecules arising from food pass over olfactory chemoreceptors to increase the magnitude of the taste perception, a fact to which you can relate if you remember how flat your favorite food tasted when you had nasal congestion. In fact, if you tightly occlude your nares and blindly take a bite of apple and then a bite of onion, you will likely not be able to taste the difference.

Olfactory sensors arise from the olfactory bulb and have the distinction of a short life and continual replacement. They last only about 60 days before being replaced by new sensors. Olfactory sensors are found within the epithelial lining of the upper posterior nasal cavity (Figure 8–10). There are small cilia protruding from the olfactory sensor, similar to the microvilli of the taste cell. These cilia are highly specialized, in that they transduce the molecular stimulant into the perception of smell that is transmitted to the olfactory bulb located within the cranial space. Recent research has revealed that although the basic structure of the odor receptors on the cilia is similar for all olfactory sensors, the specific structure of the receptor varies slightly, so that more than 1,000 different odors are decoded by the olfactory system.

After an odorant stimulates a specific receptor, information that the receptor has been activated is transmitted to the olfactory bulb, which resides within the braincase. More than 1,000 axons of sensory cells converge on each olfactory interneuron (termed a **glomerulus**) in the olfactory bulb. This information is transmitted by means of the olfactory tract to the olfactory region of the cortex, which includes the amygdala, the anterior olfactory

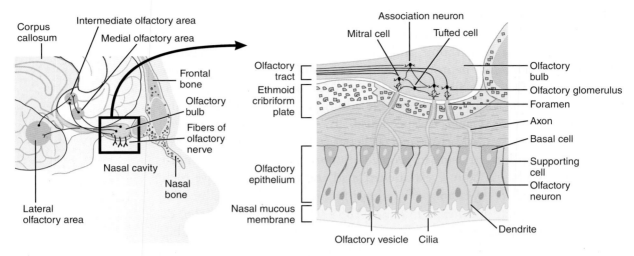

Figure 8–10. Detail of olfactory bulb. *Source:* From Seikel/Drumright/King. *Anatomy & Physiology for Speech, Language, and Hearing, 5th Ed.* ©Cengage, Inc. Reproduced by permission. *

nucleus, the piriform cortex, the olfactory tubercle, and a portion of the entorhinal cortex. Information from some of these brain centers is routed through the thalamus and subsequently relayed to the frontal lobe of the cerebral cortex, orbital region. Olfactory information from the amygdala is transmitted to the hypothalamus, whereas olfactory information from the entorhinal area terminates in the hippocampus within the temporal lobe. The functional implications are that olfaction arrives at the cerebral cortex through multiple pathways, including the thalamus, and that the information serves as a stimulus to emotion and motivation (amygdala), physiological responses (hypothalamus), and memory encoding (hippocampus). The information reaching the orbitofrontal region of the cerebral cortex appears to be involved in olfactory discrimination (i.e., conscious, discriminative processing of smell). Again, recognize that motor responses are readily mediated by reception of olfactory stimulation. Salivation may result from pleasant food odors, whereas gagging or even vomiting can be triggered by unpleasant odors.

ANAQUEST LESSON

mechanoreceptors: neural receptors designed to sense mechanical forces

glabrous: hairless

Tactile Sense

The sense of touch is mediated by a number of **mechanoreceptors**, which are sensors that are sensitive to physical contact. Generally, sensors differ based on whether the epithelium contains hair or is hairless (**glabrous** skin). Glabrous skin of the hands contains fingerprints that are, in reality, the overlay for dense collections of mechanoreceptors. Touch receptors are broadly distributed about the body and are differentiated based on the type of stimulus that causes them to respond (Figure 8–11). Hairy skin receptors are less critical to our discussion of swallowing, as the epithelial linings of the oral and pharyngeal cavities are hairless.

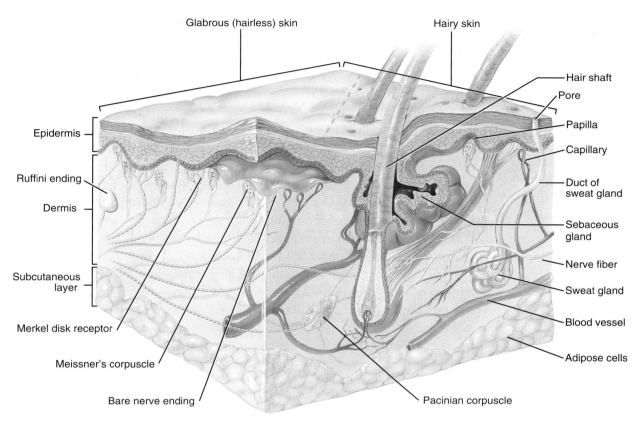

Figure 8–11. Detail of mechanoreceptors. *Source:* From Seikel/Drumright/King. *Anatomy & Physiology for Speech, Language, and Hearing, 5th Ed.* ©Cengage, Inc. Reproduced by permission.

Glabrous (hairless) skin contains **Meissner's corpuscles** and **Merkel disk receptors**. Meissner's corpuscles are physically coupled to the papillae in which they reside (similar to taste receptors) and respond to minute mechanical movement. Merkel disk receptors transmit the sense of pressure. Meissner's corpuscles adapt quickly to stimulation (i.e., they stop responding after a brief period of sustained stimulation), whereas Merkel disk receptors respond for longer periods of time to sustained stimulation. Both of these receptors are found within the superficial layer of the lingual epithelium. Both Meissner's corpuscles and Merkel disk receptors are found at the end of the papillary ridge. Deep cutaneous tissues contain **Pacinian corpuscles** and cells with the **Ruffini endings**. The Pacinian corpuscle is similar to the Meissner's corpuscle and responds to rapid deep pressure to the outer epithelium. Ruffini endings sense stretch within the deep tissues and are critical to our perception of the shape of objects perceived by touch. It is important to note that Meissner's corpuscles and Merkel disk receptors have small receptor fields, which means that their effective sensory area is more limited than those of the deeply embedded Ruffini endings and Pacinian corpuscles, which have larger receptive fields. Deep pressure has the potential to stimulate a larger field and greater array of sensors than light pressure, an issue that is important in the treatment of dysphagia.

Meissner's corpuscles: superficial cutaneous mechanoreceptors for minute movement

Merkel disk receptors: superficial cutaneous mechanoreceptors for light pressure

Pacinian corpuscles: deep cutaneous mechanoreceptors for deep pressure

Ruffini endings: deep cutaneous mechanoreceptors for tissue stretch

Vibration sense is a subclass of tactile sense. Vibration may be considered as either deep or superficial pressure, depending on the amplitude of the vibration. In both cases, vibration is sensed as individual deformation of tactile sensors. Pacinian corpuscles (deep pressure sensors) respond most efficiently to stimulation between 70 and 500 Hz (best frequency is 280 Hz), whereas Meissner's corpuscles respond best to stimulation between 10 and 100 Hz (with a shallow best frequency of 50 Hz). (**Best frequency** refers to the frequency of vibration at which a sensor responds most effectively.) Although both of these receptors are rapidly adapting sensors, Pacinian corpuscles (deep receptors) have a markedly lower threshold to vibration than Meissner's corpuscles (superficial receptors). Rapidly adapting sensors have lower thresholds of stimulation than slowly adapting receptors, meaning that Meissner's and Pacinian corpuscles respond to lower levels of stimulation than Ruffini endings and Merkel disk receptors.

The classic test for spatial density of receptors is of two-point discrimination, in which an individual is provided a pressure of calibrated force by means of two probes. The distance between the probes that can be perceived as two versus one stimulus is considered an index of the density of receptors for the structure. That is, if the two points are close enough together, they both will stimulate the same single receptor, giving the perception of a single contact point.

Thermal Receptors

Four classes of thermal stimulation are differentiated by human senses: warm, hot, cool, and cold. Thermal receptors are grossly the same as pain sensors, in that they are bare nerve endings, although the microscopic level reveals that cold receptors also have ion channels associated with thermal sense (Bouvier et al, 2018). Although it is convenient to group pain and thermal sense, the reality is that thermal sensors are functionally different from pain sensors, with different nerve endings responding to these two broad classes of stimulation.

Thermal receptors differ from mechanoreceptors in a critical manner: Mechanoreceptors respond only when stimulated, whereas thermal receptors have a tonic, ongoing discharge. The individual receptors for each of the

Sensory Examination

The clinical or bedside evaluation tests both motor and sensory functions of swallowing. Logemann (1998) provides an excellent discussion of both sensory and motor examinations. In brief, the sensory examination is designed to assess the tactile sense (two-point discrimination), thermal sense (cold, hot), and taste sense (sweet, sour, bitter, salty, and umami). As you examine these elements, you must remove visual cues to the stimulus and must remember to test multiple locations within the oral cavity. One way to test the gustatory element is to dip cotton-tipped applicators in water and then into the dry compound (salt, sugar or sugar-free sweetener, bitters, lemon, umami) and then touch a location in the oral cavity, asking what the person tastes.

four classes of temperature have **best temperature** responses to which they respond. Cold sensors increase their firing response as the temperature of stimulation drops, even as the cool-sensitive sensors drop back to their basal firing rate. Thermal receptors, apparently, are most effective at identifying thermal stimulation that differs markedly from the ambient temperature of the skin. Thus, a slow increase or decrease in stimulus temperature is more difficult to detect than a rapid change in temperature. At high temperatures, heat sensors cease firing and pain sensors fire instead. Thermal sense requires longer duration of stimulation for the perception of sensation, but the sensation is retained for longer periods of time.

Pain Sense (Nociception)

Pain sense is included in this discussion because of its importance in the development of structural disorders of swallowing. As an example, structural defects such as oral or pharyngeal lesions (e.g., cold sores) can cause pain that can interfere with swallowing responses.

Nociceptors (pain sensors) respond directly to a noxious stimulus (e.g., chemical burn), to molecules released by injured tissue (such as positive potassium ions, serotonin, and acetylcholine), to acidity caused by injury, or to direct contact with a traumatic source. Some nociceptors respond to mechanical trauma, whereas others respond to thermal stimulation. Most nociceptors respond to general destruction of tissue rather than to the specific quality of a stimulus, and the perception arising from the stimulation of these receptors (termed *polymodal nociceptors*) is a burning sensation.

nociceptors: pain sensors

Muscle Stretch and Tension Sense

Muscle stretch is sensed by muscle spindle fibers, which consist of nuclear chain fibers and nuclear bag fibers within muscle tissue itself. Stretch receptors are found predominantly in larger muscles, such as the antigravity muscles of the legs, but are also found within oral musculature. The mandibular elevators (masseter, temporalis, and lateral and medial pterygoid muscles) are richly endowed with stretch receptors, as are the deep tongue fibers of the genioglossus and the palatoglossus muscles. Facial muscles are notably deficient in stretch receptors.

Muscle spindle fibers return a muscle to its original position following passive stretching. As an example, if you were to pull sharply down on your relaxed mandible, the mandible would quickly elevate thereafter, to the point

Nociceptors

Nociceptors produce the perception of pain when they are traumatized, such as from burning. The direct trauma to a nerve ending relays this information to higher centers so that you can withdraw from the painful stimulus. If the nerve ending is destroyed entirely, there will be no perception of pain; this is one indication of the third-degree burn.

Disorders of Salivation

Disorders of salivation can occur for numerous reasons. If an individual has the reduced sensation of salivary output, it is termed **xerostomia**, or dry mouth. This condition can have numerous causes, but the most frequent cause is one of hundreds of medications, such as diuretics, antihypertensive medications, and of course antihistamines. It is also frequently caused by the irradiation of face and neck for cancer treatment, or by chemotherapy agents. Sjogren's disease is an autoimmune disorder wherein the salivary glands and tear ducts are disabled. Finally, peripheral and central nerve damage can result in the loss of salivary function.

If the submandibular and sublingual glands are affected, the person may have difficulty with bolus formation, as these two glands help to make the bolus cohesive. If the parotid gland is affected, the pharyngeal stage swallow may be affected, as the type of saliva secreted is much thinner, facilitating movement of the bolus through the pharynx.

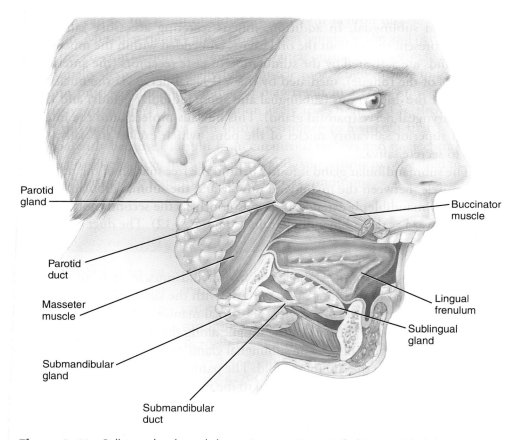

Figure 8–12. Salivary glands and ducts. *Source:* From Seikel/Drumright/King. *Anatomy & Physiology for Speech, Language, and Hearing, 5th Ed.* ©Cengage, Inc. Reproduced by permission.

Salivary flow is stimulated behaviorally by the sight, smell, and taste of food. The salivary glands produce as much as 1.2 liters of saliva per day, although the production is reduced to minute quantities during sleep.

✅ *To summarize:*

- **Gustation** (taste) is mediated by **chemoreceptors** that transmit information to the brain via the IX glossopharyngeal, X vagus, and VII facial nerves. Taste sensors are specialized for sweet, sour, salty, bitter, and umami senses.

- **Olfaction** (the sense of smell) is mediated by chemoreceptors within the nasal mucosa.

- The sense of touch (**tactile** sense) is mediated by means of **mechanoreceptors** that respond to deep or shallow touch.

- Four classes of **thermal stimulation** are differentiated by human senses: warm, hot, cool, and cold.

- Pain sense (**nociception**) is a response to a noxious stimulus.

- Muscle **stretch** is sensed by muscle spindle fibers, and muscle **tension** is sensed by Golgi tendon organs (GTOs), found within tendons and fascia.

- Tactile sense, thermal sense, pain sense, and joint and tendon sense of the face and oral cavity are mediated by the V trigeminal, IX glossopharyngeal, and X vagus nerves.

- **Salivation** occurs because of the stimulation of salivary glands.

- The type of saliva varies between glands. The **sublingual gland** produces thick **mucus** secretions, the **submandibular gland** produces both thin **serous** and mucus secretions, and the **parotid gland** secretes only serous saliva.

Reflexive Circuits of Mastication and Deglutition

ANAQUEST LESSON

The individual reflex circuits associated with mastication and deglutition are the building blocks for the normal processes associated with the intake of food and drink. Recognize that these reflexes are mediated at the level of the brain stem and do not require cortical involvement. This does not imply that there is no cortical activity associated with CSS, but rather that the cortex is not essential. We have included **expulsive reflexes** here as well (gag, retch) because of their close association with the systems of mastication and deglutition. Most of the reflexes that we will discuss are controlled by circuitry within the phylogenetically old reticular formation of the posterior brain stem (Figure 8–13).

Chewing Reflex

Chewing is a complex reflex that can be triggered by deep pressure on the roof of the mouth, as when you bite a cracker. It involves alternating left-side and right-side contraction of the muscles of mandibular elevation (masseter

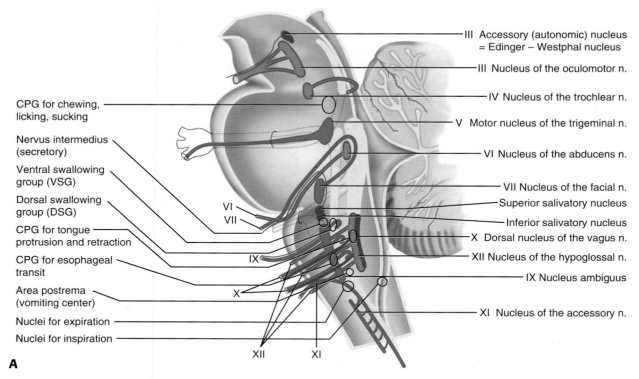

CPG for chewing, licking, sucking

Nervus intermedius (secretory)

Ventral swallowing group (VSG)

Dorsal swallowing group (DSG)

CPG for tongue protrusion and retraction

CPG for esophageal transit

Area postrema (vomiting center)

Nuclei for expiration

Nuclei for inspiration

VI
VII
IX
X
XII   XI

III Accessory (autonomic) nucleus = Edinger – Westphal nucleus

III Nucleus of the oculomotor n.

IV Nucleus of the trochlear n.

V   Motor nucleus of the trigeminal n.

VI Nucleus of the abducens n.

VII Nucleus of the facial n.
Superior salivatory nucleus
Inferior salivatory nucleus

X   Dorsal nucleus of the vagus n.

XII Nucleus of the hypoglossal n.

IX Nucleus ambiguus

XI Nucleus of the accessory n.

A

Figure 8–13. Locations of centers for swallowing, mastication/sucking, vomiting, and respiration. **A.** Lateral view of brain stem. Central pattern generator (CPG) for planning (dorsal swallowing group [DSG]) is located within the solitary nucleus and reticular formation, whereas the CPG for execution (ventral swallowing group [VSG]) is located above the nucleus ambiguus (Ertekin & Aydogdu, 2003; Jean, 2001). Motor cranial nerve nuclei involved in oropharyngeal swallowing include those of the V, VII (mastication and sucking), and XII (mastication, sucking, transport, including tongue retraction and protrusion), the nucleus ambiguus (IX and X: rostral for esophagus, pharynx, larynx; intermediate for pharynx and velum; caudal for larynx), and the dorsal motor nucleus of vagus (Jean, 2001). The CPG for inspiration is located in the reticular formation below the motor nucleus for vagus, and the CPG for expiration is located between the nucleus for vagus and the nucleus for the hypoglossal nerve (Baehr, Frotscher, & Duus, 2012). The vomiting center is located in the area postrema (dorsal reticular formation) below the hypoglossal nerve nucleus (Baehr, Frotscher, & Duus, 2012). The center for mastication, sucking, and licking is located in the pons, above the nucleus of the facial (VII) and trigeminal (V) nerves (Lund & Kolta, 2006). *continues*

and medial pterygoid muscles), such that a rotatory motion of the mandible is produced. The alternating contraction of these mandibular elevators is interspersed with the depression of the mandible, which allows the lingual musculature to move the bolus onto and off the molars. The chewing center complex is made up of a CPG for the rhythmic mandibular movement (located above the motor nuclei for the V trigeminal and VII facial nerves in the pons), as well as the nucleus pontis caudalis in the caudal reticular formation (Lund & Kolta, 2006). Hardness of food is sensed by the pressure on the teeth (periodontal afferents), and this information is fed into the central program generator to increase the force exerted by the muscles of mastication. This center is also involved in the reflexive movements of the tongue for sucking and licking (Baehr, Frotscher, & Duus, 2012; Lund & Kolta, 2006).

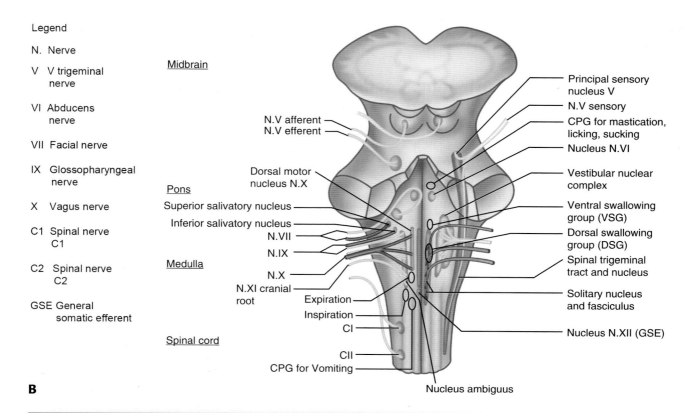

Legend

N. Nerve

V   V trigeminal
    nerve

VI Abducens
    nerve

VII Facial nerve

IX Glossopharyngeal
    nerve

X   Vagus nerve

C1 Spinal nerve
    C1

C2 Spinal nerve
    C2

GSE General
    somatic efferent

Midbrain

Pons

Medulla

Spinal cord

N.V afferent
N.V efferent

Dorsal motor
nucleus N.X

Superior salivatory nucleus
Inferior salivatory nucleus
N.VII
N.IX
N.X
N.XI cranial
root
Expiration
Inspiration
CI
CII
CPG for Vomiting

Nucleus ambiguus

Principal sensory
nucleus V
N.V sensory
CPG for mastication,
licking, sucking
Nucleus N.VI
Vestibular nuclear
complex
Ventral swallowing
group (VSG)
Dorsal swallowing
group (DSG)
Spinal trigeminal
tract and nucleus
Solitary nucleus
and fasciculus
Nucleus N.XII (GSE)

B

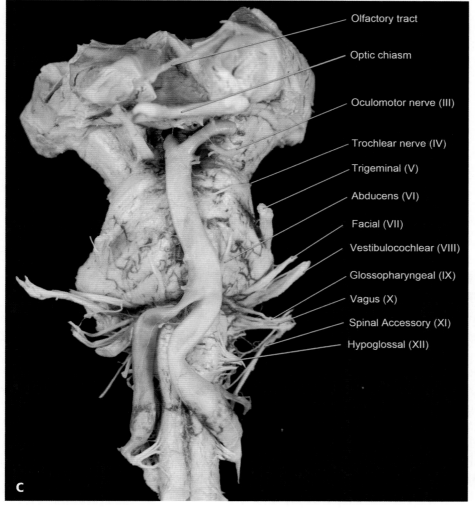

Olfactory tract

Optic chiasm

Oculomotor nerve (III)

Trochlear nerve (IV)

Trigeminal (V)

Abducens (VI)

Facial (VII)

Vestibulocochlear (VIII)

Glossopharyngeal (IX)

Vagus (X)

Spinal Accessory (XI)

Hypoglossal (XII)

C

Figure 8–13. *continued*
B. Posterior view of brain
stem, with centers located.
Source: From Seikel/
Drumright/King. *Anatomy
& Physiology for Speech,
Language, and Hearing,
5th Ed.* ©Cengage, Inc. Reproduced by permission.
C. Photograph of posterior
brain stem. Note location of
olfactory tract, optic chiasm,
and cranial nerves.

Orienting, Rooting, and Suckling/Sucking Reflexes

rooting reflex: reflexive response of infant to tactile stimulation of the cheek or lips; causes infants to turn toward the stimulus and open their mouth

The **rooting** and sucking reflexes—very functional for neonates and infants—rely on tactile stimulation of the perioral region. The suckling response is considered an earlier developmental stage of the sucking reflex. Lightly stroking the lips or cheek on one side causes the infant's mouth to open and its head to turn toward the stimulus; this is termed the rooting reflex. Light contact within the inner margin of the lips initiates a sucking response, which involves generating a labial seal (contraction of the upper and lower orbicularis oris), and alternately protruding and retracting the tongue. Tactile stimulation of the perioral region is mediated by the V trigeminal nerve, and central mediation of sucking is within the midbrain reticular formation. If the side of the newborn's tongue is touched, the infant's tongue moves in the direction of the stimulus, and this is called the **orienting reflex**. The rooting and sucking reflexes are actually composites of more basic reflexive responses (Miller, 2002).

Uvular (Palatal) Reflex

Uvular elevation occurs in response to the excitation of IX glossopharyngeal general visceral afferent (GVA) component (see Appendix G) by irritation. It appears to be mediated in a manner similar to the gag reflex (see next section), involving the palatal muscles innervated by the IX accessory and X vagus.

Gag (Pharyngeal) Reflex

The **gag reflex** is elicited by tactile stimulation of the faucial pillars, posterior pharyngeal wall, or posterior tongue near the lingual tonsils (Miller, 2002). Tactile stimulation (light or deep touch) of this region is mediated by the IX glossopharyngeal nerve GVA component. Dendrites convey sensation through the petrosal (inferior) and superior ganglia of the IX glossopharyngeal to the solitary nucleus and solitary fasciculus of the medulla oblongata in

Desensitizing the Gag Reflex

A hyperactive gag reflex can be quite problematic. Although the gag reflex for most of us is stimulated by contacting the posterior tongue, or lateral and posterior pharyngeal walls, some people experience a hyperactive gag reflex. In our clinic, we have seen children with gag reflexes that are so sensitive that simply touching the lips triggers a gag response. You may have experienced a little twinge when trying to brush your tongue when brushing your teeth, so you have a notion of how sensitive

the gag can be. This points out how important it is to desensitize the gag reflex, as well, because children with hyperactive gag reflex do not enjoy brushing their teeth.

Desensitizing the gag reflex involves slowly and systematically stimulating the oral and perioral regions, so that you never actually trigger the response itself. It is slow work that requires a lot of trust, but the benefits are great for the client, the parents, and you, the clinician.

the brain stem. Connection with the X vagus nerve via interneurons activates the muscles of general visceral efferent (GVE) lineage, including abdominal muscles and muscles of the velum and pharynx, causing the soft palate to elevate and the pharynx to elevate and constrict. Note that, as mentioned earlier, the gag reflex can be elicited by taste, specifically mediated by the IX glossopharyngeal nerve, special visceral afferent (SVA) component.

Retch and Vomit Reflex

Retching is an involuntary attempt at vomiting. **Vomiting** (emesis) refers to the oral expulsion of gastrointestinal contents. The retching reflex is a complex response mediated by noxious smells (I olfactory), tastes (IX glossopharyngeal), gastrointestinal distress (X vagus), vestibular dysfunction (VIII vestibulocochlear), or even a distressing visual or mental stimulation. Stimulation by one or more of these sensory systems activates a retching center located near the swallow center in the reticular formation of the medulla oblongata, near the motor nuclei associated with the complex of responses associated with vomiting. The vomit response includes multiple simultaneous or synchronous reflexes, including occlusion of the airway by vocal fold adduction, extreme contraction of abdominal muscles, relaxation of the upper and lower esophageal sphincters, elevation of the larynx and velum, depression of the epiglottis, elevation of the pharynx, and tongue protrusion (Miller, 2002).

Cough Reflex

The **cough** reflex is typically initiated by noxious stimulation of the pharynx, larynx, or bronchial passageway. The GVA component of the X vagus nerve transmits information concerning this stimulation to the nucleus solitarius of the medulla. Interneurons activate the expiration center of the medullary reticular formation, which causes the abdominal muscles to contract. The nucleus ambiguus, the motor nucleus of the X vagus, causes laryngeal adduction before exhalation, permitting sufficient subglottal pressure to be generated to dislodge the irritating substance from the airway. We can become hypersensitized to a stimulus, such that we will cough with a much smaller stimulus than expected (Hennel, Brozmanova, & Kollarik, 2015). You might have experienced this sensitivity following a bout of bronchitis, but individuals with chronic rhinitis or gastroesophageal reflux disorder (GERD) frequently experience it.

Pain Withdrawal Reflex

Although not technically a reflex associated with mastication or deglutition, the **pain withdrawal reflex** can have an effect on mastication and swallowing. You may remember the unpleasant sensation of having a lesion on your tongue or oral mucosa. When you masticate, you become very aware of the area and tend to avoid it if possible. This response represents a conscious

31. Cells with **RUFFINI** endings sense stretch within the deep layers of the epithelium.

32. The four classes of thermal receptors that mediate thermal events are as follows:

    A. **COOL**

    B. **COLD**

    C. **WARM**

    D. **HOT**

33. **TRUE.** Thermal sensors and pain sensors share the same morphology.

34. **NOCICEPTION** refers to the sense of pain.

35. Muscle stretch is sensed by **MUSCLE SPINDLES**.

36. **TRUE.** Facial muscles have muscle spindles.

37. **GOLGI TENDON ORGANS** sense muscle tension.

38. **SALIVATION** refers to the production and release of saliva into the oral cavity.

39. The parotid glands release **SEROUS** (type of saliva) into the posterior oral cavity and pharynx.

40. The sublingual glands release **MUCUS** (type of saliva) into the anterior oral cavity.

41. The **CHEWING** reflex involves rotary motion of the muscles of mastication.

42. The **UVULAR (PALATAL)** reflex involves elevation of the soft palate.

43. The **VOMIT** reflex involves evacuation of the contents of the stomach.

44. The **COUGH** reflex involves contracting the muscles of adduction and forcefully blowing them open to expel foreign matter from the respiratory passageway.

Bibliography

Arvedson, J. C., & Brodsky, L. (2002). *Pediatric swallowing and feeding: Assessment and management* (2nd ed.). Clifton Park, NY: Delmar.

Baehr, M., Frotscher, M., & Duus, P. (2012). *Duus' topical diagnosis in neurology: Anatomy, physiology, signs, symptoms* (5th ed.). New York, NY: Thieme.

Bouvier, V., Roudaut, Y., Osorio, N., Aimonetti, J. M., Ribot-Ciscar, E., Penalba, V., . . . Delmas, P. (2018). Merkel cells sense cooling with TRPM8 channels. *Journal of Investigative Dermatology, 138*(4), 946–956.

Broussard, D. L., & Altschuler, S. M. (2000). Brain stem viscerotopic organization of afferents and efferents involved in the control of swallowing. *American Journal of Medicine, 108*(4A), 79S–86S.

Brown, P. (1994). Pathophysiology of spasticity. *Journal of Neurology, Neurosurgery, and Psychiatry, 57,* 773–777.

Buck, L. B. (2000). Smell and taste: The chemical senses. In E. R. Kandel, J. H. Schwartz, & T. M. Jessell (Eds.), *Principles of neural science* (4th ed., pp. 625–652). New York, NY: McGraw-Hill.

Buck, L. B., & Bargmann, C. I. (2013). Smell and taste: The chemical senses. In E. R. Kandel, J. H. Schwartz, T. M. Jessell, S. A. Siegelbaum, & A. J. Hudspeth, A. J. (Eds.), *Principles of neural science* (5th ed., pp. 712–735). New York, NY: McGraw-Hill.

Bülow, M., Olsson, R., & Ekberg, O. (2003). Videoradiographic analysis of how carbonated thin liquids and thickened liquids affect the physiology of swallowing in subjects with aspiration on thin liquids. *Acta Radiologica, 44*(4), 366–372.

Bushman, J. D., Ye, W., & Liman, E. R. (2015). A proton current associated with sour taste: Distribution and functional properties. *The FASEB Journal, 29*(7), 3014–3026.

Campbell, N. A. (1990). *Biology*. Redwood City, CA: Benjamin/Cummings.

Choi, H. J., Cho, Y. K., Chung, K. M., & Kim, K. N. (2016). Differential expression of taste receptors in tongue papillae of DBA mouse. *International Journal of Oral Biology, 41*(1), 25–32.

Choi, J. H., Lee, J., Choi, I. J., Kim, Y. W., Ryu, K. W., & Kim, J. (2016). Genetic variation in the TAS2R38 bitter taste receptor and gastric cancer risk in Koreans. *Scientific Reports, 6*, 26904.

Clark, H. M., Henson, P. A., Barber, W. D., Stierwalt, J. A., & Sherrill, M. (2003). Relationships among subjective and objective measures of tongue strength and oral phase swallowing impairments. *American Journal of Speech-Language Pathology, 12*(1), 40–50.

Collings, V. B. (1974). Human taste response as a function of locus of stimulation on the tongue and soft palate. *Perception and Psychophysics, 16*(1), 169–174.

Colvin, J. L., Pullicin, A. J., & Lim, J. (2018). Regional differences in taste responsiveness: Effect of stimulus and tasting mode. *Chemical Senses, 43*(8), 645–653.

Commetto-Muñiz, J. E., Cain, W. S., & Abraham, M. H. (2004). Chemosensory additivity in trigeminal chemoreception as reflected by detection of mixtures. *Experimental Brain Research, 158*, 196–206.

Cowart, B. J. (1998). The addition of CO_2 to traditional taste solutions alters taste quality. *Chemical Senses, 23*(4), 397–402.

Crary, M. A., Carnaby-Mann, G. D., & Groher, M. E. (2006). Identification of swallowing events from sEMG signals obtained from healthy adults. *Dysphagia, 22*, 94–99.

Crow, H. C., & Ship, J. A. (1996). Tongue strength and endurance in different aged individuals. *The Journals of Gerontology Series A: Biological Sciences and Medical Sciences, 51*(5), M247–M250.

Delaney, A. L., & Arvedson, J. C. (2008). Development of swallowing and feeding: Prenatal through first year of life. *Developmental Disabilities Research Reviews, 14*(2), 105–117.

Dessirier, J. M., Simons, C. T., Carstens, M. I., O'Mahony, M., & Carstens, E. (2000). Psychophysical and neurobiological evidence that the oral sensation elicited by carbonated water is of chemogenic origin. *Chemical Senses, 25*(3), 277–284.

Ding, R., Logemann, J. A., Larson, C. R., & Rademaker, A. W. (2003). The effects of taste and consistency on swallow physiology in younger and older healthy individuals. *Journal of Speech, Language, and Hearing Research, 46*(4), 977–989.

Dodds, W. J., Stewart, E. T., & Logemann, J. A. (1990). Physiology and radiology of the normal and pharyngeal phases of swallowing. *American Journal of Roentgenology, 154*, 953–963.

Doty, R. W., & Bosma, J. F. (1956). An electromyographic analysis of reflex deglutition. *Journal of Neurophysiology, 19*, 44–60.

Ertekin, C., & Aydogdu, I (2003). Neurophysiology of swallowing. *Clinical Neurophysiology, 114*, 2226–2244.

Ertekin, C., Kiylioglu, N., Tarlaci, S., Truman, A. B., Secil, Y., & Aydogdu, I. (2011). Voluntary and reflex influences on the initiation of swallowing reflex in man. *Dysphagia, 16*, 40–47.

Fujii, N., Inamoto, Y., Saitoh, E., Baba, M., Okada, S., Yoshioka, S., . . . Palmer, K. (2011). Evaluation of swallowing using 320-detector-row multislice CT. Part I. Single- and multiphase volume scanning for three-dimensional morphological and kinematic analysis. *Dysphagia, 27*, 99–107.

Geran, L. C., & Travers, S. P. (2011). Glossopharyngeal nerve transection impairs unconditioned avoidance of diverse bitter stimuli in rats. *Behavioral Neuroscience, 125*(4), 519–528.

Glodowski, K. R., Thompson, R. H., & Martel, L. (2019). The rooting reflex as an infant feeding cue. *Journal of Applied Behavior Analysis, 52*(1), 17–27.

Goyal, R. K., Padmanabhan, R., & Sang, Q. (2001). Neural circuits in swallowing and abdominal vagal afferent-mediated lower esophageal sphincter relaxation. *The American Journal of Medicine, 111*(8A), 1–11.

Green, B. G. (2012). Chemesthesis and the chemical senses as components of a "chemofensor complex." *Chemical Senses, 37*, 201–206.

Groher, M. E. (1997). *Dysphagia* (3rd ed.). St. Louis, MO: Butterworth-Heinemann.

Guillebaud, F., Roussel, G., Félix, B., Troadec, J. D., Dallaporta, M., & Abysique, A. (2019). Interaction between nesfatin-1 and oxytocin in the modulation of the swallowing reflex. *Brain Research, 1711*, 173–182.

Gumbley, F., Huckabee, M. L., Doeltgen, S. H., Witte, U., & Moran, C. (2008). Effects of bolus volume on pharyngeal contact pressure during normal swallowing. *Dysphagia, 23*, 280–285.

Healey, J. E., & Seybold, W. D. (1969). *A synopsis of clinical anatomy*. Philadelphia, PA: Saunders.

Hennel, M., Brozmanova, M., & Kollarik, M. (2015). Cough reflex sensitization from esophagus and nose. *Pulmonary Pharmacology & Therapeutics, 35*, 117–121.

Hewitt, A., Hind, J., Kays, S., Nicosia, M., Doyle, J., Tompkins, W., . . . Robbins, J. (2008). Standardized instrument for lingual pressure measurement. *Dysphagia, 23*(1), 16–25.

Hoebler, C., Karinthi, A., Devaux, M. F., Guillon, F., Gallant, D.J.G., Bouchet, B., . . . Barry, J. L. (1998). Physical and chemical transformations of cereal food during oral digestion in human subjects. *British Journal of Nutrition, 80*, 429–436.

Hoffman, M. R., Mielens, J. D., Ciucci, M. R., Jones, C. A., Jiang, J. J., & McCulloch, T. M. (2012). High-resolution manometry of pharyngeal swallow pressure events associated with effortful swallow and the Mendelsohn maneuver. *Dysphagia, 27*, 418–426.

Hoon, M. A., Adler, E., Lindemeier, J., Battey, J. F., Ryba, N. J., & Zuker, C. S. (1999). Putative mammalian taste receptors: a class of taste-specific GPCRs with distinct topographic selectivity. *Cell, 96*(4), 541-551.

Huang, A. L., Chen, X., Hoon, M. A., Chandrashekar, J., Guo, W., Trankner, D., . . . Zuker, C. S. (2006). The cells and logic for mammalian sour taste detection. *Nature, 442*, 934–938.

Jean, A. (2001). Brain stem control of swallowing: Neuronal network and cellular mechanisms. *Physiological Reviews, 81*(2), 929–969.

Kandel, E., Schwartz, J., Jessell, T., Siegelbaum, S., & Hudspeth, A. (2013). Principles of neural science, fifth. *Journal of Chemical Information and Modeling. New York: Mc-Graw-Hill Medical*, 1689–1699.

Kochem, M. (2017). Type 1 taste receptors in taste and metabolism. *Annals of Nutrition and Metabolism, 70*(Suppl. 3), 27–36.

Koole, P., de Jongh, H. J., & Boering, G. (1991). A comparative study of electromyograms of the masseter, temporalis, and anterior digastric muscles obtained by surface and intramuscular electrodes: Raw-EMG. *Cranio, 9*(3), 228–240.

Krival, K., & Bates C. (2012). Effects of club soda and ginger brew on linguapalatal pressures in healthy swallowing. *Dysphagia, 27*(2), 228–239.

Lamster, I. B., Asadourian, L., Del Carmen, T., & Friedman, P. K. (2016). The aging mouth: Differentiating normal aging from disease. *Periodontology 2000, 72*(1), 96–107.

Lang, I. M. (2009). Brain stem control of the phases of swallowing. *Dysphagia, 24*, 333–348.

Lang, I. M., & Shaker, R. (1997). Anatomy and physiology of the upper esophageal sphincter. *American Journal of Medicine, 103*(5), 50S–55S.

Langmore, S. E., Schatz, K., & Olson, N. (1991). Endoscopic and videofluorsoscopic examination of swallowing and aspiration. *Annals of Otology, Rhinology, and Laryngology, 100*(8), 678–681.

Lau, C., Smith, E. O., & Schanler, R. J. (2003). Coordination of suck-swallow and swallow respiration in preterm infants. *Acta Paediatrica, 92*(6), 721–727.

Linden, R. W. (1993). Taste. *British Dental Journal, 175*(7), 243–253.

Lipchock, S. V., Spielman, A. I., Mennella, J. A., Mansfield, C. J., Hwang, L. D., Douglas, J. E., & Reed, D. R. (2017). Caffeine bitterness is related to daily caffeine intake and bitter receptor mRNA abundance in human taste tissue. *Perception, 46*(3–4), 245–256.

Logemann, J. A. (1995). Dysphagia: Evaluation and treatment. *Folia Phoniatrica et Logopedica, 47*(3), 140–164.

Logemann, J. (1998). *Evaluation and treatment of swallowing disorders* (2nd ed.). Austin, TX: Pro-Ed.

Logemann, J. A., & Bytell, D. E. (1979). Swallowing disorders in three types of head and neck surgical patients. *Cancer, 44*(3), 1095–1105.

Lund, J. P., & Kolta, A. (2006). Generation of the central masticatory pattern and its modification by sensory feedback. *Dysphagia, 21*, 167–174.

Martin-Harris, B., Brodsky, M. B., Michel, Y, Lee, F-S., & Walters, B. (2007). Delayed initiation of the pharyngeal swallow: Normal variability in adults swallows. *Journal of Speech-Language-Hearing Research, 50*, 585–594.

Mason, R. M. (2008). A retrospective and prospective view of orofacial myology. *International Journal of Orofacial Myology, 34*, 5–14.

Matsuo, K., & Palmer, J. B. (2013). Oral phase preparation and propulsion: Anatomy, physiology, rheology, mastication, and transport. In R. Shaker, P. C. Belafsky, G. N. Postma, & C. Eastering (Eds.), *Principles of deglutition: A multidisciplinary text for swallowing and its disorders* (pp. 117–132). New York, NY: Springer.

Mattioli, S., Lugaresi, M., Zannoli, R., Brusori, S., & d'Ovidio, F. (2003). Balloon sensors for the manometric recording of the pharyngoesophageal tract: An experimental study. *Dysphagia, 18*, 249–254.

Mazari, A., Heath, M. R., & Prinz, J. F. (2007). Contribution of the cheeks to the intraoral manipulation of food. *Dysphagia, 22*, 117–121.

McCulloch, T. M., Hoffman, M. R., & Ciucci, M. R. (2010). High-resolution manometry of pharyngeal swallow pressure events associated with head turn and chin tuck. *Annals of Otology, Rhinology, and Laryngology, 119*(6), 369–376.

McKeown, M. J., Torpey, D. A., & Gehm, W. C. (2002). Non-invasive monitoring of distinctive muscle activations during swallowing. *Clinical Neurophysiology, 113*, 354–366.

Mendell, D. A., & Logemann, J. A. (2007). Temporal sequences of swallowing events during the oropharyngeal swallow. *Journal of Speech-Language-Hearing Research, 50*, 1256–1271.

Miller, A. (2002). Oral and pharyngeal reflexes in the mammalian nervous system: Their diverse range in complexity and the pivotal role of the tongue. *Critical Reviews in Oral Biology and Medicine, 13*, 409–425.

Mishellany, A., Woda, A., Labas, R., & Peyron, M.A. (2006). The challenge of mastication: Preparing a bolus suitable for deglutition. *Dysphagia, 21*, 87–94.

Mistry, S., Rothwell, J. C., Thompson, D. G., & Hamdy, S. (2006). Modulation of human cortical motor pathways after pleasant and aversive taste stimuli. *American Journal of Physiology: Gastroentestinal and Liver Physiology, 291*, G666–G671.

Møller, A. R. (2003). *Sensory systems: Anatomy and physiology.* New York, NY: Academic Press.

Moulton, K., Seikel, J. A., Loftin, J. G., & Devine, N. (2018). Examining the effects of ankyloglossia on swallowing function. *International Journal of Orofacial Myology, 44*, 5–21.

Mountcastle, V. B. (1974). *Medical physiology* (13th ed.). Oxford, UK: C.V. Mosby.

Mueller, K. L., Hoon, M. A., Erlenbach, I., Chandrashekar, J., Zuker, C. S., & Ryba, N. J. (2005). The receptors and coding logic for bitter taste. *Nature, 434*(7030), 225.

Nelson, G., Hoon, M. A., Chandrashekar, J., Zhang, Y., Ryba, N. J., & Zuker, C. S. (2001). Mammalian sweet taste receptors. *Cell, 106*(3), 381–390.

Newman, K. D., & Randolph, J. (1990). Surgical problems of the esophagus in infants and children. In D. C. Sabiston & F. C. Spencer (Eds.), *Surgery of the chest* (5th ed., pp. 815–839). Philadelphia, PA: W. B. Saunders.

Ninomaya, Y., Imoto, T., & Sugimura, T. (1999). Sweet taste responses of mouse chorda tympani neurons: Existence of Gurmarin-sensitive and insensitive receptor components. *Journal of Neurophysiology, 81*(6), 3087–3091.

Oka, Y., Butnaru, M., von Buchholtz, L., Ryba, N. J., & Zuker, C. S. (2013). High salt recruits aversive taste pathways. *Nature, 494*(7438), 472.

Ozdemirkiran, T., Secil, Y., Tarlacı, S., & Ertekin, C. (2007). An EMG screening method (dysphagia limit) for evaluation of neurogenic dysphagia in childhood above 5 years old. *International Journal of Pediatric Otorhinolaryngology, 71*(3), 403–407.

Palmer, J. B., & Hiiemae, K. M. (1997). Integration of oral and pharyngeal bolus propulsion: A new model for the physiology of swallowing. *The Japanese Journal of Dysphagia Rehabilitation, 1*(1), 15–30.

Pauloski, B. R., Logemann, J. A., Rademaker, A. W., McConnel, F. M., Heiser, M. A., Cardinale, S., . . . Cook, B. (1993). Speech and swallowing function after anterior tongue and floor of mouth resection with distal flap reconstruction. *Journal of Speech, Language, and Hearing Research, 36*(2), 267–276.

Payne, W. S., & Ellis, F. H., Jr. (1984). Esophagus and ciaphragmatic hernias. In S. I. Schwartz, G. T. Shires, F. C. Spencer, & E. H. Storer (Eds.), *Principles of surgery* (4th ed., pp. 1063–1112). New York, NY: McGraw-Hill.

Pearson, K. G., & Gordon, J. E. (2013). Locomotion. In E. R. Kandel, J. H. Schwartz, T. M. Jessell, S. A. Siegelbaum, & A. J. Hudspeth (Eds.). *Principles of neural science* (5th ed., pp. 812–834). New York, NY: McGraw-Hill.

Pearson, W. G., Langmore, S. E., Uy, L. B., & Zumwalt, A. C. (2012). Structural analysis of muscles elevating the hyolaryngeal complex. *Dysphagia, 27*, 445–451.

Pelletier, C. A., & Dhanaraj, G. E. (2006). The effect of taste and palatability on lingual swallowing pressure. *Dysphagia, 11*, 121–128.

Pelletier, C. A., & Lawless, H. T. (2003). Effect of citric acid and citric acid-sucrose mixture on swallowing in neurogenic oropharyngeal dysphagia. *Dysphagia, 18*(4), 231–241.

Perlman, A. L., Grayhack, J. P., & Booth, B. M. (1992). The relationship of vallecular residue to oral involvement, reduced hyoid elevation, and epiglottic function. *Journal of Speech, Language, and Hearing Research, 35*(4), 734–741.

Pernambuco, L. A., Silva, H. J., Lima, L. M., Cunha, R. A., Santos, V. S., Cunha, D. A., & Leao, J. C. (2011). Electrical activity of masseter muscle in young adults during swallowing of liquid. *Jornal da Sociedade Brasileira de Fonoaudiologia, 23*(3), 214–219.

Peyron, M. A., Mishellany, A., & Woda, A. (2004). Particle size distribution of food boluses after mastication of six natural foods. *Journal of Dental Research, 83*, 573–582.

Peyron, M. A., Woda, A., Bourdiol, P., & Hennequin, M. (2017). Age-related changes in mastication. *Journal of Oral Rehabilitation, 44*(4), 299–312.

Printz, J. F., & Lucas, P. W. (1995). Swallow thresholds in human mastication. *Archives of Oral Biology, 40*(5), 401–403.

Richards, W. G., & Sugarbaker, D. J. (1995). Neuronal control of esophageal function. *Chest Surgery Clinics of North America, 5*(1), 157–171.

Robbins, J. A., Levine, R., Wood, J., Roecker, E. B., & Luschei, E. (1995). Age effects on lingual pressure generation as a risk factor for dysphagia. *The Journals of Gerontology Series A: Biological Sciences and Medical Sciences, 50*(5), M257–M262.

Roper, S. D., & Chaudhari, N. (2017). Taste buds: Cells, signals and synapses. *Nature Reviews Neuroscience, 18*(8), 485–497.

Rosenbek, J. C., Robbins, J., Fishback, B., & Levine, R. L. (1991). Effects of thermal application on dysphagia after stroke. *Journal of Speech, Language, and Hearing Research, 34*(6), 1257–1268.

Sdravou, K., Walshe, M., & Dagdilelis, L. (2012). Effects of carbonated liquids on oropharyngeal swallowing measures in people with neurogenic dysphagia. *Dysphagia, 27*(2), 240–250.

Segerstad, C. H., & Hellekant, G. (1989). The sweet taste in the calf. I. Chorda tympani proper nerve response to taste stimulation of the tongue. *Physiology and Behavior, 45*(3), 633–638.

Seikel, J. A., Ulrich, C., Evers, D., Holzer, K., Evans, L., Ellgen, L., . . . Gee, B. (2016, November). *Etiologic relation between orofacial myofunctional disorders and oropharyngeal dysphagia.* Presentation at the Annual Meeting of the American Speech-Language-Hearing Association, Philadelphia, PA.

Seong, M. Y., Oh, B. M., Seo, H. G., & Han, T. R. (2018). Influence of supraglottic swallow on swallowing kinematics: Comparison between the young and the elderly. *Journal of the Korean Dysphagia Society, 8*(1), 23–29.

Shah, A. S., Ben-Shahar, Y., Moninger, T. O., Kline, J. N., & Welsh, M. J. (2009). Motile cilia or human airway epithelia are chemosensory. *Science, 325*(5944), 1131–1134.

Simon, S. A., & S. D. Roper (1993). *Mechanisms of taste transduction.* Boca Raton, FL: CRC Press.

Stephens, J. R., Taves, D. H., Smith, R. C., & Martin, R. E. (2005). Bolus location at the initiation of the pharyngeal stage of swallowing in healthy older adults. *Dysphagia, 20*, 266–272.

Stepp, C. E. (2012). Surface electromyography for speech and swallowing systems: Measurement, analysis, and interpretation. *Journal of Speech, Language, and Hearing Research, 55*(4), 1232–1246.

Stierwalt, J. A., & Youmans, S. R. (2007). Tongue measures in individuals with normal and impaired swallowing. *American Journal of Speech-Language Pathology, 16*(2), 148–156.

Suma, S., Furuta, M., Yamashita, Y., & Matsushita, K. (2019). Aging, mastication, and malnutrition and their associations with cognitive disorder: Evidence from epidemiological data. *Current Oral Health Reports, 6*(2), 89–99.

Takeda, M., Shishido, Y., Kitao, K., & Suzuki, Y. (1982). Monoamines of taste buds in the fungiform and foliate papillae of the mouse. *Archivum Histologicum Japonicum, 45*(3), 239–246.

Tasko, S. M., Kent, R. D., & Westbury, J. R. (2002). Variability in tongue movement kinematics during normal liquid swallowing. *Dysphagia, 17*, 126–138.

Thexton, A. J., Crompton, A. W., & German, R. Z. (2007). Electromyographic activity during the reflex pharyngeal swallow in the pig: Doty and Bosma (1956) revisited. *Journal of Applied Physiology, 102*, 587–600.

Wheeler, K. M., Chiara, T., & Sapienza, C. M. (2007). Surface electromyographic activity of the submental muscles during swallow and expiratory pressure threshold training tasks. *Dysphagia, 22*(2), 108–116.

Witt, M., & Miller, I. J. (1992). Comparative lectin histochemistry on taste buds in foliate, circumvallate and fungiform papillae of the rabbit tongue. *Histochemistry, 98*(3), 173–182.

Yabunaka, K., Konishi, H., Nakagami, G., Sanada, H., Iizaka, S., Sanada, S., & Ohue, M. (2012). Ultrasonographic evaluation of geniohyoid muscle movement during swallowing: A study on healthy adults of various ages. *Radiological Physics and Technology, 5*(1), 34–39.

Yee, K. K., Sukumaran, S. K., Kotha, R., Gilbertson, T. A., & Margolskee, R. F. (2011). Glucose transporters and ATP-gated K+ (KATP) metabolic sensors are present in type 1 taste receptor 3 (T1R3)-expressing taste cells. *Proceedings of the National Academy of Sciences, 108*(13), 5431–5436.

Yoshida, M., Kikutani, T., Tsuga, K., Utanohara, Y., Hayashi, R., & Akagawa, Y. (2006). Decreased tongue pressure reflects symptoms of dysphagia. *Dysphagia, 21*, 61–65.

Zuydam, A. C., Rogers, S. N., Brown, J. S., Vaughan, E. D., & Magennis, P. (2000). Swallowing rehabilitation after oro-pharyngeal resection for squamous cell carcinoma. *British Journal of Oral and Maxillofacial Surgery, 38*(5), 513–518.

Anatomy of Hearing

The mechanisms of hearing are extraordinary in scope and complexity. In this chapter we discuss the structures of hearing. Chapter 10 will be devoted to the reasons these structures exist: the physiology of hearing.

The Structures of Hearing

ANAQUEST LESSON

The physical structures of the ear are deceptively simple, especially in light of their exquisite function. The ear is an energy **transducer**, which means that it converts acoustic energy into electrochemical energy. The details of these structures will set the stage for the discussion of the transduction process in Chapter 10.

We will talk about the ear in terms of the basic elements involved: the outer ear, the middle ear, the inner ear, and, in Chapter 10, the auditory pathways (Figure 9–1).

transducer: L., trans, across; ducer, to lead

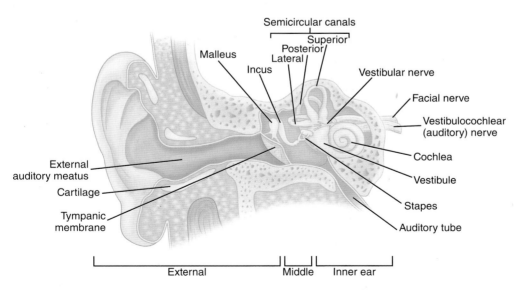

Figure 9–1. Schematic of frontal section revealing outer, middle, and inner ear structures. *Source:* From Seikel/Drumright/King. *Anatomy & Physiology for Speech, Language, and Hearing, 5th Ed.* ©Cengage, Inc. Reproduced by permission.

515

ANAQUEST LESSON

pinna: L., feather

helix: Gr., coil

Outer Ear

The outer ear is composed of two basic components with which you are quite familiar (Table 9–1). The **pinna** (or auricle) is the prominence we colloquially refer to as the ear, although it serves primarily as a collector of sound to be processed at deeper levels (e.g., the middle ear and the cochlea). The structure of the pinna is provided by a cartilaginous framework.

The pinna has several important functions, including aiding the localization of sound in space and capturing sound energy. Landmarks of the pinna are important for a number of reasons, not the least of which is their diagnostic significance for some genetic conditions (Figure 9–2). The **helix** forms the curled margin of the pinna, marking its most distal borders. The superior-posterior bulge on the helix is known as the **auricular tubercle** (or **Darwin's tubercle**). Immediately anterior to the helix is the **antihelix**, a similar fold of tissue marking the entrance to the concha. Between the

Table 9–1

Landmarks of the Outer Ear
Pinna (auricle)
Helix
Auricular tubercle (Darwin's tubercle)
Antihelix
Crura
Crura anthelicis
Triangular fossa
Scaphoid fossa
Concha
Cymba conchae
Cavum conchae
Tragus
Tuberculum supratragicum
Intertragic incisure
Antitragus
Lobule
External auditory meatus
Cartilaginous meatus
Osseous meatus
Isthmus
Tympanic membrane

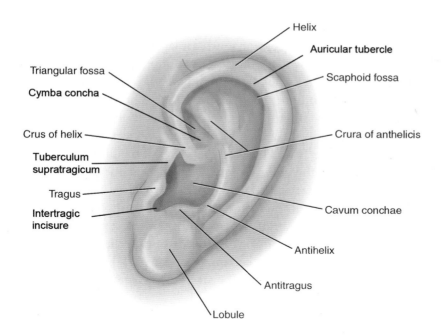

Figure 9–2. Landmarks of the auricle or pinna. *Source: From Seikel/Drumright/ King. Anatomy & Physiology for Speech, Language, and Hearing, 5th Ed.* ©Cengage, Inc. Reproduced by permission.

helix and antihelix is the **scaphoid fossa**. The antihelix bifurcates superiorly, producing the **crura anthelicis**, and the space between them forms the **triangular fossa (fossa triangularis)**. The **cymba conchae** is the anterior extension of the helix marking the anterior entrance to the concha, and the **cavum conchae** is the deep portion of the concha. The **concha** (or **concha auriculae**) is the entrance to the ear canal. The ear canal is also known as the **external auditory meatus** (abbreviated [**EAM**]; alternately **meatus acousticus externus**). A flap of epithelium-covered cartilage known as the **tragus** looks as if it could cover the entrance to the meatus (and probably did in an earlier version of the auditory mechanism). Superior to the tragus is the **tuberculum supratragicum**. Posterior and inferior to the tragus is the **antitragus** (the region between tragus and antitragus is termed the **intertragic incisure** or **incisura intertragica**), and below the antitragus is the **lobule** or **lobe**.

   If you palpate these structures on yourself, you should realize that the lobule is one of the few structures devoid of cartilage. The **auricular cartilage** is a unitary structure closely following the landmarks we have just described and is covered with a layer of epithelial tissue invested with fine hairs that are useful for keeping insects and dirt out of the ear canal.

   The **external auditory meatus** is approximately 7 mm in diameter and 2.5 cm long when measured from the depth of the concha, but you would add another 1.5 cm to its length if you chose to measure it from the tragus (Black, 2008). This is, in reality, not a trivial matter. The EAM and conchae are resonating cavities that both contribute to hearing and are a major determinant of the resonant frequency.

   The lateral third of the canal is composed of cartilage and is about 8 mm long; the medial two thirds is the bony meatus of the temporal bone. The EAM is S-shaped. If you were a fly walking toward the **eardrum** (**tympanic**

concha: Gr., konche, shell

tragus: Gr., tragos, goat

membrane [TM]), you would start out hiking generally medially, forward, and up. At the juncture of the osseous and cartilaginous meatuses of the EAM, you would take a turn down as you made your approach. During your hike you would see two constrictions. The first marks the end of the cartilaginous portion and the beginning of the osseous EAM. The second constriction, termed the **isthmus**, is about 0.5 cm from the TM itself. At the end of your hike, you would run into the TM, a thin trilaminar sheet of tissue that sits at an oblique angle in the EAM. The epithelial cover of the pinna continues into the EAM and serves as the outer layer of the tympanic membrane.

Because the adult ear canal takes a turn downward, you cannot see the medial end of the canal without some effort. If you were to look into the ear canal (you would have to manipulate the pinna and use a **speculum**, a device used to view cavities of the body), you would see that the outer third of the EAM is lined with hairs, and has **cerumen**, or ear wax. These are both quite functional additions to the canal, as they trap insects and dirt, protecting the medial-most point of the outer ear, the TM.

The TM marks the boundary between the outer and middle ear. It completely separates the two spaces, being an extremely thin three-layered sheet of tissue. The epithelial lining of the EAM continues as the external layer of the TM, while the lining of the middle ear provides the inner layer. Sandwiched between these two delicate epithelial linings is a layer of fibrous tissue that provides structure for the TM. This intermediate layer actually consists of two layers of fibers. The radial and circular fibroelastic connective tissues provide optimal strength and tension to this intermediate layer.

The TM is approximately 55 mm^2 in area and has a number of important landmarks (Figure 9–3). If you take the time to view one of your friend's TM using an otoscope (carefully), you should see the **umbo**, which is the most distal point of attachment of the inner TM to one of the bones of the middle ear, the malleus. The TM is particularly taut at this point, and the location inferior and anterior to this is referred to as the **cone of light** because it reflects the light of the audiologist's otoscope. You may be able to see the handle (or manubrium) of the malleus behind the TM, appearing as a streak on the membrane; if you are looking at the left TM, the handle of the malleus should look like the hand of a clock pointing to the 11.

The TM is slightly concave when viewed from the EAM, and the umbo is the most depressed portion of this concavity. Although most of the TM is

speculum: L., mirror

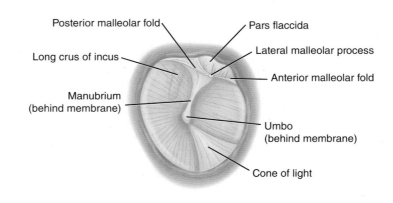

Figure 9–3. Right ear tympanic membrane, as viewed from the external auditory meatus. *Source:* From Seikel/Drumright/ King. *Anatomy & Physiology for Speech, Language, and Hearing, 5th Ed.* ©Cengage, Inc. Reproduced by permission.

Posterior malleolar fold
Pars flaccida
Long crus of incus
Lateral malleolar process
Anterior malleolar fold
Manubrium (behind membrane)
Umbo (behind membrane)
Cone of light

Otitis Externa and Cerumen

The epithelial lining of the auricle and EAM is tightly bound to the cartilage and bone of these structures, and this binding accounts for the pain involved in any swelling of the tissue. **Otitis externa** refers to inflammation of the skin of the external ear. When tissue is inflamed, it responds with **edema** (swelling). The epithelium of the EAM and pinna is tightly bound to its underlying structure, and the swelling increases the tension on the epithelium, making it quite painful.

Otitis externa may result from bacterial infection following trauma or abrasion. Failure to clean probe tips and specula could result in the transmission of the infection between clients. Otitis externa may also result from viral infection, including infection with herpes zoster virus. This painful infection may lead to facial paralysis or hearing loss if the facial or vestibulocochlear nerves are involved.

The EAM is invested with cilia and ceruminous glands, largely restricted to the cartilaginous portion of the canal. Cerumen (ear wax) is secreted by the glands into the ear canal, trapping insects and dirt that would otherwise threaten the TM. Individuals with overly active ceruminous glands may find that the EAM becomes occluded, and removal of the cerumen may be required. Attempts to remove the cerumen by the individual using cotton swabs often result in cerumen and dirt being packed against the inferior boundary of the TM, as the oblique angle forms a perfect pocket to catch the matter.

The interested student and budding audiologist would be well advised to read the descriptions of these and other conditions provided by Martin and Clark (1995, 2006).

Malformations of the Pinna and EAM

As many as 8.3 out of 10,000 live births include anomalies of the outer ear. **Auricular malformations** arise from issues in embryological development, while **deformations** arise from the effects of physical forces on the prenatal structures (Porter & Tan, 2005). The auricle develops between the fifth and ninth prenatal week, and malformations likely arise from the compounded effects of multiple genes, as well as introduction of teratogens (e.g., Wei, Makori, Peterson, Hummler, & Henrickx, 1999). Failure of cartilage to develop (failure of **chondrogenesis**) can result in auricular or **meatal atresia** (absence of the external auditory meatus), or less severely in **microtia** (small auricle). Parts of the auricle can become duplicated, referred to as **polyotia**. In this case, for instance, a person may develop a second tragus, which may occur in hemifacial microsomia (Lam & Dohil, 2007). **Preauricular tags** are prominences that form prenatally anterior to the pinna, while **cryptotia** is congenital atresia (absence) or maldevelopment of the upper portion of the ear. **Anotia** refers to complete absence of the pinna, and **Stahl's ear** refers to pointy, elfin-shaped ears.

A number of genetic syndromes manifest in auricle anomalies. Children affected by branchio-oto-renal syndrome will often have cupped ears or microtia, in conjunction with stapes disconnection and conductive or sensorineural hearing loss. A high proportion of individuals with Down syndrome (Trisomy 21) will show microtia, often have small earlobes and helix malformation, and occasionally show stenosis of the ear canal.

Many deformities require surgical intervention, although some may be treated by molding techniques postnatally (applying continued force in specific directions). The cartilage of the auricle is more malleable in the first 3 months, making molding a more attractive treatment than surgery, when applicable. Deformities of the auricle and external auditory meatus affect a person's ability to hear, but have a significant impact on appearance as well.

If the pinna is subjected to trauma, as in that inflicted during the sport of boxing, the result can be permanent deformation of its structure. Trauma can cause hemorrhaging between the epithelium and cartilage, and, if left untreated, the resulting swelling may cause a permanent distortion.

The TM is made up of three layers of tissue: the outer, intermediate, and inner layers. The **outer (cuticular) layer** is a continuation of the epithelial lining of the EAM and pinna. The **intermediate (fibrous) layer** is made up of two parts: the superficial layer is composed of fibers that radiate out from the handle of the malleus to the periphery; and the deep layer is made up of circular fibers that are found mostly in the periphery of the membrane. The **inner (mucous) layer** is continuous with the mucosa of the middle ear.

Ossicles

The bones of the ear, known as the **ossicles**, include the malleus, incus, and stapes (Figures 9–4, 9–5, and 9–6). This **ossicular chain** of three articulated bones provides the means for transmission of acoustic energy impinging on the TM to the inner ear. The **malleus** is the largest of the ossicles, providing the point of attachment with the TM.

As you can see in Figure 9–5, the **manubrium** (or handle) of the malleus is a long process, separated from the **head** by a thin neck. The **anterior** and

malleus: L., hammer

manubrium: L., handle

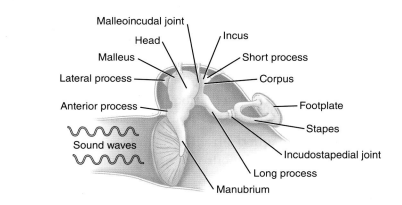

Figure 9–4. Articulated ossicular chain of the right ear in medial view (Clark & Ohlemiller, 2008). *Source:* From Seikel/Drumright/ King. *Anatomy & Physiology for Speech, Language, and Hearing, 5th Ed.* ©Cengage, Inc. Reproduced by permission.

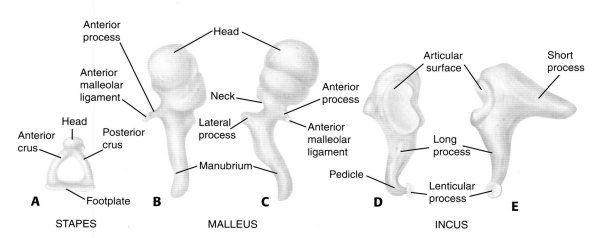

Figure 9–5. Ossicles of the middle ear and their landmarks. **A.** Stapes landmarks. **B.** Posteromedial view of malleus. **C.** Anteromedial view of malleus. **D.** Anteromedial view of incus. **E.** Posteromedial view of incus. *Source:* From Seikel/Drumright/King. *Anatomy & Physiology for Speech, Language, and Hearing, 5th Ed.* ©Cengage, Inc. Reproduced by permission. *continues*

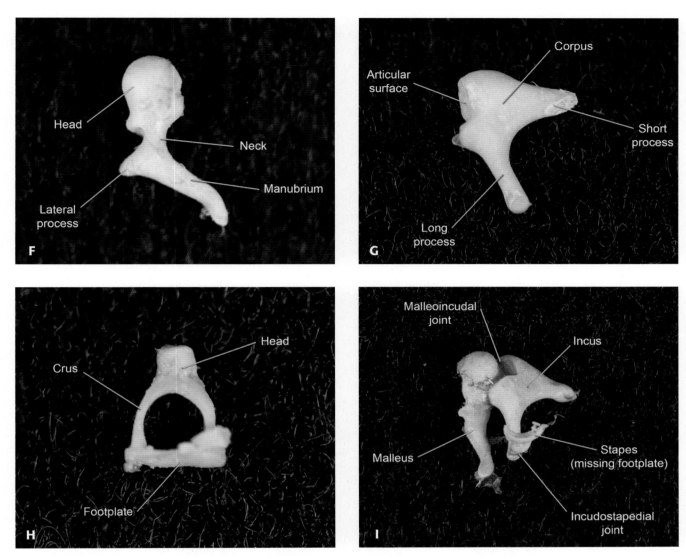

Figure 9–5. *continued* **F.** Photograph of lateral malleus. **G.** Photograph of posterior incus. **H.** Photograph of stapes. **I.** Photograph of articulated ossicles. Note that footplate is missing from stapes.

lateral processes provide points of attachment for ligaments, to be discussed. The manubrium attaches to the TM along its length, terminating with the **lateral process**. This attachment of the lateral process with the TM forms the anterior and posterior malleolar folds and the pars flaccida.

Examination of the malleus reveals that the bulk of the bone is in the head (or **caput**)—not coincidentally the articulatory facet for the incus. The head of the malleus protrudes into the epitympanic recess of the middle ear. Although the malleus is the largest of the ossicles, it is only 9 mm long and it weighs a mere 25 mg.

The **incus** (fancied to be shaped like an anvil) provides the intermediate communicating link of the ossicular chain. The **body** of the incus articulates with the head of the malleus by means of the **malleolar facet** in such a way that the **long process** of the incus is nearly parallel with the manubrium of

incus: L., anvil

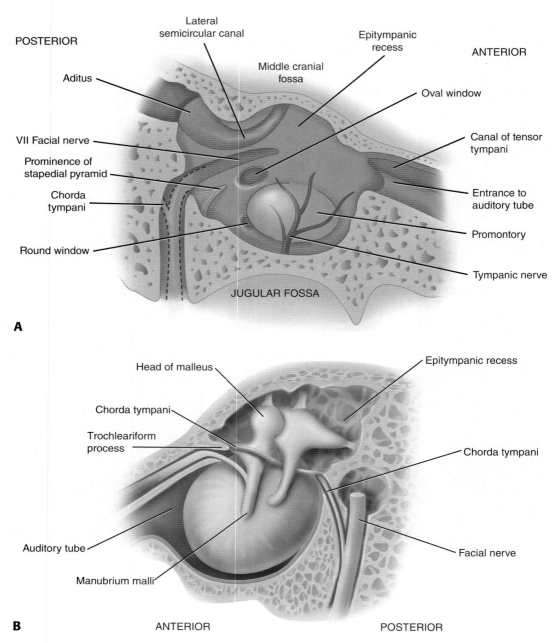

Figure 9–6. A. Schematic representation of the middle ear cavity of the right ear, as viewed from the external auditory meatus with tympanic membrane and ossicles removed. **B.** View of medial surface of tympanic membrane in situ, showing the course of the chorda tympani nerve. *Source:* From Seikel/Drumright/King. *Anatomy & Physiology for Speech, Language, and Hearing, 5th Ed.* ©Cengage, Inc. Reproduced by permission. *continues*

lenticular process: the process of the incus with which the stapes articulates

the malleus; the body is nearly entirely within the epitympanic recess. The **short process** projects posteriorly, while the end of the long process bends medially, forming the **lenticular process** with which the stapes articulates. Needless to say, this is not an accidental arrangement of nature, but we will reserve discussion of the benefits of this configuration for Chapter 10.

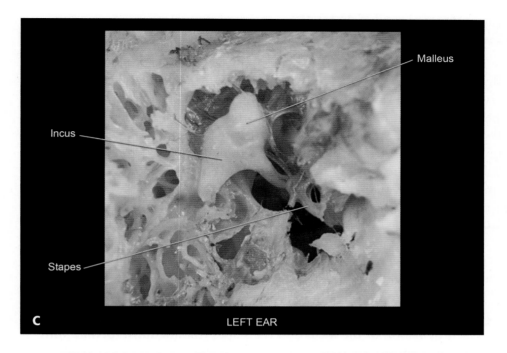

Malleus

Incus

Stapes

C   LEFT EAR

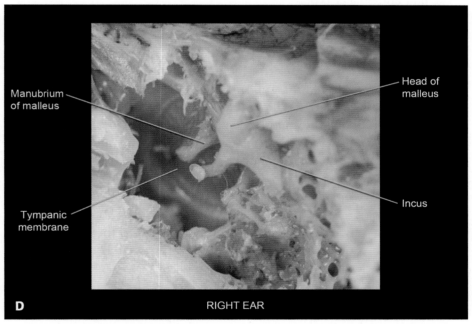

Manubrium of malleus

Head of malleus

Tympanic membrane

Incus

D   RIGHT EAR

Figure 9–6. *continued* **C.** Photograph of ossicular chain in situ, looking toward outer ear. **D.** Photograph of malleus and incus, as seen through intact tympanic membrane.

The incus weighs approximately 30 mg, and its longest process is approximately 7 mm. The malleus and incus articulate by means of a saddle joint, although it appears that the movement at the joint is quite limited. Rather, the malleus and incus appear to move as a unit upon movement of the TM.

The **stapes**, or "stirrup," is the third bone of this chain. The head (caput) of the stapes articulates with the lenticular process of the incus, and the neck of the stapes bifurcates to become the crura. The arch formed by the **anterior**

stapes: L., stirrup

Otitis Media with Effusion

Serous **(secretory)** otitis media refers to any condition in which fluid accumulates in the middle ear cavity. The typical sequence is as follows. The auditory tube stops functioning properly, allowing the middle ear space to become anaerobic as tissue within the space absorbs the available oxygen. Parallel to this, the poorly functioning auditory tube may not allow equalization of pressure between the middle ear space and the environment. In either condition, a relatively negative pressure may build in the middle ear space, pulling serous fluid from the blood of the middle ear tissues (termed **transudation**). The negative air pressure may also stimulate secretion of mucus from the middle ear tissue. This state, termed **middle ear effusion**, creates a barrier to sound transmission, in that the movement of the tympanic membrane is greatly inhibited.

and **posterior crura** converges on the **footplate** or **base** of the stapes. The footplate of the stapes rests in the oval window of the temporal bone, held in place by the **annular ligament**. This is the smallest of the ossicles, weighing approximately 4 mg, with the area of the stapes being only about 3.5 mm^2. The articulation of the incus and the stapes (the **incudostapedial joint**) is of the ball-and-socket type.

The ossicular chain is held in place by a series of strategically placed ligaments that suspend the ossicles from the walls of the middle ear cavity. The **superior ligament of the malleus** holds the head of the malleus within the epitympanic recess. An **anterior ligament of the malleus** binds the neck of the malleus to the anterior wall of the middle ear, and the **lateral ligament of the malleus** attaches the head of the malleus to the lateral wall. The **posterior ligament of the incus** suspends the incus by means of its short process, while a poorly formed **superior ligament of the incus** may be seen to bind the incus to the epitympanic recess.

Tympanic Muscles

Two important muscles of the middle ear are attached to the ossicles. These are the smallest muscles of the human body, appropriately so considering their attachment to the smallest bones (see Figure 9–6).

- **Stapedius**
- **Tensor tympani**

Stapedius Muscle

The **stapedius** muscle, approximately 6 mm long and 5 mm^2 in cross-sectional area, is embedded in the bone of the posterior wall of the middle ear, with only its tendon emerging from the **pyramidal eminence** in the middle ear space. The muscle inserts into the posterior neck of the stapes, so that when it contracts, the stapes is rotated posteriorly. Muscle spindles have been found in the stapedius muscle. Innervation of the stapedius is by means of the stapedial branch of the VII facial nerve.

Tensor Tympani Muscle

The **tensor tympani** is approximately 25 mm in length and nearly 6 mm^2 in cross-sectional area, arising from the anterior wall of the middle ear space, superior to the orifice of the auditory tube (also known as the Eustachian tube or pharyngotympanic tube). As with the stapedius, only the tendon of the tensor tympani is found in the middle ear space; the muscle itself is housed in bone. The muscle originates from the cartilaginous part of the auditory tube, as well as from the greater wing of the sphenoid, coursing through the **canal for the tensor tympani** in the anterior wall of the middle ear. The tendon for the tensor tympani emerges from the canal, courses around a bony outcropping called the **trochleariform process** (alternately **cochleari-form process**), and inserts into the upper manubrium malli. Contraction of this muscle pulls the malleus anteromedially, thereby reducing the range of movement of the TM by placing indirect tension on it. Indeed, both the tensor tympani and the stapedius muscles stiffen the middle ear transmission system, thereby reducing transmission of acoustical information in the lower frequencies. That is, contraction of these muscles reduces the strength of the signal reaching the cochlea, potentially protecting it from damage due to high signal intensity. Unfortunately, the protective function is compromised, in that the stiffening of the ossicular chain provides little barrier to transmission of the high-frequency sound so dominant in modern industrial societies. Innervation of the tensor tympani is by the V trigeminal nerve via the otic ganglion.

The arrangement of these ligament and muscle attachments is critical to the function of the middle ear. As we will see in Chapter 10, the attachments of the ossicles provide the precise tuning necessary to support vibration while prohibiting continued oscillation.

Muscle:	Stapedius
Origin:	Posterior wall of middle ear space of temporal bone
Course:	Anteriorly
Insertion:	Posterior crus of stapes
Innervation:	VII facial nerve
Function:	Rotates footplate of stapes posteriorly, thereby stiffening ossicular chain
Muscle:	Tensor tympani
Origin:	Cartilaginous portion of auditory tube and greater wing of sphenoid
Course:	Posteriorly through canal for tensor tympani and around trochleariform process
Insertion:	Manubrium malli
Innervation:	V trigeminal nerve via the otic ganglion
Function:	Pulls malleus anteromedially and stiffens ossicular chain

To summarize:

- The middle ear cavity houses the important middle ear ossicles and has a number of important landmarks.
- The **malleus** is the largest of the ossicles, providing the point of attachment with the tympanic membrane.
- The **incus** provides the intermediate communicating link for the ossicular chain, and the **stapes** is the third bone of this chain.
- The ossicular chain is held in place by a series of important ligaments; the **superior, anterior,** and **lateral ligaments of the malleus;** and the **posterior** and **superior ligaments of the incus.**
- The **stapedius muscle** inserts into the posterior neck of the stapes and pulls the stapes posteriorly.
- The **tensor tympani** muscle inserts into the upper manubrium malli and pulls the malleus anteromedially.
- Landmarks of the medial wall of the middle ear cavity include the **oval window,** the **round window,** the **promontory** of the cochlea, and the **prominence of the facial nerve.**
- The anterior wall houses the entrance to the **auditory tube,** and the posterior wall houses the **prominence of the stapedial pyramid.**

 ANAQUEST LESSON

Inner Ear

The inner ear houses the sensors for balance (the vestibular system) and hearing (the cochlea) (Table 9–3). The entryway to the cochlea is termed the **vestibule**.

Examination of Figure 9–7A will help in this preliminary discussion of the inner ear. Depicted in this figure is the **osseous** or **bony labyrinth**, representing the cavities (tunnels) within which the inner ear structures (the **membranous labyrinth**) are housed. The bony labyrinth is embedded within the petrous portion of the temporal bone, which is the densest bone in the body. The epithelial lining of the bony labyrinth secretes perilymph, the fluid that is found in the superficial cavities of the labyrinth.

The osseous labyrinth is made up of the vestibule, which is the entryway to the labyrinth the **semicircular canals**, and the **osseous cochlear canal**.

 ANAQUEST LESSON

Osseous Vestibule

The oval window is within the lateral wall of the vestibule, anterior to the semicircular canals and posterior to the cochlea. The vestibule space is continuous with both the vestibular mechanism and the cochlea (Table 9–4), although it is separated from the membranous vestibular duct and cochlear duct. The vestibule measures approximately 5 mm in the anterior-posterior dimension by 3 mm in width (Hackney, 2008). The oval window resides

Table 9–3

Landmarks of the Inner Ear

Vestibule

Saccule

Utricle

Macula

Otolithic membrane

Stereocilia

Kinocilium

Ductus reuniens

Endolymphatic duct

Semicircular canals

Lateral (horizontal) semicircular canal

Anterior vertical semicircular canal

Posterior vertical semicircular canal

Ampulla

Crista ampularis

Stereocilia

Kinocilium

Cochlea

Scala vestibuli

Scala tympani

Scala media (cochlear duct)

Reissner's membrane

Basilar membrane

Spiral ligament

Stria vascularis

Organ of Corti

    Inner and outer hair cells with stereocilia

    Deiter's cells

    Tunnel of Corti

    Spiral limbus

    Inner spiral sulcus

    Tectorial membrane

    Reticular lamina

    Hensen's cells

    Cells of Claudius

    Rods (pillars) of Corti

Osseous spiral lamina

Habenula perforata

Helicotrema

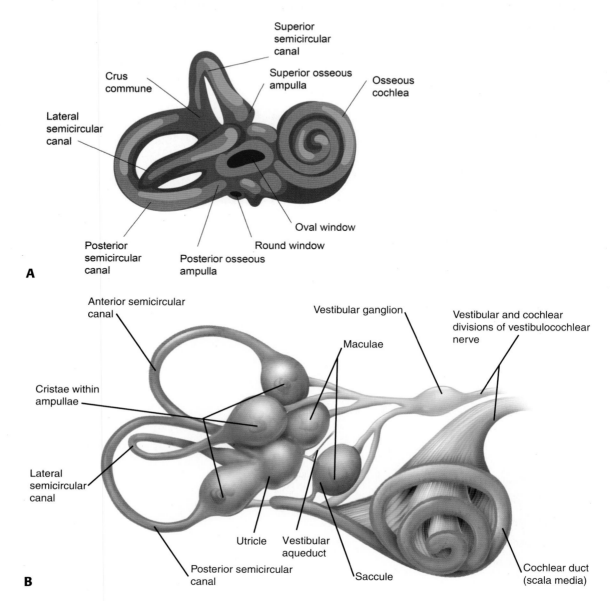

Figure 9–7. A. Lateral view schematic of the osseous labyrinth. Adapted from © Evgenil Naumov I Dreamstime.com **B.** The membranous labyrinth, revealing vestibular and cochlear ducts. Note that the vestibule is not shown because it is external to the membranous vestibular duct and is filled with perilymph. *continues*

in the lateral wall of the vestibule, and the medial wall of the vestibule houses the vestibular aqueduct, visible from the membranous labyrinth of Figure 9–7B. The interior of the osseous labyrinth (not shown) is marked by three prominent recesses, the spherical, cochlear, and elliptical recesses. The **spherical recess** of the medial wall contains minute perforations termed the **macula cribrosa media**, passages through which portions of the vestibular nerve pass to the saccule of the membranous labyrinth. The **cochlear recess** provides a similar communication between the vestibule and the basal end of the cochlear duct. The **elliptical recess** is similarly perforated, providing communication between the utricle it houses and the ampullae of the superior and lateral semicircular canals.

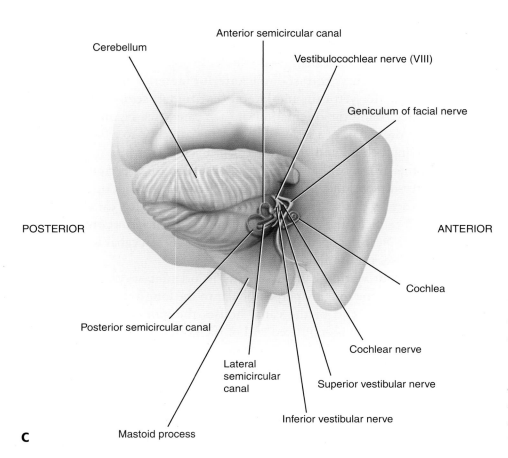

Cerebellum

Anterior semicircular canal

Vestibulocochlear nerve (VIII)

Geniculum of facial nerve

POSTERIOR

ANTERIOR

Cochlea

Posterior semicircular canal

Cochlear nerve

Lateral semicircular canal

Superior vestibular nerve

Inferior vestibular nerve

Mastoid process

C

Figure 9–7. *continued*
C. Orientation of the semi-circular canals in the erect human. *Source:* From Seikel/Drumright/King. *Anatomy & Physiology for Speech, Language, and Hearing, 5th Ed.* ©Cengage, Inc. Reproduced by permission.

Table 9–4

Critical Values of the Labyrinthine Spaces: Volumes and Lengths of Vestibular and Cochlear Spaces, as Indicated by Source		
Structure or Space	**Dimension**	**Source**
Volume of inner ear	208.26 μL	Buckingham & Valvassori (2001); Igarashi, Ohashi, & Oshii (1986); Melhem et al. (1998)
Volume of cochlear endolymph	7.7 μL	Igarashi et al. (1986)
Volume of perilymph (vestibular and cochlear)	162.45 μL	Buckingham & Valvassori (2001); Igarashi et al. (1986)
Volume of scala tympani	44.3 μL	Igarashi et al. (1986)
Length of scala tympani	28.46 mm	Thorne et al. (1999)
Volume of scala vestibuli	31.5 μL	Igarashi et al. (1986)
Area of round window	2.22 mm^2	Okuno & Sando (1988)
Length of cochlear aqueduct	6–12 mm	Gopen, Rosowski, & Merchant (1997)
Diameter of cochlear aqueduct	138 μm	Gopen et al. (1997)

Source: Derived from data compiled by A. Salt, PhD, of the Cochlear Fluids Research Lab of Washington University.

Osseous Semicircular Canals

The osseous semicircular canals house the sense organs for the movement of the body in space. These consist of the **anterior** (anterior vertical; superior), **posterior** (posterior vertical), and **lateral** (horizontal) **semicircular canals**, the names describing the orientation of each canal (see Figure 9–7A). You can envision the canals as a series of three rings attached to a ball (the vestibule) and lying behind and above that ball. Each ring is in a plane at right angles to other rings, so that the interaction of the three permits the brain to code three-dimensional space. The semicircular canals all open onto the vestibular space by means of apertures, although the vertical canals (anterior and posterior semicircular canals) share an aperture, the **crus commune** (see Figure 9–7A). Near the opening to the vestibule in each canal is an enlargement that houses the ampulla.

The anterior vertical canal is vertical in orientation, so that it senses movement in a plane roughly perpendicular to the long axis of the temporal bone. The anterior end of the canal houses the ampulla; the other end combines with the non-ampulated end of the posterior vertical canal at the crus commune.

The posterior vertical semicircular canal is vertically oriented as well, but is in the plane roughly parallel to the long axis of the temporal bone. Its ampulla is housed in the lower crus, entering the vestibule below the oval window.

The lateral (horizontal) semicircular canal senses movement roughly in the transverse plane of the body. Its ampulated end enters the vestibule near that of the anterior semicircular canal, above the level of the oval window.

Binaural orientation of the two semicircular canals is such that the anterior semicircular canal of one ear is parallel to the posterior canal of the other. The horizontal canals lie in the same plane, but the ampullae are in mirror-image locations. This horizontal orientation of the canal helps your brain differentiate rotatory movement toward the left versus right. The anterior semicircular canals sense movements of your head as it moves toward your shoulder, while the posterior semicircular canals sense the movement if you move your head to nod "yes." Shaking your head "no" is sensed by the lateral semicircular canals. The utricle and saccule are responsible for mediating the sense of acceleration of your head in space, such as in sudden movement or falling.

Osseous Cochlear Labyrinth

The osseous labyrinth has the appearance of a coiled snail shell ("cochlea" comes from the Greek word *cochlos*, meaning "snail"). The cochlea coils out from its base near the vestibule, wrapping around itself two-and-five-eighths times before reaching its **apex**. The core of the osseous labyrinth, the **modiolus**, is a finely perforated bone; fibers of the VIII vestibulocochlear nerve pass through these perforations on their way to ganglion cells within the modiolus (the modiolus is actually the combination of the core space,

modiolus: L., hub

known as Rosenthal's canal, and the spiral ganglion nerve fibers: Coleman et al., 2006). The core of the modiolus is continuous with the **internal auditory meatus** of the temporal bone, through which the vestibulocochlear nerve passes.

Figure 9–7C shows the orientation of the osseous labyrinth within the head. From this view you can see the orientation of the posterior, lateral and anterior semicircular canals, as well as the orientation of the cochlea within the skull. In the erect human depicted in this figure the lateral semicircular canal mediates motion sensation in the horizontal plane, while the anterior semicircular canal will transduce information in the vertical dimension.

The labyrinth is divided into two incomplete chambers, the **scala vestibuli** and the **scala tympani**, by an incomplete bony shelf protruding from the modiolus, the **osseous spiral lamina**. This very important structure forms the point of attachment for the scala media, which houses the sensory organ for hearing. The osseous spiral lamina becomes progressively smaller approaching the apex, such that the space between it and the opposite wall of the labyrinth increases. At the apex the two chambers formed by the incomplete lamina become hook-like (hence the name **hamulus**), forming the **helicotrema**, the region through which the scala tympani and scala vestibuli communicate.

The osseous labyrinth has three prominent openings. The round window (foramen rotundum; fenestra rotundrum) provides communication between the scala tympani and the middle ear. The oval window, upon which the stapes is placed, permits communication between the scala vestibuli and the middle ear space. The **cochlear canaliculus** or **cochlear aqueduct** is a minute opening between the scala tympani in the region of the round window and the subarachnoid space of the cranial cavity. It is hypothesized that **perilymph**, the fluid that fills the scala vestibuli and scala tympani, passes through this duct, although this has not been demonstrated. There is about 179 µL of fluid in the entire labyrinth, with only 7.7 µL of endolymph and about 162.4 µL of perilymph. The vestibule has only about 7 µL of fluid in it. To get a notion of scale, 1 mL is 1/1000 of a liter, and 1 µL is 1/1,000,000 of a liter.

✅ *To summarize:*

- The inner ear houses the sensors for balance (the vestibular system) and hearing (the cochlea).

- The entryway to these structures is termed the **vestibule**.

- The **osseous labyrinth** is made up of the entryway to the labyrinth, the vestibule, the semicircular canals, and the osseous cochlear canal.

- The osseous labyrinth has the appearance of a coiled snail shell.

- The labyrinth is divided into two incomplete chambers, the **scala vestibuli** and the **scala tympani**, by the **osseous spiral lamina**, an incomplete bony shelf protruding from the modiolus.

- The **round window** provides communication between the scala tympani and the middle ear space.

- The **oval window** permits communication between the scala vestibuli and the middle ear space.
- The **cochlear aqueduct** connects the upper duct and the subarachnoid space.

Membranous Labyrinth

The structure of the membranous labyrinth parallels that of the bony labyrinth. First, orient yourself to the oval window, recognizing its link to the stapes of the middle ear. Beneath it, but not quite visible, is the round window. The vestibule or entryway to the inner ear is a space shared by the sense organ of hearing, the cochlea, and the sense organs of balance, the semicircular canals. The same fluid flows through all of the membranous labyrinth, making balance and hearing intimately related in both function and pathology. Let us examine the sensory components of the inner ear.

Vestibular System

The membranous labyrinth (see Figure 9-7B) can be thought of as a fluid-filled sac that rests within the cavity of the osseous labyrinth. This sac does not completely fill the labyrinth but rather forms an additional space within the already fluid-filled region. The cochlear duct forms only a small portion of the membranous labyrinth and contains fluid of a slightly different composition from that of the region surrounding the duct. This fluid in the cochlear duct is termed **endolymph**.

In the vestibular system, the membranous labyrinth houses the vestibular organ. As you will recall, the **ampulla** is the expanded region of the semicircular canals near one opening to the vestibule. Each ampulla houses a **crista ampularis**, over which a gelatinous cupola lies. The **crista** is the receptor organ for movement, being made up of ciliated receptor cells and a supporting membrane. From each of the 6,000 receptor cells protrude approximately 100 **stereocilia**, minute hairs that sense movement in fluid, and one **kinocilium**. A **cupola** overlays the crista ampularis such that the cilia are embedded within the cupola.

Within the vestibule lie the **utricle** and the **saccule**, housing for the otolithic organs of the vestibular system. The utricular **macula** is the sensory organ, which is endowed with hair cells and cilia. It is covered by the **otolithic membrane**, which is invested with crystals (**otoliths**). The saccule lies near the scala vestibuli in the vestibule and is similarly endowed with macula and otolithic membrane. The saccule and utricle communicate by means of the **endolymphatic duct**, which is embedded in the dura mater. The saccule communicates with the cochlea by means of the minute **ductus reuniens**.

Cochlear Duct

The **cochlear duct** can be conceptualized as a tube suspended from the walls of the bony labyrinth, dividing the labyrinth into three spaces; the scala

crista: receptor organ for movement within vestibular mechanism

vestibuli, the scala tympani, and the **scala media**. The cochlear duct creates the middle space, and it houses the sensory apparatus for hearing.

A cross-section through the region of the scala media reveals its extraordinary structure, as shown in Figure 9–8. Note first the osseous spiral lamina, discussed previously. This shelf courses the extent of the osseous labyrinth, forming the major point of attachment for the cochlear duct. Looking at Figures 9–8 and 9–9, you can see **Reissner's membrane**, an extremely thin separation between the perilymph of the scala vestibuli and the endolymph of the scala media. One end is continuous with the **stria vascularis**, highly vascularized tissue that is firmly attached to the **spiral ligament**, and which is responsible for the potassium used by the hair cells. Disruption of the blood supply to the cochlea, such as can occur during surgery for a cerebellar tumor, results in immediate hearing loss, arising from reduced potassium output into the endolymph of the scala media (Mom, Chazal, Gabrillargues, Gilian, & Avan, 2005).

The **basilar membrane** forms the "floor" of the scala media, separating the scala media and scala tympani. It is on this membrane that the organ of hearing is found. The basilar membrane is extremely thin, because of its role in supporting the traveling wave.

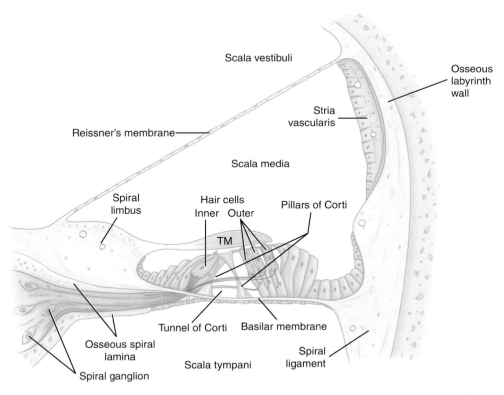

Figure 9–8. Cross-section of the cochlea, revealing scala vestibule; scala media; scala tympani; and TM, tectorial membrane. *Source:* From Seikel/Drumright/King. *Anatomy & Physiology for Speech, Language, and Hearing, 5th Ed.* ©Cengage, Inc. Reproduced by permission.

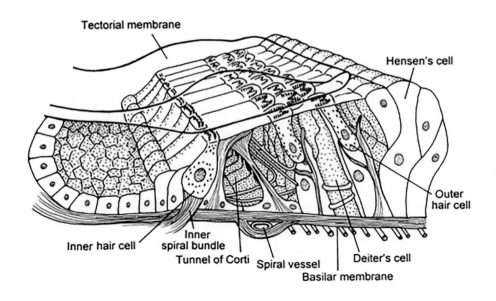

Figure 9–9. Landmarks and structures of the organ of Corti. *Source:* From Seikel/Drumright/King. *Anatomy & Physiology for Speech, Language, and Hearing, 4th Ed.* ©Cengage, Inc. Reproduced by permission.

The **organ of Corti** is grossly similar to the design of the vestibular organs. There are four rows of hair cells resting on a bed of Deiters' cells for support. The outer three rows of hair cells, known as **outer hair cells**, are separated from the single row of **inner hair cells** by the **tunnel of Corti**, the product of **pillar cells of Corti, also known as rods of Corti**. The superior surface of the outer hair cells and the phalangeal processes of Deiters' cells form a matrix termed the *reticular lamina*, through which the cilia protrude. The vascular supply for the organ of Corti arises from the labyrinthine artery (which itself arises from the basilar artery). The cochlear branch of the labyrinthine artery divides into between 12 and 14 "twigs" that serve the spiral lamina, basilar membrane, stria vascularis, and other cochlear structures (Hackney, 2008).

On the modiolar side of the cochlear duct is found the **spiral limbus**, from which arises the **tectorial membrane**. The **spiral sulcus** undergirds the spiral ligament, perhaps providing stiffness to the basilar membrane (Raftenberg, 1990). The tectorial membrane overlays the hair cells and has functional significance in the processing of acoustic stimuli. The outer hair cells are clearly embedded in this membrane, but the inner hair cells do not make physical contact with the tectorial membrane, although its proximity to the hair cells is an important contributor to hair cell excitation, as will be discussed shortly.

Inner and outer hair cells differ markedly in number. The hair cells on the modiolar side of the tunnel of Corti are termed the inner hair cells (Figure 9–10). The 3,500 inner hair cells form a single row stretching from the base to apex. The upper surface of each hair cell is graced with a series of approximately 50 **stereocilia** forming a slight "U" pattern opened toward the modiolar side. There are three rows of outer hair cells, broadening to four rows in the apical end, numbering approximately 12,000. As with the inner cells, the stereocilia protrude from the surface of each outer hair cell, but with a "W" or "V" pattern formed by approximately 150 stereocilia. In

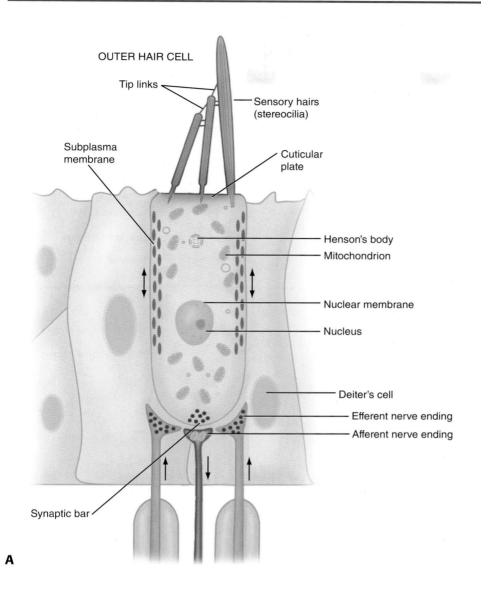

OUTER HAIR CELL

Tip links

Sensory hairs
(stereocilia)

Subplasma
membrane

Cuticular
plate

Henson's body

Mitochondrion

Nuclear membrane

Nucleus

Deiter's cell

Efferent nerve ending

Afferent nerve ending

Synaptic bar

A

Figure 9–10. Details of hair cells. **A.** Outer hair cell. *Source:* From Seikel/Drumright/ King. *Anatomy & Physiology for Speech, Language, and Hearing, 5th Ed.* ©Cengage, Inc. Reproduced by permission. *continues*

both the inner and outer hair cells, the stereocilia for a given cell are graduated in length, so that the longer cilia are distal to the modiolar side. The cilia of a hair cell are all connected by thin, filamentous links. Shorter cilia are connected to the taller cilia by "tip links," and cilia are also linked laterally, thus ensuring that movement of one cilia involves disturbance of adjacent cilia on a hair cell. Stereocilia found in the apex are longer than those found in the base.

The morphology between inner and outer hair cells differs markedly. The inner hair cells are teardrop or gourd shaped, with a broad base and narrowed neck. The outer hair cells, in contrast, are shaped like a test tube. Inner hair cells are embedded in a matrix of inner phalangeal cells for support, while outer hair cells are nested in outer phalangeal cells of Deiters', with support by cells of Claudius and Hensen's cells. Phalangeal processes apparently replace hair cells lost through acoustic trauma, thereby maintaining the delicate cuticular plate.

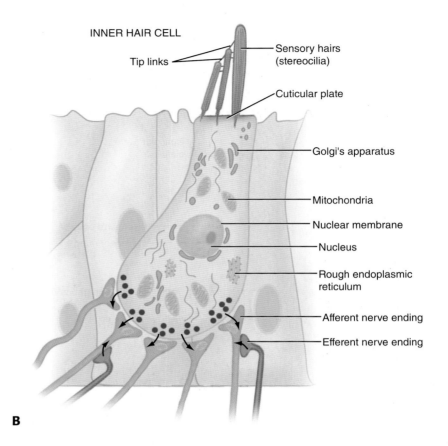

INNER HAIR CELL

Tip links

Sensory hairs (stereocilia)

Cuticular plate

Golgi's apparatus

Mitochondria

Nuclear membrane

Nucleus

Rough endoplasmic reticulum

Afferent nerve ending

Efferent nerve ending

B

Figure 9–10. *continued* **B.** Inner hair cell. Note presence of both afferent and efferent fibers innervating both types of sensory cells. (From Stach, 2008.) *Source:* From Seikel/Drumright/King. *Anatomy & Physiology for Speech, Language, and Hearing, 5th Ed.* ©Cengage, Inc. Reproduced by permission.

Innervation Pattern of the Organ of Corti

The hair cells of the cochlea receive both afferent and efferent innervation, as discussed in Chapter 12. The pattern of innervation is strikingly different between outer and inner hair cells.

Afferent Innervation

As shown in Figure 9–11, each inner hair cell is connected to as many as 10 VIII vestibulocochlear nerve fibers, referred to as *many-to-one* innervation. In contrast, each outer hair cell shares its innervation with 10 other outer hair cells, all being innervated by the same VIII nerve fiber (*one-to-many* innervation).

VIII vestibulocochlear nerve fibers consist of Type I fibers (large, myelinated fibers) and Type II fibers (small, both myelinated and unmyelinated fibers). Type I fibers, making up 95 percent of the VIII nerve, apparently innervate the inner hair cells, whereas unmyelinated Type II fibers innervate the outer hair cells. Type I fibers innervating hair cells course medially through the habenula perforata, after which point myelin will be found on the fiber. Most of the Type II outer hair cell fibers course medially to the habenula perforata as the inner radial bundle. A small portion of Type II fibers courses within the tunnel of Corti apically to join with the outer spiral bundle. The outer spiral bundle fibers innervating the outer hair cells contain both afferent and efferent fibers.

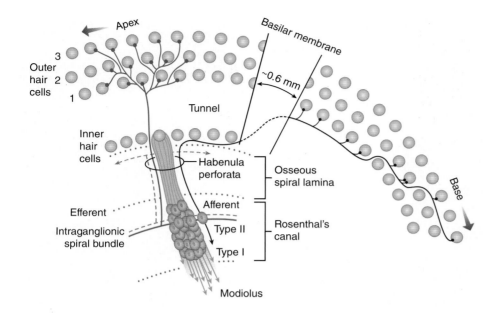

Figure 9–11. Innervation scheme of organ of Corti. Note that many nerve fibers innervate each inner hair cell, while many outer hair cells are innervated by one nerve fiber. (From Spoendlin, 1984.) *Source:* From Seikel/ Drumright/King. *Anatomy & Physiology for Speech, Language, and Hearing, 5th Ed.* ©Cengage, Inc. Reproduced by permission.

Efferent Innervation

As will be discussed in Chapter 11, the efferent innervation of the outer hair cells is inhibitory, reducing the afferent output caused by hair cell stimulation. The pathway and circuitry involved is termed the olivocochlear bundle because it arises from the region of the olivary complex of the brain stem auditory pathway. This bundle of fibers consists of about 1,600 neurons and is divided into crossed and uncrossed pathways. The crossed olivocochlear bundle (COCB) arises from a region near the medial superior olive of the olivary complex, and descends to the fourth ventricle, where the majority of the fibers decussate and proceed to innervate the outer hair cells. The uncrossed olivocochlear bundle (UCOB) originates near the lateral superior olive of the olivary complex and courses primarily ipsilaterally to the inner hair cells of the cochlea. Activation of the olivocochlear bundle appears to be controllable through cortical activity and assists in the detection of signal within a background of noise.

Figure 9–12 provides a posterior view of the brain stem with the cerebellum removed. Identify the VIII vestibulocochlear nerve and the indication of the petrous portion of the temporal bone. This is precisely the point of exit of the VIII vestibulocochlear nerve from the labyrinth, the internal auditory meatus.

✅ *To summarize:*

- The **membranous labyrinth** can be thought of as a fluid-filled sac that rests within the cavity of the osseous labyrinth and is filled with **endolymph**.

- In the vestibular system, the membranous labyrinth houses the vestibular organ.

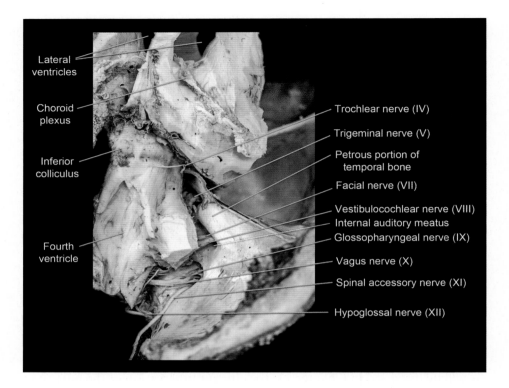

Figure 9–12. View of posterior brain stem and cranial nerves as seen from the cranial fossa.

- The **ampulla** is the expanded region of the semicircular canals containing the **crista ampularis**. Within the vestibule lie the **utricle** and the **saccule**.
- The membranous labyrinth of the cochlea resides between the scala vestibuli and scala tympani, making up the intermediate **scala media**.
- **Reissner's membrane** forms the upper boundary of the scala media, and the basilar membrane forms the floor.
- The **organ of Corti** has four rows of hair cells resting on a bed of Deiters' cells for support.
- The **outer hair cells** are separated from the **inner hair cell** row by the **tunnel of Corti**.
- The upper surface of each hair cell is graced with a series of **stereocilia** connected by tip links.
- Each inner hair cell is connected with as many as 10 VIII vestibulocochlear nerve fibers, and each outer hair cell shares its innervation with 10 other outer hair cells, all being innervated by the same VIII nerve fiber.

Chapter Summary

The outer ear is composed of the pinna and the external auditory meatus. Landmarks of the pinna include the margin of the auricle, the helix, and the auricular tubercle on the helix. The EAM has both osseous and cartilaginous parts; the cartilaginous portion makes up one third of the ear canal, while the other two-thirds are housed in bone. At the terminus of the external auditory meatus is the tympanic membrane, the structure separating the outer and middle ear.

The middle ear cavity houses the middle ear ossicles. The malleus is the largest of the ossicles, providing the point of attachment with the TM. The incus provides the intermediate communicating link of the ossicular chain, and the stapes is the third bone of this chain. The ossicular chain is held in place by a series of ligaments. The stapedius muscle inserts into the posterior neck of the stapes and pulls the stapes posteriorly; the tensor tympani muscle inserts into the upper manubrium malli, pulling the malleus anteromedially. Landmarks of the medial wall of the middle ear cavity include the oval window, the round window, the promontory of the cochlea, and the prominence of the facial nerve. The anterior wall houses the entrance to the auditory tube, and the posterior wall houses the prominence of the stapedial pyramid.

The inner ear houses the sense mechanism for balance (the vestibular system) and hearing (the cochlea). The entryway to these structures is termed the vestibule. The osseous labyrinth is made up of the entryway to the labyrinth, the vestibule, the semicircular canals, and the osseous cochlear canal.

It has the appearance of a coiled snail shell and is divided into two incomplete chambers, the scala vestibuli and the scala tympani, by the osseous spiral lamina, an incomplete bony shelf protruding from the modiolus. The round window provides communication between the scala tympani and the middle ear space. The oval window permits communication between the scala vestibuli and the middle ear space. The cochlear aqueduct connects the upper duct and the subarachnoid space.

The membranous labyrinth can be thought of as a fluid-filled sac that rests within the cavity of the osseous labyrinth and is filled with endolymph. In the vestibular system, the membranous labyrinth houses the vestibular organ. The ampulla is the expanded region of the semicircular canals containing the crista ampularis. Within the vestibule lie the utricle and saccule. The membranous labyrinth of the cochlea resides between the scala vestibuli and the scala tympani, making up the intermediate scala media. Reissner's membrane forms the distal boundary of the scala media, and the basilar membrane forms the proximal boundary. The organ of Corti has four rows of hair cells resting on a bed of Deiters' cells for support. The outer hair cells are separated from the row of inner hair cells by the tunnel of Corti. The upper surface of each hair cell is graced with a series of stereocilia. Each inner hair cell is innervated by as many as 10 VIII nerve fibers, while each outer hair cell shares its innervation with 10 other outer hair cells, all being innervated by the same VIII nerve fibers.

Chapter 9 Study Question Answers

1. The ear is a **TRANSDUCER**, in that it converts acoustical energy into electrochemical energy.

2. The **OUTER EAR** serves the function of sound collection.

3. The **EXTERNAL AUDITORY** meatus is a conduit for sound reaching the tympanic membrane.

4. The **INTERNAL AUDITORY** meatus is a conduit for the VIII nerve fibers coursing to the brain stem.

5. The tympanic membrane (or eardrum) is made up of **THREE** layers of tissue.

6. The outer layer of the tympanic membrane is continuous with the **EPITHELIUM OF THE EXTERNAL AUDITORY MEATUS**.

7. The **INTERMEDIATE** layer of the tympanic membrane is made up primarily of radiating fibers.

8. The **UMBO** is a landmark produced by the most distal part of the manubrium malli.

9. The **MALLEUS** is the bone of the middle ear directly attached to the tympanic membrane.

10. The **STAPES** is the bone of the middle ear directly communicating with the oval window.

11. The **MANUBRIUM** of the malleus attaches to the tympanic membrane.

12. The **FOOTPLATE** of the stapes articulates with the oval window.

13. The **STAPEDIUS** muscle pulls the stapes posteriorly.

14. The **TENSOR TYMPANI** muscle pulls the malleus anteromedially.

15. The entryway to the cochlea and vestibular system is via the space known as the **VESTIBULE**.

16. The **OSSEOUS LABYRINTH** is the system of cavities within bone that houses the membranous labyrinth.

17. The scala **VESTIBULI** and scala **TYMPANI** are incomplete spaces within the osseous labyrinth.

18. The **ROUND** window provides communication between the scala tympani and the middle ear.

19. The **OVAL** window permits communication between the scala vestibuli and the middle ear space.

20. The **MEMBRANOUS LABYRINTH** is a fluid-filled sac attached to the walls of the osseous labyrinth and is filled with endolymph.

21. **REISSNER'S** membrane separates the scala vestibuli and the scala media; the **BASILAR** membrane separates the scala media from the scala tympani.

22. There are **THREE** rows of outer hair cells and **ONE** row of inner hair cells.

23. The **TUNNEL OF CORTI** separates the outer and inner hair cells.

24. The hair cells are innervated by the **VIII VESTIBULOCOCHLEAR** nerve.

25. As with any other body structure, the ossicles are subject to trauma. A frequent cause of disarticulation of the ossicles is head trauma that involves the temporal bone (this may also cause a perilymph fistula, which is a tear in the basilar or Reissner's membrane that allows perilymph and endolymph to mingle). Another cause of disarticulation is noise or high-pressure trauma; the high-pressure forces associated with explosions can easily cause disarticulation.

Bibliography

Black, S. M. (2008). Head and neck: External skull. In S. Standring (Ed.), *Gray's anatomy: The anatomical and clinical basis of practice* (40th ed., pp. 409–422). London, UK: Churchill-Livingstone.

Buckingham, R. A., & Valvassori, G. E. (2001). Inner ear fluid volumes and the resolving power of magnetic resonance imaging: Can it differentiate endolymphatic structures? *Annals of Otology, Rhinology, and Laryngology*, *110*(2), 113–117.

Clark, W. W., & Ohlemiller, K. K. (2008). *Anatomy and physiology of hearing for audiologists*. Clifton Park, NY: Thomson Delmar Learning.

Coleman, B., Hardman, J., Coco, A., Epp, S., de Silva, M., Crook, J., & Shepherd, R. (2006). Fate of embryonic stem cell migration in the deafened mammalian cochlea. *Cell Transplantation*, *15*(5), 369–380.

Gleeson, M. (2008). The external and middle ear. In S. Standring (2008), *Gray's anatomy: The anatomical and clinical basis of practice* (40th ed., pp. 614–632). London, UK: Churchill-Livingstone.

Gopen, Q., Rosowski, J. J., & Merchant, S. N. (1997). Anatomy of the normal human cochlear aqueduct with functional implications. *Hearing Research*, *107*(1–2), 9–22.

Hackney, C. M. (2008). Inner ear. In S. Standring (Ed.), *Gray's anatomy: The anatomical and clinical basis of practice* (40th ed., pp. 633–650). London, UK: Churchill-Livingstone.

Igarashi, M., Ohashi, K., & Oshii, M. (1986). Morphometric comparison of endolymphatic and perilymphatic spaces in human temporal bones. *Acta Otolaryngolica*, *101*(3–4), 161–164.

Lam, J., & Dohil, M. (2007). Multiple accessory tragi and hemifacial microsomia. *Pediatric Dermatology*, *24*(6), 657–658.

Martin, F., & Clark, J. G. (1995). *Hearing care for children*. Boston, MA: Allyn & Bacon.

Martin, F., & Clark, J. G. (2006). *Elements of audiology: A learning aid with cases*. Boston, MA: Allyn & Bacon.

Melhem, E. R., Shakir, H., Bakthavachalam, S., MacDonald, C. B., Gira, J., Caruthers, S. D., & Jara, H. (1998). Inner ear volumetric measurements using high-resolution 3D T2-weighted fast spin–echo MR imaging: Initial experience in healthy subjects. *American Journal of Neuroradiology*, *19*(10), 1807–1808.

Møller, A. (2006). *Neural plasticity and disorders of the nervous system*. Boston, MA: Cambridge University Press.

Mom, T., Chazal, J., Gabrillargues, J., Gilian, L., & Avan, P. (2005). Cochlear blood supply: An update on anatomy and function. *French Oto-Rhino-Laryngology*, *88*, 81–88.

Okuno, H., & Sando, I. (1988). Anatomy of the round window. A histopathological study with a graphic reconstruction method. *Acta Otolaryngologica*. *106*(1–2), 55–63.

Porter, C. J. W., & Tan, S. T. (2005). Congenital auricular anomalies: Topographic anatomy, embryology, classification and treatment strategies. *Plastic and Reconstructive Surgery*, *115*(6), 1701–1712.

Raftenberg, M. N. (1990). Flow of endolymph in the inner spiral sulcus and the subtectorial space. *Journal of the Acoustical Society of America*, *87*(6), 2606–2620.

Spoendlin, H. (1984). Primary neurons and synapses. In I. Friedmann & J. Ballantyne (Eds.), *Ultrastructural atlas of the inner ear* (pp. 133–164). London, UK: Butterworth.

Stach, B. (2008). *Clinical audiology: An introduction*. Scarborough, ON, Canada: Nelson Education.

Thorne, M., Salt, A. N., DeMott, J. E., Henson, M. M., Henson, O. W. Jr., & Gewalt, S. L. (1999). Cochlear fluid space dimensions for six species derived from reconstructions of three-dimensional magnetic resonance images. *Laryngoscope, 109*(10), 1661–1668.

Wei, X., Makori, N., Peterson, P. E., Hummler, H., & Hendrickx, A. G. (1999). Pathogenesis of retinoic acid-induced ear malformations in primate model. *Teratology, 60*(2), 83–92.

Auditory Physiology

The auditory mechanism is responsible for processing the acoustic signal of speech. Auditory stimuli can arrive at the tympanic membrane in an amazingly wide range of sound pressures, from the whisper of a leaf blowing in the breeze to the pressures associated with painfully loud sound. Likewise, the human auditory mechanism has a frequency range of approximately 10 octaves, spanning 20 to 20,000 Hz. Within these broad requirements of transducing sounds in a range of frequencies are much finer tasks, including differentiating small increments in frequency and intensity. Even beyond these tasks are the everyday requirements of listening to a signal embedded in a background of noise and listening to extremely rapid sequences of sounds. The beauty of the auditory system is that it performs all these tasks and more with breathtaking ease. This chapter cannot provide a thorough examination of all aspects of auditory physiology, but we hope it will show you why audiologists are so excited by their field.

The field of audiology owes a great deal to the extraordinary scientist Georg von Békésy, whose work earned him a Nobel Prize in 1961 (Evans, 2003). Von Békésy (1960) performed exceedingly intricate measurements on the auditory mechanism and was at times forced to create tools where none existed. We will refer frequently to his work, which defined the basic function of the middle and inner ear, as we discuss the basic physiological principles involved in the translation of an acoustic stimulus into a form that is interpretable by the brain. The organizing principle to keep in mind is this: The outer ear collects sound and "shapes" its frequency components somewhat; the middle ear matches the airborne acoustic signal with the fluid medium of the cochlea; the inner ear performs temporal and spectral analyses on the ongoing acoustical signal; and the auditory pathway conveys and further processes that signal. The cerebral cortex interprets the signal.

An octave is a doubling in frequency.

See Chapter 5 for a discussion of frequency and periodicity.

Instrumentation in Hearing Research

There are a number of tools available for the study of hearing. Of critical importance is knowledge of the temporal and spectral characteristics of a signal being transduced by the listener, so spectral and temporal acoustic analysis tools discussed in Chapters 5 and 7 serve that purpose. Impedance of the middle ear is measured by tympanometry, and recent developments in wideband acoustic reflectance measures have become important tools for elaborating middle ear function (e.g., Sanford & Feeney, 2008). The cochlea provides significant challenges for study due to its extremely small size and the fact that it is embedded within the densest bone in the body. While the cochlea can be visualized through high-resolution magnetic resonance imaging for purposes of identifying malformations, the physical study of the cochlea relies on postmortem micrographic imaging and histological techniques. Researchers have been able to identify neural receptors and functional proteins within the cochlea (e.g., Spicer & Schulte, 1996) using ultrastructural visualizing methods.

Questions about the function of the cochlea have resulted in the development of instruments that ultimately entered the clinical realm for diagnostic purposes. You have likely been exposed to the clinical audiometer, which is a means of behaviorally assessing the hearing threshold of individuals. Otoacoustic emissions testing involves introducing tones into the ear and recording the reflection from the cochlea as a means of determining the viability of the outer hair cells. This important assessment tool began as a research instrument (e.g., Norton & Neely, 1987) and has evolved into a critically important clinical tool (e.g., Seixas et al., 2004).

Electrophysiological methods provide a window to the neurophysiology of the auditory mechanism. Research on nonhuman animals often involves direct, single-cell measurement of the auditory pathway, which gives a great deal of insight into the detail of auditory transmission (there have been a few direct measurements in humans as well). The acoustic reflex permits examination of the integrity of the early stages of the auditory pathway. For years evoked auditory brain stem responses (ABR) and electrocochleography (EcOG) have allowed researchers and clinicians to examine the integrity of the auditory pathway, and cortical auditory functioning (and even cognitive processes) can be illuminated through numerous late cortical responses to acoustic stimuli (e.g., P300, P400, contingent negative variation). Functional magnetic resonance imaging (fMRI) provides a unique window to auditory cortical functioning (although the extraordinarily high sound pressure levels of the instrument provide a particularly daunting challenge to the researcher trying to present auditory stimuli to a subject).

Instrumentation in hearing science began with the pioneering work of Georg von Békésy and Hermann von Helmholtz before him, and continues to develop as technology of acoustical, physical, and physiological measurement becomes more refined.

Outer Ear

The outer ear can be seen primarily as a collector of sound. The **pinna**, with its ridges, grooves, and dished-out regions, is an excellent funnel for sound directed toward the head from the front or side, although less effective for sound arising from behind the head.

Indeed, the crevices and crannies of the pinna are functional. If you have blown across the lip of a soda bottle and produced a tone, you know that cavities have characteristics that make them particularly responsive to specific frequencies. When a tube or bottle is excited by an input stimulus, it will tend to select energy at its resonant frequency, while tending to reject energy at frequencies other than the resonant frequency. The result is **selective enhancement** of certain frequencies (Figure 10–1).

Because the outer ear has no active (moveable) elements, it can have only a passive effect on the input stimulus. The pinna acts as a sound funnel, focusing acoustic energy into the external auditory meatus (EAM), and the EAM funnels sound to the tympanic membrane (TM). Both of these structures, however, have shapes that boost the relative strength of the signal through resonance, with the result being relatively enhanced signal intensity between 1500 and 8000 Hz.

As can be seen in Figure 10–1, the components of the pinna contribute a relatively small amount to the overall gain as compared with that of the EAM. Nonetheless, the contribution of the entire system results in a net gain reaching 20 dB at approximately 2100 Hz. Kruger (1989) showed that the resonant frequency of the outer ear changes from birth until about 3 years: The neonate has a peak resonance that is closer to 6000 Hz, but that resonance shifts down steadily as the auricle and EAM grow, reaching 2500 Hz at 37 months.

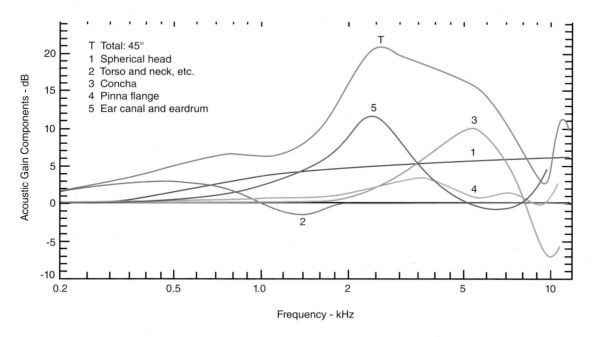

Figure 10–1. Effect of various landmarks of the outer ear upon the input acoustic signal. (Reprinted by permission from the *External Ear* by E. A. G. Shaw, 1974, p. 95. In W. D. Keidel & W. D. Neff, Eds. *Handbook of Sensory Physiology*. Copyright 1974 by Springer-Verlag, Inc. New York, NY: Springer-Verlag.) *Source:* From Seikel/Drumright/King. *Anatomy & Physiology for Speech, Language, and Hearing, 5th Ed.* ©Cengage, Inc. Reproduced by permission.

Middle Ear Function

As you remember, the primary structures of the middle ear are the TM, the ossicles, and the entry to the cochlea, the oval window. These are the players in one of the most important evolutionary dramas of the auditory mechanism.

If you can recall a dreamy summer day at a swimming pool, you may also remember that it would have been almost impossible to communicate vocally with someone in that pool if the person was submerged. When you tried to yell at your friend from above the water, nearly all of the sound energy of your speech would have reflected off the surface of the water.

The cochlea is a fluid-filled cavity, and were it not for the presence of the middle ear mechanism, talking to each other would be like trying to talk to someone under water: The sound energy would reflect off the oval window because of the vast differences in the liquid and gaseous media of perilymph and air. Somewhere in our evolution a mechanism arose to improve our plight.

The middle ear mechanism is designed to increase the pressure approaching the cochlea, thereby overcoming the resistance to flow of energy, termed **impedance**. Recall from Chapter 2 that **pressure = force/area**. That is, to increase pressure, you must either increase the force or decrease the area over which the force is being exerted. The middle ear mechanism uses the latter as the primary means of matching the impedance of the outer and inner ear. That is, the primary function of the middle ear is to match the impedance of two conductive systems, the outer ear and the cochlea.

The first mechanism of impedance matching is achieved through addressing the area parameter of the TM and the oval window. As mentioned earlier, pressure can be increased by decreasing the area over which force is distributed: A lightweight individual in a spike heel can do much more damage to floor tiles than a piano mover in sneakers. The TM has an effective area of about 55 mm^2, while the area of the oval window is about 3.2 mm^2, making the TM 17 times larger, depending on species size. Sound energy reaching the TM is "funneled" to the much smaller area of the oval window, so there is a gain of 17:1, which translates to an increase of about 25 dB.

The second impedance-matching function is achieved by a lever difference. The length of the manubrium is approximately 9 mm, while that of the long process of the stapes is about 7 mm, giving an overall gain of about 1.2. The lever effect arising from this gain is nearly 2 dB.

A third effect arises from the buckling of the TM. As it moves in response to sound, the TM buckles somewhat, such that the arm of the malleus moves a shorter distance than the surface of the TM. This results in a reduction in velocity of displacement of the malleus, with a resulting increase of force that provides a 4 to 6 dB increase in effective signal.

Combined, the area, lever, and buckling effects result in a signal gain of about 31 dB, from the TM to cochlea, depending on the stimulus frequency. Again, were the middle ear removed, a signal entering the EAM would have to be 31 dB more intense to be heard. This middle ear transformer action is very important to audition, and any process that reduces the effectiveness of this function (e.g., otitis media, otosclerosis, or glomus tumors) can have a serious impact on the conduction of sound to the inner ear.

⊘ *To summarize:*

- The outer and middle ears serve as funneling and impedance-matching devices.
- The **pinna** funnels acoustical information to the **external auditory meatus** and aids in the **localization** of sound in space.
- The **resonant frequencies** of the pinna and the external auditory meatus are those of the important components of the speech signal, between 1500 and 8000 Hz.
- Resistance to the flow of energy is termed **impedance**.
- The middle ear mechanism is an **impedance-matching device**, increasing the pressure of a signal arriving at the cochlea.
- The **area ratio** between the tympanic membrane and the oval window provides a 25 dB gain.
- The **lever advantage** of the ossicles provides a 2 dB gain.
- The buckling effect provides a 4 to 6 dB gain.

Inner Ear Function

Vestibular Mechanism

 ANAQUEST LESSON

The semicircular canals are uniquely designed to respond to rotatory movements of the body. By virtue of their orientation, each canal is at approximate right angles to the other canals, so that all movements of the head can be mapped by combinations of outputs of the sensory components, the cristae ampullares. Activation of the sensory element arises from inertia: As your head rotates, the fluid in the semicircular canals tends to lag behind. The result of this is that the cilia are stimulated by relative movement of the fluid during rotation. The utricle and saccule sense acceleration of the head rather than rotation, during body or head tilting. When you are standing erect, the macula of the utricle is roughly horizontal to the plane of movement, so straight-line acceleration in a forward or backward movement will be sensed there. The saccule, in contrast, is oriented more vertically. You can thank the macula of the utricle for the sensation associated with rapid acceleration during takeoff of a jet. In contrast, the saccule can be blamed for that sinking feeling when you hit turbulence that causes the plane to drop suddenly. Taken together, the vestibular mechanisms provide the major input to the proprioceptive system serving the sense of one's body in space. This information is integrated with joint sense, muscle spindle afferents, and visual input to form the perception of body position.

The vestibular system is our way of recognizing where our body is in space with reference to gravity, as well as when it is moving through space. It is the critical system for maintaining balance. Let's see how this works.

You'll remember that each inner ear has three semicircular canals (horizontal, anterior and superior). Each canal has a crista ampularis, and a cupola lies atop each crista. The crista has about 50 stereocilia protruding from it, embedded in the cupola. When the cupola moves, it deflects the stereocilia, and that causes the sensation of movement. (This arrangement is very similar to that of the hair cells of the cochlea, particularly the outer hair cells that are embedded in the tectorial membrane. The cupola is the correlate of the tectorial membrane, and the crista is the correlate of the hair cell.)

The horizontal canals sense movement related to head rotation, as in turning your head to signal "no," while the anterior canal senses movement in the vertical plane, as in nodding "yes." The posterior canal senses movement of the head toward the shoulders. The sensory element associated with movement depends on inertia. When you signal "no," your horizontal canal rotates with the movement, but the fluid within the canal lags the rotation by a little because of inertia. (Remember: A body at rest tends to stay at rest.) This lag actually provides the sensation that you perceive as the movement. As you rotate your head to the left, the fluid is moving relatively right with relation to the bone because of the lag. This relative movement causes deflection of the stereocilia of the crista ampularis, similar to deflection of the cilia on the hair cells in the cochlea. The left and right ears work together in this process to sense rotation in both directions. When you rotate your head to the right, the hair cells of the right crista ampularis in the horizontal canal are bent toward the kinocilium (the tallest hair cell), which opens ion channels to excite the cell. The hair cells in the left ear horizontal canal also move, but they move away from the kinocilium, hyperpolarizing the cell. In this way, activation for rotation to the left leaves the right side inhibited. You'll see this same excitation-inhibition pattern for the anterior and posterior canals. The information processed by the vestibular system is really information about change, which is specifically acceleration. The vestibular mechanism can sense very small accelerations of the head, on the order of 2 degrees per second (3 cm/sec) (Yu, Dickman, & Angelaki, 2012), but can also sense hundreds of degrees per second as well. Information about acceleration sensed by the semicircular canals is transmitted by the VIII vestibulocochlear nerve to the vestibular nuclei of the brain stem.

The otolithic organs of the utricle and saccule are sensitive to linear acceleration instead of rotational acceleration. The utricle is parallel to the horizontal canal, while the saccule is in a plane vertical to the head. The utricle and macula have hair cells supported by a macula. Like the crista ampularis, the macula have hair cells, cilia, and a kinocilium. Cilia of the utricle and saccule are embedded in a gelatinous otolithic membrane, and superficial to the membrane is a layer of otoconia. You can think of the otoconia as a gravel bed atop a gelatinous substance in which the cilia are embedded. The otoconia provide mass loading to the sensory system, again giving an inertial component that translates into an acceleration sensor. Information from the utricle and saccule combine to map any linear acceleration of the head. Utricle afferents are used to control ocular movements relative to acceleration and head position, while saccular afferents aid posture control.

You may realize that the visual and vestibular systems interact very intensely to help you maintain knowledge of your position in space. A mismatch of information can cause nausea, as in when your visual system signals movement but your vestibular system doesn't (motion sickness). Vertigo is the perception of spinning, which is translated as dizziness. Labyrinthitis is an infection of the inner ear and can cause vertigo and hearing loss. There are other causes of vertigo, such as benign paroxysmal positional vertigo (BPPV), which is sudden perception of spinning, typically upon moving the head (Labuguen, 2006). Meniere's disease (endolymphatic hydrops) is inflammation of the endolymphatic space (Minor, Schessel, & Carey, 2004), typically resulting in vertigo and sensorineural hearing loss.

Auditory Mechanism: Mechanical Events

ANAQUEST LESSON

One simply must be awed by the cochlea. This structure would neatly fit on the eraser of a pencil, and the fluid within it would be but a drop on your tabletop. The structures are astoundingly small and delicate, and yet this mechanism, given some reasonable care, can serve a lifetime of hearing without appreciable degeneration. Admittedly, the high-impact noise of modern society takes a rapid toll on such a delicate mechanism, but that is another story. Let us examine what is arguably the most amazing sensory system of the human body, the cochlea.

As we mentioned in the introduction to this chapter, the inner ear is responsible for performing spectral and temporal acoustic analyses of the

---

Clinical Manipulation of the Vestibular Mechanism

Audiologists, as you know, are involved in working with assessment and treatment of disorders of the auditory mechanism. Among those disorders are *vestibular disorders*—disorders that cause a sense of vertigo (perception of spinning or rotation) or dizziness (lightheadedness), loss of balance, and visual disturbances arising from difficulty in integrating body sense with the visual input. Benign paroxysmal positional vertigo (BPPV) is quite common, providing the patient with a spinning perception (vertigo) that occurs suddenly (paroxysmal), relative to body position (Bhattacharyya et al., 2017). The "benign" part is good news, because that means it is not associated with a degenerative or organic disease condition. Nystagmus (ratcheting oscillation of the eyes) typically occurs, resulting from the brain's perception that it needs to adjust to head movement (which is perceived, but not real). It is thought that BBPV arises because the calcium carbonate crystals of the otoliths in the semicircular canals drop into the ampulla of the posterior semicircular canal. This is where the audiologist (and physical therapist) come in.

Audiologists and physical therapists will often team up to perform the Epley maneuver. In this treatment, the client is placed in a series of positions that cause the crystals to move out of the ampulla and into the vestibule, where they no longer cause vestibular mischief. This maneuver is highly successful in alleviating the dizziness, vertigo, and cognitive distress that comes with BBPV, and all of this without requiring surgery!

incoming acoustical signal. By **spectral analysis**, we refer to the process of extracting or defining the various frequency components of a given signal. Recall from our discussion in Chapter 5 that frequency and intensity of vibration define the psychological correlates of pitch and loudness. The cochlea is specifically designed to sort out the frequency components of an incoming signal, determine their amplitude, and even identify basic temporal aspects of that signal. These processes make up the first level of auditory processing of an acoustic signal. Subsequent processing occurs as the signal works its way rapidly along the auditory pathway, ultimately to the brain. To get a notion of how this happens, we need to consider the input to the cochlea.

As you remember, sound is a disturbance in air. The airborne disturbance causes the TM to move, and that movement is translated to the oval window. When the TM moves inward, the stapes footplate in the oval window also moves in; and when the TM moves out, so does the footplate. This movement is a direct analog to the compressions and rarefactions of sound, so that, for the most part, the complexities of sound are directly translated to the cochlear fluid medial to the stapes footplate.

When the stapes compresses the perilymph of the scala vestibuli, Reissner's membrane is distended toward the scala media, and the basilar membrane is distended toward the scala tympani. That is, a compression in the fluid of the scala vestibuli is translated directly to the basilar membrane. Remember that the frequency of a sound is determined by the number of oscillations or vibrations per second. In this case, it is the number of oscillations of the TM-ossicle-footplate combination: A 100 Hz signal results in the footplate moving inward and outward 100 times per second, and that periodic vibration is translated to the basilar membrane, where it initiates a wave action known as the **traveling wave**.

Georg von Békésy discovered that the basilar membrane is particularly well designed to support wave action that directly corresponds to the frequency of vibration of the input sound. Specifically, when high-frequency sounds impinge on the inner ear, they cause vibration of the basilar membrane closer to the vestibule, the basal end of the cochlea. Low-frequency sounds result in a long traveling wave that reaches toward the apex, covering a greater distance along the basilar membrane. In this way, the traveling wave separates out the frequency components of complex sounds, because high-frequency sounds are processed in basal regions, whereas low-frequency sounds are processed nearer the apex. When a sound has both high- and low-frequency components, those components are separated out and processed at their respective portions of the basilar membrane.

If you have experienced an ocean beach, you will be familiar with wave action. Waves roll in from the ocean and swell to a large amplitude as they break on the beach. Although the analogy is not perfect, it may help you to recognize the driving force behind differentiating frequency components: The point of maximum amplitude excursion of the traveling wave on the basilar membrane is the primary point of neural excitation of the hair cells within the organ of Corti. Said another way, the traveling wave moves along the basilar membrane, growing and swelling as it travels, until it reaches a point of maximum growth. The wave very quickly damps down after that point, so there is only one truly *strong* point of disturbance from the traveling wave. In this manner, the low-frequency sound discussed earlier causes the traveling wave to "break" closer to the apex, and that place of maximum disturbance determines the frequency information that is transmitted to the brain.

Our understanding of the mechanism that determines *where* the point of maximum amplitude excursion occurs is another of von Békésy's legacies. He fashioned instruments from exotic materials such as pig bristles to measure the stiffness of the basilar membrane. As stiffness increases, the natural frequency of vibration of a body increases. (See the ANAQUEST software auditory physiology lessons to test the effects of stiffness on the traveling wave.) Von Békésy's (1960) pig bristle experiments revealed that the basal end of the basilar membrane is stiffer than the apical end, and that the stiffness decreases in a graded fashion from base to apex. (In fact, the cochlear duct is flaccid at its most apical end, where it is not connected to the bony labyrinth, to form the helicotrema.) In addition, we know that as mass of a structure increases, its resonant frequency decreases. The basilar membrane becomes increasingly massive, from base to apex. Finally, the basilar membrane becomes progressively wider from base to apex. These three components—graded stiffness, graded mass, graded width—combine to make the basilar membrane an excellent frequency analyzer. Verification of the importance of these resonance characteristics is provided by the fact that the traveling wave can be stimulated in the absence of the middle ear mechanism (as in bone conduction testing of an individual without middle ear ossicles). No matter how the traveling wave is initiated, it *always* travels from base to apex, because of the impedance gradient of the basilar membrane.

Excitation of the hair cells occurs as the result of several interacting variables. First, the cilia of the outer hair cells are embedded within the tectorial membrane (Figure 10–2). As the traveling wave moves along the basilar membrane, the hair cells are displaced relative to the tectorial membrane. This produces a **shearing action** that is, of course, greatest at the point of maximum perturbation of the basilar membrane.

ANAQUEST LESSON ▶

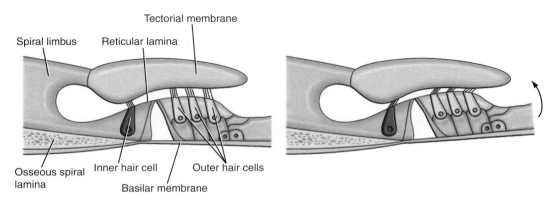

Figure 10–2. Schematic representation of shearing action of basilar membrane–tectorial membrane relationship. *Source:* From Seikel/Drumright/King. *Anatomy & Physiology for Speech, Language, and Hearing, 5th Ed.* ©Cengage, Inc. Reproduced by permission.

Tonndorf (1960) and later Møller (1973) and Dallos (1973) described another mechanism that helps to explain how the inner hair cells are excited. Recall that the inner hair cells are not embedded in the tectorial membrane, so they are not subjected to the same forces as the outer hair cells. Furthermore, their placement closer to the osseous spiral lamina gives them reduced opportunity to capitalize on shear. Rather, it appears that the inner hair cells depend on fluid movement of the endolymph to excite them. As the traveling wave moves along the basilar membrane, it effectively slides past the fluid molecules. Put another way, the fluid moves relative to the hair cell. The cilia are displaced by the fluid movement, just as grass in a riverbed is drawn by the fluid flow. If you invoke the Bernoulli principle studied in Chapter 5, you will see the final stage of excitation. At the point of maximum excursion, the basilar membrane is "humped" up, essentially protruding into the fluid stream. The Bernoulli principle states that at the constriction, velocity of fluid flow increases. This disturbance at the point of maximum excitation causes a turbulence, which produces eddies or swirls of fluid molecules. In this way, the fluid is more turbulent at the point of maximum excitation, meaning that the hair cells are more likely to be excited at that point than at other, less turbulent locations.

Stimulation of the hair cell presents a paradox, however. A hair cell is stimulated when the cilia are bent in a direction away from the modiolus, but the traveling wave produces a disturbance that is apically directed along the length of the basilar membrane, at right angles to the pattern that excites the hair cell. This dilemma is easy to resolve, however. Remember that the basilar membrane is anchored to the spiral lamina. When the traveling wave perturbs the basilar membrane, the shearing action on the cilia is produced in the medial-proximal dimension because of the hinge-like function of the lamina. Because of the nature of the traveling wave, the primary shear at the peak of the traveling wave is radial, as described, whereas the shear apical to the maximum of the wave is longitudinal, a direction that does not stimulate the hair cell (Figure 10–3).

Hair Cell Regeneration

Gene therapy is being developed to regenerate hair cells. We have known for several years that avian hair cells regenerate (Forge, Corwin, & Nevill, 1993), but researchers now identified a means for regenerating hair cells in mammals. Izumikawa et al. (2005) genetically modified a cold virus and injected it into guinea pigs, and have shown regeneration through gene therapy. Not only did new hair cells grow, but when the guinea pigs were tested using auditory brain stem responses, it was clear that the hair cells were working. The first clinical trial for hair cell regeneration in humans has been initiated by a research group at the University of Kansas Medical School. In 2013, Kraft, Hsu, Brough, and Staecker inserted Atoh1 genes into mice with cochleas that had been damaged using ototoxic drugs and found that their hearing improved 20 dB as a result of the therapy. The researchers have initiated a clinical trial on 45 humans with severe sensorineural hearing loss arising from ototoxic drugs. The research community is anxiously awaiting the results of this clinical trial. If the expanded trial proves successful it could mean return to hearing for more than 7 million people in the United States alone.

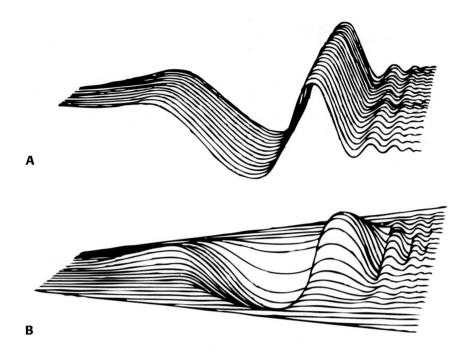

A

B

Figure 10–3. Traveling wave patterns. **A.** Pattern of oscillation in absence of lateral restraints. **B.** Pattern of vibration arising from stimulation but accounting for lateral attachment of basilar membrane. (Reproduced from Shearing Motion in Scala Media of Cochlear Models, by J. Tonndorf, 1960, *Journal of the Acoustical Society of America*, *32*(2), p. 241, with the permission of the Acoustical Society of America.)

The hinge-like arrangement of the basilar membrane and spiral limbus place the outer hair cells in a position to be activated by a lower-level stimulus than the inner hair cells. Thus, it appears that, at least for intensities less than 40 dB SPL, the outer hair cells are an important mechanism for coding intensity, although the inner hair cells are essential for frequency coding. Loss of outer hair cells does not result in complete loss of hearing, but rather elevation of the threshold of audition.

✓ To summarize:

- The inner ear is responsible for performing **spectral** (frequency) and **temporal acoustic analyses** of the incoming acoustical signal.

- Movement of the tympanic membrane is translated into an analogous movement of the stapes footplate and the fluid in the scala vestibuli.

- Compression of the fluid of the scala vestibuli is translated directly to the basilar membrane, and the disturbance at the basilar membrane initiates the **traveling wave**.

- The cochlea has a **tonotopic arrangement**, with high-frequency sounds resolved at the base and low-frequency sounds processed at the apex.

- The point of **maximum excursion** of the basilar membrane determines the frequency information transmitted to the brain.

- The traveling wave quickly **damps** after reaching its point of maximum excursion.

- The frequency analysis ability of the basilar membrane is determined by its graded **stiffness**, **thickness**, and **width**. The basilar membrane is stiffer, thinner, and narrower at the base than at the apex.

vascularis and recycled into the endolymph. In this manner, the K$^+$ rich environment of the endolymph is maintained (Spicer & Schulte, 1996). The ions move as a result of a cross-membrane ion gradient through the superficial stria vascularis and ion pumps for Na$^+$, Cl$^-$, and K$^+$. Enriching the endolymph with potassium is not a trivial matter, because the superficial cells of the stria vascularis have K$^+$ ion channels that allow osmotic movement into the endolymph. When mice are genetically engineered without the ability to move potassium via the superficial cells, they have a demonstrable hearing loss (Casimiro et al., 2001). It is precisely the establishment of the ion gradient between the intermediate cells of the stria vascularis and the endolymph that create the +80 mV potential difference that drives hearing function (Wangemann, 2006). The hair cell, in contrast, has a negative potential of –70 mV, which produces a powerful 150 mV differential between the endolymph and the hair cell.

Depolarizing the inner hair cells causes excitation of the VIII nerve as a result of glutamate release, while depolarizing the outer hair cells causes a motor response that actually moves the basilar membrane. The inner hair cells (IHC) transmit information about the site of excitation and the outer hair cells (OHC) amplify the signal by moving the basilar membrane at the site of activation, a phenomenon recorded by the audiologist as otoacoustic emissions (Musiek & Baran, 2006).

Resting Potentials

The **resting** or **standing potentials** are those voltage potential differences that can be measured from the cochlea at rest. Ions do not travel between the endolymphatic region (scala media) and those of the perilymph (scala tympani and scala vestibuli), and there are cochlear potential differences among those spaces. The scala vestibuli is slightly more positive than the scala tympani (about +5 mV), but the scala media is considerably more positive (about +80 mV). That is, the scala media has a constant positive potential (the **endocochlear potential**) relative to the scala tympani and scala vestibuli. The strong positive potential arises from passive osmosis and active ion pumping by the stria vascularis. Another resting potential, the **intracellular resting potential**, is found within the hair cells. The potential difference between the endolymph and the intercellular potential of the hair cell is –70 mV relative to the endolymph, giving a very large 150 mV difference between the hair cells and the surrounding fluid.

Potentials Arising from Stimulation

Stimulation of the hair cells results in the generation of a number of potentials, although not all of them are thought to be important in auditory processing. The **cochlear microphonic** was once thought to be the prime mover of cochlear activity, and for good reason. Wever and Bray (1930) found that the cochlear microphonic recorded from a living cat's cochlea directly followed the speech signal (Figure 10–4). It was felt that the poten-

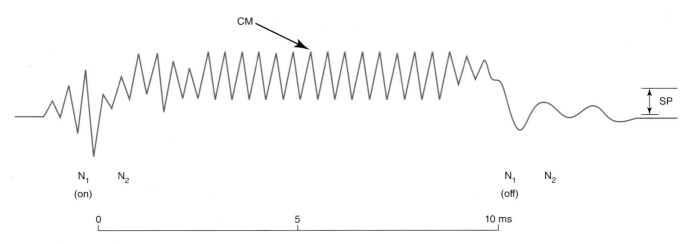

Figure 10–4. Response to tone burst, as measured from the scala tympani. Note that N1 and N2 are large negative components, marking signal onset and offset. SP refers to summating potential. CM refers to the cochlear microphonic.(Pickles, 2012, Figure 3.25.) *Source:* From Seikel/Drumright/King. *Anatomy & Physiology for Speech, Language, and Hearing, 5th Ed.* ©Cengage, Inc. Reproduced by permission.

tial was microphonic (like a microphone), directly responding to the input signal. The researchers were correct at first blush: The potential *does* directly follow the movement of the basilar membrane, and it appears to be generated by the outer hair cells or current changes at the reticular lamina in the vicinity of the outer hair cells. Although microelectrode recording of inner hair cell intracellular potentials shows an alternating current (AC) potential, the potential is not large enough to account for the microphonic. In any case, the cochlear microphonic is an AC potential that follows the movement of the input signal as it impinges upon the basilar membrane.

The **summating potential** is a sustained, direct current (DC) shift in the endocochlear potential that occurs upon stimulation of the organ of Corti by sound (see Figure 10–4). The inner hair cells are depolarized when stimulated by sound, and that results in reduced intracellular potential (a less negative potential). This potential difference between the hair cell and the endolymph may produce the summating potential. The summating potential is seen as a DC shift in electrical output that is maintained as long as an auditory stimulus is presented to the ear.

The **whole-nerve action potential** (also known as the **compound action potential**), abbreviated AP, arises directly from stimulation of a large number of hair cells simultaneously, eliciting nearly simultaneous individual action potentials in the VIII nerve, as discussed in Chapter 9. Measured extracochlearly, the whole-nerve action potential represents the sum of action potentials generated by stimulation of the hair cells. The whole-nerve action potential is best elicited using clicks with broad spectral content rather than tones, although tones certainly can be used. The AP has two major negative components, N1 (occurring around 1 ms poststimulus onset) and N2 (around 2 ms poststimulus onset), and the amplitude of the AP increases as the sound stimulus intensity increases (Musiek & Baran, 2006). The whole-nerve action potential is first detected at between 10 and 20 dB above a person's behavioral threshold (Eggermont & Odenthal, 1974), and this potential can be measured by means of the auditory brain stem response (ABR) or through ECoG. The individual action potential arising from stimulation of an individual VIII nerve fiber tells a very important story at the microscopic level. Looking at single-unit (single VIII nerve fiber) responses reveals that the cochlear mechanism has an extraordinarily fine ability to differentiate frequency components (frequency specificity), and by processing data from a large number of individual fibers we can learn a great deal about the coding of simple and complex stimuli by the auditory nervous system.

✅ *To summarize:*

- When the basilar membrane is displaced toward the scala vestibuli, the hair cells are activated, resulting in **electrical potentials**.

- **Resting** or **standing potentials** are those voltage potential differences that can be measured from the cochlea at rest.

- The scala vestibuli is 5 mV more positive than the scala tympani, but the scala media is 80 mV more positive.

- The **intracellular resting potential** within the hair cell reveals a potential difference between the endolymph and the hair cell of −70 mV, giving a 150 mV difference between the hair cells and the surrounding fluid.

- Stimulus-related potentials include the alternating current **cochlear microphonic** generated by the outer hair cells; the **summating potential**, a direct current shift in the endocochlear potential; and the **whole-nerve action potential**, arising directly from stimulation of a large number of hair cells simultaneously.

Neural Responses

There are two basic types of VIII nerve neurons: **low spontaneous rate** (high-threshold) and **high spontaneous rate** (low-threshold) fibers. High-threshold neurons require a higher level of stimulation to fire, respond to the higher end of our auditory range of signal intensity, and have little or no random background firing noise. Low-threshold fibers, in contrast, respond at very low signal intensities and display random firing even when no stimulus is present. Thus, it appears that the low-threshold neurons may be a mechanism for hearing sound at near-threshold levels, whereas high-threshold fibers may pick up where the low-threshold fibers stop, as the signal increases.

The background "chatter" of random firing poses some problems for examining neuron response, however. The task of neurophysiologists is to identify neuron responses related to a specific stimulus and to separate them from the background noise of random firing. Two basic techniques have evolved to manage that problem, and both have provided important clues to neural function. Let us look at these techniques and the results of their application.

Post-Stimulus Time Histograms

Histograms are a convenient method of looking at data that occur over time. When you are taking an anatomy exam, you know that the whole class does not finish at the same time. Rather, the first person may finish after 40 minutes, the next one at 43 minutes, then a couple more at 44 minutes, and so on. If you were interested in the *modal* finishing time for an exam, you could plot the elapsed test-taking time for each person in the form of a bar graph (**histogram**) and identify the point at which the greatest number of people left at the same time. You can also look at the response time of neurons the same way. Auditory physiologists record bursts of electrical activity of single neurons and plot their response. Because they know when the stimulus was presented (just as your instructor knows when the test started), the researcher can plot the responses relative to the onset of the stimulus—hence, post-stimulus time (PST) histogram.

Because neurons are all-or-none devices, every unit response is equal to the next in intensity and duration. Thus, the only way neurons can provide differential response is by having different rates of firing. Single-unit neural information is conveyed in the timing of its response. If you were to record the spike-rate activity of a neuron that is firing randomly, in the absence of a stimulus, there would be no real dominant mode of activity; rather, the neural response would be spread fairly evenly over the entire recording period. If you were to record that activity in response to a tonal stimulus, you would get a response more like that of Figure 10–5. When an VIII nerve fiber responds to tonal stimulation, there is an initial burst of strong activity, followed by a decline to a plateau of discharge over the duration of the tone. When the tone is terminated, the response of the fiber drops to below baseline levels, rising up to the baseline noise level after recovery.

This fairly straightforward PST histogram has provided us with very important verification of the **frequency specificity**, the ability of the cochlea to differentiate different spectral components of a signal. Figure 10–5 displays a hypothetical array of spike rate PST histograms generated for the same

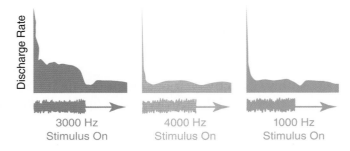

Figure 10–5. Schematic representation of post-stimulus time histogram for 3000 Hz, 4000 Hz, and 1000 Hz tones, as recorded from a nerve fiber with a characteristic frequency of 3000 Hz. *Source:* From Seikel/Drumright/King. *Anatomy & Physiology for Speech, Language, and Hearing, 5th Ed.* ©Cengage, Inc. Reproduced by permission.

neuron under different stimulus conditions. In this case, we have placed an electrode on a fiber serving the area of the cochlea in which 3000 Hz signals are processed. Look at the responses. When we deliver a 3000 Hz signal, the fiber has a strong response shortly after onset, with the characteristic plateau until the tone ends. Now see what happens when we present a 4000 Hz signal. The response is *much* weaker to that stimulation than it is to the 1000 Hz signal. As you know from the traveling wave theory, signals above 3000 Hz will not cause much disturbance on the basilar membrane at the 3000 Hz point. Likewise, the traveling wave must necessarily pass through the region of our electrode on its way to the 1000 Hz point (toward the apex, or low-frequency region), but the traveling wave has not gained much amplitude at that point so there is not much excitation. In other words, if we record the firing rate of a neuron, we can get a fair estimate of its **characteristic** or **best frequency**. The characteristic frequency (CF) of a neuron is the frequency to which it responds best. In the case shown in Figure 10–5, the CF of the neuron we were recording was 3000 Hz.

One goal of auditory physiology is to explain humans' extraordinary ability to discriminate signals in the frequency domain. Researchers who study auditory perceptual abilities as they relate to the physical mechanism (**psychoacousticians**) have found that, in general, humans can discriminate change in frequency of signals of about 1%. (Recognize that this gross generalization ignores differences in signal intensity, variations based on different stimulus frequency, signal duration, etc.) That is, if a 100 Hz tone is presented, you can hear the difference between it and a 101 Hz tone, an increase of 1%. The challenge to physiologists was to identify how the cochlea could produce such fine discriminations.

Figure 10–6 shows a tuning curve for a single-unit recording. A tuning curve is basically a composite of the responses of a single fiber at each frequency of presentation. To create a tuning curve, researchers placed an electrode on a neuron and presented different frequencies of stimulation. They then recorded the stimulus intensity at which the neuron began to fire in response to the stimulus (its threshold) and plotted that intensity. In Figure 10–6, you can see that the fiber was most sensitive to the 10,000 Hz signal. As the signal frequency decreased to 8000 Hz, the signal had to be of greater intensity to cause the neuron to fire. The signal at 5000 Hz had to be 60 dB stronger than that at the CF for that neuron, 10,000 Hz.

This tuning curve is a measure of neural specificity in one sense, but probably as much a measure of basilar membrane response. The electrode is, in effect, measuring the activity at one point on the basilar membrane (10,000 Hz, near the base), and the activity farther up the cochlea toward the apex has less and less effect on the neuron being recorded. The sharper the tuning curve, the greater the frequency specificity of the basilar membrane. Indeed, when Khanna and Leonard (1982) compared the tuning curves of the basilar membrane and the auditory nerve, they found that the two curves were quite similar. That is, the basilar membrane is a very finely tuned filter capable of fine differentiation.

sufficiently sharp, it will represent a great deal of selectivity on the basilar membrane. Think of a tuning curve as a very sharp pencil making a very thin line. That sharp, precise line is necessary for humans to be able to perceive minute differences between tones. Remember that we can perceive something in the order of a 1% change in frequency (i.e., we can hear the difference between 1000 Hz and 1010 Hz). The precision of the basilar membrane in frequency selectivity is reflected in the sharpness of the tuning curve.

Perception is actually a logarithm-based phenomenon: We can hear a 1 Hz difference at 100 Hz (1%) or a 10 Hz difference at 1000 Hz (1%) or a 100 Hz difference at 10,000 Hz (also 1%). The differential perception is a constant, but the number of cycles per second (Hz) has increased exponentially up the scale. Take a look at Figure 10–10 for the following discussion.

The top left portion of Figure 10–10 shows a tuning curve of an VIII nerve fiber from an area of the basilar membrane that is centered at 11,000 Hz. Next to it is a tuning curve that is centered at 1,100 Hz. The 11,000 Hz plot *looks* sharper than the bottom-right image. think? Looking at them you would hypothesize that the 11,000 Hz plot has greater specificity. To actually compare these two, however, we must calculate a value known as Q_{10}, which is the ratio of the center frequency divided by the bandwidth Q_{10} = cf/bw$_{10db}$. Basically, we measure up 10 dB from the tip and identify how wide the tuning curve is (bandwidth, in Hz). Then, we divide the bandwidth by the center frequency, in Hz. A higher number indicates sharper tuning. Now look at the derivation of Q_{10} for these same plots.

Calculation for the Q_{10} for the 11,000 Hz fiber is as follows:

Q_{10} = cf/bw

Q_{10} = 10,500/500

Q_{10} = 21

Calculation of Q_{10} for the 1100 Hz fiber is as follows:

Q_{10} = cf/bw

Q_{10} = 1100/20

Q_{10} = 55

Clearly, the lower-frequency fiber is sharper than the higher-frequency fiber, when you compare its precision using the Q_{10}. There is critical benefit to performing this "normalizing" process when examining tuning curves of fibers or the basilar membrane. Q_{10} allows us to put all tuning curves on common footing and to compare their sharpness relative to their response region.

⊘ To summarize:

- There are two basic types of VIII nerve neurons, and specific techniques have been developed for assessing their function.

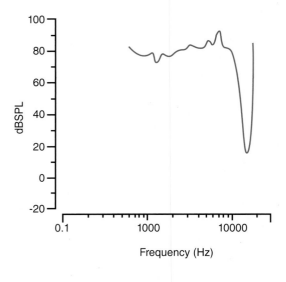

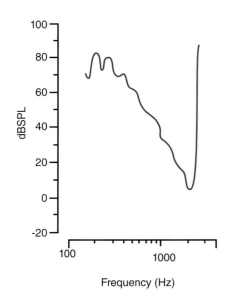

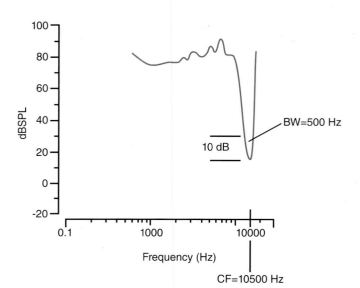

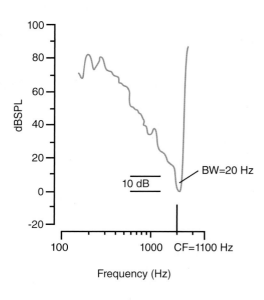

Figure 10–10. Plot of tuning curves from two different VIII nerve fibers, representing characteristic frequencies of 10,500 Hz (*top left*) and 1000 Hz (*top right*). Note that the tuning curve on the left looks sharper. Calculation of Q_{10} (*lower plots*) reveals that the low-frequency fiber is, in reality, markedly more specific (sharper) than the high-frequency fiber, as indicated by the greater Q_{10} value. (Derived from data of Acoustic Trauma in Cats, by M. C. Lieberman and N. Y. Kiang, 1978. *Otolaryngica. Supplementum, 358*, pp. 1–63. Copyright © Acta Oto-Laryngologica AB (Ltd), reprinted by permission of Informa UK Limited, trading as Taylor & Francis Group, http://www.tandfonline.com on behalf of Acta Oto-Laryngologica AB (Ltd).) *Source:* From Seikel/Drumright/King. *Anatomy & Physiology for Speech, Language, and Hearing, 5th Ed.* ©Cengage, Inc. Reproduced by permission.

- **High-threshold neurons** require a higher intensity and encompass the higher end of our auditory range of signal intensity.

- **Low-threshold fibers** respond at very low signal levels and display random firing even when no stimulus is present.

- **Low-threshold neurons** may process near-threshold sounds, whereas high-threshold fibers process higher-level sounds.

- **Frequency specificity** is the ability of the cochlea to differentiate the spectral components of a signal. It is reflected in the sharpness of the tuning curve. Humans can perceive a change in frequency of approximately 1%.

- **Poststimulus time histograms** are plots of neural response relative to the onset of a stimulus.

- The **characteristic** or **best frequency** of a neuron is the frequency to which it responds best.

- A **tuning curve** is a composite of the responses of a single fiber at each frequency of presentation.

- Q_{10} is a derived ratio that allows comparison of the sharpness of tuning curves all along the basilar membrane. Higher numbers for Q_{10} indicate sharper tuning curves.

- The sharper the tuning curve, the greater the frequency specificity of the basilar membrane.

- The **tonotopic array** of the cochlea is clearly relayed to the auditory nervous system in the form of individual nerve fiber activation.

- As the intensity of stimulation increases, **rate of firing** increases.

- When the **crossed-olivocochlear** and **uncrossed-olivocochlear bundles** are stimulated, the firing rate of neurons innervated by them is reduced dramatically.

- **Interspike interval histograms** record the interval between successive firings of a neuron, revealing phase-locking of neurons to stimulus period.

Auditory Pathway Responses

The cochlea and VIII nerve represent only the first stage of information extraction of an auditory signal. Temporal and tonotopically arrayed information is passed to progressively higher centers for further extraction of information (Figure 10–11).

Cochlear Nucleus

At the first way station in the auditory pathway, the cochlear nucleus (CN), tonotopic representation is readily observable in tuning curves. There is evidence that significant signal processing occurs at this level of the brain stem.

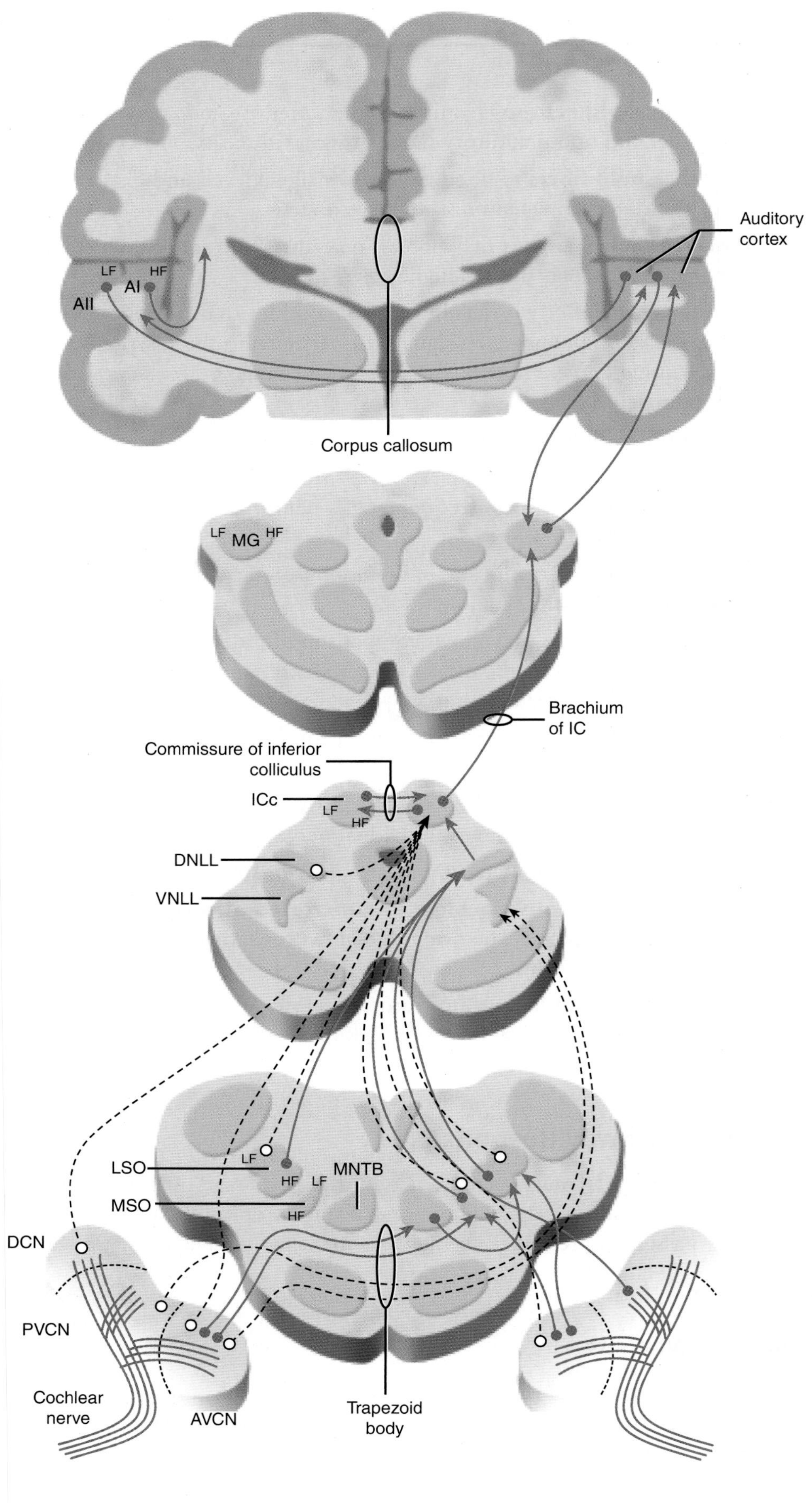

Figure 10–11. Schematic representation of auditory pathway in humans. (After Møller, 2003.) Note: DCN = dorsal cochlear nucleus; DNLL = dorsal nucleus of lateral lemniscus; VNLL = ventral nucleus of lateral lemniscus; MNTB = medial nucleus of trapezoid body; CN = cochlear nucleus; AVCN = anteroventral cochlear nucleus; ICC= Central nucleus of inferior colliculus; PVCN = postero-ventral cochlear nucleus; LSO = lateral superior olive; and MSO = medial superior olive;; AI = core; AII = auditory higher order processing areas; LF = low frequency; HF = high frequency; MG = medial geniculate body; IC = inferior colliculus. *Source:* From Seikel/Drumright/King. *Anatomy & Physiology for Speech, Language, and Hearing, 5th Ed.* ©Cengage, Inc. Reproduced by permission.

Pfeiffer (1966) demonstrated at least six different neural responses to auditory stimulation, in contrast to the single-unit response seen at the VIII nerve level (Figure 10–12). **Primary-like responses** are the firing patterns that most resemble VIII nerve responses. These responses appear to arise from bushy cells in the CN and will have identical rate functions, intensity responses, spontaneous activity, and Q_{10} values as the VIII nerve fibers they reflect. Some neurons exhibit **onset responses**, in which there is an initial response to onset of a stimulus, followed by silence. These responses will have a sharp peak at the onset of a stimulus, and then simply stop firing. They are found throughout the CN and appear to arise from octopus cells. They have a smaller Q_{10} than other responses in the cochlear nucleus (wider tuning curves), and this may represent some sort of summative function. Remember, a wider tuning curve reflects *less* specificity, and in this case that could mean that the fiber being measured is responding to multiple areas of the basilar membrane. **Chopper responses** do not seem to be related to stimulus frequency, but appear to have a periodic, chopped temporal pattern as long as a tone is present. Chopper response is marked by repeated firing when stimulated by a tone. These responses are strongest in the posteroventral cochlear nucleus (PVCN) and dorsal cochlear nucleus (DCN), although

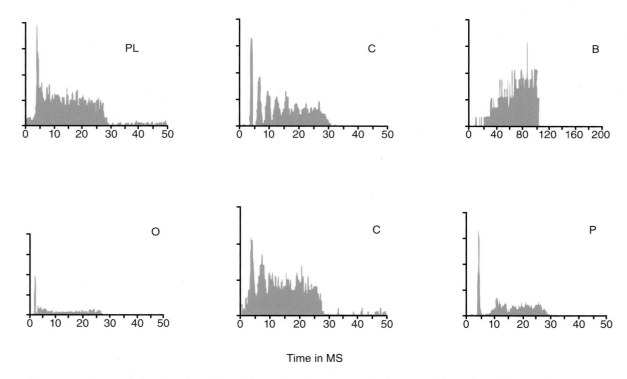

Figure 10–12. Peristimulus time histograms showing response characteristics of cochlear nucleus. Note: PL = primary-like; C = chopper type; B = buildup type; O = onset type; P = pauser type. (Reproduced from The Use of Intracellular Techniques in the Study of the Cochlear Nucleus, by W. S. Rhode, 1985, by *Journal of the Acoustic Society of America*, 78(1), p. 321, with the permission of the Acoustical Society of America.) *Source:* From Seikel/Drumright/King. *Anatomy & Physiology for Speech, Language, and Hearing, 5th Ed.* ©Cengage, Inc. Reproduced by permission.

they can be found throughout the CN. They do not seem to be related to any particular cell type, and their firing rate is not really related to the period of the stimulus. These chopper cells appear to most likely have numerous inputs and simply move through a fire–shutdown–fire cycle as long as they are stimulated. **Pausers**, found in the dorsal cochlear nucleus, take a little longer to respond than other neurons: If the signal is of higher intensity, the pauser has an initial *on*-response, is quiet, and then responds with a low-level firing rate throughout stimulation. Pausers are found mostly in the DCN and appear to arise from fusiform cells. They respond to complex stimuli and most likely represent some form of processing of complex acoustic features. **Buildup** neurons slowly increase their firing rate through the initial stages of firing.

These complex responses reflect not only different cell types within the CN, but also interactions among neurons. Although all these responses may be seen in different neurons in response to the same tonal stimulus, it would be unwise to assume that they are *simply* responses to stimulation. They are most certainly the result of complex interaction and neural processing.

Complex Interaction Within the Cochlear Nucleus

The basic neuron response types that we have just discussed have another layer of complexity we should mention. There are at least four basic types of inhibition found within the CN, which is absent in the VIII nerve that feeds it (remember that the VIII nerve does not have inhibition).

In Type II and III inhibitory patterns, one sees a rather standard tuning curve configuration in response to stimulation, but there are also inhibitory sidebands above and below the characteristic frequency. Response to a signal presented at CF is greatly sharpened if there is stimulation in the sideband, apparently by damping the off-frequency information. These fibers typically do not have spontaneous activity, so they are strictly stimulus bound.

Type IV and V fibers are almost completely inhibitory, arising from the DCN. That is, if they receive stimulation, they terminate output. Generally, there is less inhibition in the anteroventral cochlear nucleus (AVCN), and the most inhibition is found in the DCN. Indeed, it appears that fibers in the AVCN inhibit responses from the DCN. The AVCN and PVCN provide an exact, unadulterated copy of the VIII nerve response to the olivary complex for the purpose of localization of sound in space, and it appears that the DCN is responsible for performing complex acoustic analysis and forwarding that information to higher brain stem and cortical centers.

There are some other atypical responses found at the level of the CN. Pausers and buildup neurons show a specifically different response to signals that sweep up in frequency versus those sweeping down. That is, frequency modulation is a specific feature detected by these neurons: Some will be highly specific to up-sweep and blind to down-sweep, while others are specific to down-sweep and do not respond to up-sweep. This response corresponds quite well to characteristics found in the speech signal in transitions from consonants to vowels.

Similarly, some neurons are responsive to minute changes in intensity (as in pulsing intensity), producing very large responses to small changes. Møller (2003) posited that this sensitivity to pulsatile changes reflects a means of identifying the envelope of a signal, which is critical for the identification of syllable boundaries.

Superior Olivary Complex

The superior olivary complex (SOC) is the first site of binaural interaction, receiving information from the cochlear nuclei of both ears, and is specialized for localization of sound in space. There are three outputs from the CN, and two of these pathways go to the olivary complex. The dorsal stria arises from the DCN and bypasses the olivary complex. The ventral stria is made up of responses from the AVCN and PVCN, and the intermediate stria arises from the PVCN, and both of these are shunted directly to the olivary complex.

The lateral superior olive (LSO) receives high-frequency information from the ipsilateral cochlear nucleus, and the medial superior olive (MSO) receives low-frequency information. When the LSO is provided with ipsilateral (same side) stimulation, the response is entirely excitatory. The tuning curves look like VIII nerve fibers, with thresholds in the 10 to 20 dB SPL range. When the neurons are stimulated by contralateral (other side) signals, the response is entirely inhibitory, and these fibers are referred to as E–I (excitatory–inhibitory). In this way, the LSO responds to differences in intensity between the two ears. A difference in intensity between the two ears is heard when one sound has to pass around the head to reach the other ear. When the signals are high in frequency (above about 1500 Hz), there is a "head shadow" because the wavelength is too short to effectively bend around the head. The result is that a signal presented to the left ear will be louder than that presented to the right ear, and your LSO will process that difference as "location in space."

Echolocation

Animal sonar systems have been examined extensively for more than 40 years, including those in dolphins, whales, and bats. More than 800 species of bats have evolved a means of producing high-frequency (as high as 120 kHz) sounds that bounce off of objects. The reflected sound is received as an auditory echo that is processed by the superior olivary complex (SOC) to determine the spatial location of the object from which the echo was derived. When bats are flying toward an object that is getting closer, the frequency of the reflected sound shifts up (Doppler shift), resulting in a higher-frequency signal being received. This tells the bat that the object of its affection (perhaps a moth) is getting closer and may be available soon for a snack. If the object is moving away from the bat at a faster speed than the bat is flying, the frequency shifts down. Of course, moths and other insects have developed countermeasures. Moths that are preyed upon by bats have developed auditory neurons specifically tuned to the frequency of the bat's sonar, so that when they are "pinged" by a bat's echolocation system they go into a free fall that foils the bat's predictions. Other moths flutter their wings chaotically or fly upward in a spiral to defeat the sonar.

In sharp contrast to the LSO, the medial superior olive (MSO) receives input from the AVCN for both ears. It is worth remembering that the MSO receives a very clean copy of the auditory signal from the AVCN, and that copy arrives quickly because there are not any way stations between the CN and the MSO. The MSO responds to low-frequency sounds (below about 1500 Hz), being particularly tuned to timing differences in the waveforms presented to each ear. A difference in timing at low frequencies results in a phase difference between signals from the two ears. Essentially, the cells of the MSO are sensitive to the interaural delay time, which is the time difference between the two ears. That time lag is mapped by the MSO as location in space and allows us to localize sounds quite accurately. In fact, the cells of the MSO have a characteristic delay, similar to the characteristic frequency seen in other cells. This means that each cell is tuned to a specific time delay between the two ears. Most of the cells of the MSO are excited by signals from either ear (E–E, excitatory–excitatory). All cells of the MSO are binaural in nature, meaning they respond to sound from either ear. Therefore, it can be seen that two basic responses occur within the SOC. **Contralateral stimulation** (stimulation of the ear opposite the side of the SOC being studied) by high-frequency information results in excitation of the **lateral superior olive** (LSO, or S-segment) that is directly related to stimulus intensity. These so-called **E–E** (excitatory–excitatory) responses provide a means of comparing the intensity of a signal on one side of the head with that on the other side. In the MSO, when low-frequency tones are presented, an **E–I** (excitatory–inhibitory) response occurs, in which contralateral input excites neurons and **ipsilateral stimulation** causes inhibition of neurons. Said another way, a low-frequency signal arriving at the left ear causes excitation of the right-side MSO, while inhibiting the left-side MSO. In addition, some cells in the MSO respond to a **characteristic delay** in arrival time, so that the MSO detects minute changes in arrival time of a sound between the two ears. This **interaural phase (time) difference** is the primary mechanism for localization of low-frequency sounds in space; the **interaural intensity** difference is the primary means of localization of high-frequency sound in space. The neurons responding to specific characteristics or features of the stimulus are termed **feature detectors**. That is, they respond to specific features of the stimulus (e.g., interaural phase differences), extract that information from the signal, and convey the results of analysis to the cerebral cortex. In this way the complex acoustic signal can be broken into some subset of characteristics. Indeed, the different responses at the CN (e.g., pauser and onset-response) most likely represent the second level of feature extraction, the first level being at the cochlea.

Inferior Colliculus

The inferior colliculus (IC) receives bilateral innervation from the LSO, as well as indirect input from the CN via the lateral lemniscus. A wide range of responses is apparent at the IC, including those of neurons with sharp frequency tuning curves, inhibitory responses, onset and pauser responses, and intensity-sensitive units. Some neurons are sensitive to interaural time and intensity differences, apparently used for a localization function similar to the SOC. It appears that the IC may be the site at which frequency information from the CN discarded through localization processing at the SOC can be recombined with phase and intensity information.

Responses within the IC are wide-ranging. Cells of the IC have characteristic frequencies with tuning curves, but the range of sharpness (Q_{10}) of the tuning curves is dramatic, being between 25 and 40, among the best in the auditory nervous system. There are also broad tuning curves with very wide bandwidths.

Rate responses are also widely varied in the IC. About half of the cells of the IC show a monotonic rate-intensity response, which means that as intensity increases, rate increases in proportion. The other half are nonmonotonic, which is to say that the response is not a linear function of the stimulus. In fact, as intensity increases many of the neurons change from primary-type responses to pauser responses, and even to onset responses, ultimately ending in chopper responses. Some of these neurons are also highly responsive to signals sweeping either up in frequency or down in frequency (but not both), similar to those signals found in the frequency transitions of speech. Neurons of the IC are generally responsive to contralateral stimulation and appear to map auditory information based on interaural timing difference, similar to the MSO, but there are also neurons sensitive to intensity differences, similar to the LSO. This pattern implicates the MSO strongly as a mechanism for localization, but it also serves as an area of intersensory interaction.

Medial Geniculate Body

The medial geniculate body (MGB) is a relay point to the thalamus, the final sensory way station of the brain stem. The ventral portion of the MGB projects information directly to the primary auditory reception area of the temporal lobe, the medial portion projects to other regions of the temporal lobe, and the dorsal portion projects information to association regions of the cerebrum. Although a distinct tonotopic arrangement is apparent even at this level, a complex interaction of response types is also apparent. Surprisingly, these include neurons responsive to minute interaural intensity differences, much like the SOC and IC.

The MGB shows sharp tuning curves similar to those of the VIII nerve fibers. Responses of the MGB neurons include onset responses, as well as sustained excitatory responses. Most neurons within the MGB respond to stimuli from both ears and have nonmonotonic rate-intensity functions. Some of the neurons of the MGB respond to intensity differences much as the LSO does, and, in fact, some neurons are so sensitive to interaural intensity difference that they reach 80% of their response rate with as little as 2 dB difference between the ears.

Cerebral Cortex

The cerebral cortex receives input primarily from the contralateral ear via the ipsilateral MGB. A full tonotopic map is found at the primary reception area of the temporal lobe, Heschl's gyrus. In addition, the auditory reception area is organized in columns, with each column having similar CFs, but different tuning curve widths. Furthermore, different neurons within the columns respond to different stimulus parameters, such as frequency up-glides, down-glides, intensity up-glides and intensity down-glides, and so on. It is clear that the neurons of the cerebral cortex use the ipsilateral and contralateral temporal and spectral information extracted at earlier processing stages for identification of the features of speech. For example, neurons that are sensitive to frequency up-glides would be very useful in encoding information concerning formant frequency transitions, whereas the vocal fundamental frequency would be readily coded from the temporal information arising from the phase-locking at the cochlear level and presented, intact, to the cortex.

The brain stem is clearly responsible for initial coding of the neural signal representing the auditory stimulus, but there remain significant challenges to understanding the true mechanism involved in that coding. Work by Gollisch and Meister (2008) with the visual system revealed that the initial spike latencies of the retinal ganglion cells provided very clear spatial coding, despite the rapidly changing nature of the visual system as a result of saccadic eye movements. This unexpected coding mechanism from bipolar cells, in a system that has the benefit of longer sensory memory (i.e., afterimage), may provide a fruitful research path for the auditory system.

While quite complex and daunting, the auditory pathway is simple when compared with the cerebral cortex. Take a look at Figures 10–13 and 10–14. Figure 10–13A is an elaborated illustration of the auditory pathway from Kaas and Hackett (2000), taking into consideration the known direct pathways for audition (we have not mentioned the indirect pathways yet). The area to focus on in this diagram is the top four or so layers. The lower areas, from the cochlea up through the thalamus, are quite familiar to you by now. The representation of Heschl's gyrus may be new to you, so let us discuss that a bit before we talk about physiology.

Typically, we state that Heschl's gyrus is located in the superior aspect of the temporal lobe, at the sylvian fissure. Brodmann (Brodmann & Garey, 2007) actually described the superior temporal gyrus (STG) as consisting of four distinct regions, based on cell type: areas 22 (most of the lateral surface of the STG), 41 (typically considered to be Heschl's gyrus), 42 (lateral to Heschl's gyrus, being a higher processing region), and 52 (on the medial, and, typically, hidden surface of the STG). If one pulls out the temporal lobe and rotates it out a bit, areas 41, 42, and 52 are revealed in more detail. With the medial surface of the temporal lobe revealed, you would see the planum temporale, which is posterior to Heschl's gyrus. The planum polare (also known as the temporal pole) is anterior to Heschl's gyrus.

Kaas and Hackett (2000) have laid to rest the notion that the auditory cortex consists of a simple receptive zone and an adjacent higher-order processing area. Instead, the auditory cortex is seen as consisting of a medially placed core, a more distal belt, and a surrounding parabelt (see Figure 10–13). A great deal of research has elaborated its function in primates, and some research has elucidated its function in humans. First, look at the elaboration

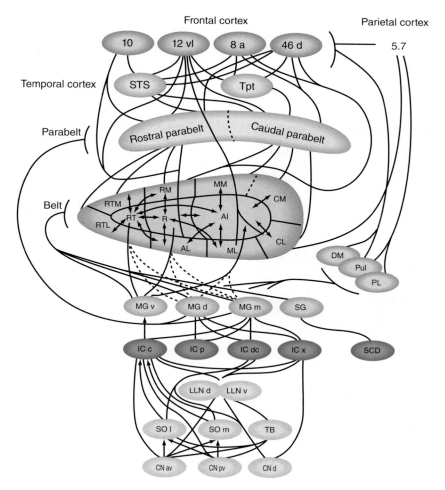

A

Figure 10–13. A. Primate auditory pathway, based upon physiological studies (Kaas & Hackett, 2000). *Note:* CNav = Cochlear nucleus, anterioventral; CNpv = postero-ventral cochlear nucleus; CNd = dorsal cochlear nucleus; Sol = lateral superior olive; SOm = medial superior olive; TB = trapezoid body; LLNd = dorsal nucleus of lateral lemniscus; LLv = ventral nucleus of lateral lemniscus; ICc = Central nucleus of inferior colliculus; ICp = pericentral nucleus of inferior colliculus; ICx = external nucleus of inferior colliculus; MGv = ventral medial geniculate body (thalamus); MGd = dorsal medial geniculate body (thalamus); MGm = magnocellular nucleus of medial geniculate body; Sg = suprageniculate nucleus of medial thalamus; DM = dorsome-dial nucleus of thalamus; Pul = Pulvinar; PL = posterolateral nucleus of thalamus; AI = auditory core of cortex; R = Rostral portion of core, cortex; RT = rostrotemporal aspect of core; CL = caudolateral area of belt, cortex; CM = caudomedial area of belt, cortex; ML = middle lateral area of belt, cortex; MM = middle medial area of belt, cortex; RM = rostromedial area of belt, cortex; AL = anterolateral area of belt, cortex; RTL = rostrotemporal area of belt, cortex; RTM = rostrotemporal area of belt, cortex; CPB = caudal parabelt; R = rostral parabelt; Tpt = temporoparietal area of temporal lobe; STS = superior temporal sulcus of temporal lobe; STS = superior temporal sulcus, temporal lobe; 8 = Brodmann area 8a (frontal eye field); 46 = Brodmann area 46d (working memory area); 12vl = Brodmann area 12, prefrontal cortex; 10 = Brodmann area 10, frontal pole. *Source:* From Seikel/Drumright/King. *Anatomy & Physiology for Speech, Language, and Hearing, 5th Ed.* ©Cengage, Inc. Reproduced by permission. *continues*

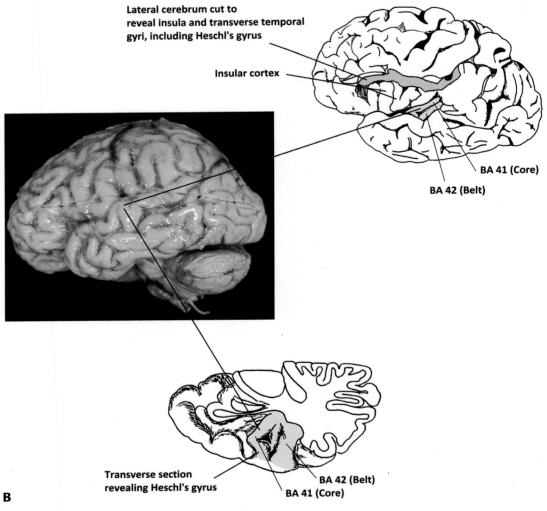

Lateral cerebrum cut to
reveal insula and transverse temporal
gyri, including Heschl's gyrus

Insular cortex

BA 41 (Core)

BA 42 (Belt)

Transverse section
revealing Heschl's gyrus

BA 42 (Belt)

BA 41 (Core)

B

Figure 10–13. *continued* **B.** Elaboration of auditory reception area as core, belt, and parabelt.
continues

of the receptive region (see Figures 10–13B and C). This receptive region consists of the core, belt, and parabelt.

Core

The core in Figure 10–13A represented by areas AI, R, and RT, and makes up most of Heschl's gyrus in humans. The classical notion of auditory reception is represented by AI. The tonotopic relationship that we have been observing throughout the auditory pathway is retained. Low frequency processed on AI is in the distal or rostral end of the area, while high frequencies are processed more medially (closer to Wernicke's area). To the left of AI is the rostral portion of the core (R): The tonotopic array is reversed for this portion of the core, so that the high frequencies are processed closer to the temporal pole (anterior aspect). Finally, the rostro-temporal (RT) portion of the core appears to have the tonotopic relationship seen in AI. Essentially then, auditory information arises at this core region in one or more of these three locations. All three of them appear to receive input from the MGB.

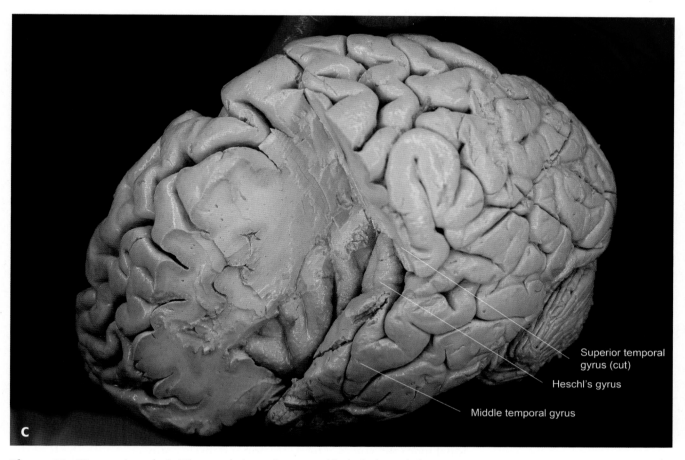

Figure 10–13. *continued* **C.** Dissected view of core and belt, in lateral view.

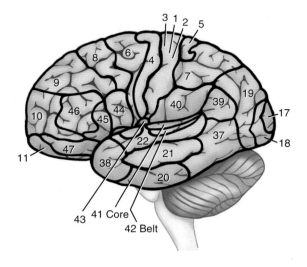

Figure 10–14. Brodmann areas for auditory reception, including areas BA41 (core) and BA42 (belt). *Source:* From Seikel/Drumright/King. *Anatomy & Physiology for Speech, Language, and Hearing, 5th Ed.* ©Cengage, Inc. Reproduced by permission.

Belt

The belt is a 2- to 3-mm region consisting of eight areas surrounding the core. The names simply represent the location of the region. Neurons in the caudomedial (CM) region have some identifiable CFs, but do not really respond well to tones. Note that CM also displays a tonotopic processing scheme but is reversed relative to its neighbor, AI. Neurons in the CM respond not only to auditory information but also to somatosensory stimulation of the neck and head. The caudolateral (CL) region has the same tonotopic array as the CM, but responds generally better to high-frequency information. This region appears to be sensitive to the location of sound in space. The mediolateral (ML) region is also tonotopically arrayed, but parallel to AI. The ML is strongly linked with AI, but only weakly linked with the rostral core (R). The ML projects its output to the area 46 of the frontal lobe, an area involved in visual processing. This region receives its input from the MGB, supergeniculate limitans, and the pulvinar nuclei of the thalamus. Importantly, the pulvinar is involved in language processing. The middle medial (MM) region is not really well defined but appears to represent the AI portion of the core. Output of the MM is to the rostral parabelt and then to the frontal eye region (8) of the cortex, just as with the ML (Clarke, Adriani, & Tardif, 2005).

The anterior lateral (AL) region (indicated as RL in this figure) has broadly tuned neurons that respond to tones and has a general tonotopicity. The AL region has a special function: It is responsive to tones, but it is more responsive to complex signals. In fact, it is specifically responsive to species-specific calls. For the macaque monkey, this region would be most responsive to macaque calling. For the human, it is most responsive to human speech. Significantly, the region is not particularly involved in the location of the calls, but their nature (Belin & Zatorre, 2005). In fact, Petkov et al. (2008) found that this area in macaque monkeys can differentiate individual macaque voices. The AL region is densely connected with the R of the core, and less so with AI. The input of this region is from the posteromedial portion of the thalamus, including the nucleus limitans, medial portion of the MGB, and dorsal portion of the MGB. Ouput of AI projects to the visual region (46) and polysensory region (12) of the frontal lobe.

The rostromedial portion of the belt (RM) appears to be important for both identification and localization of a sound. It communicates with the AL and ML of the belt and has a stronger connection with the R of the core than with AI. The RM region also projects to the parabelt region (to be discussed next). The rostromedial (RTM) and lateral rostrotemporal regions (LRT) both project to the rostral parabelt (RPB).

Parabelt

The parabelt region is lateral to the belt and makes up the third level of processing of the input auditory signal at the reception area. The parabelt is closely linked to the belt. It appears that the RPB is most closely interconnected with the rostral belt, and the caudal parabelt (CPB) is most closely connected with the caudal portion of the belt. The parabelt appears to receive its input from disparate regions of the thalamus, including the dorsal and medial portions of the MGB, suprageniculate nucleus, nucleus limitans, and the posteromedial nucleus. The parabelt projects to area 8 of the frontal lobe, responsible for some high-level visual processing, and may assist in directing vision toward an auditory stimulus. It also projects to area 46 of the frontal lobe, which appears to be an important region for visual-spatial memory processing. The RPB also connects with area 10, which is part of the orbital portion of the cortex. This area appears to be important for the integration of visual and auditory information. The RPB is also responsive to species-specific vocalization (i.e., in humans it is responsive to the human voice), so this region may be involved in identifying the nature of sounds, perhaps helping to define them as linguistic in nature.

It is important to realize that all of the core, belt, and parabelt projects to other regions of the temporal lobe. If you once again look at the pathways of Figure 10–13, you should see rich connections running from the core, belt, and parabelt to the rest of the superior temporal gyrus, the superior temporal sulcus, and the temporoparietal region.

Highest-Level Processing

The highest level of auditory processing occurs throughout the rest of the superior temporal gyrus (STG) and the superior temporal sulcus (STS), as well as the temporo-parieto-occipital association area (the area that includes Wernicke's area in humans). Auditory processing is also performed in the prefrontal and orbital regions of the brain, as well as in the temporal pole (anterior temporal lobe). The middle temporal gyrus, just inferior to the STG, is activated more by the recognition of a stimulus than by its location. In nonhumans, the left auditory cortex is necessary for discriminating species-specific vocalizations.

It appears that AI and the lateral belt region of humans are sensitive to human voices. Physiological studies reveal that the largest responses to human vocalizations are in the superior temporal sulcus, and the responses are strongest when the speech is linguistically interpretable as opposed to scrambled. This pattern implies that it is not simply the acoustic elements that are triggering a response, but rather the acoustic elements of a meaningful stimulus. In macaque monkeys this function is lateralized to the left hemisphere, just as it is in humans. The left hemisphere response to speech by humans is very robust in the left planum temporale, medial to the core.

There are other, noncortical processing sites as well for auditory stimuli. The cerebellum has been implicated as a contributor to the millisecond-level timing required for speech processing. We have already discussed the role of the SOC and IC of the brain stem for localization of sound in space, but it appears that an intact cortex is a requirement for adequate localization function. Unilateral lesion of the cerebral cortex causes severe localization deficit. We already know that the superior colliculus has a very well-defined map of the external visual space it processes, and that map is integrated with auditory information so that an auditory-visual map is developed. Is there such a map in the cerebrum for auditory stimuli? That remains to be seen. It does appear that there are two paths taken by stimuli relative to localization and identification. One stream of information courses from the thalamus to AI, and it seems specialized for identification of a stimulus. A posterior stream appears to process the localization information.

A dual stream model of speech processing posits that auditory information arises bilaterally at the STS and STG, where spectral and temporal information is defined. This information is delivered to the phonological processing center in the middle and posterior STS. At that point the information is sent to the dorsal and ventral streams. The dorsal stream information, which is strongly left-hemisphere dominated, is translated to the left parietal-temporal junction at the sylvian fissure (corresponding to Wernicke's area of the temporal lobe and the supramarginal gyrus of the parietal lobe), and subsequently to the area around and including Broca's area and the anterior insula. This dorsal stream also projects information to the supplementary motor area. Conceptually, this dorsal stream dominates the motor patterning associated with articulatory production. The ventral stream similarly arises from the STG and STS (and perhaps the middle temporal gyrus) and is also projected bilaterally to the middle and posterior STS. The ventral stream is much more bilateral, projecting to the middle temporal gyrus and anterior portion of the inferior temporal sulcus to lexical processing areas. This projection allows phonological information to combine with areas related to word meaning bilaterally, and appears to be essential for processing speech (Hickok & Poeppel, 2007). As you can see from Figure 10–15, the strongly left-hemisphere dorsal stream is involved in translating the speech acoustics into spatial articulatory representations within the frontal lobe, and is involved in a type of auditory-to-motor transformation. Hickok and Poeppel 2007) posited that speech perception is processed by the dorsal stream, but speech recognition involves the ventral system. The dorsal stream (speech perception) is a left-hemisphere function, but the ventral stream is bilaterally represented (speech recognition).

According to this dual-stream model, the auditory cortex first performs a spectral or temporal analysis bilaterally, by means of the core, belt, and parabelt. The middle and posterior aspects of the bilateral superior temporal sulcus is involved in phonological processing and phonological representation. From there the dorsal stream converts the phonological and sensory information into linguistically meaningful units (lexicon). The dorsal stream may or may not be involved in spatial processing of speech information but certainly appears to be important for mapping linguistic information to the motor system.

The cortical processing of stimuli is complex but becoming more apparent. There are at least three locations that receive direct input from the thalamus, and projections from these regions reach frontal, temporal, and parietal lobes of the cerebrum. The core consists of three regions with their own tonotopic maps. The belt is made up of at least eight regions, all of which have unique response characteristics. The parabelt region is the highest-input processing region, projecting to other levels of the cortex. The belt and parabelt appear to be critical for recognition of species-specific calls, as well as for localization of sound in space. They also appear to be important for the identification of the nature of a sound, and perhaps the identification of a sound as speech versus nonspeech. Information is projected to an area of the STS that processes phonological information. A dorsal stream projects to motor planning areas and is involved in speech perception, while a ventral stream projects to lexical regions for speech recognition.

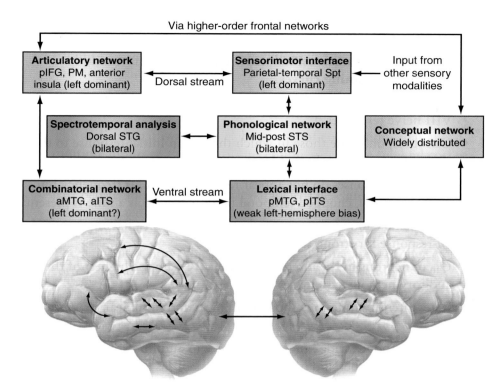

Figure 10–15. Graphic illustration of the proposed pathways of the dual stream model of auditory processing. Hickok and Poeppel (2007) proposed stages of speech processing as follows. Speech information arises at area 41 (bilateral Heschl's gyrus, superior temporal sulcus, *green*) where spectral and temporal analysis occurs in both hemispheres. Bilateral phonological processing (*yellow*, probably dominated by left-hemisphere function) occurs in the superior temporal sulcus (middle and posterior). The flow of processing divides into ventral (*pink*) and dorsal (*blue*) streams. The left-hemisphere dorsal stream maps the phonological representations to articulatory processing regions (peri-Broca's region and supplementary motor area, left hemisphere). The ventral pathway maps phonological representations to linguistic or lexical processing regions (region around Spt, the parietal-temporal boundary of the sylvian fissure, particularly adjacent to and including Wernicke's area and inferior temporal lobes). This area synthesizes sensory and motor information related to language. *Note:* STS = superior temporal sulcus; STG = superior temporal gyrus; aITS = anterior inferior temporal sulcus; aMTG = anterior middle temporal gyrus; pIFG = posterior inferior frontal gyrus; PM = premotor region; Spt = sylvian fissure at parietal-temporal lobe boundary (near Wernicke's area); pMTG=posterior middle temporal gyrus; pITS = posterior inferior temporal sulcus. (Based on figure, data, and description of Hickok and Poeppel, 2007. Redrawn by permission from Macmillan Publishers Ltd. The cortical organization of speech processing. *Nature Reviews: Neuroscience, 8,* pp. 393–402. Copyright 2007.) *Source:* From Seikel/Drumright/King. *Anatomy & Physiology for Speech, Language, and Hearing, 5th Ed.* ©Cengage, Inc. Reproduced by permission.

The auditory nervous system is a complex processor of sound that defies simplistic description. The audiologist and speech-language pathologist must recognize that this most astounding of the sensory systems provides the raw material for the development of speech and language.

administered. The pressure associated with Meniere's will result in loss of hearing (typically high frequency first), as well as dizziness and vertigo.

Viral or bacterial infection may cause labyrinthitis, an inflammation of the inner ear. The effects of labyrinthitis include dizziness, balance problems, and tinnitus, potentially remitting at the end of the infection course. Other problems include perilymph fistula, in which one of the cochlear membranes (typically Reissner's) is torn so that perilymph and endolymph mix, producing a relatively localized sensorineural loss.

Congenital Problems

A number of conditions that affect hearing are present at birth. Congenital atresia of the external auditory meatus results in an absent meatus, while congenital stenosis is narrowing of the ear canal. The pinna may be congenitally absent as well, or it may be deformed. Preauricular pits and ear tags may be present on the pinna or area anterior to the pinna, but they do not affect hearing. They do, however, signal the possibility of the presence of a number of genetic conditions, including branchio-oto-renal syndrome. Low-set auricles are also indicators of a number of genetic syndromes, such as Apert syndrome. Posteriorly rotated auricles are one component of fetal alcohol syndrome. Cleft palate is a significant cause of conductive hearing loss in children. In cleft palate the muscles of the velum are often affected, causing dysfunction of velar elevation, as well as of auditory tube function. The tensor tympani is a dilator of the auditory tube, and if it is involved in cleft palate the auditory tube will fail to aerate, causing otitis media. Similarly, if the auditory tube is patent (open), bacteria, liquid, and food can enter the middle ear space during swallowing, promoting infection. Children with cleft palate very likely have chronic otitis media.

Traumatic Lesions

Trauma to the ear can have an effect on hearing. A blow to the head or acoustic shock from an explosion may cause the middle ear ossicles to become disarticulated, producing a significant conductive hearing loss. The temporal bone is vulnerable to fracturing in lateral injuries, such as those sustained in a side-impact motor vehicle accident or other lateral trauma to the skull. Besides cochlear damage, traumatic impact to the temporal bone can result in cerebrospinal fluid otorrhea, which is leakage of cerebrospinal fluid into the middle ear space. When the cranial space is breeched in this fashion, there is significant opportunity for bacteria to enter the brain case, resulting in meningitis or encephalitis, which is inflammation of the meninges or brain.

Neoplastic Changes

Tumors and other neoplastic changes can also affect hearing. Glomus jugulare tumors can be mistaken for a host of other otologic conditions. If the tumor contacts the tympanic membrane, it provides objective, pulsatile movement of the ear drum; if it contacts the ossicles, it can cause what appears to be otosclerosis. The degree of hearing impairment is typically related to the degree to which structures of the middle ear conduction mechanism are involved. Acoustic neuroma is a benign tumor typically arising within the internal auditory meatus. A sign indicating presence of the tumor is unilateral hearing loss. The loss will typically begin as affecting high frequencies, because the high frequency fibers of the VIII vestibulocochlear nerve are on the outside of the nerve. Ultimately all frequencies will be affected. Removal of the tumor results in permanent unilateral sensorineural hearing loss. If the tumor is outside of the internal auditory meatus, it will likely be a cerebellopontine angle tumor. In this type, growth of the tumor will compress the brain stem and cerebellum, affecting not only the VIII vestibulocochlear nerve, but also potentially the V trigeminal and VII facial nerves.

Bone Changes

Otosclerosis is a bone disorder that results in bony growth that fixates the footplate of the stapes in the oval window, resulting in conductive hearing loss. Otosclerosis can also result in vestibular difficulties, such as vertigo, arising from disturbance of the function of the vestibular mechanism. Rheumatoid arthritis can also result in conductive loss as well as sensorineural loss. Conductive loss appears to occur as a result of ossification of the ossicular joints, while sensorineural loss may be the result of ototoxicity of medications used to treat the disease.

Semicircular Canal Dehiscence

Sometimes the superior semicircular canal of the vestibular mechanism can develop a fistula, making the vestibular space continuous with the cerebrospinal fluid of the brain. Remember that the footplate of the stapes communicates sound to the vestibule, which excites the perilymph of the scala vestibuli and, by association, the endolymph of the scala media. This excitation is facilitated by the round window, which actually protrudes into the middle ear space as the footplate pushes into the vestibule. In contrast, the vestibular mechanism does not have an outlet akin to the round window, so that pressure changes on any of the entryways to the semicircular canals are balanced. When there is an opening into the brain cavity, the mechanical pressure from sound that impinges on the vestibule by means of the stapes footplate is translated as a compression not only to the scala tympani but also to the semicircular canal with the fistula. The fistula acts as a third window, and the result is that a person with third-window syndrome (semicircular canal dehiscence) will have a vestibular response to sounds. This is a nontrivial problem, because our world is full of loud and unpredictable sounds, all of which have the potential to cause vertigo in the patient.

Chapter Summary

The outer and middle ears serve as funneling and impedance-matching devices. The pinna funnels acoustical information to the external auditory meatus and aids in localization of sound in space. Resistance to the flow of energy is termed impedance. The middle ear plays the role of an impedance-matching device, increasing the pressure of a signal arriving at the cochlea. The area ratio between the tympanic membrane and the oval window provides a significant gain of 25 dB in output over input, and the lever advantage of the ossicles provides a smaller gain of 2 dB. The buckling effect grants another 4 to 6 dB gain.

The inner ear is responsible for performing spectral (frequency) and temporal acoustic analyses of the incoming acoustical signal. Movement of the tympanic membrane is translated into parallel movement of the stapes footplate and the fluid in the scala vestibuli. Movement of the fluid of the scala vestibuli is translated directly to the basilar membrane, and the disturbance at the basilar membrane causes the initiation of the traveling wave. The cochlea has a tonotopic arrangement, with high-frequency sounds resolved at the base and low-frequency sounds processed toward the apex. The point of maximum displacement of the basilar membrane determines the frequency information transmitted to the brain. The traveling wave quickly damps after reaching its point of maximum displacement. The frequency analysis ability of the basilar membrane is determined by graded stiffness, thickness, and width. The basilar membrane is stiffer, thinner, and narrower at the base than at the apex. Excitation of the outer hair cells occurs primarily as a result of a shearing effect on the cilia. Excitation of the inner hair cells is caused by the effect of fluid flow and turbulence of endolymph.

When the basilar membrane is displaced toward the scala vestibuli, the hair cells are activated, resulting in electrical potentials. Resting or standing potentials are those voltage potential differences that can be measured from the cochlea at rest. The scala vestibuli is 5 mV more positive than the scala tympani, but the scala media is 80 mV more positive. The intracellular resting potential in the hair cells reveals a negative potential difference between the endolymph and the hair cell of 70 mV, giving a 150 mV difference between the hair cells and the surrounding fluid. Stimulus-related potentials include the alternating current cochlear microphonic, generated by the outer hair cells; the summating potential, a direct current shift in the endocochlear potential; and the whole-nerve action potential, arising directly from stimulation of a large number of hair cells simultaneously.

There are two basic types of VIII nerve neurons, and specific techniques have been developed for assessing their function. High-threshold neurons require a higher intensity for response and encompass the higher end of our auditory range of signal intensity. Low-threshold fibers respond at very low signal levels and display random firing even when no stimulus is present. Low-threshold neurons may process near-threshold sounds, whereas high-threshold fibers process higher-level sounds. Frequency specificity is the ability of the cochlea to differentiate the various spectral components of a signal. Post-stimulus time histograms are plots of neural response relative to the onset of a stimulus. The characteristic or best frequency of a neuron is the frequency to which it responds best. A tuning curve is a composite of the responses of a single fiber at each frequency of presentation. The sharper the tuning curve, the greater the frequency specificity of the basilar membrane. The tonotopic array of the cochlea is clearly maintained within the auditory nervous system in the form of individual nerve fiber activation. As the intensity of stimulation increases, the rate of firing increases. When the crossed-olivocochlear and uncrossed-olivocochlear bundles are stimulated, the firing rate of neurons innervated by them is reduced dramatically.

Interspike interval histograms record the interval between successive firings of a neuron, revealing phase-locking of neurons to stimulus period.

Temporal and tonotopically arrayed information progresses to higher centers for further extraction of information. The cochlear nucleus reveals tonotopic representation, with a wide variety of neuron responses. Primary-like responses most resemble VIII nerve firing, onset responses show an initial response to the onset of a stimulus followed by silence, and chopper responses show a periodic, chopped temporal pattern as long as a tone is present. Pauser responses take longer to respond than other neurons. Buildup responses slowly increase in firing rate through the initial stages of firing.

The superior olivary complex (SOC) is the primary site of localization of sound in space. Contralateral stimulation of the SOC by high-frequency information results in excitation related to stimulus intensity. Low-frequency stimuli presented binaurally to the SOC result in interaural time difference detection. A wide array of responses is seen at the inferior colliculus, including neuron inhibitory responses, onset and pauser responses, intensity-sensitive units, and interaural time- and intensity-sensitive responses. The medial geniculate body is a relay of the thalamus. The cerebral cortex receives input primarily from the contralateral ear via the ipsilateral medial geniculate body (MGB). A full tonotopic map on the cortex may be seen at the primary reception area. The auditory reception area is organized in columns, with each column having a similar characteristic frequency. Different neurons within the columns respond to different stimulus parameters, such as frequency up-glides and down-glides, intensity up-glides and down-glides, and so on. Hickok and Poeppel (2007) proposed stages of speech processing that are differentiated based on the level of complexity of the stimulus. Sublexical information appears to be bilaterally processed in the superior temporal gyrus by a ventral stream, whereas lexical information is processed by a left-hemisphere dorsal stream.

❓ Chapter 10 Study Questions

1. The _____ of the outer ear is important for the localization of sound in space.

2. Resistance to the flow of energy is termed _____.

3. The area ratio between the tympanic membrane and the oval window provides a _____ dB gain, and the lever advantage gives a _____ dB gain.

4. The cochlea performs both _____ analysis and _____ analysis.

5. Compression of the fluid of the scala vestibuli is translated directly to the basilar membrane, and the disturbance at the basilar membrane causes the initiation of a _____ wave.

6. High-frequency sounds are resolved at the base of the cochlea, with progressively lower-frequency sounds processed at progressively higher positions on the cochlea. This array is termed _____.

7. The frequency analysis ability of the basilar membrane is determined by graded _____ and _____.

8. T/F At the apex, the basilar membrane is thicker than at the base.

9. T/F At the apex, the basilar membrane is narrower than at the base.

10. T/F The cilia of the outer hair cells are embedded in the tectorial membrane.

11. T/F The cilia of the inner hair cells are embedded in the tectorial membrane.

12. T/F The scala vestibuli is 5 mV more positive than the scala tympani, but the scala media is 80 mV more positive than the scala vestibuli.

13. The _____ arises directly from the stimulation of a large number of hair cells simultaneously.

14. _____ neurons require a higher intensity and encompass the higher end of our auditory range of signal intensity, whereas _____ neurons respond at very low signal levels and display random firing even when no stimulus is present.

15. _____ refers to the ability of the cochlea to differentiate the various spectral components of a signal.

16. The _____ frequency of a neuron is the frequency to which it responds best.

17. The tuning curves are composites of the responses of a single fiber at each frequency of presentation. The sharper the tuning curve, the greater the _____ of the basilar membrane.

18. The rate of firing of neurons increases as the _____ increases.

19. Stimulation of the _____ bundle and the _____ bundle reduces the firing rate of neurons innervated by them.

20. _____ are those firing patterns that most resemble VIII nerve responses.

21. The _____ is the primary site of localization of sound in space.

22. Comparative anatomy provides insights into function. What changes in the cochlea would you predict when comparing the cochlea of a human with that of a mammal, such as a fruit bat, that used ultra-high-frequency sound to echolocate? What changes would you predict that you would find when comparing an elephant's cochlea with that of a human?

23. The _____ is the primary brain stem location for localization of sound in space.

24. The _____ of the brain stem is involved in both localization and intersensory interaction.

25. The _____ of the auditory cortex is responsible for primary reception of the auditory signal and is divided into three portions.

26. The planum _____ is posterior to Heschl's gyrus.

27. The planum _____ is anterior to Heschl's gyrus.

28. The _____ region of the auditory cortex surrounds the core area for auditory reception.

29. The _____ of the thalamus is the primary source of input to the core of the auditory cortex.

? Chapter 10 Study Question Answers

1. The **PINNA** of the outer ear is important for the localization of sound in space.

2. Resistance to the flow of energy is termed **IMPEDANCE**.

3. The area ratio between the tympanic membrane and the oval window provides a **25** dB gain, and the lever advantage gives a **2** dB gain.

4. The cochlea performs both **SPECTRAL** analysis and **TEMPORAL** analysis.

5. Compression of the fluid of the scala vestibuli is translated directly to the basilar membrane, and the disturbance at the basilar membrane causes the initiation of a **TRAVELING** wave.

6. High-frequency sounds are resolved at the base of the cochlea, with progressively lower frequency sounds processed at progressively higher positions on the cochlea. This array is termed **TONOTOPIC**.

7. The frequency analysis ability of the basilar membrane is determined by graded **WIDTH**, **STIFFNESS**, and **THICKNESS**.

8. **TRUE** At the apex, the basilar membrane is **THICKER** than at the base.

9. **FALSE** At the apex, the basilar membrane is **WIDER** than at the base.

10. **TRUE** The cilia of the outer hair cells are embedded in the tectorial membrane.

11. **FALSE** The cilia of the inner hair cells are **NOT** embedded in the tectorial membrane.

12. **TRUE** The scala vestibuli is 5 mV more positive than the scala tympani, but the scala media is 80 mV more positive than the scala vestibuli.

13. The **WHOLE-NERVE ACTION POTENTIAL** arises directly from the stimulation of a large number of hair cells simultaneously.

14. **HIGH-THRESHOLD** neurons require a higher intensity and encompass the higher end of our auditory range of signal intensity, whereas **LOW-THRESHOLD** neurons respond at very low signal levels and display random firing even when no stimulus is present.

15. **FREQUENCY SPECIFICITY** refers to the ability of the cochlea to differentiate the various spectral components of a signal.

16. The **CHARACTERISTIC** frequency of a neuron is the frequency to which it responds best.

17. The tuning curves are composites of the responses of a single fiber at each frequency of presentation. The sharper the tuning curve, the greater the **FREQUENCY SPECIFICITY** of the basilar membrane.

18. The rate of firing of neurons increases as the **INTENSITY** increases.

19. Stimulation of the **CROSSED-OLIVOCOCHLEAR** bundle and the **UNCROSSED-OLIVOCOCHLEAR** bundle reduces the firing rate of neurons innervated by them.

20. **PRIMARY-LIKE** are those firing patterns that most resemble VIII nerve responses.

21. The **SUPERIOR OLIVARY COMPLEX** is the primary site of localization of sound in space.

22. The fruit bat cochlea is, naturally enough, smaller than that of the human. In addition, the cochlea of the bat is extremely sensitive to ultra-high frequencies (above human range of hearing), because high-frequency sounds are more efficient for echolocation. Elephants, in contrast, have larger cochleas than humans. They process sounds that are lower than those we can hear.

23. The **SUPERIOR OLIVARY COMPLEX** is the primary brain stem location for localization of sound in space.

24. The **INFERIOR COLLICULUS** of the brain stem is involved in both localization and intersensory interaction.

25. The **CORE** of the auditory cortex is responsible for primary reception of the auditory signal and is divided into three portions.

26. The planum **TEMPORALE** is posterior to Heschl's gyrus.

27. The planum **POLARE** is anterior to Heschl's gyrus.

28. The **BELT** region of the auditory cortex surrounds the core area for auditory reception.

29. The **MEDIAL GENICULATE BODY** of the thalamus is the primary source of input to the core of the auditory cortex.

Bibliography

Anderson, D. J., Rose, J. E., Hind, J. E., & Brugge, J. F (1980). Temporal position of discharges in single auditory nerve fibers within the cycle of a sine-wave stimulus: Frequency and intensity effects. *Journal of the Acoustical Society of America, 49,* 1131–1138.

Banerjee, A., & Nikkar-Esfahani, A. (2011). Occlusion of the round window: A novel way to treat hyperacusis symptoms in superior canal dehiscence syndrome. *Otolaryngology–Head and Neck Surgery, 145*(2 Suppl.), P89–P99.

Belin, P., & Zatorre, R. J. (2005). Voice processing in human auditory cortex. In R. Konig, P. Heil, E. Budinger, & H. Scheich (Eds.), *The auditory cortex* (pp. 163–180). Mahwah, NJ: Lawrence Erlbaum.

Bhattacharyya, N., Gubbels, S. P., Schwartz, S. R., Edlow, J. A., El-Kashlan, H., Fife, T., . . . Seidman, M. D. (2017). Clinical practice guideline: Benign paroxysmal positional vertigo (update). *Otolaryngology–Head and Neck Surgery, 156*(3 Suppl.), S1–S47.

Brodmann, K., & Garey, L. J. (2007). *Brodmann's: Localisation in the cerebral cortex.* New York, NY: Springer.

Casimiro, C. C., Knollmann, B. C., Ebert, S. N., Vary, J. C., Greene, A. E., Franz, M. R., . . . Pfeifer, K. (2001). Targeted disruption of the Kcnq1 gene produces a mouse model of Jervell and Lange-Nielsen syndrome. *Proceedings of the National Academy of Sciences, USA, 98*(5), 2526–2531.

Clarke, S., Adriani, M., & Tardif, E. (2005). "What" and "where" in human audition: Evidence from anatomical, activation, and lesion studies. In R. Konig, P. Heil, E. Budinger, & H. Scheich (Eds.), *The auditory cortex* (pp. 77–94). Mahwah, NJ: Lawrence Erlbaum.

Dallos, P. (1973). *The auditory periphery.* New York, NY: Academic Press.

Eggermont, J. J., & Odenthal, D. W. (1974). Electrophysiological investigation of the human cochlea: Recruitment, masking and adaptation. *Audiology, 13*(1), 1–22.

Evans, R. B. (2003). Georg von Bekesy: Visualization of hearing. *American Psychologist, 58*(9), 742–746.

Forge, A., Li, L., Corwin, J. T., & Nevill, G. (1993). Ultrastructural evidence for hair cell regeneration in the mammalian inner ear. *Science, 259*(5101), 1616–1619.

Gollisch, T., & Meister, M. (2008). Rapid neural coding in the retina with relative spike latencies. *Science, 319,* 1108–1111.

Haralabidis, A. S., Dimakopoulou, K., Vigna-Taglianti, F., Giampaolo, M., Borgini, A., Dudley, M. L., . . . Jarup, L. (2008). Acute effects of night-time noise exposure on blood pressure in populations living near airports. *European Heart Journal, 29*(5), 658–664.

Hickok, G., & Poeppel, D. (2007). The cortical organization of speech processing. *Nature Reviews of Neuroscience, 8*, 393–402.

Izumikawa, M., Minoda, R., Kawamoto, K., Abrashkin, K. A., Swiderski, D. L., Dolan, D. F., . . . Raphael, Y. (2005). Auditory hair cell replacement and hearing improvement by Atoh1 gene therapy in deaf mammals. *Nature Medicine, 11*, 271–276.

Javel, E. (1980). Coding of AM tones in the chinchilla auditory nerve: Implications for the pitch of complex tones. *Journal of the Acoustical Society of America, 68*(1), 133–146,

Kaas, J. H., & Hackett, T. A. (2000). Subdivisions of auditory cortex and processing streams in primates. *Proceedings of the National Academy of Sciences, USA, 97*(22), 11793–11799.

Khanna, S. M., & Leonard, D. G. B. (1982). Basilar membrane tuning in the cochlea. *Science, 215*, 305–306.

Kiang, N. Y., Liberman, M. C., Sewell, W. F., & Guinan, J. J. (1986). Single unit clues to cochlear mechanisms. *Hearing Research, 22*, 171–182.

Kraft, S., Hsu, C., Brough, D. E., & Staecker, H. (2013). Atoh1 induces hair cell recovery in mice with ototoxic injury. *Laryngoscope, 123*(4), 992–999.

Kruger, B. (1989). An update on external ear resonance in infants and young children. *Ear and Hearing, 8*(6), 333–336.

Labuguen, R. H. (2006). Initial evaluation of vertigo. *American Family Physician, 73*(2), 244–251.

Liberman, M. C., & Kiang, N. Y. (1978). Acoustic trauma in cats. *Acta Otolarygnolgica. Supplementum, 358*, 1–63.

Minor, L. B., Schessel, D. A., & Carey, J. P. (2004). Meniere's disease. *Current Opinion in Neurology, 17*(1), 9–16.

Møller, A. R. (1973). *Basic mechanisms in hearing* (pp. 593–619). Cambridge, MA: Academic Press.

Moller, A. R. (2003). *Sensory systems: Anatomy, physiology and pathophysiology*. Houston, TX: Gulf Professional Publishing.

Musiek, F. E., & Baran, J. A. (2006). *The auditory system: Anatomy, physiology, and clinical correlates*. Glenview, IL: Allyn & Bacon.

Norton, S., & Neely, S. T. (1987). Tone-burst otoacoustic emissions from normal hearing adults. *Journal of the Acoustical Society of America, 81*(6), 1860–1872.

Petkov, C. I., Kayser, C., Steudel, T., Whittingstall, K., Augath, M., & Logothetis, N. K. (2008). A voice region in the monkey brain. *Nature Neuroscience 11*, 367–374.

Pfeiffer, R. R. (1966). Classification of response patterns of spike discharges for units in the cochlear nucleus: Tone-burst stimulation. *Experimental Brain Research, 1*, 220–235.

Pickles, J. O. (2012). *An introduction to the physiology of hearing* (4th ed.). London, UK: Emerald Group.

Rhode, W. S. (1985). The use of intracellular techniques in the study of the cochlear nucleus. *Journal of the Acoustical Society of America, 78*(1), 320–327.

Sanford, C. A., & Feeney, M. P. (2008). Effects of maturation on tympanic wideband acoustic transfer function in human infants. *Journal of the Acoustical Society of America, 124*(4), 2106–2122.

Seikel, J. A., Konstantopoulos, K., & Drumright, D. G. (2020). *Neuroanatomy and neurophysiology for speech and hearing sciences*. San Diego, CA: Plural Publishing.

Seixas, N. S., Kujawa, S. G., Norton, S., Sheppard, L., Neitzel, R., & Slee, A. (2004). Prediction of hearing threshold levels and distortion product otoacoustic emissions among noise-exposed young adults. *Occupational Environmental Medicine, 61*(11), 899–907.

Shaw, E. A. G. (1974). The external ear. In W. D. Keidel & W. D. Neff (Eds.), *Handbook of sensory physiology* (pp. 455–490). New York, NY: Springer-Verlag.

Spicer, S. S., & Schulte, B. A. (1996). The fine structure of spiral ligament cells relates to ion return to the stria and varies with place-frequency. *Hearing Research, 100*, 80–100.

Tonndorf, J. (1960). Shearing motion in scala media of cochlear models. *Journal of the Acoustical Society of America, 32*(5), 238–244.

Von Bohlen und Halbach, O., & Dermietzel, R. (2006). *Neurotransmitters and neuromodulators*. Weinheim, Germany: Wiley-VCH.

Von Békésy, G. (1960). *Experiments in hearing*. New York, NY: McGraw-Hill.

Wangemann, P. (2006). Supporting sensory transduction: Cochlear fluid homeostasis and the endocochlear potential. *Journal of Neurophysiology, 576*(1), 11–21.

Watson, S. R. D., Halmagyi, M., & Colebatch, J. G. (2000). Vestibular hypersensity to sound (Tullio phenomenon). *Neurology, 54*(3), 213–225.

Wever, E. G., & Bray, C. W. (1930). Action currents in the auditory nerve in response to acoustical stimulation. *Proceedings of the National Academy of Sciences, USA, 16*(5), 344–350.

Winslow, R. L., & Sachs, M. B. (1988). Single tone intensity discrimination based on auditory nerve rate responses in backgrounds of quiet, noise, and with stimulation of the crossed olivocochlear nerve. *Hearing Research, 35*(2–3), 165–189.

Yost, W. A. (2007). *Fundamentals of hearing: An introduction* (5th ed.). New York, NY: Elsevier Academic Press.

Yu, X. J., Dickman, J. D., & Angelaki, D. E. (2012). Detection thresholds of macaque otolith afferents. *Journal of Neuroscience, 32*(24), 8306–8316.

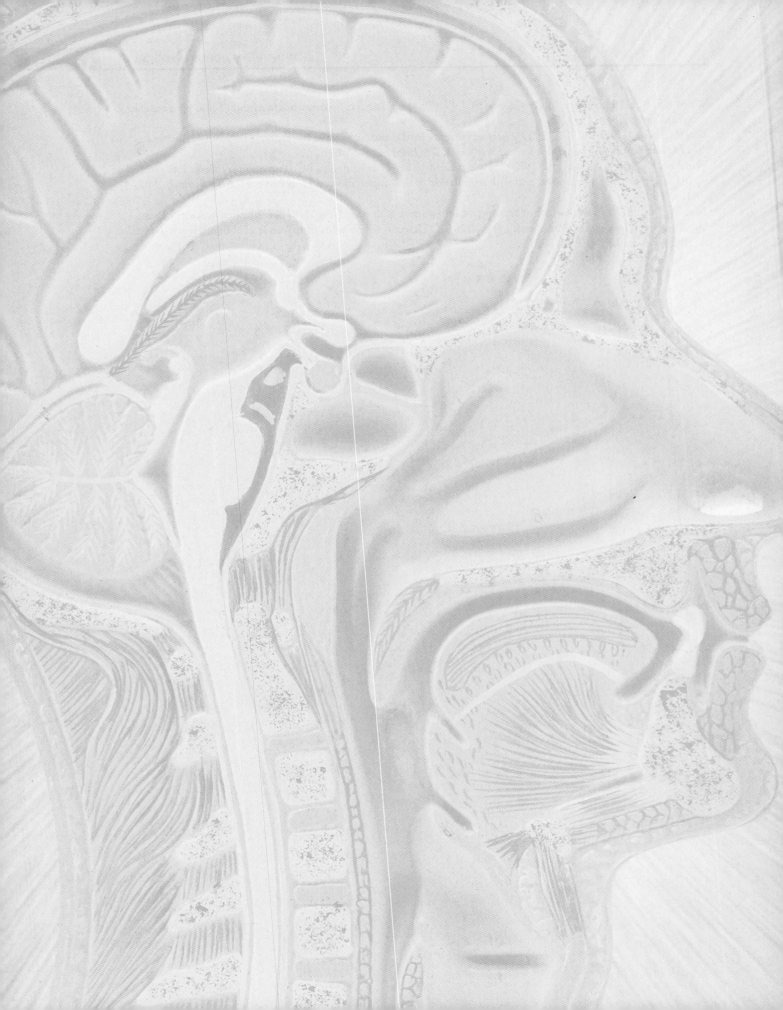

Neuroanatomy

There is nothing in nature as awe-inspiring as the nervous system. Despite centuries of study, humans have only begun to gain understanding of this extraordinarily complex system. The brain contains approximately 86 billion neurons, with the cerebral cortex being the home to 17 billion of them (Azevado et al., 2009; Karlsen & Pakkenberg, 2011). Neurons are densely interconnected so that each neuron may communicate directly with as many as 2,000 other neurons. There are on the order of 190 trillion **synapses** (points of communication) within the brain. We tell you these extraordinary numbers so that you can get a notion of the vastness of the nervous system. The tremendous challenge of neuroscience is, and always has been, to figure out how these elements interact to produce all the complex processes involved in thought, language, and speech. As before, we discuss both the structure and function of this system.

Synapse is a noun, but is often used as a verb, indicating the action of communication between two neurons.

Overview

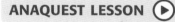

ANAQUEST LESSON

During our discussion of human anatomy associated with speech and language, we have been quite concerned with the voluntary musculature and the supporting framework associated with it. Communication is, by and large, voluntary. Nonetheless, the term *voluntary* takes on new meanings when seen in the context of automaticity and background. **Automaticity** refers to the development of patterns of responses that no longer require highly specific motor control but rather are relegated to automated patterns. **Background** activity is the muscular contraction that supports action or movement, providing the form against which voluntary movement is placed. Voluntary activities are generally considered to be conscious activities, but they are, in reality, largely automated responses. To prove this to yourself, try washing the dishes and actually thinking about the act of dishwashing. The movements and responses to this act are so automated that you probably feel you do them without thinking. In fact, your brain receives a vast number of signals from body sensors every second (including information about soap suds and water temperature), but you need not respond to all of it, because your brain monitors and alerts you to dangers or alterations from expectations. You can think about other things while your hands do the dishes.

Speech capitalizes on similar automaticity, as you can see in your ability to speak easily while riding a bike or while walking. You no more think of every movement of the extraordinary number of muscles contracting for the simple speech act than you do during dishwashing. This automaticity changes when the mechanism changes, however. When your mouth is numb from the dentist's anesthesia, you become very aware of your lack of feedback from that system, and inaccurate speech results. When an individual suffers a cerebrovascular accident, the result is often a loss of previously attained automaticity in speech. When a child is born with developmental apraxia of speech, a condition that limits the ability of a child to plan articulatory function, achieving automaticity may be a lifelong struggle. You might want to revisit our Chapter 7 discussion of motor control, feedback systems, and feed-forward systems as you think about these "automatic" functions of speech.

Automatic functions are supported by a background **tonicity**, a partial contraction of musculature to maintain muscle tone. All action occurs within an environment, and the environment of your musculature is the tonic contraction of supporting muscles. As you extend your arm to reach for a coffee cup, the action of your fingers to grasp the object is supported by the rotation of your shoulder and the extension of your arm. Without these background support movements, the act of grasping would not occur in the graceful, fluid manner to which you are accustomed. Your body works as a unit to meet your needs.

Voluntary functions are the domain of the **cerebral cortex**, the core of a new structure by evolutionary standards that makes up the bulk of the human brain. It is the seat of consciousness, and sensory information that does not reach the level of the cerebrum does not reach consciousness. The cerebrum is also the source of voluntary movement, although many lower brain centers are involved in the execution of commands initiated by the cerebrum (Figure 11–1).

Phylogeny *refers to the evolution of a species, whereas* ontogeny *is the development of an individual organism. The statement that "Ontogeny recapitulates phylogeny" refers to the notion that structures that are phylogenetically oldest tend to emerge earliest in the developing organism, whereas later evolutionary additions, such as the cerebral cortex, will emerge later in development.*

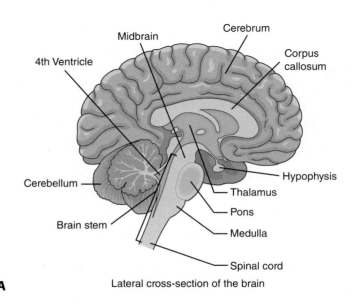

Figure 11–1. A. Medial view of cerebrum, brain stem, and cerebellum. *Source: From Seikel/Drumright/ King. Anatomy & Physiology for Speech, Language, and Hearing, 5th Ed.* ©Cengage, Inc. Reproduced by permission. *continues*

A   Lateral cross-section of the brain

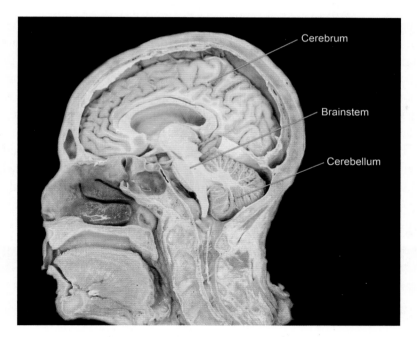

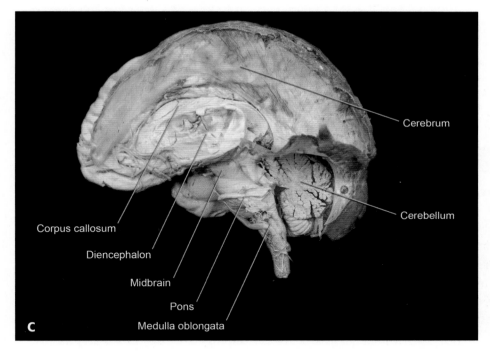

Figure 11–1. *continued*
B. Sagittal section showing relationship among cerebrum, cerebellum, and brain stem.
C. Sagittal view with dissection to show subcortical structures.

Movement requires coordination, and that is one of the responsibilities of the **cerebellum**. Information from peripheral sensors is coordinated with the motor plan of the cerebrum to provide the body with the ability to make finely tuned motor gestures. The output from the cerebrum is modified by the **basal ganglia**, a group of nuclei (cell bodies) with functional unity deeply involved in background movement.

Motor commands are conveyed to the periphery for execution by neural pathways termed **nerves** or **tracts**. Sensory pathways transmit information concerning the status of the body and its environment to the brain for evaluation. This information permits the cerebrum and lower centers to act on changing conditions to protect the systems of the body and to adjust to the body's environment. For instance, information that tells your brain that it is cold outside is transmitted to the cerebrum and hypothalamus—the result being shivering and goose bumps as well as a conscious effort to retrieve your ski parka from the car.

The brain can communicate with its environment only through sensors and effectors (Møller, 2003; Table 11–1). Sensors are the means by which your nervous system translates information concerning the internal and

Table 11–1

Classes of Sensation	
Superficial Sensations	**Deep Sensations**
Temperature	Muscle tension and length
Pain	Joint position
Touch	Proprioception
	Muscle pain
	Pressure
	Vibration

Coming to Your Senses

Thanks to Aristotle, we have come to know the five senses as stereotypes: touch, taste, vision, hearing, and smell. The reality is far different, however. Physiologists now state that there are at least 21 senses, and some place the number much higher. Here is how they come to this conclusion.

There are certainly basic senses: vision, hearing, olfaction (smell), gestation (taste), tactile sense (touch), nociception (pain), mechanoreception, thermal sense, and interoception (senses associated with internal, subconscious processes such as blood pressure, CO_2 in the blood). That said, each of these basic senses can be further subdivided. For instance, vision can be divided into light and color, but some say it should be divided into light, red sense, green sense, and blue sense. This makes "sense," in that the receptors for these colors are mutually exclusive. You could make the same argument for taste. Taste consists of sweet, salty, bitter, sour, and umami. Smell is smell, right? Wrong. We can sense more than 2,000 different and highly specific smells, and there is evidence that the olfactory receptors are highly specialized.

Mechanoreception diversifies in the same way (Table 11–2). We have the sense of balance and acceleration (rotational and linear) mediated by the vestibular mechanism, but we also have joint sense (proprioception), body movement sense (kinesthesia), and muscle tension (Golgi tendon organs [GTO]), and stretch (muscle spindle) senses.

Finally, there are at least five basic interoceptors, including sensors for blood pressure, arterial pressure, venous pressure, oxygen content, acid balance of cerebrospinal fluid, and stomach distension. So, it looks as if Aristotle needs an update.

Table 11–2

Sense, Sensor, and Stimulation		
Sense	**Sensor type**	**Stimulus**
Pain	Nerve endings	Aversive stimulation
Temperature	Thermoreceptors	Heat and cold
Mechanical stimulation (including tactile sense)	Pacinian corpuscles Golgi tendon organs Muscle spindle	Light and deep pressure Vibration Joint sense Muscle stretch
Kinesthetic sense	Labyrinthine (vestibular) hair receptors	Motion of body
Vision	Photoreceptors	Light stimulation
Olfactory	Chemoreceptors	Chemical stimulation
Audition	Labyrinthine (cochlear) hair receptors	Acoustical stimulation
Gustatory	Chemoreceptors	Chemical stimulation

external environment into a form that is usable by the brain, whereas effectors are the means by which your body responds to changing conditions. Broadly speaking, **superficial sensation** (temperature, pain, touch) is a sensation arising from the stimulation of the surface of the body. **Deep sensation** includes muscle tension, muscle length, joint position sense, proprioception, muscle pain, pressure, and vibration. **Combined sensation** integrates both multiple senses to process stimulation. This involves integration of many pieces of sensory information to determine a quality, such as **stereognosis** (the ability to recognize the form of an object through touch).

Within each of these broad classes are specific types of sensation. **Somatic sense** is that sensation related to pain, thermal sensation (temperature sense), and mechanical stimulation. Mechanical stimulation takes the form of light and deep pressure, vibration (which is actually pressure that is perceived to change over time), and changes in joints and muscles, particularly stretch. **Kinesthetic sense**, or *kinesthesia*, is the sense of the body in motion. **Special senses** are those designed to **transduce** (change one form of energy into another) specific exteroceptive information. For example, in the **visual sense**, light from external sources is transduced into electrochemical energy by the photoreceptors of the retina; in **hearing**, acoustical disturbances in the air are transduced by the hair cells of the cochlea. Other special senses are **olfaction** (sense of smell), **tactile sense** (sense of touch), and **gustation** (sense of taste).

Sensor types vary by the stimulus to which they respond. Sensors communicate with the nervous system by means of dendritic connection with bipolar first-order sensory neurons. Axons of these first-order neurons **synapse**, or make neurochemical connection, within the central nervous system. A graded **generator potential** arises from adequate stimulation of the sensor, and adequate stimulation causes the generation of an action potential.

Receptors may be mechanoreceptors, chemoreceptors, photoreceptors, or thermoreceptors. **Mechanoreceptors** respond to physical distortion of tissue. Pressure on the skin, for example, results in the distension of **Pacinian corpuscles**, whereas hair follicles have mechanoreceptors to let you know that something has disturbed your hair. **Muscle spindle** and **Golgi tendon organs** and the **labyrinthine hair receptors** of the inner ear are also mechanoreceptors. In contrast, olfaction (smell) and gustation (taste) are mediated by **chemoreceptors** because they depend on contact with molecules of the target substance. Visual stimulation by light is transduced by highly specialized **photoreceptors**, and temperature sense arises from **thermoreceptors**. Visual and auditory sensors are also termed **telereceptors** because their respective light and sound stimuli arise from a source that does not touch

When Sensation Goes Bad

Sensations are processed by the nervous system as a means of relating the real world with our "inner world." These sensations are required for normal function, including motor coordination and protective action. When sensory systems fail, any valuable information required by the nervous system is lost. The most obvious sensory losses for those of us in the fields of speech-language pathology and audiology are those associated with hearing and vestibular function. Prenatal loss of hearing has a significant impact on the development of speech and language, whereas postnatal loss results in significant communication problems. Vestibular dysfunction, as in that seen in Meniere's disease (endolymphatic hydrops), results in significant balance difficulties and vertigo.

One can also have a disruption of sensory systems related to joint perception, which can cause errors in motor execution. Similarly, a deficit in sensory feedback drives the muscle spindle into hyperfunction when upper motor neuron lesion limits the inhibition of that reflexive system. Diseases such as diabetes can cause loss of pain sense, which may result in failure to recognize a wound until it has become seriously infected. Loss of appropriate sensory input to the cerebellum, which coordinates motor function (including correction of the motor plan), will result in cerebellar ataxia, which is reduction of coordinated movement.

Finally, sometimes our senses can fool us. There are well-known illusions that can be elicited relative to sensation. For instance, if you are seated so that you cannot see your right arm, but *can* see an artificial limb that could be your arm, you will perceive the artificial limb as your own arm if an experimenter stimulates both your hidden "real" arm and the visible artificial arm, an apparent function of the premotor cortex (Ehrsson, Spence, & Passingham, 2004). In this illusion, you perceive the touch sensation as occurring to the artificial arm. This very real and robust phenomenon is mirrored in several versions of the phantom limb phenomenon. In this condition, people who have undergone amputation of a limb sometimes perceive the presence of that limb, despite all evidence to the contrary. As Kandel (2012) noted, a person with phantom limb syndrome may feel the amputated limb move and even perceive it extending to shake another person's hand.

Locked-in Syndrome

Locked-in syndrome is a condition that typically arises because of brain stem stroke (cerebrovascular accident, or CVA). The condition results in complete paralysis of all musculature except the ocular muscles. The condition typically has no effect on sensory or cognitive function, so the individual is left with intact mental function but no means of communication. A system of eye blinks is typically established with the individual as a means of alternative communication.

the body (olfactory sense is stimulated directly by molecules of the material being sensed).

Another way to categorize receptors is by the region of the body receiving stimulation. **Interoceptors** monitor events within the body, such as distention of the lungs during inspiration or blood acidity. **Exteroceptors** respond to stimuli outside of the body, such as tactile stimulation, audition, and vision. Contact receptors are exteroceptors that respond to stimuli that touch the body (e.g., tactile, pain, deep and light pressure, temperature). **Proprioceptors** are sensors that monitor change in a body's position or the position of its parts, and these include muscle and joint sensors, such as muscle spindles and Golgi tendon organs (GTOs). Vestibular sense falls into this category because it provides information about the body's position in space.

Despite our rich communicative ability, we can know our environment *only* by means of the sensory receptors of our skin, muscles, tendons, eyes, ears, and so forth. Without sensation, a perfectly functioning brain would be worthless as a communicating system. Likewise, communication *requires* some sort of muscular activity or glandular secretion. The absence of *all* motor activity would likewise signal the end of communication. Fortunately, the extraordinary number of sensors in the human body permits us to use alternate pathways for receiving communication (e.g., tactile, or touch, communication) or for passing information to another person (e.g., use of eye-blink code). We are rarely completely cut off from communication with others. Let us now examine the components of this system.

Divisions of the Nervous System

The **nervous system** can be viewed and categorized in a number of ways. It is important to develop a framework for the discussion of this system, lest the volume of components become overwhelming. In the overview, we discussed an informal **functional view** of nervous system organization, assessing the components in terms of their relationship to the systems of communication. We can view the nervous system as being composed of two major components (central nervous system and peripheral nervous system) or as having two major functions (autonomic nervous system and somatic nervous system) (Table 11–3). We can also view the nervous system in developmental terms, differentiating based on embryonic structures.

Table 11–3

Divisions of the Nervous System From Anatomical and Physiological Perspectives
Anatomical Divisions of the Nervous System
Central nervous system: cerebrum, cerebellum, brain stem, spinal cord, thalamus, subthalamus, basal ganglia, and other structures
Peripheral nervous system: spinal nerves, cranial nerves, sensory receptors
Functional Divisions of the Nervous System
Autonomic nervous system: involuntary bodily function
Sympathetic nervous system: expends energy (e.g., vasoconstriction when frightened)
Parasympathetic nervous system: conserves energy (e.g., vasodilation upon removal of feared stimulation)
Somatic nervous system: voluntary bodily function

Central Nervous System and Peripheral Nervous System

The nervous system may be divided anatomically into central and peripheral nervous systems (see Table 11–3). The **central nervous system (CNS)** includes the brain (cerebrum, cerebellum, subcortical structures, brain stem) and spinal cord. The **peripheral nervous system (PNS)** consists of the 12 pairs of cranial nerves and 31 pairs of spinal nerves as well as the sensory receptors. All the CNS components are housed within bone (skull or vertebral column), whereas most of the PNS components are outside of bone. We will spend a great deal of time within this organizational structure as we discuss the anatomy of the nervous system.

Autonomic and Somatic Nervous Systems

A functional view of the nervous system categorizes the brain into autonomic and somatic nervous systems (see Table 11–3). The **autonomic nervous system (ANS)** governs involuntary activities of the visceral muscles or **viscera**, including glandular secretions, heart function, and digestive function. You have little control over what happens to that triple chili cheeseburger once you make the commitment to eat it, although you will admit that occasionally you are *aware* of the digestive process. You can also view the enteric nervous system (ENS) as a subsystem of the ANS. The enteric nervous system governs how that cheeseburger is processed (Horn & Swanson, 2012). The ENS contains more than 900,000 neurons (compared with 120,000 neurons in the spinal cord) that govern the stomach, heart, bladder, intestines, and vascular system all in the background.

The ANS may be further divided into two subsystems. The subsystem that responds to stimulation through energy expenditure is called the **sympathetic system** or **thoracolumbar system**, and the system that counters these responses is known as the **parasympathetic system** or **craniosacral system**. You feel the result of the sympathetic system when you have a close call in an automobile or hear a sudden, loud noise. Sympathetic responses include **vasoconstriction** (constriction of blood vessels), increase in blood pressure, dilation of pupils, cardiac acceleration, and goose bumps. If you attend for a few more seconds, you will notice the glandular secretion of sweat under your arms. All these fall into the category of "flight, fight, or fright" responses. Your body dumps the hormone norepinephrine into your system to provide you with a means of responding to danger, although the speed of modern emergencies such as automobile accidents clearly outstrips the rate of sympathetic responses (wear your seatbelt).

You may be less aware of the parasympathetic system response. This system is responsible for counteracting the effects of this preparatory act, because extraordinary muscular activity requires extraordinary energy. Parasympathetic responses include slowing of the heart rate, reduction of blood pressure, and pupillary constriction. While this view of the ANS as a pair of subsystems continually counteracting each other is useful, the reality is that the ANS is a system designed to create homeostasis rather than compensation. The ANS helps us respond to our internal and external environments in useful ways and is charged with maintaining an optimal "operating system" of the body. We do, however, encounter problems with this system when we live in highly charged, stressful environments, because our ANS will respond to those environments in a way to maximize our survival at the moment, even at the cost of our long-term viability. The CNS component of the ANS arises from the prefrontal region of the cerebral cortex, as well as from the hypothalamus, thalamus, hippocampus, brain stem, cerebellum, and spinal cord. The viscera are connected to these loci of control by means of **afferent** (ascending, typically sensory) and **efferent** (descending, typically motor) tracts.

The PNS components of the ANS include paired **sympathetic trunk ganglia** running parallel and in close proximity to the vertebral column, **plexuses** (networks of nerves), and **ganglia** (groups of cell bodies having functional unity and lying outside the CNS).

The **somatic nervous system** (voluntary component) is of major importance to speech pathology. This system involves the aspects of bodily function that are under our conscious and voluntary control, including control of all skeletal or **somatic muscles**. CNS control of muscles arises largely from the precentral region of the cerebral cortex, with neural impulses conveyed through descending motor tracts of the brain stem and spinal cord. Communication with the cranial nerves of the brain stem and with the spinal nerves of the spinal cord permits activation of the periphery of the body. Likewise, the sensory component of the somatic nervous system monitors information about the function of the skeletal muscles, their environment, and other "non-visceral" activities.

afferent: L., ad ferre, to carry toward

efferent: L., ex ferre, to carry away from

somatic: Gr., soma, body

The motor component of the somatic system may be subdivided into **pyramidal** and **extrapyramidal** systems, although defining all the anatomical correlates of this functional division is difficult. The pyramidal system arises from pyramidal cells of the motor strip of the cerebral cortex and is largely responsible for the initiation of voluntary motor acts. The extrapyramidal system also arises from the cerebral cortex (mostly from the premotor region of the frontal lobe) but is responsible for the background tone and movement supporting the primary acts. The extrapyramidal system is referred to as the **indirect system**, projecting to the basal ganglia and reticular formation.

There is one more important way of categorizing structures within the nervous system, and it is developmental in nature. The anatomical and developmental organizations overlap, and both sets of terminology are often used together.

Development Divisions

During the fourth week of embryonic development, the brain (**encephalon**) is composed of the **prosencephalon** (forebrain), **mesencephalon** (midbrain), and **rhombencephalon** (hindbrain). As the encephalon develops, further differentiation results in the telencephalon, rhinencephalon, diencephalon, metencephalon, and myelencephalon (Table 11–4). The **telencephalon** refers to the "extended" or "telescoped" brain and includes the cerebral hemispheres, the white matter immediately beneath it, the basal ganglia, and the olfactory tract. The **rhinencephalon** refers to structures within the telencephalon. The name arises from the relationship of the structures to olfaction (remember that *rhino* refers to "nose"). These are parts of the brain that developed early in our evolution and include the olfactory bulb, tract, and striae; pyriform area; intermediate olfactory area; paraterminal area; hippocampal formation; and fornix. The **diencephalon** is the next descending level and includes the thalamus, hypothalamus, pituitary gland (hypophysis), third ventricle, and optic tract. The **mesencephalon** is the midbrain of the brain stem, but also includes the cerebral peduncles, cerebral aqueduct, and the corpora quadrigemina. The **metencephalon** includes the pons, cerebellum, and a portion of the 4th ventricle. The **myelencephalon** refers to the medulla oblongata, the lowest level of the encephalon, as well as the central canal and the remainder of the 4th ventricle. The term **bulb** or **bulbar** refers technically to the pons and medulla but is nearly always used to refer to the entire brain stem, including the midbrain.

Let us examine the nervous system, beginning with the building block of the nervous system. The basic units of the nervous system are neurons, from which all larger structures arise.

Anatomy of the CNS and PNS

Although it is an understatement to say that the CNS is extremely complex, it may be a comfort to realize that there is a common denominator to all

telencephalon: Gr., telos enkephalos, end or distant brain

rhinencephalon: Gr., rhis enkephalos, nose brain

Table 11–4

Development and Elements of the Encephalon	
Development of Encephalon	
Structure	*Differentiates into*
Prosencephalon	Telencephalon (including rhinencephalon)
	Diencephalon
Mesencephalon	Mesencephalon
Rhombencephalon	Metencephalon
	Myelencephalon
Components of Levels of Encephalon	
Telencephalon	Cerebral hemispheres
	Basal ganglia
	Olfactory tract
	Rhinencephalon, including olfactory bulb, tract, and striae; pyriform area; intermediate olfactory area; paraterminal area; hippocampal formation; and fornix
	Lateral ventricle, part of third ventricle
Diencephalon	Thalamus
	Hypothalamus
	Pituitary gland (hypophysis)
	Optic tract
	Third ventricle
Mesencephalon	Midbrain
	Cerebral aqueduct
	Cerebral peduncles
	Corpora quadrigemina
Metencephalon	Pons
	Cerebellum
	Portion of fourth ventricle
Myelencephalon	Medulla oblongata
	Portion of fourth ventricle and central canal

the structures of the nervous system: All structures are made of neurons. Functionally, the smallest organizational unit of the nervous system is also the neuron and other cellular components such as glial cells, followed in complexity by the spinal arc reflex and higher reflexes and aggregates of neurons referred to as ganglia and nuclei (Table 11–5). Tracts are a means

Table 11–5

Hierarchical Order of Complexity for the Structures of the Nervous System	
Structure	**Function**
Glial cells	Nutrients to neurons, support, phagocytosis, myelin
Neuron	Communicating tissue
Reflexes	Subconscious response to environmental stimuli
Ganglia/nuclei	Aggregates of cell bodies with functional unity
Tracts	Aggregates of axons that transmit functionally united information; spinal cord
Structures of the brain stem	Aggregates of ganglia, nuclei, and tracts that mediate high-level reflexes and mediate the execution of cortical commands
Diencephalon and other subcortical structures	Aggregates of nuclei and tracts that mediate sensory information arriving at cerebrum and provide basic somatic and autonomic responses for body maintenance
Cerebellum	Aggregates of nuclei, specialized neurons, and tracts that integrate somatic and special sensory information with motor planning and command for coordinated movement
Cerebrum	All conscious sensory awareness and conscious motor function, including perception, awareness, motor planning and preparation, cognitive function, attention, decision making, voluntary motor inhibition, language function, speech function

of connecting disparate structures made up of all the smaller components, and the brain stem is made up of aggregates of the smaller structures, including nuclei and tracts. The brain stem provides the next level of complexity, followed by subcortical structures (including the diencephalon) and the cerebellum, and finally the most complex aggregate of tissue, the cerebral cortex. Let us begin with the discussion of the most basic component of the nervous system, the neuron.

Neurons

The nervous system is composed of the communicating elements, **neurons**, and support tissue, **glia** or **glial cells**. Neurons (nerve cells) are the functional building blocks of the nervous system and are unique among tissue types in that they are *communicating* tissue. Their function is to transmit information. Recently, however, the glial cell has come under close scrutiny, and it looks as if its original role as a support system for neurons grossly understates its function. Some scientists have demonstrated that without glial cells the neurons would be virtually incapable of storing information in long-term memory (e.g., Sajja, Hlavac, & VandeVord, 2016; also see Fields, 2004). Glial cells are also critical players in the development of synapses. Astrocytes secrete thrombospondin, which supports the development of synapses, so that without astrocytes there would be no communication between neurons (Allen & Eroglu, 2017).

The general structure of most neurons includes the **soma**, or cell body; a **dendrite**, which transmits information toward the soma; and an axon, which transmits information away from the soma (Table 11–6 and Figure 11–2).

Neurons respond to stimulation, and the neuron's response is the mechanism for transmitting information through the nervous system. A neuron can have one of two types of responses: excitation or inhibition. **Excitation** refers to stimulation that causes an increase of activity of the tissue stimulated. That is, if a neuron is stimulated, it increases its activity in response. It is as if you were at a traffic signal in your car, and when the light changed, the person behind you honked. Your response to this stimulation is to take off from the light (excitation). **Inhibition**, in contrast, refers to stimulation of a neuron that reduces the neuron's output. That is, when a neuron is inhibited, it reduces its activity. Again, using the traffic analogy, if you hear a siren while at the traffic light, you know that there is an emergency vehicle coming. The siren inhibits your activity, and you decide *not to move* because of that stimulation. That is an inhibitory response. Neurons with excitatory responses give an active output when stimulated, whereas those with inhibitory responses *stop* responding when they are stimulated.

Table 11–6

Basic Components of the Neuron	
Component	**Function**
Soma	Contains metabolic organelles
Dendrite	Receptor region
Axon	Transmits information from neuron
Hillock	Generator site for action potential
Myelin sheath	Insulator of axon
Schwann cells	Form myelin in PNS
Oligodendrocytes	Form myelin in CNS
Nodes of Ranvier	Permit saltatory conduction
Telodendria	Processes from axon
Terminal (end) boutons	Contain synaptic vesicles
Synaptic cleft	Region between pre- and postsynaptic neurons
Neurotransmitter	Substance that facilitates synapse

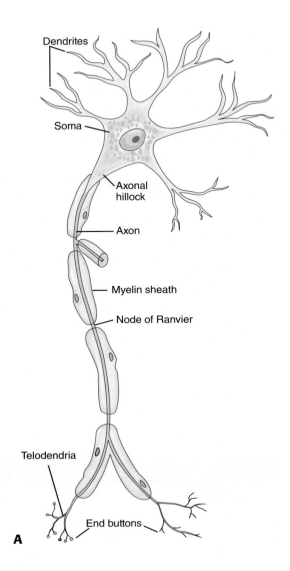

Figure 11–2. A. Schematic of basic elements of a neuron. *continues*

A

Morphology Characteristics

There are several important landmarks of the neuron (see Figures 11–1 and 11–3). A neuron may have many dendrites, often referred to as the "dendritic tree" because it looks "bushy," but it will typically have only one axon. The **axon hillock** is the junction of the axon and the soma. Many axons are covered with a white fatty wrapping called the **myelin sheath**. Myelin is made up of **Schwann cells** in the PNS and of **oligodendrocytes** in the CNS, but in both cases myelin serves a very important function: it speeds up neural conduction. This means that axons (fibers) that have myelin wrapping around them are capable of conducting impulses at a much greater rate than those that do not have myelin. This will be very important when you study diseases that destroy the myelin, such as multiple sclerosis.

Myelin is segmented, so that it resembles a series of hot dog buns linked together. The areas between the myelinated segments are known as **nodes of Ranvier**, and we will see that these are important in conduction as well. If you follow the axon to its end point, you can see **telodendria**, which are

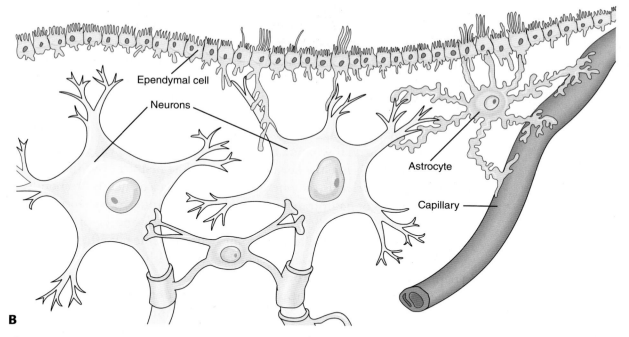

Figure 11–2. *continued* **B.** Astrocyte, a glial cell that supports the transport of nutrients to the neuron while shielding it from toxins via the blood-brain barrier. *Source:* From Seikel/Drumright/King. *Anatomy & Physiology for Speech, Language, and Hearing, 5th Ed.* ©Cengage, Inc. Reproduced by permission.

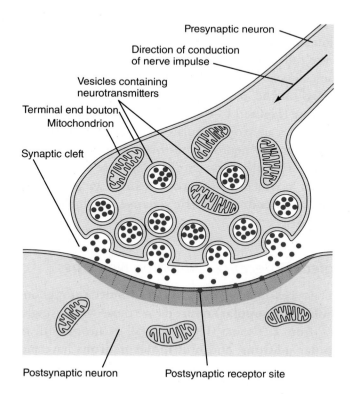

Figure 11–3. Schematic of elements of synapse. Note that the synapse consists of the terminal end bouton, synaptic cleft, and postsynaptic receptor sites. *Source:* From Seikel/Drumright/King. *Anatomy & Physiology for Speech, Language, and Hearing, 5th Ed.* ©Cengage, Inc. Reproduced by permission.

long, thin projections. The telodendria have **terminal (end) boutons** (or **buttons**), and within the boutons are **synaptic vesicles**. Synaptic vesicles contain a special chemical known as neurotransmitter substance (or simply *neurotransmitter*). **Neurotransmitters** are compounds that are responsible for activating the next neuron in a chain of neurons. As we will discuss later on in this chapter, neurotransmitter is released into the gap between two neurons (the **synaptic cleft**). The boutons also contain **mitochondria**, organelles responsible for energy generation and protein development. Groups of cell bodies appear gray and are referred to as **gray matter**, whereas **white matter** refers to myelin.

The synapse deserves special discussion. When a neuron is sufficiently stimulated, the axon discharges neurotransmitter into the synaptic cleft. The neurotransmitter is like the key to your door: The neurotransmitter released into the synaptic cleft is the one to which the adjacent neuron responds. If some other class of neurotransmitter makes its way into that synaptic region, it will have no effect on the adjacent neuron. This lock-and-key arrangement lets neurons have specific effects on some neurons while not affecting others.

We speak of the neurons in a chain as being either presynaptic or postsynaptic. **Presynaptic neurons** are those "upstream" from the synapse and are the ones that stimulate the **postsynaptic neurons** (the ones following the synapse). This makes sense when you realize that information passes in only one direction from a neuron: Information enters generally at the dendrite and exits at the axon.

Neurotransmitter released into the synaptic cleft stimulates **receptor sites** on the postsynaptic neuron. When the postsynaptic neuron is stimulated, ion channels in its membrane open up and allow ions to enter, and this leads to a discharge, or firing, of that neuron as well. Dendrites are the typical location for synapse on the receiving neurons, and the synapses in this location are called **axodendritic synapses**. Synapse may also occur on the soma: These are called **axosomatic synapses** and are usually inhibitory. If synapse occurs on the axons of the postsynaptic neuron, it is called an **axoaxonic synapse** (Figure 11–4), and these synapses tend to be modulatory in nature. Sometimes an axon stimulates a neuron secondarily on its way to the synapse with another neuron, and this is referred to as ***en passant*** ("in passing") synapse. Two other less common synapse formations are **somato-somatic synapse**, in which the soma of a neuron synapses with the soma of another neuron, and **dendrodendritic synapse**, in which communication is between two dendrites.

Morphological Differences Between Neurons

There are several types or *forms* of neurons distributed throughout the nervous system. **Unipolar (monopolar) neurons** are those with a single, bifurcating process arising from the soma (Figure 11–5). Neurons with two processes are called **bipolar neurons**, and **multipolar neurons** have more than two processes. Sensory neurons are generally unipolar or pseudo-unipolar. The exception is neurons that transmit information about smell (olfaction), hearing (**audition**), and vestibular senses: These are bipolar.

Glial cells make up approximately half of the brain tissue (Azevado et al., 2009), providing support and nutrients to the neurons. **Astrocytes**

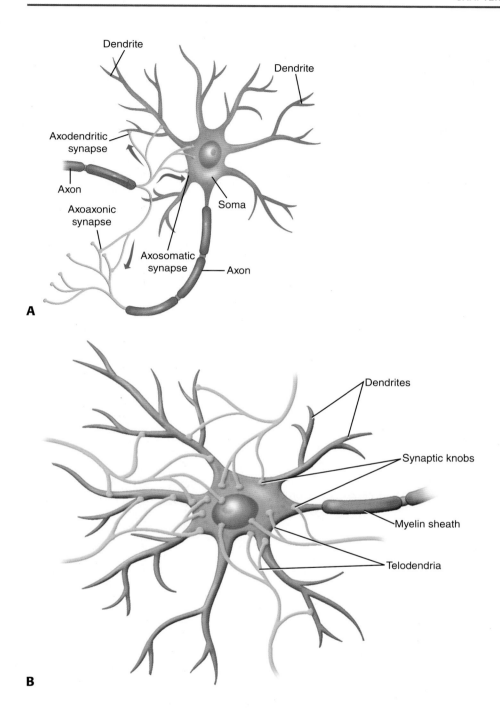

Figure 11–4. A. Types of synapses, including axodendritic (excitatory), axosomatic (inhibitory), and axoaxonic (modulatory). **B.** Illustration of excitatory and inhibitory synapses on a postsynaptic neuron. Note that excitatory axons synapse on the dendrite, while inhibitory axons synapse at the cell body. *Source:* From Seikel/Drumright/King. *Anatomy & Physiology for Speech, Language, and Hearing, 5th Ed.* ©Cengage, Inc. Reproduced by permission.

appear to be largely structural, separating neurons from one another and adhering to capillaries. They play a role in supplying nutrients to neurons, as well as in ion and neurotransmitter regulation at the synapse. Oligodendrocytes are glial cells that make up the CNS myelin, and **Schwann cells** are glia constituting the myelin of the PNS. Although technically not neurons, glial cells are an important component of the nervous system tissue. Astrocytes provide the primary support for neurons, aid in the suspension of neurons, and transport nutrients from the capillary supply. They also provide the important **blood–brain barrier**, a membranous filter system that prohibits

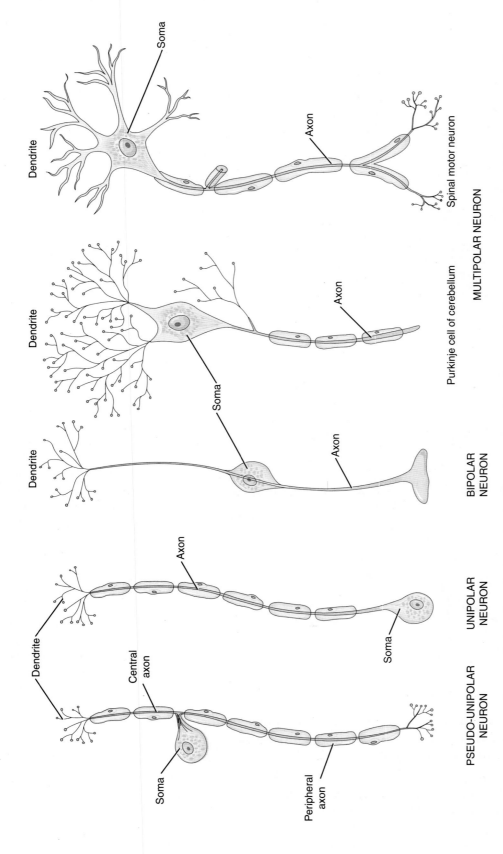

Soma

Dendrite

Axon

Spinal motor neuron

MULTIPOLAR NEURON

Dendrite

Axon

Soma

Purkinje cell of cerebellum

Dendrite

Soma

Axon

BIPOLAR NEURON

Axon

Soma

UNIPOLAR NEURON

Dendrite

Central axon

Peripheral axon

Soma

PSEUDO-UNIPOLAR NEURON

Figure 11–5. Types of neurons. Pseudo-unipolar and unipolar neurons are primarily somatic afferent neurons, whereas bipolar neurons mediate special senses. Multipolar neurons, which are primarily efferent, include spinal motor neurons, Purkinje cells of the cerebellum, and pyramidal cells (not shown). *Source:* From Seikel/Drumright/King. *Anatomy & Physiology for Speech, Language, and Hearing, 5th Ed.* ©Cengage, Inc. Reproduced by permission.

some toxins from passing from the cerebrovascular system to neurons (de Vries, Kuiper, de Boer, Van Berkel, & Breimer, 1997; O'Brown, Pfau, & Gu, 2018).

Yet another type of glial cell, **microglia**, performs the housekeeping process known as *phagocytosis* (e.g., Tremblay, Cookson, & Civiero, 2019). Microglia scavenge necrotic tissue formed by a lesion in the nervous system. Astrocytes assist by forming scarring around necrotic tissue, effectively isolating it from the rest of the brain tissue.

Neuroscience is now taking a very hard look at the role of astrocytes. We have long known that they had an important role in support of neurons, including nutrient delivery, but only recently has evidence emerged to indicate that glial cells are critical to the creation of long-term memory, as well as to the formation of synapses (Suzuki et al., 2011).

Functional Differences Between Neurons

There are *functional* differences between neurons as well. **Interneurons** make up the largest class of neurons in the brain. The job of interneurons is to provide communication between other types of neurons, and interneurons do not exit the central nervous system. Another type of neuron is the **motor neuron**. Motor neurons are efferent in nature, and they are typically bipolar neurons that activate muscular or glandular response. These neurons usually have long axons that are myelinated. Motor neurons are further differentiated based on size, **conduction velocity** (how fast they can conduct an impulse), and the degree of myelination. Generally speaking, a neuron with a wider axon and thicker myelin will have more rapid conduction of neural impulses.

Neuronal fibers are classified in terms of conduction velocity as being A, B, or C class fibers. The A and B fibers are myelinated. The **A fibers** are further broken down, based on conduction velocity, into **alpha, beta, gamma**, and **delta fibers** (Table 11–7). **Alpha motor neurons** have high conduction velocities (50–120 m/s) and innervate the majority of skeletal muscle, called **extrafusal muscle fibers**. Slower-velocity **gamma motor neurons** innervate **intrafusal muscle fibers** within the muscle spindle, the sensory apparatus responsible for maintaining muscle length. Thus, alpha motor neurons activate the prime movers of the motor act; gamma motor neurons are responsible for maintaining muscle tone and muscle readiness for the motor act.

Sensory alpha fibers are identified by a Roman numeral and a lowercase letter (**type Ia, Ib, II, III, or IV fibers**), reflecting a different classification scheme. The Ia neurons are the primary afferent fibers from the muscle spindle, whereas the Ib neurons send sensory information generated at the Golgi tendon organs, sensors that respond to the stretching of the tendon. Type II afferent fibers are secondary muscle spindle afferents of the beta class and convey information from touch and pressure receptors. The type III afferent fibers are delta class, conducting pain, pressure, touch, and coolness sensations. Type IV fibers convey pain and warmth senses. Again, some sensory neurons are essential for movement, and these include types Ia, Ib,

Table 11–7

Type A, B, and C Sensory and Motor Fibers			
Fiber Class	**Velocity (m/s)**	**Motor Function**	**Sensory**
Class A			
A α (alpha)	50–120	Large alpha motor neurons innervating extrafusal muscle	
A α Ia	120		Primary muscle spindle afferents
A α Ib	120		Golgi tendon organs; touch and pressure receptors
A β (beta)	70	Motor axons serving extrafusal and intrafusal fibers	
A β II	70		Secondary afferents of muscle spindles; secondary afferents for touch, pressure, vibration
A γ (gamma)	40	Gamma motor neurons serving muscle spindles	
A δ III (delta)	15		Touch, pressure, pain, temperature sensation
Class B			
B	14	Unmyelinated, pre-ganglion autonomic fibers	
Class C			
C	2	Unmyelinated post-ganglion autonomic fibers	
C IV	2		Unmyelinated pain, temperature fibers

Source: Data from Winans, Gilman, Manter, and Gatz (2002).

and II. Types III and IV are important for transmitting other body senses (pain, temperature, pressure) but are not essential to movement.

✅ To summarize:

- The **nervous system** is a complex, hierarchical structure made up of **neurons**.
- Many **motor functions** become automated through practice.
- **Voluntary movement**, **sensory awareness**, and **cognitive function** are the domain of the **cerebral cortex**, although we are capable of sensation and response without consciousness.

- The communication links of the nervous system are **spinal nerves, cranial nerves**, and **tracts** of the **brain stem** and **spinal cord**.

- The nervous system may be divided functionally as **autonomic** and **somatic nervous systems** serving involuntary and voluntary functions, respectively.

- The nervous system may be divided anatomically as **central** and **peripheral nervous systems** as well.

- **Developmental divisions** separate the brain into the **prosencephalon** (which is further divided into telencephalon and diencephalon), the **mesencephalon** or midbrain, and the **rhombencephalon**, which includes the metencephalon and myelencephalon.

- **Neurons** are widely varied in morphology but may be broadly categorized as **unipolar**, **bipolar**, or **multipolar**.

- Neurons communicate through **synapse** by means of **neurotransmitter** substance, and the response by the postsynaptic neuron may be **excitatory** or **inhibitory**.

- The size and type of axon is related to the conduction of neural impulse.

- **Glial cells** provide the fatty sheath for **myelinated axons**, support structure for neurons, and long-term memory potentiation.

Anatomy of the Cerebrum

The cerebrum is the mostly highly evolved and organized structure of the human body. This is the largest structure of the nervous system, weighing approximately 3 pounds and made up of billions of neurons and glial cells. The cerebrum is divided into grossly similar left and right hemispheres and is wrapped by three meningeal linings that protect and support the massive structure of the brain. We will discuss those meningeal linings first and then introduce you to the most important structure of your body.

The brain remains one of the most complex structures in the known universe. The cells of the brain are packed to extraordinary density: one cubic centimeter (1 cm × 1 cm × 1 cm) contains on the order of 44 million neurons (Pakkenberg & Gunderson, 2011), and for every cubic centimeter of gray matter, there are nearly 90 billion synapses. This is some very dense tissue.

Meningeal Linings

The CNS is invested with a triple-layer meningeal lining serving important protective and nutritive functions. There are three meningeal linings covering the brain. The **dura mater** is a tough bi-layered lining, which is the most superficial of the meningeal linings (Figure 11–6). The dura mater itself is made up of two layers that are tightly bound together. The outer layer is more inelastic than the inner layer, and meningeal arteries course through this

dura mater: L., tough mother

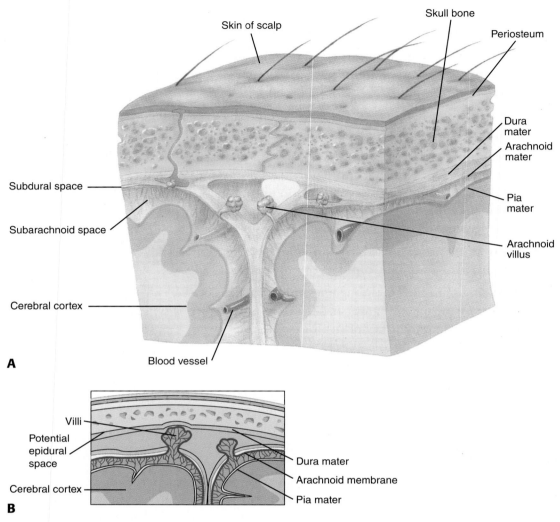

Figure 11–6. A. Meningeal linings of the brain. **B.** Schematic of meningeal linings. *Source: From Seikel/Drumright/King. Anatomy & Physiology for Speech, Language, and Hearing, 5th Ed.* ©Cengage, Inc. Reproduced by permission. *continues*

layer. Whereas the layers making up the dura mater are bound together, the potential space superficial to the dura mater is called the **epidural space**, a term that will gain meaning when discussing vascular lesions that can release blood into the areas of the brain (e.g., *epidural hematoma* is a hemorrhagic release of blood into the space between the two layers of the dura mater). The epidural space doesn't really exist until it is filled with blood from a hemorrhage.

The **arachnoid mater** is a covering through which many blood vessels for the brain pass. The arachnoid lining is a lacey, spiderlike structure separating the dura mater from the innermost meningeal lining, the **pia mater**. The pia mater is a thin, membranous covering that closely follows the contour of the brain. The major arteries and veins serving the surface of the brain course within this layer.

pia mater: L., pious mother; so named because of its gentle but faithful attachment to the cerebral cortex

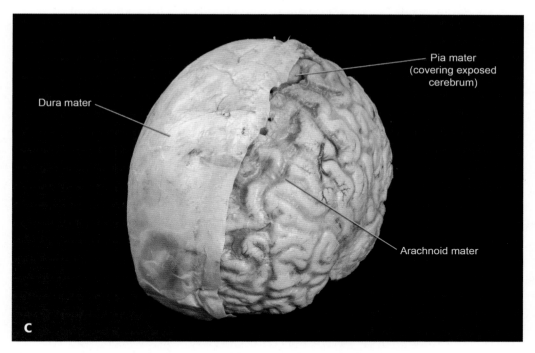

Figure 11–6. *continued* **C.** Meningeal linings on the cerebral cortex.

The function of the meningeal linings is to protect the brain, holding structures in place during movement and providing support for those structures. To provide this protection, the linings must conform to the structure of the brain. As part of this support, the dura mater takes on four major infoldings, which separate the major structures of the brain, providing some isolation. The four infoldings are the falx cerebri, falx cerebelli, tentorium cerebelli, and diaphragma sella. The falx cerebri and falx cerebelli are sagittal dividers, separating left and right structures of the brain, while the tentorium cerebelli and diaphragma sella separate brain structures by means of a transversely posed membrane.

The **falx cerebri** separates the two cerebral hemispheres with a vertical sheath of dura, running from the crista galli of the ethmoid to the tentorium cerebelli. The falx cerebri completely separates the two hemispheres down to the level of the **corpus callosum**. The **falx cerebelli** performs the same function for the cerebellum, separating the left and right cerebellar hemispheres for protection and isolation (Figure 11–7).

The **tentorium cerebelli** is a horizontal dural shelf at the base of the skull that divides the cranium into superior (cerebral) and inferior (cerebellar) regions. The **diaphragma sella** forms a boundary between the pituitary gland and the hypothalamus and optic chiasm. The dura mater encircles the cranial nerves as they exit the brain stem. Because of its placement, the tentorium cerebelli supports the cerebrum and keeps its mass from compressing the cerebellum and brain stem, as would most certainly happen if the dural lining was absent. The dural shelves can be liabilities when trauma results in **subdural hematoma**, a release of blood through hemorrhage beneath the

corpus callosum: L., large (or hard) body

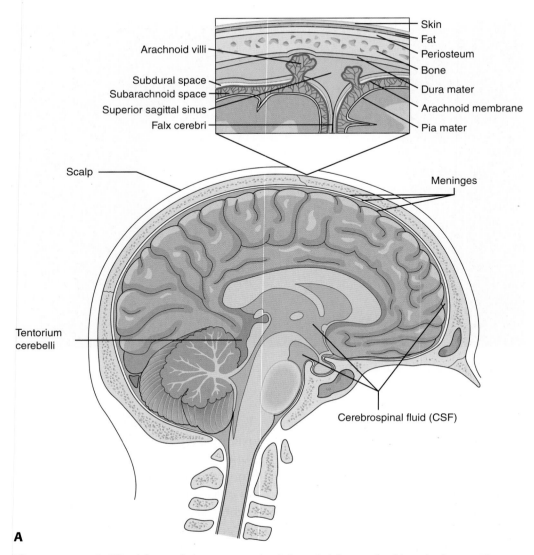

Arachnoid villi

Subdural space
Subarachnoid space
Superior sagittal sinus
Falx cerebri

Skin
Fat
Periosteum
Bone
Dura mater
Arachnoid membrane
Pia mater

Scalp

Meninges

Tentorium
cerebelli

Cerebrospinal fluid (CSF)

A

Figure 11–7. A. The falx cerebri separates the left and right cerebral hemispheres. The tentorium cerebelli separates the cerebellum from the cerebrum. The falx cerebelli (not shown) separates the cerebellar hemispheres. (Data from Winans, Gilman, Manter, & Gatz, 2002.) *Source:* From Seikel/Drumright/King. *Anatomy & Physiology for Speech, Language, and Hearing, 5th Ed.* ©Cengage, Inc. Reproduced by permission. *continues*

dura that can push on the cerebrum, causing the temporal lobe to herniate under the tentorium. Subdural hematoma may also cause a life-threatening herniation of the brain stem into the foramen magnum.

There are meningeal linings of the spinal cord as well, paralleling the structure and function of the cerebral meninges. At the foramen magnum, the meningeal linings are continuous with the **spinal meningeal linings**. The spinal meninges are broadly similar to those of the brain, with some exceptions. The dura of the brain adheres to the bone, but the dura of the spinal cord does not adhere to the vertebrae. As with the brain meninges, cerebrospinal fluid flows through the subarachnoid space. Likewise, the pia

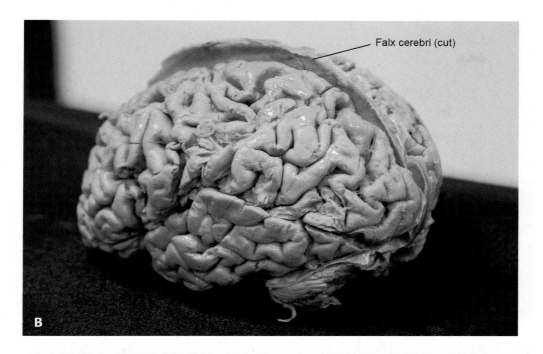

Falx cerebri (cut)

B

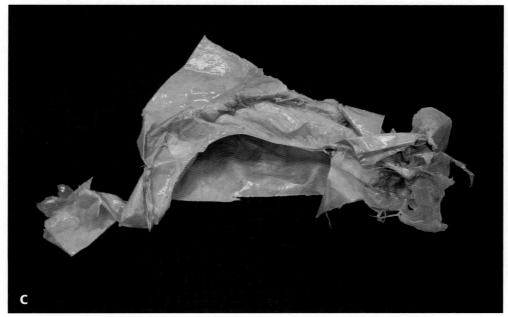

C

Figure 11–7. *continued* **B.** Falx cerebri as seen in situ between hemispheres. **C.** Excised falx cerebri. *continues*

mater closely follows the surface of the spinal cord but serves an anchoring function as well. The cord is attached to the dura by means of 22 pairs of **denticulate ligaments** arising from the pia. The dura extends laterally to encapsulate the dorsal root ganglion. At the inferior cord, the pia is continuous with the filum terminale, which is attached to the first segment of the coccyx (Figure 11–8).

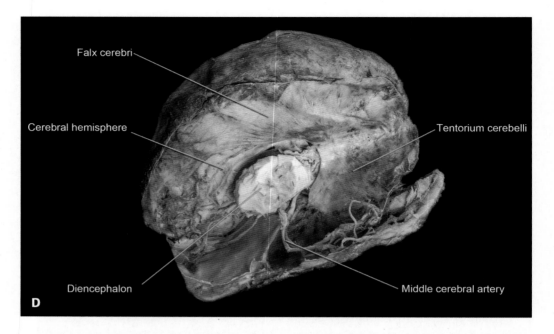

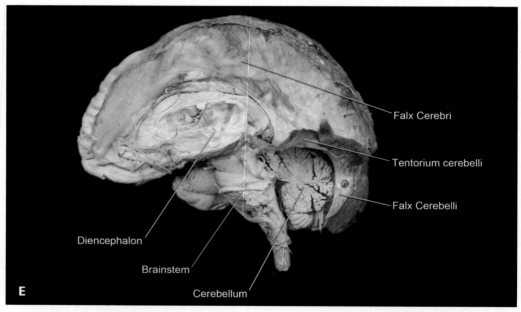

Figure 11–7. *continued* **D.** Falx cerebri and tentorium cerebelli. **E.** Falx cerebelli and tentorium cerebelli in relation to cerebellum and falx cerebri.

Arnold–Chiari Malformation

Arnold–Chiari malformation (or simply Chiari malformation) is a condition in which the space within the posterior skull is too small for the structures. Essentially, the cerebellum and the brain stem can herniate through the foramen magnum, causing a number of signs. Included in the problems associated with Chiari malformation are dizziness, ataxia (gait problems of cerebellar origin), hydrocephaly (increased cerebrospinal fluid pressure from the occlusion of the cerebral aqueduct), and muscular weakness.

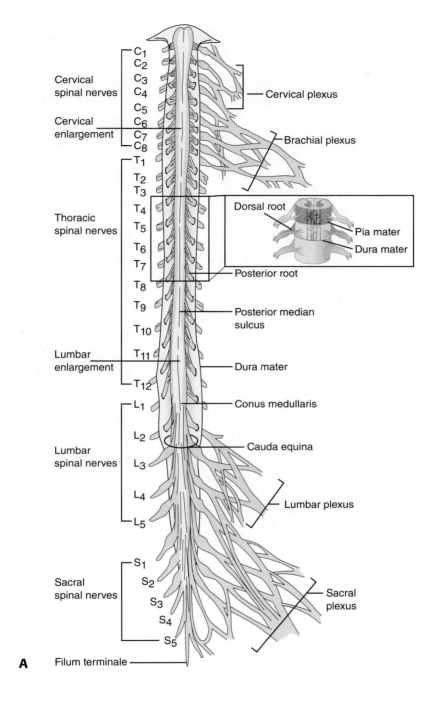

Cervical spinal nerves

C1
C2
C3
C4
C5
C6

Cervical enlargement

C7
C8

Cervical plexus

Brachial plexus

Thoracic spinal nerves

T1
T2
T3
T4
T5
T6
T7
T8
T9
T10

Dorsal root

Pia mater

Dura mater

Posterior root

Posterior median sulcus

Lumbar enlargement

T11
T12

Dura mater

L1

Conus medullaris

L2

Cauda equina

Lumbar spinal nerves

L3
L4
L5

Lumbar plexus

Sacral spinal nerves

S1
S2
S3
S4
S5

Sacral plexus

A Filum terminale

Figure 11–8. A. Spinal cord and emerging spinal nerves. Note the inset showing the meningeal linings of the spinal cord. *Source:* From Seikel/Drumright/King. *Anatomy & Physiology for Speech, Language, and Hearing, 5th Ed.* ©Cengage, Inc. Reproduced by permission. *continues*

Together, the meningeal linings provide an excellent means of nurturing and protecting the CNS structures. The dura is a tough structure that provides a barrier between the bone of the skull and the delicate neural tissue, and to which blood vessels can be anchored as they pass to the cerebrum. The delicate pia mater completely envelopes the cerebrum, supporting the blood vessels as they serve the surface of the brain. Between the dura and pia is the arachnoid lining, through which a cushioning fluid, cerebrospinal fluid, flows. A similar network supports the spinal cord within the vertebral column. Thus, the meninges support the brain, separate major structures, and maintain the brain in its fluid suspension. In this manner, the brain is

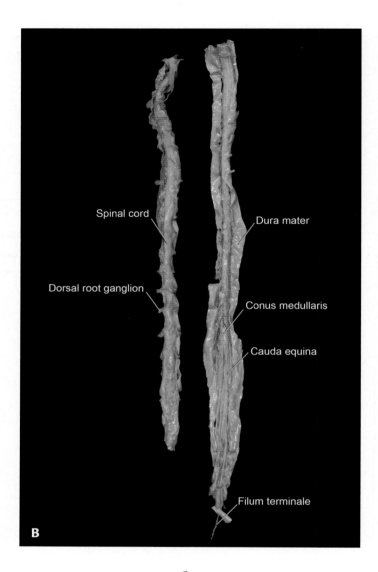

B

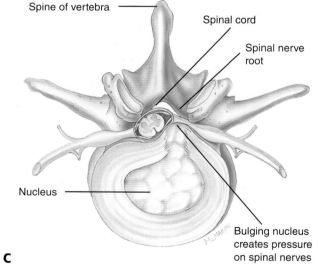

C

Figure 11–8. *continued* **B.** Photograph of excised spinal cords. *Source:* From *Neuroanatomy & Neurophysiology for Speech and Hearing Sciences* by Seikel, J. A., Konstantopoulos, K., & Drumright, D. G. Copyright © 2020 Plural Publishing, Inc. **C.** Illustration of herniated vertebral disc and subsequent compression of spinal nerves. *Source:* From Seikel/Drumright/King. *Anatomy & Physiology for Speech, Language, and Hearing, 5th Ed.* ©Cengage, Inc. Reproduced by permission.

Hematoma

Hematoma is a pooling of blood, typically arising from the breakage of a blood vessel. Subdural hematoma involves intracranial bleeding beneath the dura mater caused by the rupture of cortical arteries or veins, usually because of trauma to the head. Pressure from the pooling blood displaces the brain, shifting and compressing the brain stem, forcing the temporal lobe under the tentorium cerebelli, and compressing cerebral arteries. This critically dangerous condition may not be immediately recognized, because it may take several hours before pooling blood sufficiently compresses the brain to produce symptoms such as reduced consciousness, hemiparesis, pupillary dilation, and other symptoms associated with compressed cranial nerves. **Epidural hematoma**, hematoma occurring above the dura mater, may result in a patient being initially lucid but displaying progressively decreasing levels of consciousness, reflecting compression of the brain.

Hematomas are characterized by the location of insult. **Frontal epidural hematomas** arise from blows to the frontal bone and may result in personality changes. **Posterior fossa epidural hematomas** arise from blows to the back of the head, producing visual and coordination deficits.

able to overcome many otherwise dangerous shocks from external acceleration, such as those experienced during falls or blunt trauma. You may wish to read the Clinical Note "An Ounce of Prevention" for a brief discussion of what happens when these protective measures are not enough.

The Ventricles and Cerebrospinal Fluid

The CNS is bathed in **cerebrospinal fluid (CSF)**, which provides a cushion for the delicate and dense neural tissue as well as some nutrient delivery and waste removal. Examining the system of ventricles and canals through which the CSF flows will help you as we describe the cerebral cortex and subcortical structures. You will want to refer to Figure 11–9 for this discussion.

An Ounce of Prevention

Should you choose to work in a trauma center, a significant portion of your caseload will arise from traumatic brain injury (TBI). TBI is one of the leading causes of death in individuals under 24 years of age, with transportation-related brain injury far exceeding all other causes (falls, assaults, sport, firearms). The addition of seat and lap belts to automobiles has resulted in a reduction of death in automobile accidents arising from brain injury by nearly 50%. Unfortunately, use of alcohol is related to reduced seatbelt use and increased death arising from head injury during accidents. Mandatory use of helmets has reduced the frequency of brain injury in motorcycle accidents by 20% to 50% and up to 85% for bicycle riders.

Gunshot wounds to the head result in most deaths attributable to firearms, and handguns are involved in more than 60% of homicides. More than 40,000 people in the United States are killed by firearms annually. Whereas laws that restrict access to firearms are hotly debated as a constitutional issue, the ability to eliminate accidental firearm deaths through trigger lock systems could greatly reduce the carnage that occurs in the United States, a country in which nearly 50% of the households have firearms. You will want to refer to Mackay, Chapman, and Morgan (1997) for a thorough review of the causes and treatment in TBI.

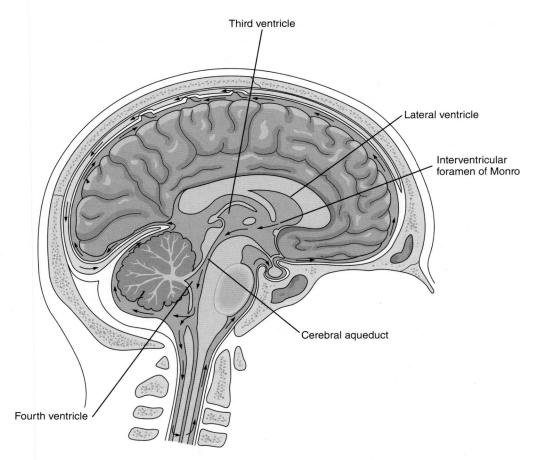

Figure 11–9. Ventricles of the brain. *Source:* From Seikel/Drumright/King. *Anatomy & Physiology for Speech, Language, and Hearing, 5th Ed.* ©Cengage, Inc. Reproduced by permission.

The ventricles of the brain are spaces within the brain through which CSF flows. They are cavities that are, in reality, remnants of the embryonic neural tube. The system of ventricles consists of four cavities: the right lateral ventricle, the left lateral ventricle, the third ventricle, and the fourth ventricle. Within each ventricle is a **choroid plexus**, an aggregate of tissue that produces CSF. Whereas all ventricles produce CSF, the plexuses of the lateral ventricles produce the bulk of the fluid. The cavities are ideally suited to act as buffers for the delicate brain tissue. If you remember the discussion of the meningeal linings, you will recall that the cerebrum is supported by the tough dura and delicate pia and that CSF flows between these two linings within the arachnoid space. That CSF buffers the cerebral hemispheres and structures from sudden movements of the head (accelerations), and the addition of CSF within the brain by means of ventricles further buoys up the brain against trauma.

There are two **lateral ventricles**, which are the largest of the ventricles. These ventricles are composed of four spaces bounded superiorly by the corpus callosum that extend into each of the lobes of the cerebrum. The lateral ventricles are shaped somewhat like horseshoes opened toward the front, but with posterior horns attached. The **anterior horn** of the lateral ventricles projects into the frontal lobe to the genu of the corpus callosum. The medial wall is the septum pellucidum, and the inferior margin is the head of the caudate nucleus. The **central portion**, located within the parietal lobe, includes the region between the **interventricular foramen of Monro** and the splenium, with the superior border being the corpus callosum, the medial boundary being the septum pellucidum, and the inferior being portions of the caudate nucleus. The **posterior** or **occipital horn** extends into the occipital lobe to a tapered end, with its superior and lateral surfaces being the corpus callosum. The **inferior horn** extends into the temporal lobe, curving down behind the thalamus to terminate blindly behind the temporal pole. The hippocampus marks the lower margin of the inferior horn. The lateral ventricles communicate with the third ventricle via the interventricular foramen of Monro.

The **third ventricle** is the unpaired medial cavity between the left and right thalami and hypothalami. The roof of the third ventricle is the tela choroidea, and the ventricle extends inferiorly to the level of the optic chiasm. The prominent **interthalamic adhesion** (massa intermedia or intermediate mass) bridges the ventricle, connecting the two thalami. The CSF of the lateral ventricle passes into the third ventricle by means of left and right interventricular foramina.

The **fourth ventricle** is shaped roughly like a diamond, projecting upward from the central canal of the spinal cord and lower medulla. This ventricle is difficult to envision because it is the space between the brain stem and cerebellum. One must remove the cerebellum to see the fourth ventricle. The floor of the fourth ventricle is the junction of the pons and the medulla, and the cerebellum forms the roof and posterior margin. The fourth ventricle has three openings or **apertures**. The **median aperture (foramen of Magendie)** and the paired left and right **lateral apertures (foramina of Luschka)** permit CSF to flow into the subarachnoid space behind the brain stem and beneath the cerebellum.

Circulation of CSF depends upon a pressure gradient. In this case, CSF is created in the ventricles, and the increased pressure causes CSF to flow toward the periphery. CSF is the clear, fluid product of the choroid plexus in each of the ventricles. It provides an excellent cushion to protect the brain against trauma and also serves a transport function, as mentioned previously. The volume of CSF in the nervous system is approximately 125 mL, which is replenished every 7 hours. The fluid is under a constant pressure that changes with body position, and life-threatening conditions can develop should something occlude the pathway for CSF.

Circulation of CSF begins in each of the lateral ventricles, coursing through the interventricular foramina of Monro to the third ventricle. From there, the fluid flows through the minute cerebral aqueduct to the fourth ventricle, where it drains into the subarachnoid space through the foramen of Luschka and the foramen of Magendie to the cerebellomedullary cistern beneath the cerebellum. From there the fluid freely circulates around the brain and spinal cord. CSF then can course around the cerebellum and cerebrum to exit through the arachnoid granulation in sinuses of the dura mater, ultimately absorbed by the venous system. Alternatively, the CSF courses downward through the foramen magnum and subarachnoid space around the spinal cord.

✅ To summarize:

- The **cerebral cortex** is protected from physical insults by **cerebrospinal fluid** and the **meningeal linings**, the **dura**, **pia**, and **arachnoid mater**.

- The meninges provide support for delicate neural and vascular tissue, with the dura dividing into regions that correspond to the regions of the brain supported.

- The **spinal meningeal linings** similarly protect the spinal cord from movement trauma.

- Cerebrospinal fluid originating within the **ventricles** of the brain and circulating around the spinal cord cushions these structures from trauma associated with rapid acceleration.

ANAQUEST LESSON ▶

Layers of Cerebrum

The cerebrum consists of two **cerebral hemispheres** or roughly equal halves of the brain (Figure 11–10). The term **cortex** means "bark," referring to the bark or outer surface of a tree, and the cerebral cortex is the outer surface of the brain. The cortex is between 2 and 4 mm thick, being comprised of six cell layers.

The layers of the cortex consist of two basic cell types: pyramidal and non-pyramidal cells. **Pyramidal cells** are large, pyramid-shaped cells that are involved in motor function. Pyramidal cells are oriented so that the apex of the pyramid is directed toward the surface of the cortex, with the base directed medially. A single apical dendrite projects through cortex layers toward the surface, whereas multiple basal dendrites course laterally through the layer in which the cell body resides. Axons of pyramidal cells typically project to the white matter beneath the cortex or beyond, although they have branches within the cortex itself.

Non-pyramidal cells are small and often stellate (star shaped) and are involved in sensory function or intercommunication between brain regions. Their axons typically project only a short distance, either within a cortex layer or adjacent layers. Functionally, these non-pyramidal cells connect local regions, whereas pyramidal cells project to more distant regions.

The outermost layer of the cerebral cortex consists mostly of glial cells and axons from neurons of succeeding layers. The second and third layers consist of small and large pyramidal cells, respectively, and are thus highly involved in motor function. The fourth layer receives sensory input from the thalamus and consists of non-pyramidal cells, whereas the fifth layer is made up of large pyramidal cells that project to motor centers beyond the cerebrum

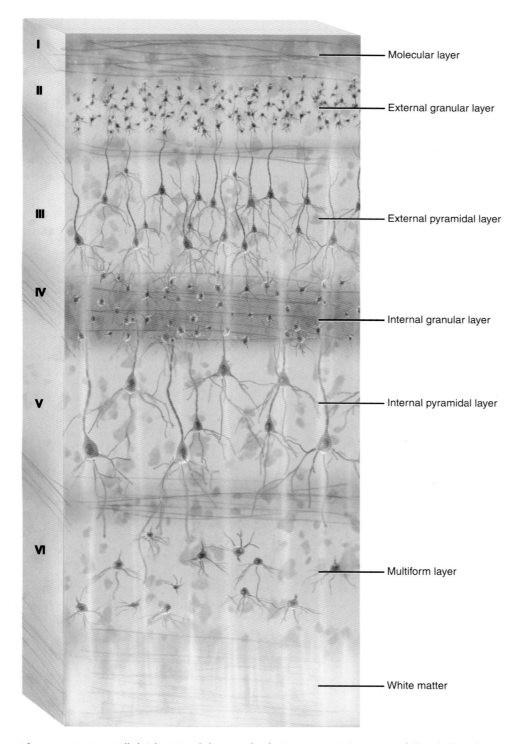

Molecular layer

External granular layer

External pyramidal layer

Internal granular layer

Internal pyramidal layer

Multiform layer

White matter

Figure 11–10. Cellular layers of the cerebral cortex. Layer I is termed the molecular layer, consisting of glial cells and axons from neurons. Layer II is the external granular layer, made up of small pyramidal cells. Layer III is the external pyramidal layer, made up of large pyramidal cells. Layer IV is the internal granular layer, which receives sensory input from the thalamus. Layer V is the internal pyramidal layer, and the cells from this layer project to distant motor sites. Layer VI is the multiform layer, consists of pyramidal cells that project to the basal ganglia, brain stem, and spinal cord. *Source:* From Seikel/Drumright/King. *Anatomy & Physiology for Speech, Language, and Hearing, 5th Ed.* ©Cengage, Inc. Reproduced by permission.

(basal ganglia, brain stem, and spinal cord). The sixth layer also consists of pyramidal cells, although these project to the thalamus.

The layers have varying densities within the cerebrum, corresponding to the dominant function for a specific region. For instance, the pyramidal layers are thickest in the areas of the cortex responsible for motor function, whereas the granular layers are most richly represented in the areas of the brain that process predominantly sensory input. The region of primary motor output (the motor strip) has extremely rich representation of the fifth layer, with a very thin fourth layer, while the primary sensory areas have a rich layer fourth with a few cells in the pyramidal layers. Areas involved in the association of sensory and motor functions have representation of both sensory and motor layers.

Much of our early knowledge concerning the cell structure of the cortical layers arose from the work of Korbinian Brodmann in the early part of the twentieth century (Kandel, 2012). His microscopic examination of the cerebral cortex revealed the dominant cell types of the cortical layers, and his keen analysis showed that the localized areas of the brain were dominated by specific cell types, as discussed. From his work came what has become known as the "Brodmann map" of the cerebrum (Figure 11–11 and Table 11–8), a tool that remains a mainstay for navigating the regions of the cerebrum.

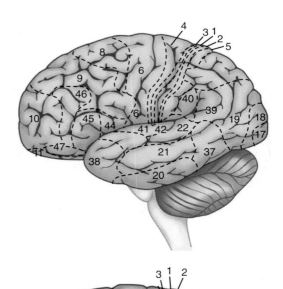

Figure 11–11. A. Brodmann map of lateral and medial cerebrum. *Source:* From Seikel/Drumright/King. *Anatomy & Physiology for Speech, Language, and Hearing, 5th Ed.* ©Cengage, Inc. Reproduced by permission. *continues*   **A**

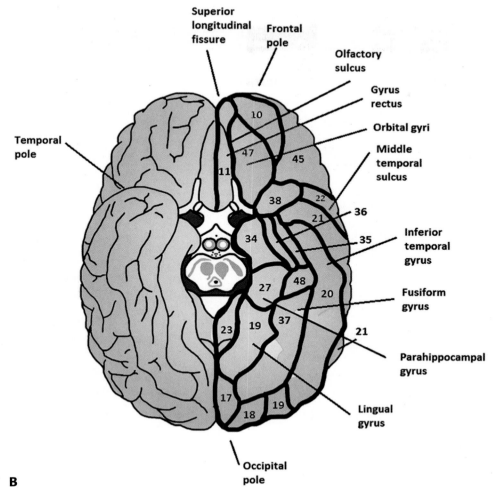

Figure 11–11. *continued* **B.** Brodmann map of inferior cerebrum. *Source:* From *Neuroanatomy & Neurophysiology for Speech and Hearing Sciences* by Seikel, J. A., Konstantopoulos, K., & Drumright, D. G. Copyright © 2020 Plural Publishing, Inc.

Brodmann's observations proved to be quite important, and his notation has served many decades of neuroscience study. You will want to refer to this figure as we discuss landmarks of the superficial cortex.

Landmarks of Cerebrum

The **cerebral longitudinal fissure** (also known as the **superior longitudinal fissure** and the **interhemispheric fissure**) separates the left and right cerebral hemispheres, as can be seen in Figure 11–12 and the photographs in Figure 11–13. Remember from our discussion of the meningeal linings that the falx cerebri runs between the two hemispheres through this space. The cerebral longitudinal fissure completely separates the hemispheres down to the level of the corpus callosum, a major group of fibers providing communication between the two hemispheres. Within the cerebral longitudinal fissure reside the anterior cerebral artery and its collaterals.

Table 11–8

Locations Associated With Brodmann Areas (Ba)

Brodmann Number	Name and Putative Function	Location
3	Rostral postcentral gyrus (somatic sense reception area; a.k.a. *area postcentralis oralis*)	Rostral postcentral gyrus
1	Intermediate postcentral gyrus (somatic sense integration; a.k.a. *area postcentralis intermedia*)	Postcentral gyrus
2	Caudal postcentral gyrus (somatic sense integration; a.k.a. *area postcentralis caudalis*)	Caudal postcentral gyrus
4	Precentral gyrus (motor strip or primary motor cortex; a.k.a. gigantopyramidal; *area gigantopyramidalis*)	Precentral gyrus
5	Preparietal (a.k.a. *area preparietalis*)	Dorsal parietal lobe; part of superior parietal lobule
6	Premotor cortex (premotor area; a.k.a. agranular frontal; *area frontalis agranularis*)	Anterior to precentral gyrus in frontal lobe
7	Superior parietal (a.k.a. *area parietalis superior*)	Part of superior parietal lobule and some of precuneus in medial cerebral surface
8	Intermedial frontal (a.k.a. *frontalis intermedia*)	Part of superior frontal gyrus, with extension into cingulate gyrus; functionally part of frontal eye field controlling conjugate eye movement
9	Granular frontal area (part of dorsolateral prefrontal cortex DPFC or DLPC; a.k.a. granular frontal; *area frontalis granularis*)	Superior frontal gyrus and middle frontal gyrus
10	Anterior prefrontal cortex (a.k.a. frontal pole; frontopolar region; *area frontopolaris*)	Anterior-most frontal lobe
11	Straight gyrus (part of prefrontal cortex; a.k.a. orbitofrontal cortex; *area praefrontalis*)	Anterior-inferior frontal pole
12	Prefrontal area; part of orbitofrontal cortex (a.k.a. *area praefrontalis*)	Anterior-inferior medial cortex
13	Insular cortex	Deep to operculum (BA 44, 45)
15	Anterior insular cortex (not originally identified by Brodmann in humans, but subsequently identified in humans by Fischer et al., 1998)	Deep to operculum (BA 44, 45)
16	Posterior Insular cortex (not defined in humans by Brodmann)	Deep to operculum (BA 44, 45)
17	Striate cortex (a.k.a., calcarine sulcus; *area striata*; primary visual cortex)	Posterior aspect of occipital lobe, bounded by calcarine sulcus

Table 11–8

	continued	
Brodmann Number	**Name and Putative Function**	**Location**
18	Parastriate area (higher-order processing area for visual cortex; sometimes called secondary visual cortex; a.k.a. *area parastriata*)	On medial cortex, in posterior aspect including parts of the cuneus and lingual gyrus; on lateral cortex, includes areas surrounding striate cortex
19	Lingual gyrus (higher-order processing area for visual cortex; a.k.a. *area parastriata*)	On inferior surface of cortex, medial to fusiform gyrus
20	Inferior temporal gyrus (a.k.a. *area temporalis inferior*)	Visible on lateral and inferior surface of temporal lobe
21	Middle temporal gyrus (a.k.a. *area temporalis media*)	Immediately superior to inferior temporal gyrus
22	Superior temporal gyrus (includes Wernicke's area in posterior aspect; a.k.a., *area temporalis superior*)	Forms superior lateral margin of temporal lobe
23	Ventral posterior cingulate gyrus (a.k.a. ventral posterior cingulate; posterior cingulate cortex [PCC]; *area cingulate posterior ventralis*)	Visible on medial view in posterior, adjacent to BA 17; visible as medial most aspect in posterior-inferior cerebrum
24	Ventral anterior cingulate gyrus (a.k.a. anterior cingulate cortex, [ACC]); *area cingularis anterior ventralis*)	Anterior aspect of cingulate gyrus, visible on medial view only
25	Subgenual area (portion of ventral prefrontal cortex; referring to genu of corpus callosum; a.k.a. *area subgenualis*)	Inferior cerebrum, in medial view, beneath genu of corpus callosum
26	Ectosplenial area (a.k.a. *area ectosplenialis*)	Posterior-most aspect of cingulate gyrus
27	Parahippocampal gyrus	On inferior surface, medial-most structure that is immediately lateral to cerebral peduncles
28	Entorhinal area (a.k.a. *area entorhinalis*)	On medial surface, inferior to uncus
29	Granular retrolimbic (a.k.a., *area retrolimbica granularis*)	In medial view, posterior to cingulate gyrus
30	Agranular retrolimbic (a.k.a. *area retrolimbica agranularis*)	In medial view, posterior to cingulate gyrus
31	Dorsal posterior cingulate (a.k.a. *area cingularis posterior dorsalis*)	In medial view, posterior-superior cingulate cortex
32	Dorsal anterior cingulate (a.k.a. *area cingularis anterior dorsalis*)	In medial view, anterior aspect of cingulate gyrus
33	Pregenual (a.k.a. *area praegenualis*)	Anterior-inferior aspect of cingulate gyrus
34	Dorsal entorhinal (a.k.a. uncus; *area entorhinalis dorsalis*)	Inferior surface, anterior to parahippocampal gyrus and lateral to cerebral peduncles

continues

Table 11–8

	continued	
Brodmann Number	**Name and Putative Function**	**Location**
35	Perirhinal (a.k.a. *area perirhinalis*)	In posterior medial view, posterior to uncus and anterior to visual reception area
36	Ectorhinal (a.k.a. *area ectorhinalis*)	In posterior medial view, anterior to visual association areas 18 and 19
37	Occipitotemporal (a.k.a. fusiform gyrus, *area occipitotemporalis*)	On inferior surface, lateral to lingual gyrus, extending to lateral surface of temporal lobe
38	Temporopolar (a.k.a. *area temporopolaris*)	On inferior surface, lateral and anterior surfaces, anterior-most region of temporal lobe
39	Angular gyrus (a.k.a. *area angularis*)	On lateral cortex, posterior to superior temporal gyrus in parietal lobe
40	Supramargingal gyrus (a.k.a. *area supramarginalis*)	On inferior-lateral surface of parietal lobe, bordering temporal lobe
41	Heschl's gyrus (a.k.a. anterior transverse temporal; *area temporalis transversa anterior*)	On medial surfaces of temporal lobe, within lateral sulcus at mid-anterior region of temporal lobe
42	Posterior transverse temporal area; Higher-order processing area for audition (part of belt) (a.k.a. posterior transverse temporal; *area temporalis transversa posterior*)	Region in lateral sulcus anterior to Heschl's gyrus
43	Subcentral (a.k.a. *area subcentralis*)	Inferior-lateral cerebrum in post-central gyrus
44	Pars operculum (a.k.a. opercular; *area opercularis*; with BA 45, makes up Broca's area)	On inferior-lateral surface of cerebrum, posterior to precentral gyrus
45	Pars triangularis (a.k.a. *area triangularis*; with BA 44, makes up Broca's area)	On inferior-lateral surface of cerebrum, adjacent to pars operculum
46	Middle frontal gyrus (part of dorsolateral prefrontal cortex; a.k.a. middle frontal gyrus; *area frontalis media*)	On lateral surface, superior to pars triangularis (BA 45)
47	Orbital area (a.k.a. *area orbitalis*)	On lateral-inferior surface in anterior cortex, and medial aspect of inferior surface
52	Parainsular cortex (a.k.a. *area parainsularis*)	Located in lateral sulcus, superior aspect of temporal lobe

Note that if an area does not have a specific name, it is referred to in parentheses. Alternate names are also given in parentheses. Note that there are gaps in the numbering (for instance, BA 48 is missing). These gaps reflect the presence of Brodmann areas in nonhumans, but absent in humans. Sources for nomenclature: Brodmann and Garey, 2007; Kaiser, 2010; NeuroNames Ontologies (BrainInfo, 1991–present), National Primate Research Center, University of Washington, http://www.brainfo.org; Mark Durban, PhD, University of Colorado, http://spot.colorado.edu/~dubin/talks/brodmann/neuronames.html.

Source: Seikel, Konstantopoulos, and Drumright, 2020.

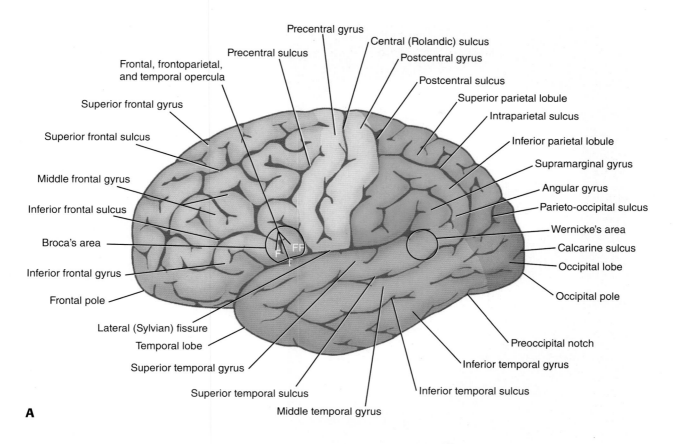

A

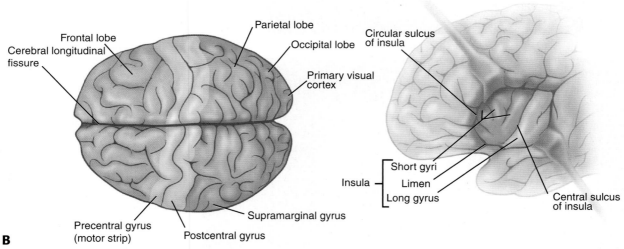

B

Figure 11–12. A–B. Major landmarks of the cerebrum as seen from above and the side. Note that the insular cortex (insula, *bottom right*) is typically hidden from view. *Source:* From Seikel/Drumright/King. *Anatomy & Physiology for Speech, Language, and Hearing, 5th Ed.* ©Cengage, Inc. Reproduced by permission. *continues*

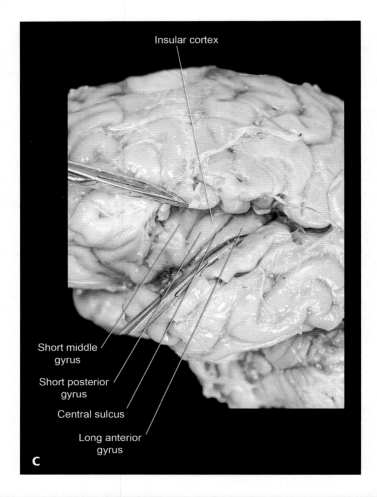

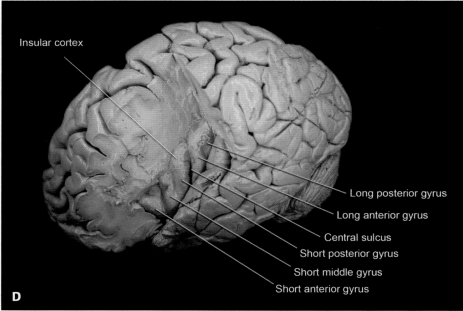

Figure 11–12. *continued*
C. Insular cortex revealed by deflecting the operculum.
D. Gyri and sulci of insular cortex revealed through dissection of the operculum.

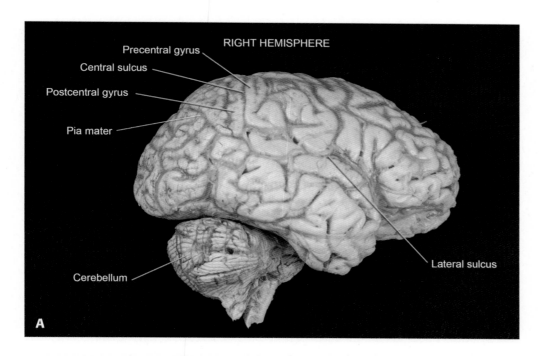

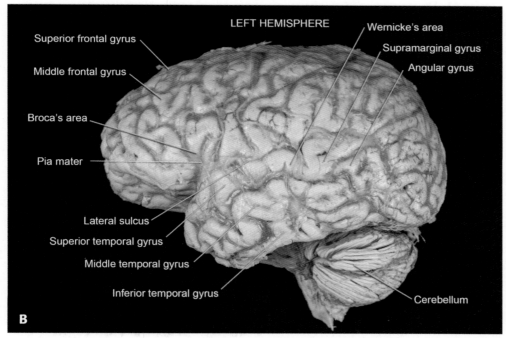

Figure 11–13. A. Lateral view of right cerebral cortex. *continues* **B.** Lateral view of left cerebral cortex. *continues*

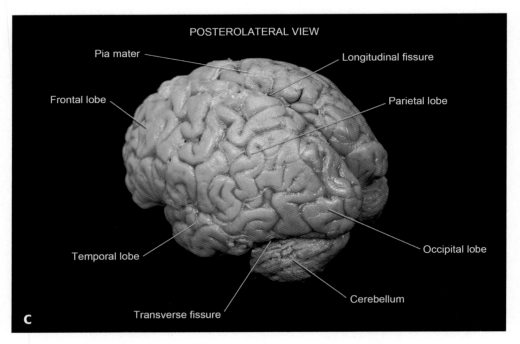

POSTEROLATERAL VIEW

Pia mater

Longitudinal fissure

Frontal lobe

Parietal lobe

Temporal lobe

Occipital lobe

Cerebellum

Transverse fissure

C

Figure 11–13. *continued* **C.** Oblique view of cerebral cortex. Note that the pia mater may be seen in portions of all photographs. *continues*

As you can also see in the photographs of Figure 11–13, the surface of the brain is quite convoluted. Early in development, the cerebral cortex has few of these furrows and bulges, but as the brain growth outstrips the skull growth, the cerebral cortex doubles in on itself. The result of this is greatly increased surface area, translating into more neural horsepower. You can think of the surface as a topographical map with mountains and valleys. The mountains (**convolutions**) in this case are called **gyri** (singular, **gyrus**) and the infolding valleys that separate the gyri are called **sulci** (singular, **sulcus**). If the groove is deeper and more pronounced, it is termed a **fissure**. These sulci, fissures, and gyri provide the major landmarks for navigating the cerebral cortex.

We divide the cerebral cortex into five lobes. Four of them are reasonably easy to see and are named after the bones with which they are associated (see Figures 11–13 and 11–14), but one of these lobes (**insular**) requires some thought and imagination. The five lobes are the frontal, parietal, occipital, temporal, and insular lobes.

Before differentiating the lobes of the brain, it will help to identify some major landmarks. Figure 11–13 shows the dominant landmarks of the cerebrum. Figure 11–13a shows two prominent sulci that serve as benchmarks in our study of the cerebral cortex. The **lateral sulcus** (also known as the **sylvian fissure**) divides the temporal lobe from the frontal and anterior parietal lobes. The **central sulcus** (also known as the **Rolandic sulcus** or **Rolandic fissure**) separates the frontal and parietal lobes entirely. The central sulcus is the very prominent vertical groove running from the cerebral longitudinal fissure to the lateral sulcus, terminating in the inferior parietal lobe.

insular: L., island

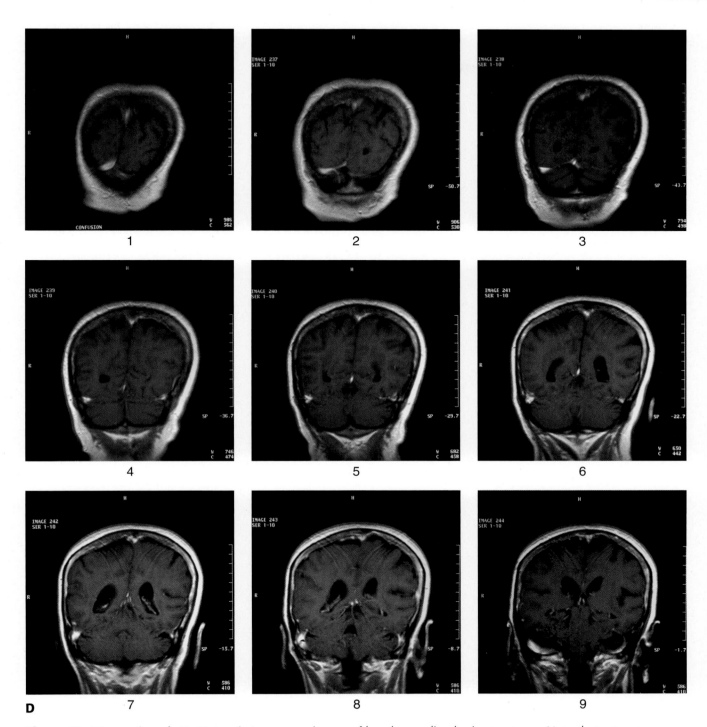

Figure 11–13. *continued* **D.** Magnetic resonance image of head, revealing brain structures. Note that a tumor emerges in the 12th slice, appearing lighter (denser) than the surrounding tissue. *Source:* From Seikel/Drumright/King. *Anatomy & Physiology for Speech, Language, and Hearing, 5th Ed.* ©Cengage, Inc. Reproduced by permission. *continues*

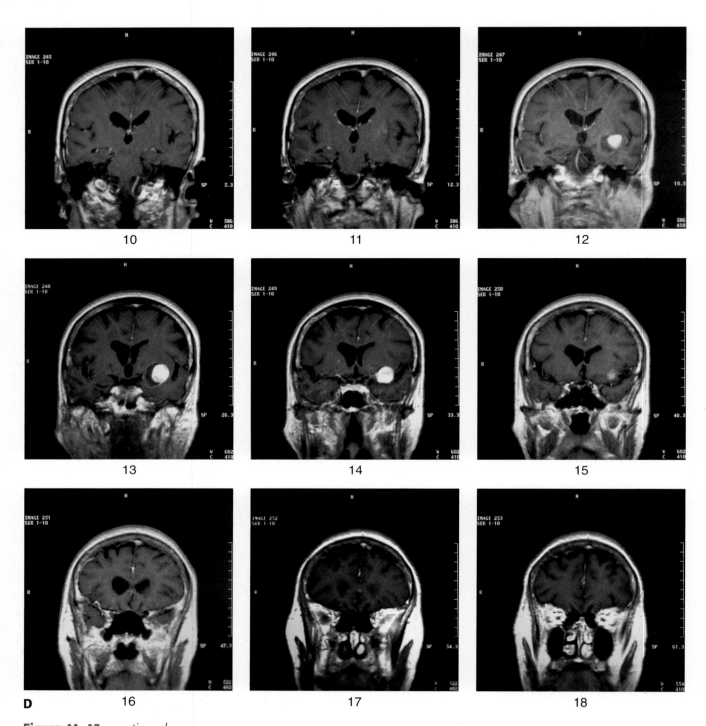

D

Figure 11–13. *continued*

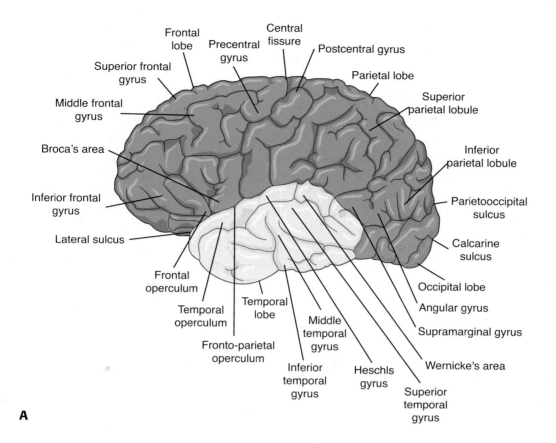

A

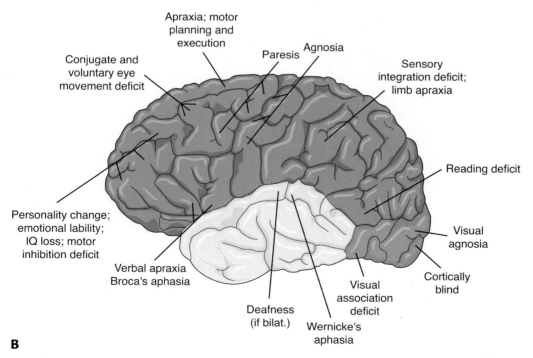

B

Figure 11–14. A. Landmarks of the left cerebral hemisphere. **B.** Effects of lesion at different cerebral locations. *Source:* From Seikel/Drumright/King. *Anatomy & Physiology for Speech, Language, and Hearing, 5th Ed.* ©Cengage, Inc. Reproduced by permission.

When the cerebrum is viewed in sagittal section (Figure 11–15) you can see that the central sulcus does not extend far down the medial surface.

Frontal Lobe

The frontal lobe is the largest of the lobes, making up one third of the cortex (see Figure 11–14). This lobe predominates in planning, initiation, and inhibition of voluntary motion, as well as cognitive function, as we will see in Chapter 12. The frontal lobe is the anterior-most portion of the cortex and is bounded posteriorly by the central sulcus. The inferior boundary is the lateral sulcus, and the medial boundary is the longitudinal fissure.

Three gyri run parallel to the longitudinal fissure in the frontal lobe. The **superior frontal gyrus** borders the longitudinal fissure and is separated from the **middle frontal gyrus** by the superior frontal sulcus. The **inferior frontal gyrus** includes an extremely important region known as the **pars opercularis** or simply the **frontal operculum** (see Figure 11–14). This area overlies one of the "hidden lobes," the insular cortex. The frontal operculum (BA 44, 45) is more commonly referred to as **Broca's area**, an extremely important region for speech motor planning within the dominant hemisphere, as will be discussed in Chapter 12. Another important

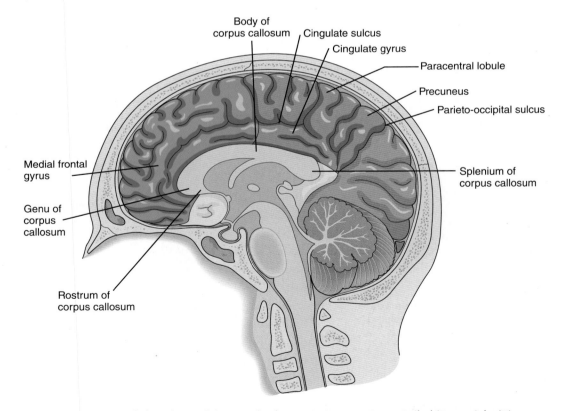

Figure 11–15. Medial surface of the cerebral cortex. *Source:* From Seikel/Drumright/King. *Anatomy & Physiology for Speech, Language, and Hearing, 5th Ed.* ©Cengage, Inc. Reproduced by permission.

region of the inferior frontal gyrus is the **pars orbitale** or **orbital region**, the region of the inferior frontal gyrus overlying the eyes. The pars orbitale and anterior regions of the upper frontal lobe are associated with memory, emotion, motor inhibition, processing of reward and punishment, and intellect (Kringelbach & Rolls, 2004).

Another important landmark of the frontal lobe is the **precentral gyrus** or **motor strip**. It is anterior to the central sulcus (thus the name "*precentral*") and is the site of initiation of voluntary motor movement. Anterior to the motor strip is the premotor region, generally involved in motor planning (but see the earlier note "When Sensation Goes Bad" for yet another function of the prefrontal cortex). The premotor cortex includes portions of the superior, middle, and inferior frontal lobes but is indicated functionally as area 6 on the Brodmann map. The upper and medial portions of BA 6 are called the **supplementary motor area (SMA)**. Axons from the motor strip and the SMAs give rise to the corticospinal and corticobulbar tracts, the major motor tracts of voluntary movement on the side of the body opposite to the area of the cortex giving the command. That is, a command arising from the left hemisphere to move the little finger will cause the finger of the right hand to twitch. We will discuss the mechanism for this **contralateral innervation** when we discuss the pathways of the brain.

The areas of the motor strip serving regions of the body have been well mapped, thanks in large part to the pioneering direct brain stimulation work of Penfield and Roberts (1959) and Woolsey (Schaltenbrand & Woolsey, 1964). As you can see from Figure 11–16, different regions of the motor strip

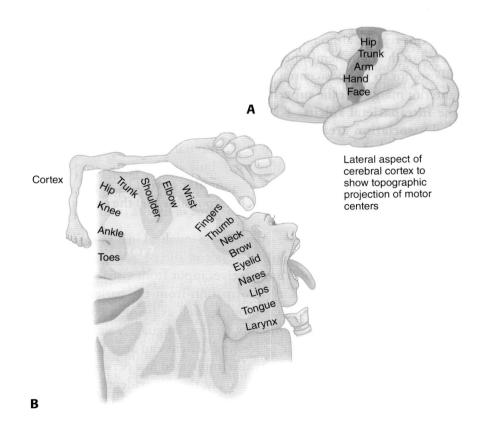

Lateral aspect of cerebral cortex to show topographic projection of motor centers

Figure 11–16. A. Left hemisphere, displaying regions of motor strip governing activation of specific muscle groups. **B.** Homunculus revealing areas of representation on the motor strip. Note that this represents a frontal section through the cerebral cortex. Size of structure drawn represents the degree of neural representation of the given structure (i.e., neural density). *Source:* From Seikel/Drumright/King. *Anatomy & Physiology for Speech, Language, and Hearing, 5th Ed.* ©Cengage, Inc. Reproduced by permission.

occipital lobe rests on the tentorium cerebelli discussed previously, with its anterior margin being the parieto-occipital sulcus. The regions surrounding the **calcarine sulcus** are the primary reception areas for visual information. The calcarine sulcus and parieto-occipital sulcus mark the boundaries of the wedge-shaped **cuneus**. Lateral to the calcarine sulcus is the **lingual gyrus**.

cuneus: L., wedge

Insula

Find the insular cortex on the lower right in Figure 11–12. The insular lobe (also known as the **insular cortex**, the **island of Reil**, or simply **insula**) is located deep to a region of the cerebrum known as the operculum. The operculum consists of regions of the temporal lobe (medial BA 38, 41, 42), parietal lobe (inferior BA 1, 2, 3, and 40), and frontal lobes (BA 44, 45, and inferior 6) along the lateral sulcus. These regions, which overlie the insular cortex, are known as the **temporal operculum**, **fronto-parietal operculum**, and **frontal operculum**.

To see the insular cortex, you would have to pull the temporal lobe laterally and lift up the frontal and parietal opercula, as displayed in Figure 11–12. Upon doing that, you would see the **circular sulcus** that surrounds the insula, deep in the lateral sulcus. The **central sulcus of the insula** divides the insula into anterior short gyri and a single posterior long gyrus. The insula is a fascinating structure that appears to be intimately involved in motor speech planning (Di Cesare, Marchi, Errante, Fasano, & Rizzolatti, 2017; Dronkers, 1996; but see Uddin, Nomi, Hebert-Seropian, Ghaziri, & Boucher, 2017 for alternate interpretations to Dronkers), perception of taste (gustation: Kobayashi, 2006), processing emotion (Dalgleish, 2004), our perception of self (Craig, 2002), and even our development of compassion and empathy (Lutz, Greischar, Perlman, & Davidson, 2009). Damage to the insula has even been shown to completely disrupt craving cigarettes (Naqvi, Rudrauf, Damasio, & Bechara, 2007).

Limbic System

The limbic system is not an anatomically distinct region, but one arising from functional relationships associated with motivation, sex drive, emotional behavior, and affect. The limbic system includes the uncus (formed by the amygdala), parahippocampal gyrus, cingulate gyrus, and olfactory bulb and tract, as well as the hippocampal formation, orbitofrontal cortex, and the **dentate** gyrus, structures we will discuss again when we talk about the hippocampus later in this chapter (Figure 11–17).

dentate: L., referring to tooth; notched, toothlike

✔ To summarize:

- The **cerebrum** is divided into two grossly similar, mirror-image **hemispheres** that are connected by means of the massive **corpus callosum**.

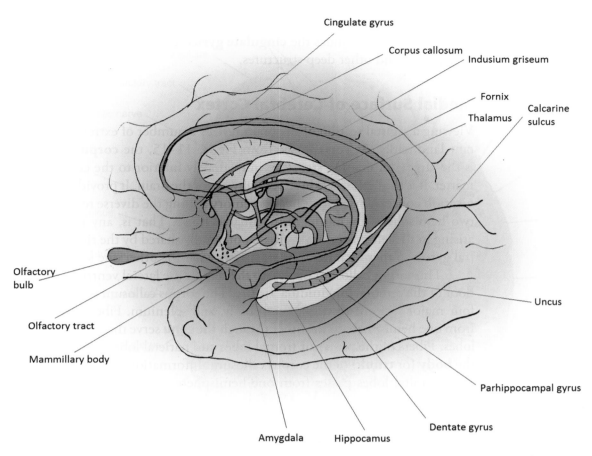

Cingulate gyrus

Corpus callosum

Indusium griseum

Fornix

Thalamus

Calcarine sulcus

Olfactory bulb

Olfactory tract

Mammillary body

Uncus

Parhippocampal gyrus

Dentate gyrus

Amygdala Hippocamus

Figure 11–17. Schematic of components of the limbic system in context of the hippocampal formation. *Source:* From *Neuroanatomy & Neurophysiology for Speech and Hearing Sciences* by Seikel, J. A., Konstantopoulos, K., & Drumright, D. G. Copyright © 2020 Plural Publishing, Inc.

- The **gyri** and **sulci** of the hemispheres provide important landmarks for lobes and other regions of the cerebrum.
- The **temporal lobe** is the site of **auditory reception** and **Wernicke's area**.
- The temporal lobe is the prominent lateral lobe separated from the parietal and frontal lobes by the **lateral fissure**.
- The anterior-most region is the **frontal lobe**, the site of most voluntary **motor activation** and the important speech region known as **Broca's area**.
- Adjacent to the frontal lobe is the **parietal lobe**, the region of **somatic sensory reception**.
- The **occipital lobe** is the most posterior of the regions, the site of **visual input** to the cerebrum.
- The **insular lobe** is revealed by deflecting the temporal lobe and lies deep in the **lateral sulcus**.

Multiple Sclerosis

There are a number of demyelinating diseases, conditions that cause degeneration of the brain myelin. Multiple sclerosis (MS) is a disease in which an individual's immune system attacks the myelin of the brain. As the name indicates, multiple areas of the brain myelin are affected, causing diffuse symptoms. The myelin is damaged or destroyed, and replaced with a scarlike plaque (sclerotic plaque), which greatly inhibits neural conduction. Early signs are often vestibular or balance dysfunction and optic neuritis (inflammation of the optic nerve). A subtype of MS is relapsing-remitting, in which an individual undergoes periods of disease activity followed by periods of remission in which signs and symptoms are greatly reduced.

Projection Fibers

The tracts running to and from the cortex, brain stem, and spinal cord are made up of **projection fibers**. Projection fibers connect the cortex with distant locations. The **corona radiata** is a mass of projection fibers running from and to the cortex (Figure 11–19). It condenses as it courses down, forming an L-shape as it reaches a location known as the **internal capsule**. The **anterior limb** (frontopontine fibers) of the internal capsule separates the caudate nucleus and the putamen of the basal ganglia and serves the frontal lobe. The **posterior limb** (corticospinal tract) includes the **optic radiation (reticulolenticular tract)**, which is a group of fibers projecting to the calcarine sulcus for vision. Nearly all the *afferent* fibers within the corona radiata arise from the thalamus, the major sensory relay of the brain. The point of juncture of the anterior and posterior limbs is called the **genu,** which marks the location of the corticobulbar tracts. *Efferent* fibers from the cortex make up the motor tracts. We will discuss these tracts shortly.

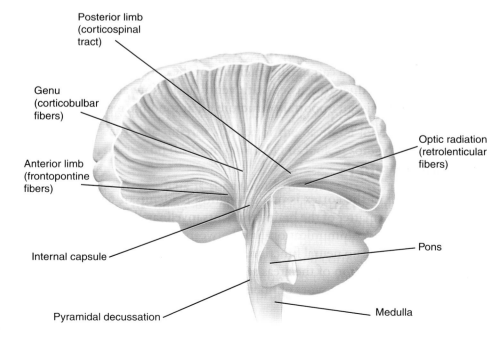

Figure 11–19. Corona radiata as it passes through the internal capsule. The anterior limb of the internal capsule includes fibers from the frontal lobe, and the genu of the internal capsule includes fibers of the corticobulbar tract. The corticospinal tract passes through the posterior limb of the internal capsule. *Source: From Seikel/Drumright/ King. Anatomy & Physiology for Speech, Language, and Hearing, 5th Ed.* ©Cengage, Inc. Reproduced by permission.

Association Fibers

The second group of fibers consists of **association fibers**. Association fibers provide communication between regions of the same hemisphere. For example, they may connect the superior temporal gyrus with the middle temporal gyrus within the left hemisphere.

There are both long and short association fibers. **Short association fibers** connect neurons of one gyrus to the next, traversing the sulcus. The **long association fibers** interconnect the lobes of the brain within the same hemisphere. The **uncinate fasciculus** connects the orbital portion, inferior, and middle frontal gyri with the anterior temporal lobe. The extremely important **arcuate fasciculus** permits the superior and middle frontal gyri to communicate with the temporal, parietal, and occipital lobes. The arcuate fasciculus has long been held to be the dominant pathway between Broca's and Wernicke's areas. We now know that the inferior parietal lobule connects the two portions of the arcuate fasciculus, apparently within the supramarginal gyrus (Ffytch, 2005). A lesion of the arcuate fasciculus can result in **conduction aphasia**, in which expressive language and receptive language remain essentially intact but the individual remains unable to repeat information presented auditorily. The **cingulum**, the white matter of the cingulate gyrus, connects the frontal and parietal lobes with the parahippocampal gyrus and temporal lobe. At birth only a small number of axons are myelinated. Myelination begins in earnest after birth, and is completed around 30 years of age. It correlates well with the development of cognitive and motor functions in various parts of the brain, beginning in the posterior brain and working forward as you grow. Thus, the occipital and parietal lobes will have completed myelin before the frontal lobes, which are the final lobes to become myelinated. It has been hypothesized that this slow myelination process is responsible for the poor judgment shown by teenagers at times.

Commissural Fibers

The third group of fibers is the **commissural fibers**. The corpus callosum is the major group of commissural fibers. Commissural fibers run from one location on a hemisphere to the corresponding location on the other hemisphere, such as from the supramarginal gyrus of the left parietal lobe to that of the right parietal lobe. We have already discussed one of the groups of commissural fibers, the corpus callosum. Another important group of fibers makes up the **anterior commissure**. The anterior commissure crosses between hemispheres to connect the right and left olfactory areas as well as portions of the inferior and middle temporal gyri.

Anatomy of the Subcortex

ANAQUEST LESSON

Basal Ganglia

The basal ganglia (or basal nuclei) are a group of cell bodies intimately related to the control of background movement and initiation of movement patterns. The ganglia included under the broader term of basal ganglia

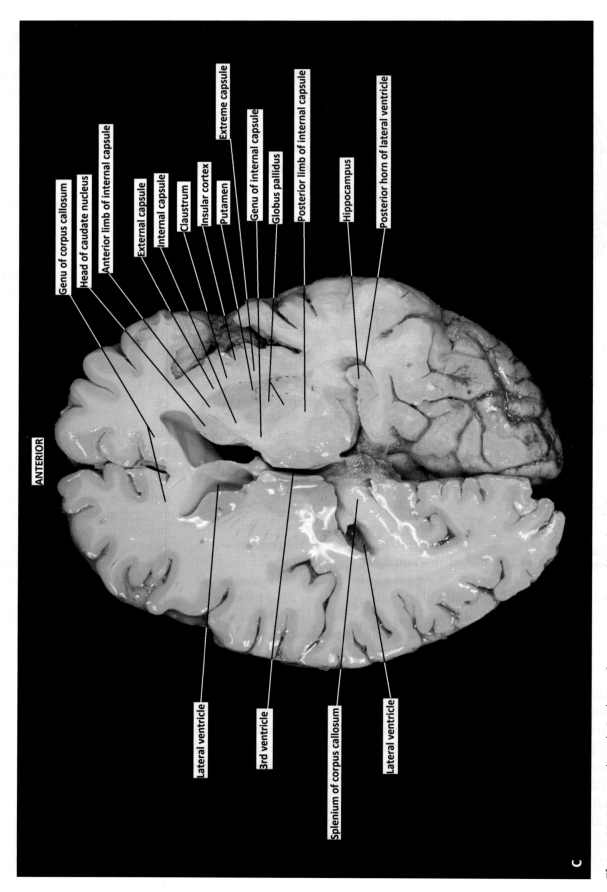

Figure 11–20. *continued* **C.** Photo of transverse view of basal ganglia structures. *Source:* From Neuroanatomy & Neurophysiology for Speech and Hearing Sciences by Seikel, J. A., Konstantopoulos, K., & Drumright, D. G. Copyright © 2020 Plural Publishing, Inc.

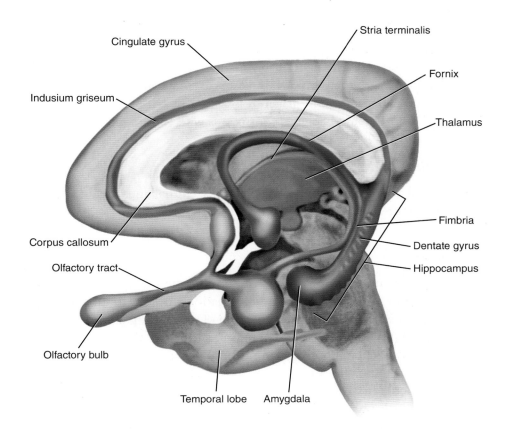

Figure 11–21. Orientation of the hippocampal formation. *Source:* From Seikel/Drumright/King. *Anatomy & Physiology for Speech, Language, and Hearing, 5th Ed.* ©Cengage, Inc. Reproduced by permission.

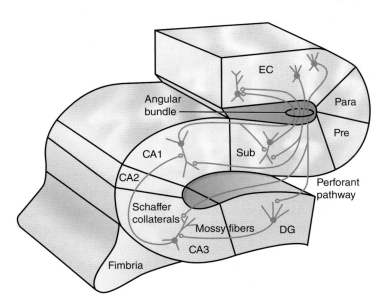

Figure 11–22. Cross-section through the hippocampus. Note the following: CA1 = cornu ammonis area 1; CA2 = Cornu ammonis area 2; CA3 = cornu ammonis area 3; Para = parasubiculum; Pre = presubiculum; Sub = subiculum; EC = entorhinal cortex; and DG = dentate gyrus. *Source:* From Seikel/Drumright/King. *Anatomy & Physiology for Speech, Language, and Hearing, 5th Ed.* ©Cengage, Inc. Reproduced by permission.

level of CA1 that there is reciprocal projection back to the entorhinal cortex. The hippocampus consists of six cell layers, much as the cerebral cortex.

The **pes hippocampus** ("foot of the hippocampus") is the anterior projection of the hippocampus, and the **fimbria** of hippocampus is a medial layer of white fibers that are continuous with the fornix. The **fornix** is a near-circle of myelinated fibers terminating in the **mammillary body** and provides most of the communication between the hippocampus and the

pes hippocampus: L., foot of hippocampus

fimbria: L., fringe

fornix: L., arch

mammillary body: L., mamillia, nipple

hypothalamus. It contains commissural fibers that permit communication with the opposite hippocampus.

The **dentate gyrus** (dentate fascia) lies between the fimbria of the hippocampus and the parahippocampal gyrus and continues as the indusium griseum. The **indusium griseum** is a layer of cell bodies that overlies the corpus callosum and becomes continuous with the cingulate gyrus.

Diencephalic Structures

The diencephalon is composed of the thalamus, epithalamus, hypothalamus, and subthalamus. This is a small and compact region.

Thalamus

The paired thalami are the largest structures of the diencephalon and are the final, common relay for sensory information directed toward the cerebral cortex. All sensation, with the exception of olfaction, passes through the thalamus, making it an exceedingly important region of the brain. Of those sensations, only pain (and possibly temperature) sense is consciously perceived at the thalamus, but pain cannot be localized without cortical function.

The **reticular activating system** that arises from the intralaminar nuclei of the thalamus is the functional system responsible for arousing the cortex and perhaps for focusing cortical regions to heightened awareness. In addition, the thalamus is the primary bridge for information from the cerebellum and globus pallidus to the motor portion of the cerebral cortex. Each of the nuclei that communicate with a cortical region also receives efferent, corticothalamic projections from the same region.

The thalami form a portion of the lateral walls of the third ventricle and are separated from the globus pallidus and putamen by the internal capsule. Fibers from the thalamus project to the cortex via the internal capsule and corona radiata. The thalamus is composed of 26 nuclei in three regions defined by the internal medullary lamina.

Thalamic nuclei may be organized into functional categories (Figure 11–23). Specific thalamic nuclei communicate with specific regions of the cerebral cortex. **Association nuclei** communicate with association areas of the cortex. **Subcortical nuclei** have no direct communication with the cerebral cortex. There are some critically important nuclei for those of us in speech-language pathology and audiology. The **pulvinar** is a critically important nucleus related to language function, and damage to this nucleus can result in aphasia, an acquired language deficit. The **lateral geniculate body** is a visual relay, whereas **the medial geniculate body** is the last auditory relay of the auditory pathway before reaching the cerebral cortex.

Epithalamus

The most prominent structures of the epithalamus include the pineal body, which is a gland involved in the development of gonads, the **habenular**

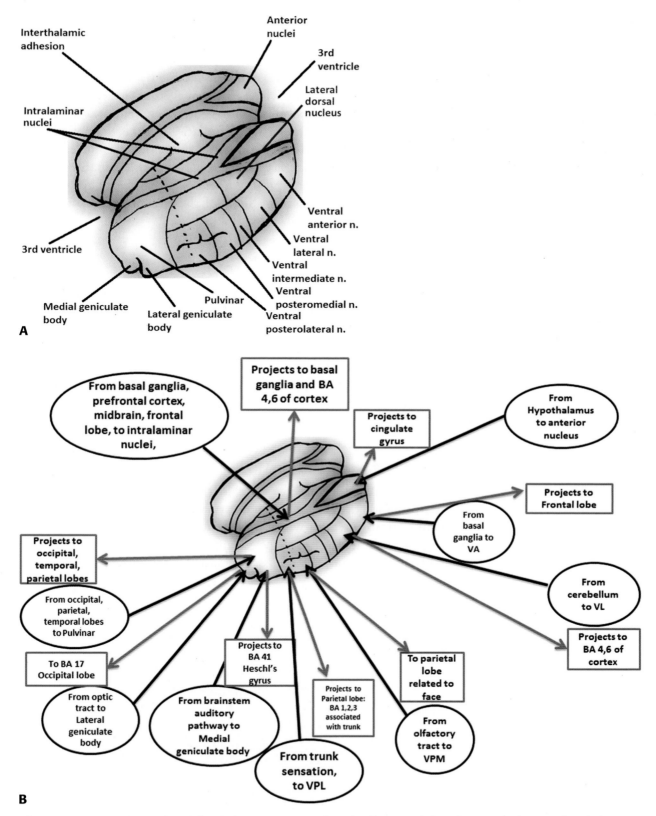

Figure 11–23. Major nuclei of the thalamus. **A.** Critical nuclei for speech-language pathology and audiology include the medial geniculate body (input to the core of the auditory cortex), lateral geniculate body (input to visual cortex), pulvinar (language function), ventral posteriomedial nucleus (input to anterolateral belt auditory cortex), and lateral dorsal nucleus (input to the parabelt of the auditory cortex). **B.** Schematic showing afferent and efferent projections of the thalamic nuclei. *Source:* From *Neuroanatomy & Neurophysiology for Speech and Hearing Sciences* by Seikel, J. A., Konstantopoulos, K., & Drumright, D. G. Copyright © 2020 Plural Publishing, Inc.

nuclei and habenular commissure, the stria medularis, and the posterior commissure. The habenular nuclei receive input from the septum, hypothalamus, brain stem, raphe nuclei, and ventral tegmental area via the habenulopeduncular tract and stria medullaris. Connections with the thalamus, hypothalamus, and septal area from the habenular nuclei are via the habenulopeduncular tract (fasciculus retroflexus), terminating in the interpeduncular nucleus, which projects to those structures. The posterior commissure consists of decussating fibers of the superior **colliculi**, nuclei associated with visual reflexes.

colliculi: L., mounds

Subthalamus

The major landmark of the subthalamus is the **subthalamic nucleus**, a lentiform structure on the inner surface of the internal capsule. Many fibers project through the subthalamus on their way to the thalamus. The subthalamus receives input from the globus pallidus and the motor cortex and is involved in the control of striated muscle. Lesions to the subthalamus have been known to produce the uncontrolled flailing movements of arms and legs known as **ballism** (e.g., Albin, 1995). Unilateral lesion produces **hemiballism** of the contralateral side.

Hypothalamus

The hypothalamus makes up the floor of the third ventricle. The hypothalamus provides the organizational structure for the **limbic system**. The hypothalamus interacts with other components of the limbic system, including the parahippocampal gyrus, amygdala, and hippocampus (see Figures 11–17 and 11–24), as well as the cingulate gyrus and septal region

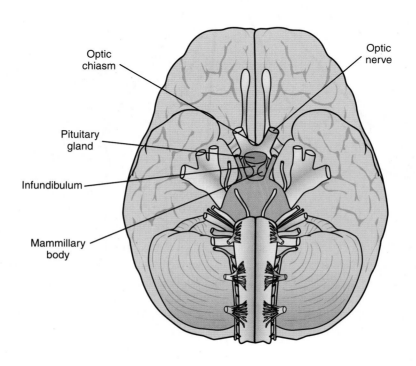

Figure 11–24. Structures of the hypothalamus visible from an inferior view. *Source: From Seikel/Drumright/ King. Anatomy & Physiology for Speech, Language, and Hearing, 5th Ed.* ©Cengage, Inc. Reproduced by permission.

(not shown in figures). The hypothalamus regulates reproductive behavior and physiology, desire or perception of need for food and water, perception of satiation, control of digestive processes, and metabolic functions (including the maintenance of water balance and body temperature). Damage to the hypothalamus can result in the loss of appropriate autonomic responses, such as heart-rate acceleration and sweating, shivering when cold, or even moving to a warmer environment when cold. Damage to the **satiety center** will result in voracious eating, whereas damage to the **feeding center** will result in starvation and dehydration. The hypothalamus is involved in the behavioral manifestations associated with emotion (tearing, heart-rate acceleration, sweating, gooseflesh, flushing, and mouth dryness), although it is assumed that cortical function is an important intermediary in normal emotional response.

✅ To summarize:

- The structures underlying the cerebral cortex are vital to the modification of information arriving at or leaving the cerebral cortex.

- The **basal ganglia** are subcortical structures involved in the control of **movement**, whereas the **hippocampal formation** of the inferior temporal lobe is deeply implicated in **memory** function.

- The **thalamus** of the **diencephalon** is the final relay for **somatic sensation** directed toward the cerebrum and for other diencephalic structures.

- The **subthalamus** interacts with the globus pallidus to control **movement**, and the **hypothalamus** controls many bodily functions and desires.

- The regions of the cerebral cortex are interconnected by means of a complex network of **projection fibers**, connecting the cortex with other structures; **association fibers**, which connect regions of the same hemisphere; and **commissural fibers**, which provide communication between the corresponding regions of the two hemispheres.

Cerebrovascular System

Although the brain makes up only 2% of the body weight, it consumes an enormous 20% of the oxygen transported by the vascular system to meet the high metabolic requirements of nervous tissue. The vascular system of the brain (the **cerebrovascular system**) maintains the constant circulation required by the nervous system (e.g., Jespersen & Ostergaard, 2012). Disruption of this supply for even a few seconds will lead to cellular changes in neurons, and longer vascular deprivation results in cell death.

The vascular supply of the brain arises from the carotid and vertebral branches, both of which originate from the aorta. The **carotid division** arises from the left and right **internal carotid arteries**, which enter the brain lateral

cerebrovascular system: vascular supply of brain

Venous Drainage

The blood supply for the brain requires a return route for blood that has circulated and exchanged its nutrients. The **venous system** is the system of blood vessels called *veins* that provides the means of draining carbon-dioxide-laden blood to the lungs for reoxygenation.

Venous drainage is accomplished by means of a series of superficial and deep cisterns. Superficial drainage empties into the superior sagittal sinus and transverse sinus. Deep drainage is by means of the inferior sagittal sinus, the straight sinus, transverse sinuses, and the sigmoid sinus. Blood returns to the general bloodstream by means of the jugular veins, and spinal cord drainage is by means of radicular veins.

Obstruction of the cerebrovascular supply typically occurs in one of two ways. A **thrombus** is a foreign body (such as a blood clot or bubble of air) that obstructs a blood vessel, and such obstruction is called a **thrombosis**. If the thrombus breaks loose from its site of formation and floats through the bloodstream, it becomes an **embolus**, or floating clot. An **embolism** is an obstruction of a blood vessel by that foreign body brought to the point of occlusion by blood flow. **Aneurysm** is a dilation or ballooning of a blood vessel because of weak walls. When an intracranial aneurysm ruptures, the blood is released into the space surrounding the brain, in most cases because most aneurysms occur in arteries rather than capillaries. The pressure associated with both the development of the ballooning aneurysm and the sudden release of blood into the cranial cavity is life-threatening, with sites of neural damage being related to the location of the rupture.

Occlusion of the anterior cerebral artery is infrequent, but may result in hemiplegia, loss of some sensory function, and personality change. Occlusion of the middle cerebral artery is the most common and can result in severe disability because of the critical nature of the areas served. In addition to severe unilateral or bilateral motor and sensory deficit, left-hemisphere damage to Broca's area, Wernicke's area, and association areas may produce profound aphasia. Posterior cerebral artery occlusion produces variable deficit that may include memory dysfunction.

☑ To summarize:

- The **cerebrovascular system** is the literal lifeblood of the brain.
- The **anterior cerebral arteries** serve the medial surfaces of the brain, whereas the **middle cerebral artery** serves the lateral cortex, including the temporal lobe, motor strip, Wernicke's area, and much of the parietal lobe.
- The **vertebral arteries** branch to form the anterior and posterior spinal arteries, with ascending components serving the ventral brain stem.
- The **basilar artery** gives rise to the **superior** and **anterior inferior cerebellar arteries** to serve the cerebellum, whereas the **posterior inferior cerebellar artery** arises from the **vertebral artery**.

- The basilar artery divides to become the **posterior cerebral arteries**, serving the inferior temporal and occipital lobes, upper midbrain, and diencephalon.

- The **circle of Willis** is a series of communicating arteries that provides redundant pathways for blood flow to regions of the cerebral cortex, equalizing pressure and flow of blood.

- Obstruction of the blood supply is always critical. A foreign body within the blood vessel (**thrombus**) creates an obstruction to blood flow (**thrombosis**) or becomes an **embolus** when released into the bloodstream.

- An **aneurysm** is a ballooning of a blood vessel, and rupture of an aneurysm results in blood being released into the region of the brain.

- The **middle cerebral artery** is the most common site of occlusion; the result may be significant language and speech deficit if the occlusion involves the dominant cerebral hemisphere.

Cerebellum

The cerebellum is the largest component of the hindbrain, resting within the posterior cranial fossa, immediately inferior to the posterior cerebral cortex. The cerebellum is the heavy hitter of the nervous system in terms of neurons: While the cerebral cortex is home to 18 billion neurons, the cerebellum has 69 billion neurons, which is 80% of the total number in the brain (Azevado et al., 2009). Needless to say, this neuron density speaks to the critical nature of the cerebellum as an integration center. The cerebellum is responsible for coordinating motor commands with sensory inputs to control movement, and it communicates with the brain stem, spinal cord, and cerebral cortex by means of superior, middle, and inferior cerebellar peduncles. The cerebellum also plays a significant role as memory for motor function and even cognitive processing (Akshoomoff & Courchesne, 1992). It has connections with the limbic system, reticular activating system, and cortical association areas; and clinical studies of individuals with cerebellar lesions confirm its role in cognitive executive function and memory.

From behind, one can see that the cerebellum is composed of two hemispheres and is prominently invested with horizontal grooves. As you can see from the inferior view of Figure 11–26, the **primary fissure** separates the cerebellar cortex into two lobes (this is a good time to realize that the term "cortex" doesn't apply only to the cerebral cortex, since there is also a cerebellar cortex). The **anterior lobe** is often referred to as the *superior lobe*, and the **middle lobe** is known also as the *inferior lobe*. The **vermis** separates the two hemispheres and aids in defining the **intermediate** and **lateral** cerebellar regions of the posterior surface.

To view the cerebellum from the front, you must remove it from the brain stem. The anterior surface reveals the third lobe of the cerebellum, the **flocculonodular lobe**, made up of the right and left **flocculi** and central

vermis: L., worm

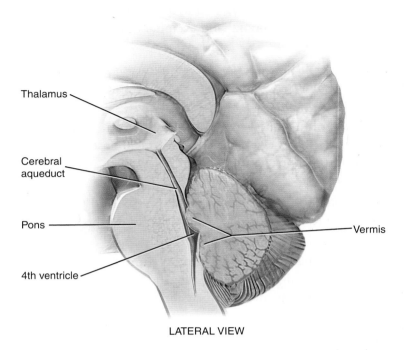

Thalamus

Cerebral
aqueduct

Pons

4th ventricle

Vermis

LATERAL VIEW

4th ventricle   Anterior lobe   Middle cerebellar
peduncle

Superior cerebellar
peduncle

Inferior
cerebellar
peduncle

Primary
fissure

Flocculus

Nodulus of
vermis

Vermis

Middle lobe

INFERIOR VIEW

Figure 11–26. Cerebellum
as seen in sagittal section
and from beneath. *Source:*
From Seikel/Drumright/
King. *Anatomy & Physiology
for Speech, Language, and
Hearing, 5th Ed.* ©Cengage,
Inc. Reproduced by permission.

nodulus. The prominent **middle cerebellar peduncle** is between the **superior** and **inferior cerebellar peduncles**.

The cerebellum may be divided functionally into three regions. The flocculonodular lobe is functionally referred to as the **vestibulocerebellum** (or **archicerebellum**), whereas the **spinocerebellum** (or **paleocerebellum**) is the anterior lobe and the portion of the posterior lobe associated with the arm and leg. The posterior lobes and the intermediate vermis make up the **neocerebellum** (or **pontocerebellum**).

The inner cerebellum is faintly reminiscent of the cerebral cortex. The outer cortex is a dense array of neurons, and beneath this is a mass of white communicating axons. At the center of the white fibers is a series of nuclei serving as relays between the cerebellum and the communicating regions of the body.

The cerebellar cortex is composed of three layers: the outer **molecular layer**, the intermediate **Purkinje layer**, and the deep **granular layer** (Figure 11–27). The outer molecular layer contains **basket, stellate, and Golgi cells** (not shown in figure), and the intermediate layer contains **Purkinje cells**. Purkinje cells are large neurons forming the boundary between the molecular and granular layers of the cortex. Axons of the 15 million Purkinje cells project to the central cerebellar nuclei. Excitation of a Purkinje cell causes inhibition of the nucleus with which it communicates. Golgi cells project their dendrites into the molecular layer and their axons into the granular layer. Their soma receive input from both climbing fibers and Purkinje cells, and the axons synapse with granule cell dendrites. Basket cells and stellate cells arborize to communicate with Purkinje cells.

Climbing fibers arising from the inferior olivary nuclei pass through the inner granular layer to communicate with the Purkinje cells. These fibers are strongly excitatory to Purkinje cells. Granule cells within this inner layer project axons to the outer layer where they divide into a T-form. The branches course at roughly right angles to the base of the axon, synapsing with the dendritic arborization of the Purkinje cells. Activation of these granule cells excites basket and stellate cells but inhibits Purkinje cells. Projections from non-cerebellar regions (spinal cord, brain stem, cerebral cortex) terminate in mossy fibers.

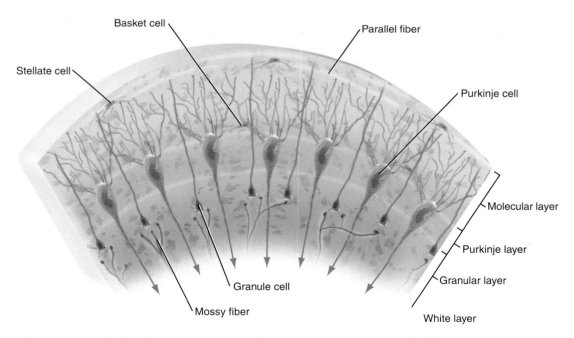

Figure 11–27. Cellular layers of the cerebellar cortex. *Source:* From Seikel/Drumright/King. *Anatomy & Physiology for Speech, Language, and Hearing, 5th Ed.* ©Cengage, Inc. Reproduced by permission.

There are four pairs of nuclei within the cerebellum, all of which receive input from the Purkinje cells of the cortex (Figure 11–28). The **dentate nucleus** has the appearance of a serrated sac, opening medially. Projections from this nucleus route through the superior cerebellar peduncle to synapse in the ventrolateral nucleus of the thalamus and from there ascend to the cerebral cortex by means of thalamocortical fibers. The **emboliform** and **globular nuclei** (also known as globose nuclei, and collectively referred to as the **nucleus interpositus**) project to the red nucleus, providing input to the **rubrospinal** tract. The **fastigial nucleus** communicates with the vestibular nuclei of the brain stem, the reticular formation of the pons and medulla, and the inferior olive.

rubrospinal: L., ruber spina, red thorn; referring to the tract arising from the red nucleus

Tracts of the Cerebellum

The **dorsal spinocerebellar tract** communicates sensation of temperature, proprioception (muscle spindle), and touch from the lower body and legs to the ipsilateral cerebellum. Afferents arise from the nucleus dorsalis (Clarke's column) in the spinal cord and project to both the anterior and posterior lobes of the cerebellum. The **cuneocerebellar tract** serves the same function for the arms and upper trunk, originating in the external cuneate nucleus of the cervical region and entering the cerebellum through the inferior cerebellar peduncle.

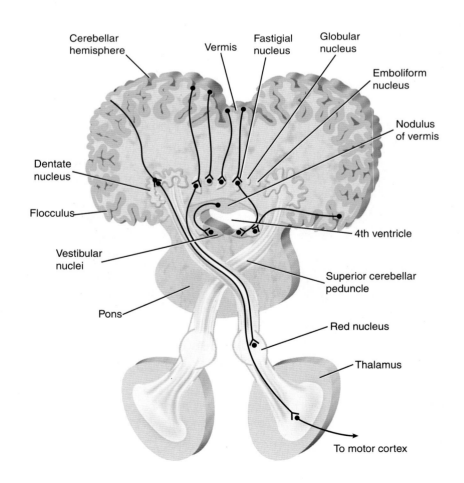

Figure 11–28. Schematic of cerebellar nuclei and interaction between cerebellum and cerebral cortex. *Source:* From Seikel/Drumright/King. *Anatomy & Physiology for Speech, Language, and Hearing, 5th Ed.* ©Cengage, Inc. Reproduced by permission.

The **ventral spinocerebellar tract** transmits proprioception information (GTOs) and pain sense from the legs and lower trunk to the ipsilateral cerebellar cortex. Fibers decussate (cross the midline) within the spinal cord, ascend, enter through the superior cerebellar peduncle, and then decussate again to project to the cortex. The **rostral spinocerebellar tract** is the cervical parallel of the ventral spinocerebellar tract, serving the upper trunk and arm region.

Pontocerebellar fibers from the pontine nuclei provide the greatest input to the cerebellum as they cross midline and ascend as the middle cerebellar peduncle to terminate as mossy fibers. **Olivocerebellar fibers** from the inferior olivary and medial accessory olivary nucleus of the medulla project to the contralateral cerebellum, terminating as climbing fibers. The olive receives input from the spinal cord, cerebral cortex, and red nucleus, as well as visual information. All other tracts of the cerebellum terminate on mossy fibers. The **vestibulocerebellar** tract provides input from the vestibular nuclei to the flocculonodular lobe via the inferior cerebellar peduncles.

The **corticopontine** projection is an important feedback system for the control of voluntary movement. Projections from parietal, occipital, temporal, and frontal lobes (including the motor cortex) synapse on the pontine nuclei, projecting via pontocerebellar fibers to the opposite cerebellar cortex. The mossy fiber terminations synapse with granule cells, the branches of which synapse with Purkinje cell dendrites. The Purkinje cells synapse with the dentate nucleus, which projects back to the cerebellar cortex as well as to the motor cortex of the cerebrum via the superior cerebellar peduncle and thalamus. In this way, the command for voluntary movement can be modified relative to body position, muscle tension, muscle movement, and so on.

Cerebellar Peduncles

The superior cerebellar peduncle (brachium conjunctivum) arises in the anterior cerebellar hemisphere, coursing through the lateral wall of the fourth ventricle to decussate within the pons at the level of the inferior colliculi. Many tracts are served by this peduncle. **Dentatothalamic** fibers arise from the dentate nucleus and synapse in the opposite red nucleus and thalamus. The ventral spinocerebellar tract ascends within this peduncle, and fibers from the fastigial nucleus descend in conjunction with this peduncle as they course to the lateral vestibular nucleus. The **middle cerebellar peduncle** (brachium pontis) is made up of fibers projecting from the contralateral pontine nuclei. The inferior cerebellar peduncle (restiform body) communicates input from the spinocerebellar tracts to the cerebellum, exiting the brain stem at the upper medulla.

Cerebellar Control Function

Cerebellar control function may be reasonably partitioned according to the portions of the cerebellum. The flocculonodular lobe (archicerebellum) is the oldest component and is responsible for the perception of orientation

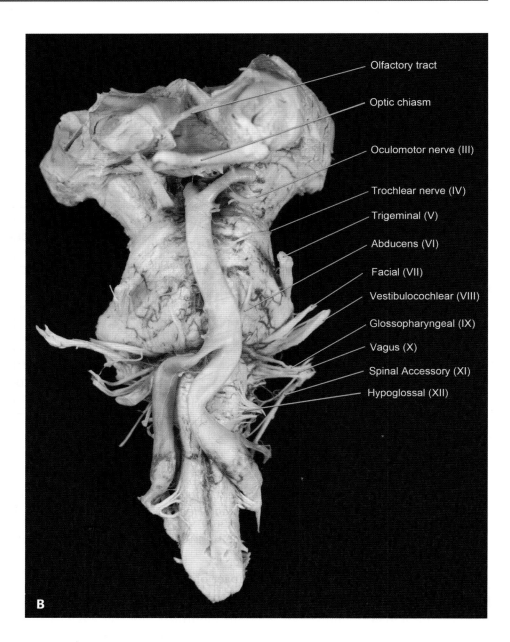

Olfactory tract

Optic chiasm

Oculomotor nerve (III)

Trochlear nerve (IV)

Trigeminal (V)

Abducens (VI)

Facial (VII)

Vestibulocochlear (VIII)

Glossopharyngeal (IX)

Vagus (X)

Spinal Accessory (XI)

Hypoglossal (XII)

B.

Figure 11–30. *continued*
B. Photograph of anterior brain stem, showing cranial nerves.

obex: L., band

calamus scriptorius: L., reed cane (calligraphy) pen

brain stem; and by removing the cerebellum, we can see several structures on the dorsal side of the brain stem that are otherwise hidden from view.

On Figure 11–31 you can see that the inferior-most point on the ventricle is the **obex**. The obex is a point that marks the beginning of a region known as the **calamus scriptorius**, so named because it looks like the point of a calligraphy pen. Lateral to the obex is the **clava** or **gracilis tubercle**, a bulge caused by the **nucleus gracilis**. As you will see, one of the important afferent pathways is the fasciculus gracilis, and it terminates in the brain stem at the nucleus gracilis. To the side and a little above the clava is the **cuneate tubercle**, which is the prominence that marks the end point of the fasciculus cuneatus. Information concerning touch pressure, vibration, muscle stretch, and tension from the upper and lower extremities terminates at these two

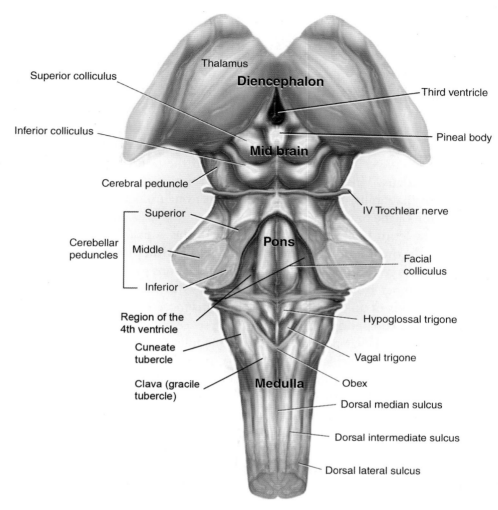

Figure 11–31. Posterior view of the brain stem. *Source: From Seikel/Drumright/King. Anatomy & Physiology for Speech, Language, and Hearing, 5th Ed.* ©Cengage, Inc. Reproduced by permission.

locations in the brain stem. As you can well imagine, focal damage to this region would affect sensation for the entire body.

The calamus scriptorius includes the **vagal trigone**, a bulge marking the dorsal vagal nucleus of the X vagus nerve, as well as the **hypoglossal trigone**, a prominence caused by the XII hypoglossal nucleus. You will remember the importance of the vagus nerve for phonation, because this is the nerve responsible for adducting, abducting, tensing, and relaxing the vocal folds (and so much more). You will also remember that the hypoglossal nerve activates the tongue muscles. A little reflection is all that is needed to realize the importance of the medulla for speech.

Superficial Pons

The pons is above the medulla, serving as the "bridge" between medulla and midbrain, as well as to the cerebellum. The significant anterior bulge of the pons is an obvious landmark for this structure. The pons is the site of four cranial nerve nuclei and is the origin of the middle and superior cerebellar peduncles, as we mentioned earlier. These peduncles serve as superhighways for communication with the cerebellum. At the junction of the medulla and the pons, the inferior cerebellar peduncle has expanded in diameter to its maximum and is entering the cerebellum.

Look once again at Figure 11–29. The anterior pons is marked by a prominent band of transverse fibers, giving it a bulging appearance. Underlying that bulge is the **pontocerebellar tract**, proving communication between the cerebellum and the pons. The **basal sulcus** is a prominent anterior landmark, because it marks the course of the vital basilar artery. The VI abducens nerve exits at the inferior border of the pons, from the **inferior pontine sulcus**. This nerve is important for rotating the eye outward, and a deficit in that ability serves as an indication to neurologists of the location of a lesion of the brain stem.

Now let us look at the lateral surface of the pons (see Figure 11–30). You can see the middle **cerebellar peduncle (brachia pontis)**, which is the intermediate communicating attachment of the pons to the cerebellum. You may remember from your audiology coursework that one of the important functions of an audiologist is to help diagnose cerebellopontine angle tumors. The **cerebellopontine angle** is the space created by the cerebellum, the middle cerebellar peduncle, and the medulla oblongata. The VII facial and VIII vestibulocochlear nerves emerge from the cerebellopontine angle, so tumors at this location may cause sensorineural hearing loss as well as facial paralysis. Also you will notice that the V trigeminal nerve exits the pons from the middle cerebellar peduncle of the lateral pons. The trigeminal nerve is responsible for facial sensation and the activation of the muscles of mastication.

The surface of the posterior pons marks the upper limit of the fourth ventricle. As can be seen in Figure 11–31, the **superior cerebellar peduncles (brachia conjunctiva)** form the upper lateral surface of the fourth ventricle, and the **superior** and **inferior medullary veli** and cerebellum provide the superior border. On either side of the median sulcus are the paired **facial colliculi**. The facial colliculus represents the location of the nucleus of the VI abducens nerve as well as the place where the fibers of the VII cross that nucleus.

Superficial Midbrain

The superior-most structure of the brain stem is the midbrain. As you can see in Figure 11–31, the lower surface of the midbrain is dominated by the prominent paired **crus cerebri**. These crura represent the **cerebral peduncles**, which house the communicating pathways leading to and from the cerebrum. Again, if you stop and think about it, a lesion to a small area in the midbrain could have devastating effects on the function of the entire body, because all the motor fibers must pass through this crus.

Between the cerebral peduncles is an indentation known as the **interpeduncular fossa**. The III oculomotor nerve exits from this fossa, at the juncture between the pons and midbrain. The **optic tracts**, an extension of the optic nerve, course around the crus cerebri following the decussation at the **optic chiasm**. Once again, problems in visual function following stroke provide vital information to the neurologist about the site of a lesion, as we will discuss shortly.

Now turn your attention to the posterior midbrain (see Figure 11–31). The posterior midbrain is the **tectum**. The tectum is behind the cerebral aqueduct, which is the upper extension of the fourth ventricle. There are four important landmarks on the tectum, known as the **corpora quadrigemina**. The corpora quadrigemina (literally "four bodies") are made up of the left and right **superior** and **inferior colliculi**. As shown in this figure, the IV trochlear nerve emerges near the inferior colliculus and courses around the crus cerebri.

corpora quadrigemina: L., body of four parts

Deep Structure of the Brain Stem

An examination of the deep structure of the brain stem requires some patience and a good imagination. Like the spinal cord, the brain stem is organized vertically. It is made up of columnar nuclei and tracts that serve the periphery, spinal cord, cerebral, cerebellar, and subcortical structures. Referring to Figure 11–32 may help you with orientation as we discuss the brain stem. We will once again take you from the medulla to the level of the midbrain, this time looking at the deep structures of the brain stem.

Deep Structures of Medulla Oblongata

The deep structure of the medulla represents an expansion on the developments that started in the spinal cord (Figure 11–33). At the lowest regions

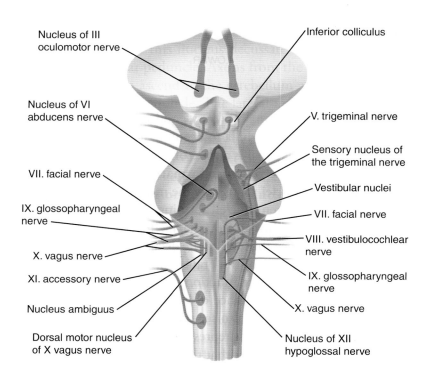

Figure 11–32. Posterior view of the brain stem revealing orientation of major nuclei and cranial nerves supplied by those nuclei. *Source:* From Seikel/Drumright/King. *Anatomy & Physiology for Speech, Language, and Hearing, 5th Ed.* ©Cengage, Inc. Reproduced by permission.

movement of the tongue and muscles of mastication, as well as pathways mediating the vestibular sense, all motor function in the periphery, and all sensations that reach the cerebrum or cerebellum. Take just an instant to realize that all these extraordinarily important functions and processes are housed within an area about the size of the first joint of your thumb. Once again, ponder the danger associated with a lesion to this region, and we promise to tell you a story with a surprisingly happy ending related to a brain stem stroke.

Deep Structures of the Pons

The pons is classically divided into two parts: the posterior **tegmentum** and the anterior **basilar portion**. Look at Figures 11–34 and 11–35 as we discuss the pons.

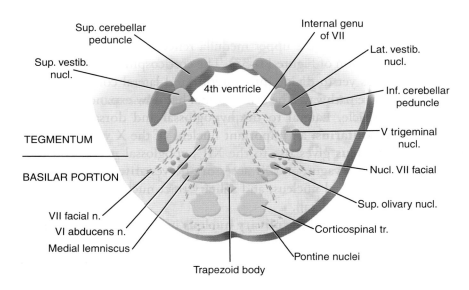

Figure 11–34. Schematic of a transverse section through the pons. *Source:* From Seikel/Drumright/King. *Anatomy & Physiology for Speech, Language, and Hearing, 5th Ed.* ©Cengage, Inc. Reproduced by permission.

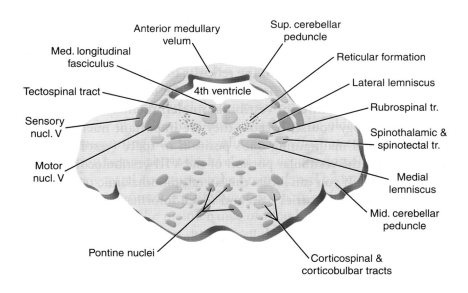

Figure 11–35. Schematic of a transverse section through the middle pons. *Source:* From Seikel/Drumright/King. *Anatomy & Physiology for Speech, Language, and Hearing, 5th Ed.* ©Cengage, Inc. Reproduced by permission.

First, let us examine the basilar (anterior) portion of the pons. Orient yourself by finding the corticospinal and corticobulbar tracts. At the level of the lower pons, the tracts are beginning to become organized for their medulla decussation and course through the spine. At higher levels of the pons, you would see that the tracts are less well defined and more diffusely distributed. Near these tracts are the **pontine nuclei**. The pontine nuclei are important because they receive input from the cerebrum and spinal cord, with that information being relayed to the cerebellum by means of the axons of the pontine nuclei that make up the pontocerebellar tract. This tract ascends to the cerebellum as the middle cerebellar peduncle. The transmission of information from the cerebrum to the pontine nuclei and pontocerebellar tract is an extremely important conduit between the cerebrum and cerebellum.

Locate the **medial lemniscus** on Figure 11–34. The lemniscal pathway begins to coalesce within the medulla, becoming the medial lemniscus within the pons. This is an important pathway for somatic (body) sense.

In the section on spinal cord anatomy, we will discuss the medial longitudinal fasciculus (MLF), which is responsible for the maintenance of flexor tone. Most of the ascending fibers of the MLF shown in Figure 11–35 arise from the vestibular nuclei and project to muscles of the eye for the regulation of eye movement with relation to head position in space. Note the relationship between the vestibular nuclei (see Figure 11–34) and the MLF (see Figure 11–35), and you can see the important interaction between the vestibular system and ocular tracking. Without the vital information from the vestibular system, the eyes would interpret every movement as external to the body. As it is, the vestibular system can notify the visual system of how the head is moving (for instance, bumping up and down as you drive on a country road) so that the ocular muscles can adjust for these changes in head position.

You will also certainly remember that we discussed the vestibular nuclei as being part of the medulla. In reality, only the inferior vestibular nucleus is within the medulla. The lateral and superior vestibular nuclei are shown in Figure 11–34, although the medial vestibular nucleus is not visible in this view. Another center of the auditory system, the **trapezoid body**, is a mass of small nuclei and fibers seen at this level. The trapezoid body is a relay within the auditory pathway. Lateral and posterior to the trapezoid body is the **superior olivary complex**, containing auditory relays associated with the localization of sound in space, as well as with the efferent component of the auditory pathway.

The posterior **pontine tegmentum** is actually a continuation of the reticular formation of the medulla. Projections from the reticular formation ascend to the thalamus and hypothalamus. As you can see from Figure 11–34, the tegmentum houses nuclei for cranial nerves V, VI, VII, as well as relays of the VIII vestibular nerve, the vestibular nuclei To remind you, within this small space are the control centers for mastication, ocular abduction, facial musculature, and portions of the auditory pathway. The ventral pons is made up largely of fibers of the corticospinal, corticobulbar, and corticopontine tracts. At this level, those fibers are less compactly bundled than they are at

- The **midbrain** contains the important **cerebral peduncles** and gives rise to the **III** and **IV cranial nerves**.

- The deep structure of the brain stem reflects the level of the brain stem's phylogenetic development.

- At the **decussation** of the pyramids, the **descending corticospinal tract** has condensed from the less-structured form at higher levels to a well-organized tract.

- The **reticular formation** is a phylogenetically old set of nuclei essential for life function.

- In the dorsal medulla, the expansion to accommodate the **fourth ventricle** is apparent, marking a clear divergence from the minute central canal of the spinal cord and lower medulla.

- The levels of the pons and midbrain set the stage for communication with the higher levels of the brain, including the cerebellum and cerebrum.

- This communication link permits not only complex motor acts but also consciousness, awareness, and volitional acts.

Cranial Nerves

Working knowledge of the cranial nerves is vital to the speech-language pathologist or audiologist. You may wish to refer to Appendixes F and G as we discuss them. Although not all cranial nerves are involved with speech or hearing, knowledge of cranial nerves is of great assistance in assessment. Figure 11–37A might help you organize these nerves.

Cranial Nerve Classification

Cranial nerves are referred to by name, number, or both. By convention, Roman numerals are used when discussing cranial nerves, and the number represents inverse height in the brain stem. Cranial nerves I through IV are found at the level of the midbrain, V through VIII are pons-level cranials, and IX through XII are found in the medulla. When we discussed the spinal cord, we pointed out that the nuclei of sensory neurons reside in dorsal root ganglia and that their axons enter the spinal cord for synapse. This pattern is followed in the brain stem as well, in which axons of sensory nuclei enter the brain stem for synapse and motor nuclei are within the brain stem.

Unlike spinal nerves, cranial nerves are differentiated based on seven defining characteristics or categories. Cranial nerve functions are divided into *general* and *special*, with areas of service being *somatic* and *visceral*. Nerves can be efferent, afferent, or mixed efferent/afferent. Thus, you will see the notation *general somatic afferent* for one component of the V trigeminal nerve that combines all three functional categories (Table 11–9).

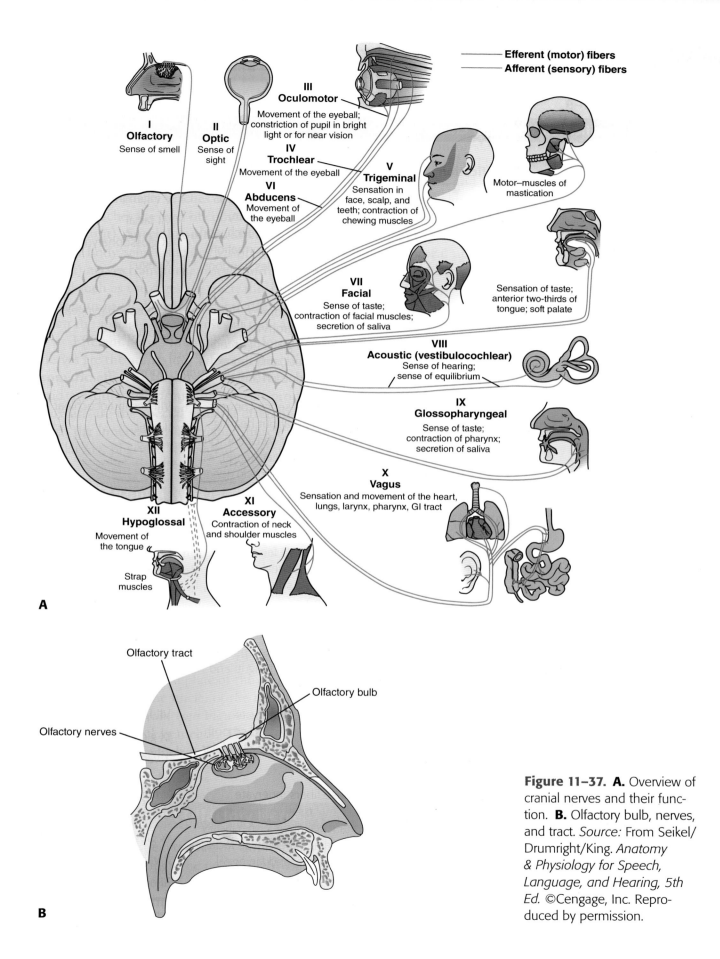

Figure 11–37. A. Overview of cranial nerves and their function. **B.** Olfactory bulb, nerves, and tract. *Source:* From Seikel/Drumright/King. *Anatomy & Physiology for Speech, Language, and Hearing, 5th Ed.* ©Cengage, Inc. Reproduced by permission.

Table 11–10

Summary of Cranial Nerve Function

Cranial	Function	Classification	Primary Nucleus
I olfactory	Sense of smell	SVA	Mitral cells, olfactory bulb
II optic	Vision	SSA	Retinal ganglion cells
III oculomotor	Innervation of all extrinsic ocular muscles except superior oblique and lateral rectus	GSE	Oculomotor nucleus, midbrain
	Light accommodation reflexes of iris	GVE	Edinger-Westphal nucleus, midbrain
IV trochlear	Superior oblique eye muscles	GSE	Trochlear nucleus, pons
V trigeminal	Exteroceptive sensation, including pain, tactile, and thermal sense from face and forehead, mucous membrane of mouth, upper teeth, gums, temporomandibular joint, stretch receptors of mastication	GSA	Sensory nucleus of trigeminal, pons
	Motor innervation to muscles of mastication (temporalis, masseter, medial and lateral pterygoids), tensor veli palatini, tensor tympani, mylohyoid & anterior digastricus	SVE	Motor nucleus of trigeminal, pons
VI abducens	Motor innervation of lateral rectus ocular muscle	GSE	Abducens nucleus, pons
VII facial	Motor innervation of facial muscles	SVE	Motor nucleus of VII, pons
	Taste, anterior two-thirds of tongue	SVA	Solitary nucleus, medulla
	Tactile sense of external auditory meatus and epithelium of pinna	GSA	Solitary tract nucleus, pons
	Lacrimal glands for tearing; sublingual and submandibular glands for saliva; mucous membrane of nose and mouth	GVE	Superior salivatory and lacrimal nuclei, pons
VIII vestibulocochlear	Auditory nerve	SSA	Spiral ganglion of auditory branch
	Vestibular nerve	SSA	Vestibular ganglion of vestibular branch
IX glossopharyngeal	Somatic sense (pain, tactile, and thermal) from posterior one-third of tongue, pharynx (mediation of gag reflex), tonsils, mastoid cells	GVA	Solitary nucleus, medulla

Table 11–10

continued			
Cranial	**Function**	**Classification**	**Primary Nucleus**
	Taste in posterior one-third of tongue	SVA	Inferior salivatory nucleus, pons
IX glossopharyngeal continued	Somatic sense (pain, thermal, tactile), auditory tube, faucial pillars, nasopharynx, uvula, middle ear	GSA	Trigeminal nuclei, pons
	Motor innervation, stylopharyngeus and superior pharyngeal constrictor	SVE	Inferior salivatory nucleus, pons
	Motor innervation of parotid gland	GVE	Inferior salivatory nucleus, pons
X vagus	Cutaneous sensation, external auditory meatus	GSA	Trigeminal nuclei, pons
	Sensory information from pharynx, larynx, trachea, esophagus, viscera of thorax, abdomen	GVA	Solitary nucleus, medulla
	Taste sensors of epiglottis, laryngeal aditus, valleculae	SVA	Solitary nucleus, medulla
	Motor innervation of parasympathetic ganglia, thorax, abdomen	GVE	Dorsal motor nucleus of vagus, medulla
	Striated muscle of larynx and pharynx	SVE	Nucleus ambiguus, medulla
XI accessory	Anastomoses with X vagus to form recurrent laryngeal nerve; motor innervation of laryngeal muscles (except cricothyroid) and cricopharyngeus	SVE, cranial component	Nucleus ambiguus, medulla
	Motor innervation, sternocleidomastoid and trapezius	SVE, spinal component	Anterior horn, C1–C5 spinal cord
XII hypoglossal	Motor innervation of muscles of the tongue	GSE	Nucleus of hypoglossal nerve, medulla

Source: Seikel, Konstantopoulos, and Drumright, 2020.

II Optic Nerve (SSA)

Although not technically related to speech, hearing, or language, the optic nerve provides valuable clinical insight into the extent of damage arising from cerebrovascular accident. The optic nerve is the *special somatic afferent* component associated with the visual system. Motor function of the eye is accommodated through other nerves.

The retinal cells receive stimulation from light, and output from the rod and cone cells of the retina (first-order neurons) is relayed to bipolar cells and

Crossed and uncrossed information passes through the optic tract to the LGB. Dendrites of fourth-order neurons synapse and course via the optic radiation (geniculostriate projection) to the occipital lobe (Brodmann's area 17), the primary receptive area of the cerebral cortex. Branches from the LGB course to the **superior colliculus** of the midbrain, an apparent point of interaction between visual and auditory information received at the inferior colliculus and the relay involved in orienting to visual stimuli. The image from the retina is neurally projected onto the occipital lobe, inverted from the real-world object it represents.

III Oculomotor Nerve (GSE, GVE)

The III oculomotor is comprised of two components. The *general somatic efferent* component serves the extrinsic ocular muscles ipsilaterally, including the superior levator palpebrae; superior, medial, and inferior rectus muscles; and inferior oblique muscle. The only ocular muscles not innervated by the III oculomotor nerves are the superior oblique and lateral rectus muscles (Figure 11–39). The oculomotor nuclei are found within the midbrain at the level of the superior colliculus, an important relay for the visual system. Axons from the nuclei course through the red nucleus and medial to the cerebral peduncles, exiting the brain stem to differentiate into inferior and superior branches. Activation of muscles served by the oculomotor nucleus results in the eye being turned up and out (temporally), inward (nasally), or down and out.

The *general visceral efferent* component arising from the Edinger–Westphal (accessory oculomotor) nucleus provides light and accommodation reflexes associated with pupil constriction and focus. The nuclei reside ventral to the cerebral aqueduct, emerge medial to the cerebral peduncle, and pass into the orbit via the superior orbital fissure.

IV Trochlear Nerve (GSE)

The IV trochlear is broadly classed as a *general somatic efferent* nerve. It arises from the trochlear nucleus of the midbrain and innervates the ipsilateral superior oblique muscle of the eye, which turns the eye down and slightly out. Fibers of the trochlear nerve course around the cerebral peduncles and enter the orbit.

V Trigeminal Nerve (GSA, SVE)

The V trigeminal nerve is an extremely important mixed nerve for speech production, as it provides motor supply to the muscles of mastication and transmits sensory information from the face. As Figure 11–40 indicates, the nerve arises from the motor trigeminal nucleus and sensory nucleus of the trigeminal within the upper pons, emerging from the pons at the level of the superior margin of the temporal bone. An enlargement in the nerve

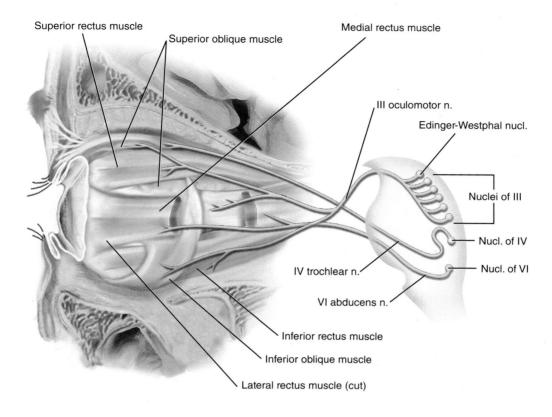

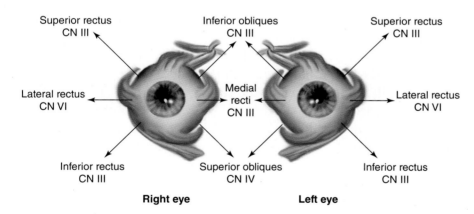

Figure 11–39. Schematic of III oculomotor, IV trochlear, and VI abducens nerve and muscle innervated. *Source:* From Seikel/Drumright/King. *Anatomy & Physiology for Speech, Language, and Hearing, 5th Ed.* ©Cengage, Inc. Reproduced by permission.

indicates the trigeminal ganglion containing pseudounipolar cells, and there the nerve divides into three components: the ophthalmic, maxillary, and mandibular nerves.

The **ophthalmic nerve** is the small, superior nerve of the trigeminal, and is entirely sensory. The *general somatic afferent* component of the

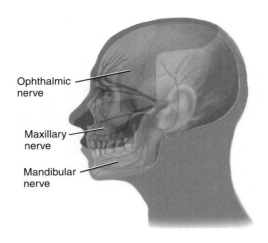

Figure 11–40. Areas served by the nerves arising from the V trigeminal nerve. *Source:* From Seikel/Drumright/King. *Anatomy & Physiology for Speech, Language, and Hearing, 5th Ed.* ©Cengage, Inc. Reproduced by permission.

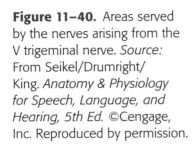

ophthalmic branch transmits general sensory information from the skin of the upper face, forehead, scalp, cornea, iris, upper eyelid, conjunctiva, nasal cavity mucous membrane, and lacrimal gland.

Lesion to the III Oculomotor, IV Trochlear, and VI Abducens Nerves

These three nerves provide motor control of the eye, eyelid, and iris. The III oculomotor nerve passes near the circle of Willis and is subject to compression from tumors, aneurysms, or hemorrhage. It serves the muscles responsible for adducting the eye (superior rectus, medial rectus, inferior rectus, and inferior oblique muscles), for elevating the eyelid (levator palpebrae), and for pupil constriction. A lower motor neuron (LMN) lesion of one of the oculomotor nerves will result in ipsilateral paralysis, because decussation occurs before this level. Because of the unopposed activity of the lateral rectus (which rotates the eye out) oculomotor paralysis will result in abduction (outward deviation, or **divergent strabismus**) of the eye and inability to turn the eye in, **ptosis** (drooping of the eyelid), and **mydriasis** (abnormal dilation of the pupil). Control of the III nerve arises predominantly from area 8 of the frontal lobe, with a projection to the superior colliculus, and from there to the contralateral pontine reticular formation and nuclei for the III, IV, and VI nerves. Because of the extreme coordination of movements of the two eyes for **convergence** (bringing the eyes together) and **conjugate movement** (moving the eyes together to look toward the same side),

hemispheric damage affecting ocular movements will result in contralateral involvement. That is, right hemisphere damage results in an inability to turn the eyes to the left side, because the right hemisphere controls movements of the eyes to the left. In other words, the patient with upper motor neuron (UMN) lesion will "look at the lesion."

LMN lesion of the IV trochlear nerve affects the superior oblique muscle. When an eye rotates medially, the superior oblique is able to pull the eye down, and paralysis will result in loss of this ability. The VI abducens nerve controls the lateral rectus, which rotates the eye out. An LMN lesion to this nerve results in **internal strabismus** (eye is rotated in). The concomitant inability to fuse the visual images from both eyes is called **diplopia**, or double vision.

Traumatic injury to the IV trochlear and VI abducens is more frequent than damage to the III oculomotor nerve. Surgical intervention to remedy the diplopia is typically attempted after 9 months, giving the nerves an opportunity to recover function and stabilize. Surgery is performed to eliminate double vision in the reading position (see Mackay et al., 1997).

The **maxillary nerve** is only sensory, being *general somatic afferent* in nature (Figure 11–41). It transmits information from the lower eyelid, skin on the sides of the nose, upper jaw, teeth, lip, mucosal lining of buccal and nasal cavities, maxillary sinuses, and nasopharynx.

The **mandibular nerve** is both *general somatic afferent* and *special visceral efferent*. This largest branch of the trigeminal nerve exits the skull via the foramen ovale of the sphenoid and gives rise to a number of branching nerves. The afferent component conducts general somatic afferent information from a region roughly encompassing the mandible, including the skin, lower teeth, gums, and lip; a portion of the skin and mucosal lining of the cheek; the external auditory meatus and auricle; the temporomandibular joint; and the region of the temporal bone, as well as kinesthetic and proprioceptive sense of muscles of mastication. The **lingual nerve** conducts somatic sensation from the anterior two thirds of the mucous membrane of the tongue and floor of the mouth.

The *special visceral efferent* component arises from the trigeminal motor nucleus of the pons, innervates the muscles of mastication (masseter, medial and lateral pterygoids, temporalis), the tensor tympani, the mylohyoid, the anterior digastricus, and the tensor veli palatini muscles. Note that taste is *not* mediated by the trigeminal, but the pain from biting the tip of your tongue is.

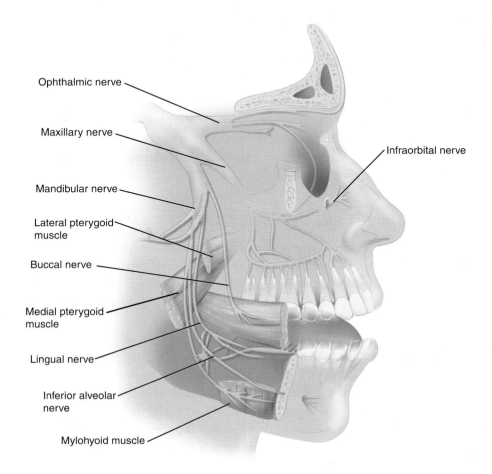

Figure 11–41. Ophthalmic, maxillary, and mandibular branches of the V trigeminal nerve. *Source:* From Seikel/Drumright/King. *Anatomy & Physiology for Speech, Language, and Hearing, 5th Ed.* ©Cengage, Inc. Reproduced by permission.

Lesions of the V Trigeminal Nerve

The V trigeminal nerve has both motor and sensory components, and all have the potential to be affected by lesions. UMN damage to the V trigeminal will result in minimal motor deficit because of strong bilateral innervation by each hemisphere. With UMN lesion, you may see increased **jaw jerk reflex** (elicited by pulling down on the passively opened mandible). LMN damage will result in **atrophy** (wasting) and weakness on the affected side. When your patient closes the mouth, the jaw will deviate toward the side of the lesion because of the action of the intact internal pterygoid muscle. The jaw will hang open with bilateral LMN damage, which has an extreme effect on speech. The tensor veli palatini is also innervated by the trigeminal, and weakness or paralysis may result in hypernasality because of the role of this muscle in maintaining the velopharyngeal sphincter.

Damage to the sensory component of the V cranial nerve will result in loss of tactile sensation for the anterior two-thirds of the tongue, loss of the corneal blink reflex elicited by touching the cornea with cotton, and alteration of sensation at the orifice of the eustachian tube, external auditory meatus, tympanic membrane, teeth, and gums. Sensation of the forehead, upper face, and nose region will be lost with ophthalmic branch lesion, and the sensation to the skin region roughly lateral to the zygomatic arch and over the maxilla will be lost with maxillary branch lesion. Damage to the mandibular branch will affect sensation from the side of the face down to the mandible. **Trigeminal neuralgia (tic douloureux)** may also arise from damage to the V cranial nerve. The result of this is severe and sharp shooting pain along the course of the nerve, which may be restricted to areas served by only one of the branches.

VI Abducens Nerve (GSE)

As the name implies, the **VI abducens** (or **abducent**) is an abductor, providing *general somatic efferent* innervation to the lateral rectus ocular muscle. It arises from the abducens nucleus of the pons, which is embedded in the wall of the fourth ventricle and emerges from the brain stem at the junction of the pons and medulla. The abducens enters the orbit via the superior orbital fissure to innervate the lateral rectus.

VII Facial Nerve (SVE, GVE, SVA, GSA)

The facial nerve is quite important to any discussion of speech musculature. This nerve supplies efferent innervation to the facial muscles of expression and tear glands, as well as sense of taste for a portion of the tongue. It communicates with the X vagus, V trigeminal, VIII vestibulocochlear, and IX glossopharyngeal nerves.

The *special visceral efferent* component arises from the motor nucleus of the facial nerve within the reticular formation of the inferior pons. As you may see in Figure 11–42, fibers from both hemispheres of the cerebral cortex terminate on this nucleus. The motor nucleus is divided, so that not all muscles are innervated bilaterally. The upper facial muscles receive bilateral cortical input, whereas those of the lower face receive only contralateral innervation. Unilateral damage to the cerebral cortex will produce contralateral deficit in the lower facial muscles, but no noticeable deficit of the upper

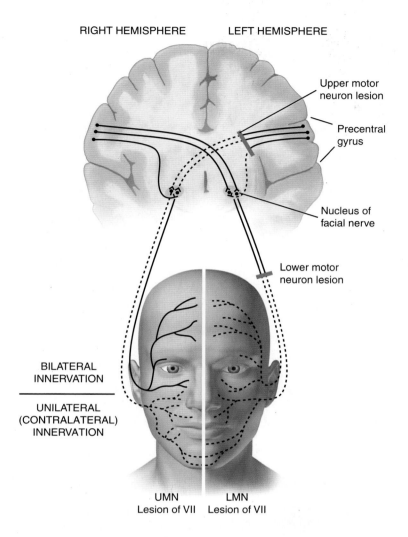

RIGHT HEMISPHERE   LEFT HEMISPHERE

Upper motor
neuron lesion

Precentral
gyrus

Nucleus of
facial nerve

Lower motor
neuron lesion

BILATERAL
INNERVATION

UNILATERAL
(CONTRALATERAL)
INNERVATION

UMN
Lesion of VII

LMN
Lesion of VII

Figure 11–42. Effects of upper and lower motor neuron lesion of the VII facial nerve on facial muscle function. (After view of Gilman & Winans, 2002.) *Source:* From Seikel/Drumright/King. *Anatomy & Physiology for Speech, Language, and Hearing, 5th Ed.* ©Cengage, Inc. Reproduced by permission.

muscles, because those receive innervation from both cerebral hemispheres. That is, left hemisphere damage could result in right facial paralysis of the oral muscles, but spare the ability to wrinkle the forehead, close the eye, and so forth.

A schematic of the innervation pattern of the motor component of the VII facial nerve can be seen in Figure 11–43. The motor component of the VII facial nerve continues to exit at the stylomastoid foramen of the temporal bone, coursing between and innervating the stylohyoid and posterior digastricus muscles. The nerve branches into **cervicofacial** and **temporofacial** divisions. The cervicofacial division further gives off the buccal, lingual, marginal mandibular (not shown), and cervical branches, whereas the temporofacial division gives rise to the temporal and zygomatic branches.

The *general visceral efferent* component of the facial nerve arises from the **salivatory nucleus** of the pons, forming the **nervus intermedius**. Fibers from the nervus intermedius innervate the **lacrimalgland** for tearing (not shown), the **sublingual gland** beneath the tongue, and the **submandibular gland**.

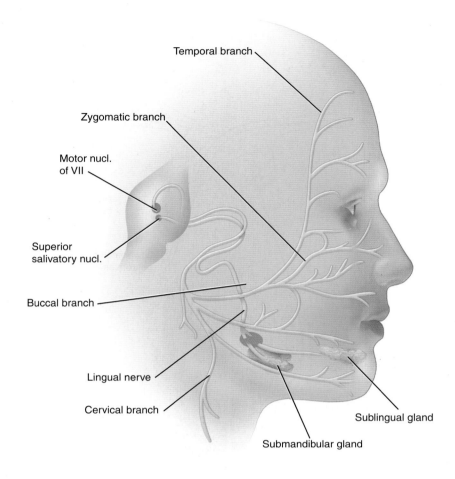

Figure 11–43. General course of the motor component of the VII facial nerve. *Source:* From Seikel/Drumright/ King. *Anatomy & Physiology for Speech, Language, and Hearing, 5th Ed.* ©Cengage, Inc. Reproduced by permission.

Lesions of the VII Facial Nerve

Lesions of the facial nerve may significantly affect articulatory function. Because the upper motor neuron supply to the upper face is bilateral, unilateral UMN damage will not result in upper face paralysis. It may, however, paralyze all facial muscles below the eyes. Even then, muscles of facial expression (**mimetic muscles**) may be contracted involuntarily in response to emotional stimuli, because these motor gestures are initiated at regions of the brain that differ from those of speech.

LMN damage will cause upper and lower face paralysis on the side of the lesion. This may involve the inability to close the eyelid and will result in muscle sagging, loss of tone, and reduction in wrinkling around the lip, nose, and forehead. When the individual attempts to smile, the affected corners of the mouth will be drawn toward the unaffected side. Your patient may drool because of loss of the ability to impound saliva with the lips, and the cheeks may puff out during expiration because of a flaccid buccinator.

Bell's palsy (palsy means "paralysis") may result from any compression of the VII nerve, or even from cold weather. It results in the paralysis of facial musculature, which remits in most cases within a few months.

Damage to the facial nerve following penetrating facial or cranial trauma is quite common. Damage to the middle ear or skull fractures involving the temporal bone will both result in facial nerve damage. Most fractures of the temporal bone occur along the long axis of the temporal bone, although facial paralysis is much more likely if the fracture is transverse (see Mackay et al., 1997).

The *special visceral afferent* sense of taste (gustation) arising from the anterior two-thirds of the tongue is mediated by the facial nerve. The facial nerve exits the pons at the cerebellopontine angle to enter the internal auditory meatus, coursing laterally through the facial canal of the temporal bone. At the geniculate ganglion, the nerve turns to continue as a medial prominence in the middle ear cavity. An afferent twig of the facial nerve, the **chorda tympani**, enters the cavity and passes medial to the malleus and tympanic membrane. It ultimately conveys taste sense from the anterior 2/3 of the tongue to the solitary tract nucleus of the brain stem. Information is transmitted via the chorda tympani to the nervus intermedius, and ultimately to the **solitary tract nucleus**.

The *general somatic afferent* component of the facial nerve communicates tactile sense via the posterior auricular nerve. Sensation arising from the posterior external auditory meatus and region the concha cava is transduced to the solitary tract nucleus of the pons.

VIII Vestibulocochlear Nerve (SSA)

The vestibulocochlear nerve is extremely important for both the speech-language pathologist and the audiologist because it mediates both auditory information and sense of movement in space. The nerve consists of both afferent and efferent components, although the efferent component is not yet classified as SVE. The special somatic afferent portion mediates information concerning hearing and balance, whereas the efferent component appears to assist in selectively damping the output of hair cells (see Figures 11–44 and 10–11).

Lesions of the VIII Vestibulocochlear Nerve

Clearly, damage to the VIII nerve will result in ipsilateral hearing loss, reflecting the degree of trauma. Damage to the VIII nerve may arise from a number of causes, including physical trauma (skull fracture), tumor growth compressing the nerve (benign but life-threatening tumors of the myelin sheath will result in slow-onset unilateral hearing loss and other symptoms as compression of the brain stem increases), or vascular incident. Damage to the vestibular component of the VIII nerve may result in disturbances of equilibrium arising from the loss of information concerning position in space.

Traumatic injury to the VIII vestibulocochlear nerve usually arises from fracture of the temporal bone or penetrating injury, such as that from gunshot wounds. A fracture along the long axis of the temporal bone will often result in sensorineural loss and vertigo without VIII nerve compression or apparent damage to the labyrinth. If the fracture is in the transverse dimension, the VII and VIII nerves may well be sheared or compressed. Vertigo and nystagmus in head injury often occur when the head position is changed (as in turning the head, looking up or down, or turning a corner when walking). In the absence of evidence of physical damage to the labyrinth, it is hypothesized that the vertigo and nystagmus arise from the disturbance of calcium particles used within the sensory mechanisms of the vestibular system. Fortunately, most trauma-induced vertigo remits over time (see Mackay et al., 1997).

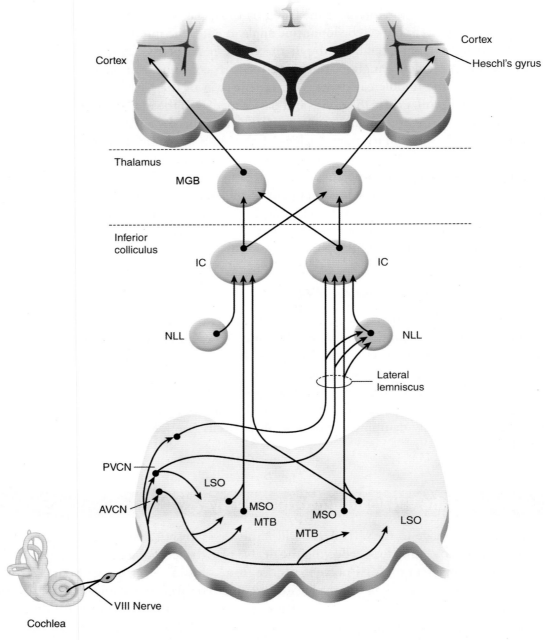

Figure 11–44. The auditory pathway, showing the nuclei of the brain stem involved in audition. Note: AVCN = anteroventral cochlear nucleus; PVCN = posteroventral cochlear nucleus; LSO = lateral superior olive; MSO = medial superior olive; MTB = medial nucleus of trapezoid body; NLL = nucleus of lateral lemniscus; IC = inferior colliculus; MGB = medial geniculate body. (Based on Pickles, 2012.) *Source:* From Seikel/Drumright/King. *Anatomy & Physiology for Speech, Language, and Hearing, 5th Ed.* ©Cengage, Inc. Reproduced by permission.

Acoustic Branch

Information concerning acoustic stimulation at the **cochlea** is transmitted via short dendrites to the spiral ganglion within the modiolus of the bony labyrinth. The spiral ganglion consists of bodies of bipolar cells whose axons project through the internal auditory meatus, where the nerve joins with the vestibular branch of the VIII nerve. The nerve enters the medulla oblongata at the junction with the pons to synapse with the **dorsal cochlear nucleus (DCN)** and the **ventral cochlear nucleus (VCN)**, lateral to the inferior cerebellar peduncle.

Vestibular Branch

The vestibular branch of the VIII cranial nerve transmits information concerning acceleration and position in space to the bipolar cells of the **vestibular ganglion** within the internal auditory meatus. From within the pons, fibers branch to synapse in the nuclei of the pons and medulla, as well as directly to the flocculonodular lobe of the cerebellum. Within the pons and medulla, the vestibular branch communicates with the superior, medial, lateral, and inferior vestibular nuclei. Vestibular nuclei project to the spinal cord, cerebellum, thalamus, and cerebral cortex.

Efferent Component

Although considered to be a sensory device, the cochlea is served by efferent fibers of the **olivocochlear bundle**. Despite the fact that this pathway has only about 1,600 fibers (compared with the 30,000 fibers of the afferent VIII), activation of the bundle has a significant attenuating effect on the output of the hair cells with which they communicate.

The **crossed olivocochlear bundle (COCB)** arises from a region near the **medial superior olive** (MSO) of the olivary complex. Fibers descend, and most of them decussate near the fourth ventricle and communicate with **outer hair cells**. The **uncrossed olivocochlear bundle (UCOB)** originates near the **lateral superior olive** of the olivary complex, with most of the fibers projecting ipsilaterally to the **inner hair cells** of the cochlea. It is believed that the olivocochlear bundle can be controlled through cortical activity and may be active in signal detection within noise.

Auditory Pathway

The auditory pathway to the cerebral cortex is illustrated in Figure 11–44 (see also Chapter 10, Figures 10–11 and 10–13). Dendrites of VIII nerve fibers synapsing on cochlear hair cells become depolarized following adequate mechanical stimulation via the cochlear traveling wave. Axons of the bipolar cells of the VIII vestibulocochlear nerve project to the cochlear nucleus, which is functionally divided into the dorsal cochlear nucleus (DCN), anteroventral cochlear nucleus (AVCN), and posteroventral cochlear nucleus (PVCN) of the pons. (Some anatomists distinguish only two nuclei, the DCN and the ventral cochlear nucleus.) Projections from the VIII nerve are arrayed **tonotopically** within the cochlear nucleus, reflecting the organization of the cochlear partition. That is, there is an orderly array of fibers representing the information processed within the cochlea, from low to high frequency. This order is maintained throughout the auditory nervous system.

Projections from the cochlear nucleus take the form of **acoustic striae**. The **dorsal acoustic stria** arises from the DCN, coursing around the inferior cerebellar peduncle. It decussates, bypasses the superior olivary complex

(SOC) and lateral lemniscus, and makes synapse at the inferior colliculus (IC). Fibers of the **ventral acoustic stria** course anterior to the inferior cerebellar peduncle and terminate in the contralateral superior olivary nuclei. The **intermediate acoustic stria** arises from the PVCN and terminates at the ipsilateral superior olivary complex.

The medial superior olive (MSO) and lateral superior olive (LSO, also known as the **s-segment**) are major auditory nuclei of the superior olivary complex within the pons. Localization of sound in the environment is processed primarily at this level. High-frequency information at the LSO provides the binaural intensity cue for the location of sound in space, whereas low-frequency information projected to the MSO provides the interaural phase (frequency) cue for localization. In addition, the crossed and uncrossed olivocochlear bundles arise from cells peripheral to the MSO and LSO nuclei.

As you can see from the schematic of the auditory pathway, fibers from the SOC ascend to the lateral lemniscus and inferior colliculus, structures apparently involved in localization of sound. You may also notice that there are ample decussations throughout the pathway, following cochlear nucleus synapse. Indeed, the auditory pathway is primarily crossed, although a small ipsilateral component is retained. Unilateral deafness will result from cochlea or VIII nerve damage, but not from unilateral damage to the auditory pathway above the level of the auditory nerve. Although much hearing function will be retained because of the redundant pathway, interaction of the two ears is essential for localization of sound in space, and damage to the brain stem nuclei will result in loss of discrimination function. Of course, complete bilateral sectioning of the pathway would result in complete loss of auditory function.

The medial geniculate body (MGB), a thalamic nucleus, is the final auditory relay. The **auditory radiation** (also known as the **geniculotemporal radiation**) projects from the MGB to Heschl's gyrus (area 41) of the temporal lobe. This segment of the dorsal surface of the superior temporal convolution is partially hidden in the sylvian fissure, and projections to the auditory cortex retain tonotopic organization. The adjacent area 42 is an auditory association area, which projects to other areas of the brain, as well as to the contralateral auditory cortex via the corpus callosum (see Chapter 10 for a discussion of the architecture of the auditory reception region.)

IX Glossopharyngeal Nerve (SVA, GVA, GSA, SVE, GVE)

The IX glossopharyngeal nerve serves both sensory and motor functions (Figure 11–45). The motor component arises from the nucleus ambiguus and inferior salivatory nucleus of the medulla, whereas axons of the sensory component terminate in the medulla at the **solitary tract nucleus** and **spinal tract nucleus** of the V trigeminal. The rootlets emerge in the ventrolateral aspect of the medulla, converge, and exit the skull through the jugular foramen of the temporal bone. The nerve courses deep to the styloid process of the temporal bone and beside the stylopharyngeus muscle. It enters the

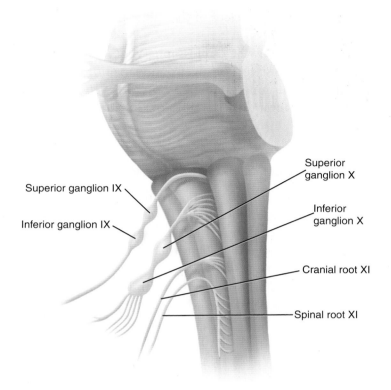

Superior ganglion IX

Inferior ganglion IX

Superior ganglion X

Inferior ganglion X

Cranial root XI

Spinal root XI

Figure 11–45. Relation of glossopharyngeal nerve to vagus and accessory nerves. *Source:* From Seikel/Drumright/King. *Anatomy & Physiology for Speech, Language, and Hearing, 5th Ed.* ©Cengage, Inc. Reproduced by permission.

base of the tongue after penetrating the superior constrictor muscle. The nerve has **superior and inferior (petrosal) ganglia**.

The *special visceral afferent* function of the nerve mediates sensation from taste receptors of the posterior one third of the tongue and a portion of the soft palate, with this information delivered to the solitary tract nucleus. Impulses from **baroreceptors** within the carotid sinus convey information concerning arterial pressure within the common carotid artery to the same nucleus. The *general visceral afferent* component provides sensation of touch, pain, and temperature from the posterior one-third of the tongue, as well as from the faucial pillars, upper pharynx, and eustachian tube to the inferior ganglion.

General somatic afferent information from the region behind the auricle and external auditory meatus is transmitted by the superior branch of the

Lesions of the IX Glossopharyngeal Nerve

The IX glossopharyngeal nerve works in concert with the X vagus, making its independent function difficult to determine. Damage to the IX nerve will result in paralysis of the stylopharyngeus muscle and may result in the loss of general sensation (**anesthesia**) for the posterior one-third of the tongue and pharynx, although the vagus may support these functions as well. The cooperative innervation with the vagus results in little effect on the pharyngeal constrictors, although reduced sensation of the auricle and middle ear may indicate IX nerve damage. IX nerve damage may also cause reduced or absent gag reflex, although absence of the reflex does not guarantee that a lesion exists.

IX glossopharyngeal to the nucleus of the spinal trigeminal via the superior ganglion.

Efferent innervation by the IX glossopharyngeal includes *special visceral efferent* activation of the stylopharyngeus and superior constrictor muscles by means of the nucleus ambiguus. *General visceral efferent* innervation of the parotid gland for salivation arises from the inferior salivatory nucleus via the otic ganglion.

X Vagus Nerve (GVE, GSA, GVA, SVA, SVE)

The vagus nerve is both complex and important. Let us examine both motor and sensory components of this nerve. The vagus arises from the lateral medulla oblongata and exits from the skull through the jugular foramen along with the IX glossopharyngeal and the cranial and spinal roots of the XI accessory nerves (Figure 11–46).

The vagus is served by several nuclei and ganglia. The dorsal vagal nucleus (dorsal motor nucleus) gives rise to visceral efferent fibers for para-

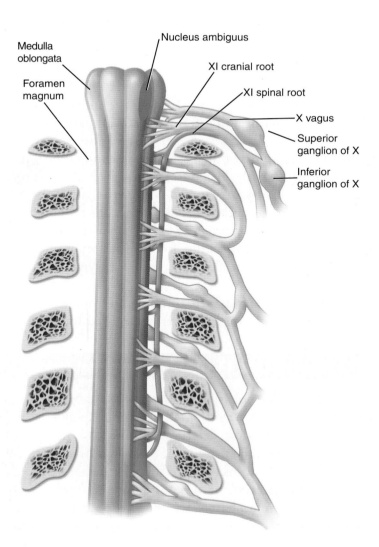

Figure 11–46. Spinal accessory nerve origins. *Source:* From Seikel/Drumright/King. *Anatomy & Physiology for Speech, Language, and Hearing, 5th Ed.* ©Cengage, Inc. Reproduced by permission.

Lesions of the X Vagus Nerve

The X vagus is the most extensive of the cranial nerves, presenting an important constellation of clinical manifestations. Damage to the pharyngeal branch will result in deficit in swallowing, potential loss of gag through interaction with the IX glossopharyngeal nerve, and hypernasality arising from weakness of the velopharyngeal sphincter (all velopharyngeal muscles are innervated by the vagus, with the exception of the tensor veli palatini, which is innervated by the trigeminal). Unilateral pharyngeal branch damage will result in failure to elevate the soft palate on the involved side (asymmetrical elevation), producing hypernasality. Bilateral lesion will produce absent or reduced (but symmetrical) movement of the soft palate, causing hypernasality, **nasal regurgitation** (loss of food and liquid through the nose), dysphagia, and paralysis of the pharyngeal musculature.

Lesions of the superior laryngeal nerve may result in loss of sensation of the upper larynx mucous membrane and stretch receptors, as well as paralysis of the cricothyroid muscle. Recurrent laryngeal nerve damage will alter sensation below the level of the vocal folds and stretch receptor information from the intrinsic muscles. Unilateral recurrent laryngeal nerve lesion typically results in a flaccid vocal fold on the side of the lesion, accompanied by hoarse and breathy voice. In bilateral lesion, the vocal folds may rarely be paralyzed in the adducted position, which is life-threatening because of airway occlusion. More commonly, the vocal folds are paralyzed in the paramedian position, compromising the airway by risk of aspiration. Paralysis in the adducted position will result in **laryngeal stridor** (harsh, distressing phonation upon inspiration and expiration). Paralysis in the paramedian position may permit limited breathy and hoarse phonation with limited pitch range arising from loss of tensing ability of the vocalis. Vocal intensity range will be extremely limited by the loss of adductory ability.

---

sympathetic innervation and receives information from the inferior vagal ganglion. The solitarius tract and nucleus serve taste, whereas the nucleus ambiguus provides motor innervation to laryngeal musculature and mucosa. As with the glossopharyngeal nerve, the vagus has inferior (nodose) and superior ganglia.

The *general visceral efferent* component of the vagus arises from the dorsal motor nucleus of the X vagus, providing parasympathetic motor innervation of intestines, pancreas, stomach, esophagus, trachea, bronchial smooth muscle and mucosal glands, kidneys, liver, and heart. This branch is responsible for inhibiting heart rate. The striated muscles of the larynx, as well as most pharyngeal and palatal muscles, are innervated by the *special visceral efferent* portion of the vagus, served by the nucleus ambiguus.

The *general somatic afferent* component of the vagus delivers pain, touch, and temperature sense from the skin covering the eardrum, posterior auricle, and external auditory meatus to the superior vagal ganglion, and subsequently to the spinal nucleus of the V trigeminal. It is this innervation that triggers nausea or vomiting when the eardrum is touched by external stimuli.

Pain sense from the mucosal lining of the lower pharynx, larynx, thoracic and abdominal viscera, esophagus, and bronchi is conveyed by means of the *general visceral afferent* component, with soma in the inferior ganglion, and with axons terminating in the caudal nucleus solitarius and dorsal vagal nucleus. Sensations of nausea and hunger are mediated by the vagus. This GVA component supports the maintenance of heartbeat, blood pressure (via baroreceptors), respiration (stretch receptors in the lung signal fully distended tissue to terminate inspiration), and digestion.

Taste sense from the epiglottis and valleculae is mediated by the *special visceral afferent* component of the vagus, with some of these afferent fibers residing in the inferior ganglion (Gilman & Winans, 2002). Axons from this component terminate in the caudal nucleus solitarius.

These functions are served through four important branches of the vagus. The auricular branch arises from the superior ganglion, whereas the pharyngeal, recurrent laryngeal, and superior laryngeal branches arise from the inferior ganglion.

The right **recurrent laryngeal nerve** courses under and behind the subclavian artery and ascends between the trachea and the esophagus. The left recurrent laryngeal nerve loops under the aortic arch to ascend between the trachea and esophagus. After entering the larynx between the cricoid and thyroid cartilages, tracheal and esophageal branches provide GVA innervation to the laryngeal mucosa beneath the vocal folds, and SVE innervation serves the intrinsic muscles of the larynx and the inferior pharyngeal constrictor. The auricular branch conveys sensory information from the tympanic membrane and external auditory meatus.

The **pharyngeal branch** of the vagus mediates the SVA taste sense and GVA sensation from the base of the tongue and upper pharynx. It also mediates SVE innervation of the upper and middle pharyngeal constrictors, palatopharyngeus, palatoglossus, salpingopharyngeus, levator veli palatini, and musculus uvulae. The only soft-palate muscle not innervated by the vagus is the tensor veli palatini.

The **superior laryngeal nerve** has both internal and external branches. The internal branch enters the larynx through the thyrohyoid membrane, receiving GVA information from the laryngeal region above the vocal folds. The external branch provides SVE innervation of the cricothyroid muscle.

XI Accessory Nerve (SVE)

The XI accessory nerve consists of both cranial and spinal components. It provides *special visceral efferent* innervation directly to the sternocleidomastoid and trapezius muscles and works in conjunction with the vagus to

---

Lesions of the XI Accessory Nerve

Lesion to the XI accessory nerve may have an effect on the trapezius and sternocleidomastoid muscles. Unilateral lesion affecting the sternocleidomastoid will result in the patient being unable to turn the head away from the side of the lesion. (The left sternocleidomastoid rotates the head toward the right side when contracted.) Lesions resulting in the paralysis of trapezius will result in restricted ability to elevate the arm and a drooping shoulder on the side of the lesion.

innervate the intrinsic muscles of the larynx, pharynx, and soft palate. The exceptions to this are the tensor veli palatini, which is innervated by the V trigeminal, and the cricothyroid muscles, which are innervated by the superior laryngeal nerve of the vagus (see Figure 11–45).

The cranial root arises from the caudal portion of the nucleus ambiguus, where it is joined by the spinal root, to exit through the jugular foramen with the vagus. On exiting the skull, the internal branch of the accessory nerve joins the inferior ganglion of the vagus. The accessory nerve serves both recurrent laryngeal and pharyngeal nerves of the vagus.

The spinal root emerges from the first five spinal segments between the dorsal and ventral rootlets, ascends to enter the skull through the foramen magnum, and joins the cranial accessory nerve before exiting the skull (see Figure 11–45). The spinal root makes up the external root of the accessory nerve and innervates the sternocleidomastoid and trapezius muscles.

XII Hypoglossal Nerve (GSE)

As the name implies, this nerve provides the innervation to motor function of the tongue. *This general somatic efferent* nerve arises from the hypoglossal nucleus of the medulla, exits the skull through the hypoglossal canal, and courses with the vagus. The hypoglossal nerve descends and branches to innervate all intrinsic muscles of the tongue, and all the extrinsic muscles of the tongue except the palatoglossus, which is innervated via the XI accessory nerve through the pharyngeal plexus.

Each hypoglossal nucleus is served primarily by the contralateral corticobulbar tract, which means that *left* upper motor neuron (UMN) damage will result in *right* tongue weakness. Damage to the lower motor neurons (LMNs) will result in ipsilateral deficit, because the fibers of the corticobulbar tract decussate before reaching the hypoglossal nucleus. Thus, left UMN damage or right LMN damage will affect muscles of the right side of the tongue. When the tongue is protruded, it will point to the side of the paralyzed muscles, because contraction of the posterior genioglossus is bilaterally unequal.

Lesions of the XII Hypoglossal Nerve

Lesions affecting the XII hypoglossal will have a profound impact on articulation function and speech intelligibility. This nerve provides efferent innervation of intrinsic and extrinsic muscles of the tongue, as well as afferent proprioceptive supply. Unilateral LMN lesion will result in loss of movement on the side of the lesion. Muscular weakness and atrophy on the affected side will result in deviation of the tongue toward the side of the lesion (function of the normal contralateral genioglossus will cause this). **Fasciculations**, or abnormal involuntary twitching or movement of muscle fibers, may occur before atrophy, arising from damage to the cell body. At rest, the tongue may deviate toward the unaffected side because of the tonic pull of the normal styloglossus muscle. Upper motor lesion may result in muscle weakness and impaired volitional movements with accompanying spasticity.

Cranial Nerve 0: The Terminal Nerve

The final nerve we wish to discuss is also the first one. The terminal nerve (cranial nerve 0) was first discovered in sharks in the early 20th century and is known to mediate pheromones that are used for sexual-partner selection and identification (Whitlock, 2004). Recent discussion reveals that it may be functional in humans. Cranial nerve 0 terminates in the vomeronasal organ, located on either side of the nasal septum. It is clearly evident in sharks and other animals, but the field is divided on whether it exists *functionally* in humans. Fuller and Burger (1990) found positive evidence of the terminal nerve in adult humans, and recent studies indicate that, indeed, humans may use this nerve as a subconscious but very real means of mate selection. Although many feel that it is most likely vestigial, it is found in almost half of humans, dependent upon the study. An article by Fields (2007) showed strong evidence that not only is the terminal nerve present in humans, but we use that information for mate selection.

✓ To summarize:

- **Cranial nerves** are extremely important to the speech-language pathologist.

- Cranial nerves may be **sensory**, **motor**, or **mixed sensory-motor** and are categorized based on their function as being **general** or **specialized** and as serving **visceral** or **somatic** organs or structures.

- The **I olfactory nerve** serves the sense of smell, and the **II optic nerve** communicates visual information to the brain.

- The **III oculomotor**, **IV trochlear**, and **VI abducens nerves** provide innervation for eye movements.

- The **V trigeminal nerve** innervates muscles of **mastication** and the **tensor veli palatini** and communicates sensation from the face, mouth, teeth, mucosal lining, and tongue.

- The **VII facial nerve** innervates muscles of **facial expression**, and the sensory component serves taste of the anterior two thirds of the tongue.

- The **VIII vestibulocochlear nerve** mediates auditory and vestibular sensation.

- The **IX glossopharyngeal nerve** serves the **posterior tongue taste** receptors, as well as somatic sense from the tongue, fauces, pharynx, and eustachian tube.

- The **stylopharyngeus** and **superior pharyngeal constrictor** muscles receive motor innervation via this nerve.

- The **X vagus nerve** is extremely important for autonomic function as well as somatic motor innervation.

- Somatic sensation of **pain**, **touch**, and **temperature** from the region of the **eardrum** is mediated by the vagus, as well as pain sense from **pharynx**, **larynx**, **esophagus**, and many other regions.

- The **recurrent laryngeal nerve** and **superior laryngeal nerves** supply motor innervation for the intrinsic muscles of the larynx.

- The **XI accessory nerve** innervates the **sternocleidomastoid** and **trapezius** muscles and collaborates with the vagus in the activation of palatal, laryngeal, and pharyngeal muscles.

- The **XII hypoglossal nerve** innervates the **muscles of the tongue** with the exception of the **palatoglossus**.

Anatomy of the Spinal Cord

ANAQUEST LESSON

The spinal cord is the information lifeline to and from the periphery of the body. Movement of axial skeletal muscles occurs by means of information passed through this structure, and sensory information from the periphery must pass through it as well. The spinal cord is a long mass of neurons, with both cell bodies and projections from (and to) those neurons. If you can imagine taking many long lengths of rope, stretching them out and banding them together so it made a long cable, you will have the basic concept of the spinal cord. The spinal cord is the aggregation of many single-nerve fibers into bundles (called tracts) of fibers. These bundles provide communication between the peripheral body and the brain, and each bundle has unique properties. Because of this, the spinal cord can be viewed in its length (vertical anatomy) and in cross-section (transverse anatomy). Both of these views are important, because discussion of the spinal cord provides an understanding of how the brain communicates with the rest of the body. Without that communication, there would be no reason to have a brain.

Vertical Anatomy

The spinal cord is a longitudinal mass of columns. The columns consist of neurons: gray portions are neuron cell bodies within the spinal cord, whereas white portions are the myelinated fibers of tracts that communicate information to and from the brain. The spinal cord is wrapped in **meningeal linings** (meninges), which are thin coverings that were discussed earlier in this chapter (see Figure 11–8).

The spinal cord begins at the foramen magnum of the skull (the superior margin of the atlas or C1) and courses about 46 cm through the vertebral canal produced by the vertebral column (you may want to refresh your memory of the vertebral column by reviewing Figure 2–4). You can think of the spinal cord as being safely contained within a long tube made up of connective tissue (the meningeal linings). The spinal cord is suspended within the tube by means of denticulate ligaments that pass through the meningeal linings and attach the spinal cord to the vertebral column. The lower portion of the spinal cord ends in a cone-shaped projection known as the **conus medullaris**, so that the spinal cord is present down to the level of the first lumbar vertebra. There is a fibrous projection from the conus medullaris called the **filum terminale** ("end filament"), and this joins with the toughest part of the tube surrounding the spinal cord (the **dural tube**: Figure 11–47) and then becomes the **coccygeal ligament** (Figure 11–47B). The coccygeal ligament attaches to the posterior coccyx. Thus, the spinal cord is wrapped in meningeal linings, is attached to the vertebral column laterally by denticulate ligaments, and is firmly attached to the coccyx by means of the coccygeal ligament.

What you can also see from Figure 11–47 and Tables 11–11 and 11–12 is that there are nerves arising at regular intervals along the cord. The 31 pairs of **spinal nerves** arise from regions related to each vertebra, with the first

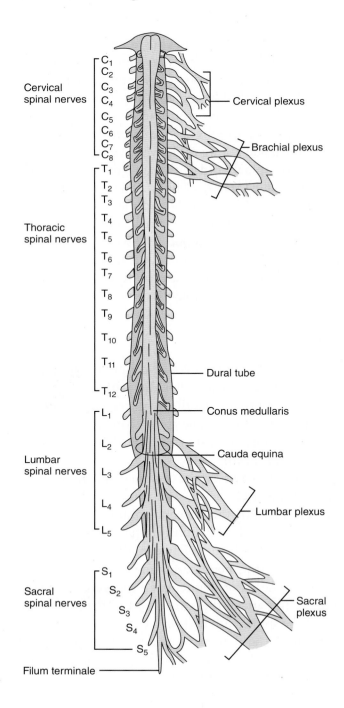

Figure 11–47. A. Arrangement of spinal nerves relative to vertebral segment. *Source:* From Seikel/Drumright/ King. *Anatomy & Physiology for Speech, Language, and Hearing, 5th Ed.* ©Cengage, Inc. Reproduced by permission. *continues*

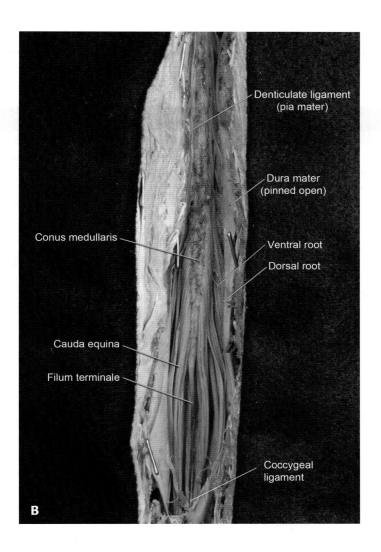

Labels on figure:
- Denticulate ligament (pia mater)
- Dura mater (pinned open)
- Conus medullaris
- Ventral root
- Dorsal root
- Cauda equina
- Filum terminale
- Coccygeal ligament
- B

Figure 11–47. *continued*
B. Photograph of spinal cord in situ.

Table 11–11

Segments of Spinal Cord and Muscles Served

Segment	Function	Muscles Innervated
C3–C4	Respiration	Diaphragm, via cervical plexus
C2–C7	Head and neck stability and respiration	Sternocleidomastoid (with XI spinal accessory)
		Scalenus anterior, medius, posterior (C3–C8)
		Serratus anterior (C5–C7)
		Subclavius (C5–C6)
		Levator scapulae (C1–C4)
		Trapezius (XI accessory, C2–C5)
C1–T1	Arm and hand function	Pectoralis major
		Pectoralis minor
		Levator scapulae (C1–C4)
		Rhomboideus major and minor (C5)

continues

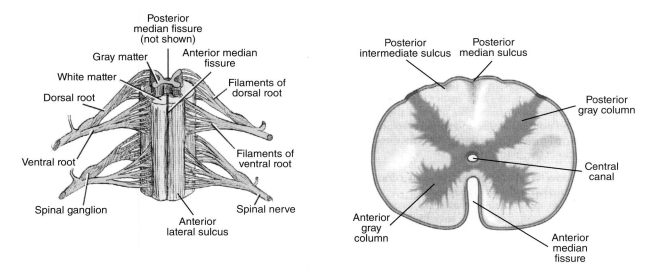

Figure 11–49. Transverse section through spinal cord, with landmarks. *Source:* From Seikel/Drumright/King. *Anatomy & Physiology for Speech, Language, and Hearing, 5th Ed.* ©Cengage, Inc. Reproduced by permission.

Figure 11–50. Transverse section through spinal cord and vertebral segment. Note the dorsal root ganglion and ventral root. *Source:* From Seikel/Drumright/King. *Anatomy & Physiology for Speech, Language, and Hearing, 5th Ed.* ©Cengage, Inc. Reproduced by permission.

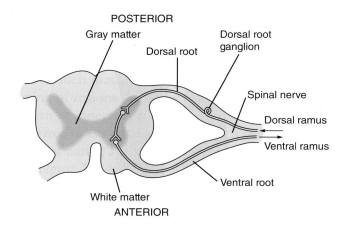

Sensory information enters the spinal cord by means of the afferent neurons, the **dorsal root fibers**. The cell bodies of these sensory neurons combine into the **dorsal root ganglia**, which lie outside the spinal cord (see Figures 11–49 and 11–50). Motor information leaves the spinal cord through the ventral root, but there are no "ventral root ganglia" because the cell bodies of motor neurons are housed within the spinal cord instead of outside of the cord. The dorsal and ventral roots combine to form the spinal nerve, so that each spinal nerve has both a sensory and a motor component. The spinal nerves divide into posterior and anterior parts (**dorsal** and **ventral rami**) to serve posterior and anterior portions of the body, respectively. Branches of the ventral rami course anteriorly to communicate with the sympathetic ganglia, nuclei of the autonomic nervous system. Efferent neurons of the dorsal and ventral rami communicate with muscle by means of a **motor endplate**. The motor endplate is analogous to the synapse seen as the communication between two neurons. Afferent fibers that enter the spinal cord receive their stimulation from sensors that are peripheral to the spinal cord. We now have all the elements in place for the most basic unit of interaction with the environment, the segmental reflex arc.

The Reflex Arc

The **segmental spinal reflex arc** is the simplest stimulus–response system of the nervous system and is the most basic means that the nervous system has of responding to its environment (Figure 11–51). Although we use the term *basic* to imply simplicity, it is not too early to let you know that many speech-language pathologists involved in oral motor therapy recognize that this "basic" response is an essential element of their therapy, because it is a critical component of adequate muscle tone.

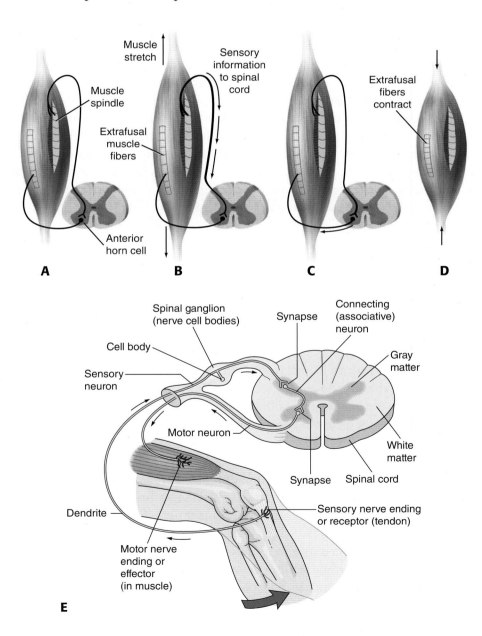

Figure 11–51. Schematic of segmental spinal reflex arc. **A.** The muscle is in a stable state. **B.** The muscle has been passively stretched. Information from the muscle spindle concerning muscle length is transmitted to the spinal cord via the dorsal root ganglion. **C.** Synapse with motor neuron causes efferent activation of muscle fiber. **D.** Extrafusal muscle fibers contract, shortening the muscle to its original length. **E.** Patellar tendon reflex. Note that the blue arrow indicates extension of the lower leg as a result of the muscle contraction. *Source:* From Seikel/Drumright/King. *Anatomy & Physiology for Speech, Language, and Hearing, 5th Ed.* ©Cengage, Inc. Reproduced by permission.

Muscle length and tension must be continually monitored by the nervous system. Your brain needs to know where its muscles are in space and what degree of tone each muscle has. As importantly, a muscle that is supposed to hold a static or stable posture for long periods of time needs to have a system that keeps its length constant. The nervous system has a means of monitoring length and tension that fulfills both of these important functions. The muscle spindle unit senses muscle length, and that information is transmitted to the brain for the purposes of programming movement. The muscle spindle also provides a way to monitor muscle length without having to bother the brain with that detail (Bowman, 1971).

Look at Figure 11–51. Sensory information concerning the length of the muscle is transmitted by means of dorsal root fibers to the spinal cord. The dorsal root fibers synapse with the motor neuron in the ventral cord, and the motor fiber exits the cord to innervate muscle fibers that are being sensed by the muscle spindle. Therefore, if the muscle spindle senses that a muscle has been passively stretched, that information causes the muscle that became longer passively to contract to its original length. The purpose of this reflex is to maintain the length of a muscle fiber that is not being actively contracted, typically for maintenance of posture. If, for instance, you are standing and lean forward slightly, the muscles that are stretched by your leaning will be reflexively contracted until they return to their original length. In this way, you can maintain tonic posture without voluntary effort. This is not a trivial or academic detail, because we have muscle spindles in some of the speech musculature, and that makes a very big difference in neuropathology. Let us examine the sequence of the reflex arc in detail.

As you can see in Figure 11–51B, at rest the muscle is not being stretched and the reflex arc is quiet. In Figure 11–51E, the muscle is being stretched, and a highly specialized sensor, the muscle spindle, senses that stretching process. This information is passed along the neuron to the cell body in the dorsal root ganglion. The information is then passed to a synapse within the anterior horn cells of the spinal cord. The axon synapses with the cell body of a motor neuron in the dorsal gray area of the spinal cord, and that causes the muscle it innervates to contract. Thus, when a muscle is passively stretched, it contracts to return to its original length.

To make this muscle contract, an efferent neuron had to be excited. This neuron within the gray matter of the ventral gray matter is known as the **final common pathway** or **lower motor neuron** (**LMN**), a very functional unit to remember (Figure 11–52). The LMN consists of the dendrites and soma within the spinal cord as well as the axon and components that communicate with the muscle fiber. In contrast, upper motor neurons (**UMNs**) are efferent fibers descending from upper brain levels. UMNs bring commands from the upper brain levels that activate or inhibit muscle function by synapsing with LMNs.

Damage to LMNs results in muscle weakness or complete paralysis, just as if you cut the power line leading to your radio. Damage to the UMNs will cause muscle weakness or paralysis because the information from the brain

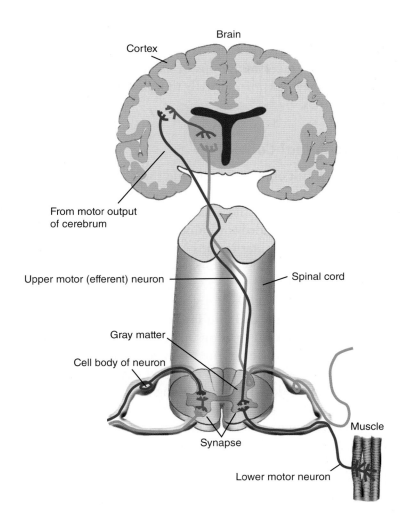

Brain

Cortex

From motor output
of cerebrum

Upper motor (efferent) neuron —

— Spinal cord

Gray matter

Cell body of neuron

Muscle

Synapse

Lower motor neuron

Figure 11–52. Schematic representation of upper motor neuron arising from precentral gyrus of cerebral cortex and projecting through corticospinal tract. *Source:* From Seikel/ Drumright/King. *Anatomy & Physiology for Speech, Language, and Hearing, 5th Ed.* ©Cengage, Inc. Reproduced by permission.

to the LMN is lost; but this UMN damage will leave reflexes intact because the spinal arc reflex is an LMN process. This has great clinical significance, which will become clearer in Chapter 12 when we examine function.

These reflexive responses are certainly important and provide a basic response to the environment. For instance, you reflexively withdraw your hand upon touching the hot burner on a stove. However, for you to make *decisions* about the information, it must reach the cerebral cortex, the seat of conscious thought. You might recall that when you touched the burner on that stove, you retracted your hand well before you felt the heat and pain. This is the hallmark of interaction between the cerebrum and the reflex. Reflexes "put out the brush fire," but neural circuitry also lets the cerebrum know that something has happened so that other action may be taken (such as putting ice on the burn). The time lag between retracting your hand and feeling the burn is an important reminder that reflexes provide nearly instant, automated response well before the cortex could ever respond. On the other hand, the simple reflex is never going to win you the Nobel Prize. These neurons will not produce conscious thought or mediate cognitive processes.

There must be a system of pathways for information to reach the higher centers or to come from those centers. Within the CNS, such pathways are referred to as tracts. Tracts are groups of axons with a functional and anatomical unity (i.e., they transmit generally the same information to generally the same locations).

Pathways of the Spinal Cord

The spinal cord is a conduit of information, and the channels are built along the longitudinal axis. The spinal cord is compartmentalized, so that it is actually subdivided into functionally and anatomically distinct areas. The gray matter of the spinal cord is divided into nine **laminae** or regions, based on cell-type differences. These laminar regions correspond well with the nuclei and regions identified anatomically within the spinal gray.

As you can see from Figure 11–53, a transverse section of the spinal cord is divided into **dorsal, lateral,** and **ventral funiculi** (a *funiculus* is a large column), which are subdivided into **fasciculi** or tracts of white matter. The size and presence of a tract depend on the level of the spinal cord. Tracts that must serve the muscles of the entire body, for instance, will certainly be larger in the upper spinal cord than in the lower cord. Similarly, the gray matter of the cord will be wider in regions serving more muscles, specifically in the cervical and thoracic segments serving the neck (segments C3 to T2) and thoracic segments serving the arms (segments T9 to T12). Those regions have more cell bodies to serve the extremities. Tracts of white matter are widest in the cervical region because all descending and ascending fibers must pass through those segments. Sensory pathways tend to be in the posterior portion of the spinal cord, and motor pathways tend toward the anterior aspect, reflecting the dorsal and ventral orientation of the spinal roots.

Figure 11–53. Transverse section of a spinal cord segment revealing dorsal, lateral, and anterior funiculi and major ascending tracts. *Source:* From Seikel/Drumright/King. *Anatomy & Physiology for Speech, Language, and Hearing, 5th Ed.* ©Cengage, Inc. Reproduced by permission.

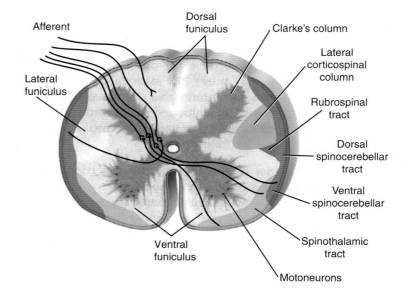

Ascending Pathways

The major ascending sensory pathways include the fasciculus gracilis, fasciculus cuneatus, anterior and lateral spinothalamic tracts, and the anterior and posterior spinocerebellar tracts (Figure 11–54 and Table 11–13). Neurons are referred to as first-order, second-order, and so on to indicate the number of neurons in a chain. Thus, the afferent neuron transmitting information from the sensor is the first-order neuron, the next neuron in the chain following synapse is the second-order neuron, and so forth up to the terminal point in the neural chain.

Posterior Funiculus

The **fasciculus gracilis** and **fasciculus cuneatus** are separated by the posterior intermediate septum of the posterior funiculus. These tracts convey information concerning touch pressure and **kinesthetic sense** (sense of movement), as well as vibration sense, which is actually a temporal form of touch pressure. These columns convey information from group Ia muscle spindle sensors and GTOs as well. The Ia spindle fibers convey information about rate of muscle stretch, whereas the GTOs appear to respond to stretch of the tendon.

Information concerning sensation in the periphery is conducted by the unipolar, first-order neuron of the dorsal root ganglion to the spinal cord. The axons of those neurons ascend on the same side of entry, so that the information is conveyed toward the brain. (The same information remains at the level of entry to form the spinal reflex.) The fasciculus gracilis serves the lower extremities, whereas the fasciculus cuneatus arises from the cervical regions.

The fibers of these tracts ascend **ipsilaterally** (on the same side they entered the cord) until they reach the level of the medulla oblongata of the brain stem to synapse with the nucleus gracilis and **nucleus cuneatus**. The

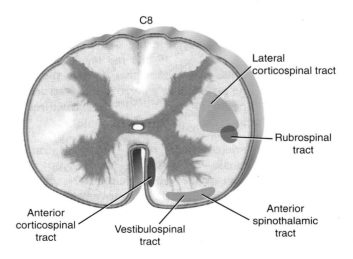

Figure 11–54. Major efferent tracts of the spinal cord as seen in a transverse segment of the cervical spinal cord. *Source:* From Seikel/Drumright/King. *Anatomy & Physiology for Speech, Language, and Hearing, 5th Ed.* ©Cengage, Inc. Reproduced by permission.

Table 11–13

Major Ascending and Descending Pathways			
Afferent Pathways			
Tract	**Origin**	**Termination**	**Function**
Fasciculus gracilis (lemniscal pathway)	Posterior funiculus	Nuc. gracilis	Touch pressure, vibration, kinesthetic sense, muscle stretch (spindles), muscle tension (GTOs), proprioception for lower extremities
Fasciculus cuneatus (lemniscal pathway)	Posterior funiculus	Nuc. cuneatus	Touch pressure, vibration, kinesthetic sense, muscle stretch (spindles), muscle tension (GTOs), proprioception for upper extremities
Anterior spinothalamic (anterior white commissure and medial lemniscus)	Anterior funiculus	Ventral posterolateral nucleus of thalamus	Light touch
Lateral spinothalamic	Anterior funiculus	Ventral posterolateral nucleus of thalamus	Pain, thermal sense
Anterior spinocerebellar	Lateral funiculus	Vermis of cerebellum	Muscle tension from Golgi tendon organ
Posterior spinocerebellar	Lateral funiculus	Vermis of cerebellum	Muscle tension from Golgi tendon organ
Efferent Pathways			
Tract	**Origin**	**Termination**	**Function**
Corticospinal	Frontal lobe, cerebrum	Spinal cord	Activation of skeletal muscle of extremities
Corticobulbar	Frontal lobe, cerebrum	Brain stem	Activation of muscles served by cranial nerves
Tectospinal	Superior colliculus, midbrain	C1–C4 spinal cord	Orienting reflex to visual input
Rubrospinal	Red nucleus, midbrain	Spinal cord	Flexor tone
Vestibulospinal	Lateral vestibular nuclei, pons, and medulla	Spinal cord	Extensor tone, spinal reflexes
Pontine reticulospinal	Medial tegmentum, pons	Spinal cord	Voluntary movement
Medullary reticulospinal	Medulla oblongata	Spinal cord	Voluntary movement

axons of the second-order neuron arising from those nuclei combine and **decussate** (cross the midline) to ascend **contralaterally** (on the other side) as the medial lemniscus to the **thalamus**, and from the thalamus to the precentral gyrus, which is the major sensory relay of the brain (for this reason, the pathway is also referred to as the **lemniscal pathway**). **Spatiotopic** information (information about the specific region of the body stimulated) is maintained throughout the process.

Damage to these pathways will cause problems in touch discrimination, especially in the hands and feet. Patients may lose **proprioceptive sense** (sense of body position in space), which can greatly impair gait.

Anterior Funiculus

The **anterior spinothalamic tract** conveys information concerning light touch, such as the sense of being stroked by a feather, conveyed from the spinal cord to the thalamus (Figure 11–55). Afferent axons of the first-order neuron synapse with anterior spinothalamic tract neurons, the axons

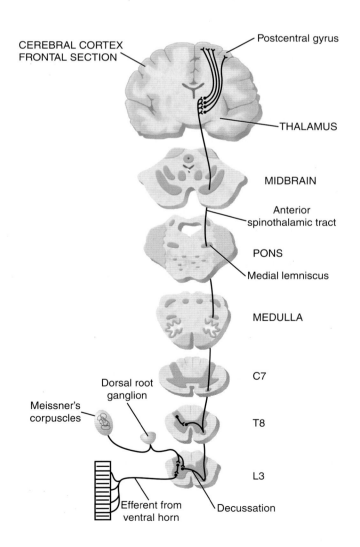

Figure 11–55. Anterior spinothalamic tract, transmitting information concerning the sense of light touch. *Source:* From Seikel/Drumright/King. *Anatomy & Physiology for Speech, Language, and Hearing, 5th Ed.* ©Cengage, Inc. Reproduced by permission.

of which decussate in the **anterior white commissure** of the spine at the level of entry, or perhaps two or three segments higher. The second-order tract neurons ascend to the pons of the brain stem, where fibers enter the **medial lemniscus** to terminate at the ventral posterolateral (VPL) nucleus of the thalamus.

Lateral Funiculus

The last time you stubbed your toe, the information concerning that pain traveled through the **lateral spinothalamic tract**. This important tract transmits information concerning pain and thermal sense. Dorsal root fibers synapse with second-order interneurons that subsequently synapse with third-order tract neurons. These decussate in the anterior white commissure to ascend to the VPL of the thalamus and reticular formation. If the spinal cord is cut unilaterally, the result will be *contralateral* loss of pain and thermal sense beginning one segment below the level of the trauma.

Anterior and Posterior Spinocerebellar Tracts

These important tracts convey information concerning muscle tension to the cerebellum. The **posterior spinocerebellar tract** is an uncrossed tract, meaning that information from one side of the body remains on that side during its ascent through the pathway. Afferent information from GTOs and muscle spindle stretch receptors enters the spinal cord via the dorsal root ganglion where axons of these neurons synapse with the second-order tract fibers. Branches of these first-order neurons ascend and descend, so that synapse occurs at points above and below the site of entry as well. The second-order neurons arise from the dorsal nucleus of Clarke, located in the posterior gray of the cord. Upon reaching the medulla oblongata, the second-order neurons enter the inferior cerebellar peduncle, the lower pathway to the cerebellum. These axons terminate in the rostral and caudal vermis of the cerebellum.

None of the information transmitted by this tract reaches consciousness, although the result of damage to the pathway would. Information from muscles concerning length, rate of stretch, degree of muscle and tendon stretch, and some pressure and touch sense would all be impaired, causing deficit in movement and posture.

The **anterior spinocerebellar tract** is a crossed pathway. Information from Ib afferent fibers serving the Golgi apparatus enters the spinal cord via the dorsal root, where it synapses with the second-order tract neurons. Tract fibers decussate at the same level and ascend through the anterolateral portion of the spinal cord. The tract enters the superior cerebellar peduncle, the superior pathway to the cerebellum from the brain stem. Most of the fibers cross to enter the cerebellum on the opposite side of the tract (but the same side as initial stimulation), with the information presumably serving the same function as that of the posterior spinocerebellar tract.

Descending Pathways

Descending motor pathways are the conduits of information commanding muscle contraction that will result in voluntary movement, modification of reflexes, and visceral activation. The most important of these arise from the cerebral cortex, although there are tracts originating in the brain stem as well. The major pathways include the **pyramidal pathways**. These pathways include the corticospinal tract of Figure 11–56 and corticobulbar tract of Figure 11–57, as well as the tectospinal, rubrospinal, vestibulospinal, pontine reticulospinal, and medullary reticulospinal tracts.

Corticospinal Tract

As the name implies, this extraordinarily important tract runs from the cortex to the spine, providing innervation of skeletal muscle (see Figure 11–56). Myelination of the axons of these fibers occurs after birth and is normally complete by a child's second birthday. The corticospinal tract is made up

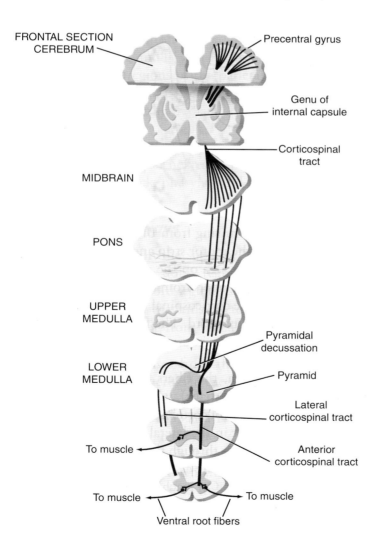

Figure 11–56. Corticospinal pathway as traced from cerebral cortex to spinal cord. *Source:* From Seikel/Drumright/King. *Anatomy & Physiology for Speech, Language, and Hearing, 5th Ed.* ©Cengage, Inc. Reproduced by permission.

Terms of Paralysis

Paralysis refers to temporary or permanent loss of motor function. Paralysis is **spastic** in nature if the lesion causing it is of a UMN. In this type of paralysis, voluntary control is lost through the lesion, but hyperactive reflexes will remain, producing seemingly paradoxical **hyperreflexia** (brisk and overly active reflex responses) and **hypertonia** (muscle tone greater than appropriate) coupled with muscular weakness. **Flaccid** paralysis arises from lesion to the LMN, and results in **hypotonia** (reduced muscle tone) and **hyporeflexia** (reduced or absent reflex response), with co-occurring muscle weakness.

Paralysis of the lower portion of the body, including legs, is termed **paraplegia**. **Tetraplegia (also known as quadriplegia)** refers to the paralysis of all four limbs, usually arising from damage to the spinal cord above C5 or C6. Spinal cord cut above C3 causes death. If lesions produce paralysis of the same part on both sides of the body, it is referred to as **diplegia**, whereas **triplegia** involves three limbs. **Monoplegia** refers to paralysis of only one limb or group of muscles. **Hemiplegia** arises from UMN damage, resulting in loss of function in one side of the body.

The **pontine reticulospinal tract** arises from nuclei in the medial tegmentum of the pons and descends, primarily ipsilaterally, near the MLF in the spinal cord. The **medullary reticulospinal tract** is formed in the medulla oblongata near the inferior olivary complex and descends in the lateral funiculus. Activity of these neurons has both facilitating and inhibiting effects on motor neurons and hence on voluntary movement.

✓ *To summarize:*

- The **spinal cord** is comprised of tracts and nuclei.
- The 31 pairs of **spinal nerves** arise from spinal segments, serving sensory and voluntary motor function for the limbs and trunk.
- **Sensory nerves** have their cell bodies within the dorsal root ganglia, whereas **motor neuron** bodies lie within the gray matter of the spinal cord.
- The **spinal reflex arc** is the simplest motor function, providing an efferent response to a basic change in muscle length.
- Several landmarks of the transverse cord assist in identifying the **funiculi** and **fasciculi** of the spinal cord.
- **Upper motor neurons** have their cell bodies rostral to the segment at which the spinal nerve originates, whereas **lower motor neurons** are the final neurons in the efferent chain.
- **Efferent tracts**, such as the corticospinal tract, transmit information from the brain to the spinal nerves.
- **Afferent tracts**, such as the spinothalamic tract, transmit information concerning the physical state of the limbs and trunk to higher brain centers.
- The **corticobulbar tract** is of particular interest to speech-language pathologists because it serves the motor **cranial nerves** for speech.

Chapter Summary

The nervous system is a complex, hierarchical structure. Voluntary movement, sensory awareness, and cognitive function are the domain of the cerebral cortex. The communication links of the nervous system are spinal nerves, cranial nerves, and tracts of the brain stem and spinal cord. Several organizational schemes characterize the nervous system. The autonomic and somatic nervous systems control involuntary and voluntary functions. We may divide the nervous system into central and peripheral nervous systems. Developmental characterization separates the brain into prosencephalon (telencephalon and diencephalon), the mesencephalon (midbrain), and the rhombencephalon (metencephalon and myelencephalon). Unipolar, bipolar, or multipolar neurons communicate through synapse by means of neurotransmitter substance. Responses may be excitatory or inhibitory. Glial cells provide the fatty sheath for myelinated axons, as well as the support structure for neurons. They also are implicated in long-term memory facilitation.

The cerebral cortex is protected from physical insult by cerebrospinal fluid and the meningeal linings, the dura, pia, and arachnoid mater. Cerebrospinal fluid originating within the ventricles of the brain and circulating around the spinal cord cushions these structures from trauma associated with rapid acceleration. The cerebrum is divided into two hemispheres connected by the corpus callosum. The gyri and sulci of the hemisphere provide important landmarks for lobes and other regions of the cerebrum. The temporal lobe is the site of auditory reception and auditory comprehension; the frontal lobe is responsible for most voluntary motor activation and cognitive function, and is the site of the important speech region known as Broca's area. The parietal lobe is the region of somatic sensory reception. The occipital lobe is the site of visual input to the cerebrum. The insular lobe is revealed by deflecting the temporal lobe and lies deep in the lateral sulcus. The operculum overlies the insula. The functionally defined limbic lobe includes the cingulate gyrus, uncus, parahippocampal gyrus, and other deep structures.

The basal ganglia are subcortical structures involved in the control of movement, and the hippocampal formation of the inferior temporal lobe is deeply implicated in memory function. The thalamus of the diencephalon is the final relay for somatic sensation directed toward the cerebrum and other diencephalic structures. The subthalamus interacts with the globus pallidus to control movement, and the hypothalamus controls many bodily functions and desires. The regions of the cerebral cortex are interconnected by means of a complex network of projection fibers that link the cortex with other structures; association fibers, which connect regions of the same hemisphere; and commissural fibers, which provide communication between corresponding regions of the two hemispheres.

The anterior cerebral arteries serve the medial surfaces of the brain, and the middle cerebral artery serves the lateral cortex, including the temporal lobe, motor strip, Wernicke's area, and much of the parietal lobe. The vertebral arteries branch to form the anterior and posterior spinal arteries, with ascending components serving the ventral brain stem. The basilar artery gives rise to the superior and anterior inferior cerebellar arteries to serve the cerebellum, whereas the posterior inferior cerebellar artery arises from the vertebral artery. The basilar artery divides to become the posterior cerebral arteries, serving the inferior temporal and occipital lobes, upper midbrain, and diencephalon. The circle of Willis is a series of communicating arteries that provide redundant pathways for blood flow to regions of the cerebral cortex, equalizing pressure and flow of blood.

The cerebellum coordinates motor and sensory information, communicating with the brain stem, cerebrum, and spinal cord. It is divided into anterior, middle, and flocculonodular lobes and communicates with the rest of the nervous system via the superior, middle, and inferior cerebellar peduncles. Position in space is coordinated via the flocculonodular lobe, and adjustment against gravity is mediated by the anterior lobe. The posterior lobe mediates fine motor adjustments. The superior cerebellar peduncle enters the pons and serves the dentate nucleus, red nucleus, and thalamus. The middle cerebellar peduncle communicates with the pontine nuclei, whereas the inferior cerebellar peduncle receives input from the spinocerebellar tracts.

The brain stem is divided into medulla, pons, and midbrain. It is more highly organized than the spinal cord and mediates higher-level body functions such as vestibular responses. The pyramidal decussation of the medulla is the point at which the motor commands originating in one hemisphere of the cerebral cortex cross to serve the opposite side of the body. The IX, X, XI, and XII cranial nerves emerge at the level of the medulla. The pons contains three cranial nerve nuclei, the V, VI, and VII nerves. The midbrain contains the important cerebral peduncles and gives rise to the III and IV cranial nerves. The reticular formation is a phylogenetically old set of nuclei essential for life function. The pons and midbrain set the stage for communication with the higher levels of the brain, including the cerebellum and cerebrum. This communication link permits not only complex motor acts but also consciousness, awareness, and volitional acts.

Cranial nerves are extremely important to the speech-language pathologist. Cranial nerves may be sensory, motor, or mixed sensory-motor and are categorized based on their function as being general or specialized, and as serving visceral or somatic organs or structures. The V trigeminal innervates muscles of mastication, the tensor veli palatini, and the tensor tympani, and communicates sensation from the face, mouth, teeth, mucosal lining, and tongue. The VII facial nerve innervates muscles of facial expression, and the sensory component serves taste of the anterior two-thirds of the tongue. The VIII vestibulocochlear nerve mediates auditory

and vestibular sensation. The IX glossopharyngeal nerve serves the posterior tongue taste receptors, as well as somatic sense from the tongue, fauces, pharynx, and eustachian tube. The stylopharyngeus and superior pharyngeal constrictor muscles receive motor innervation via this nerve. The X vagus serves autonomic and somatic functions, mediating pain, touch, and temperature from the ear drum and pain sense from the pharynx, larynx, and esophagus. The recurrent laryngeal nerve and superior laryngeal nerves supply motor innervation for the intrinsic muscles of the larynx. The XI accessory nerve innervates the sternocleidomastoid and trapezius muscles and collaborates with the vagus in the activation of palatal, laryngeal, and pharyngeal muscles. The XII hypoglossal nerve innervates the muscles of the tongue with the exception of the palatoglossus.

The spinal cord is composed of tracts and nuclei. The 31 pairs of spinal nerves serve the limbs and trunk. Sensory nerves have cell bodies in dorsal root ganglia, and motor neuron bodies lie within the spinal cord. Upper motor neurons have their cell bodies above the segment at which the spinal nerve originates. Lower motor neurons are the final neurons in the efferent chain. Efferent tracts, such as the corticospinal tract, transmit information from the brain to the spinal nerves. Afferent tracts, such as the spinothalamic tract, transmit information concerning the physical state of the limbs and trunk to higher brain centers. The corticobulbar tract is of particular interest to speech-language pathologists because it serves motor cranial nerves for speech.

This overview of neuroanatomy should give you some feel for the complexity of this system. The interaction of these systems provides us with the smooth motor function required for speech, as well as the cognitive and linguistic processes required for the comprehension of the spoken word and formulation of a response. Chapter 12 examines some of those processes.

Chapter 11 Study Questions

1. The _____ governs voluntary actions.

2. The _____ is responsible for coordinating movement.

3. _____ is the sense of muscle and joint position.

4. _____ are groups of cell bodies in the PNS with functional unity.

5. _____ sense is the sense of the body in motion.

6. Special senses include _____, _____, _____, and _____.

7. The _____ system includes the cerebrum, cerebellum, subcortical structures, brain stem, and spinal cord.

8. The _____ consists of the 12 pairs of cranial nerves and 31 pairs of spinal nerves, as well as the sensory receptors.

9. The _____ governs involuntary activities of involuntary muscles.

10. The _____ governs voluntary activities.

11. Information directed toward the brain is termed _____ whereas information directed from the brain is termed _____.

12. Developmental divisions: Identify the division referred to by each statement.

   A. _____ refers to the "extended" or "telescoped" brain and includes the cerebral hemispheres, the white matter immediately beneath it, the basal ganglia, and the olfactory tract.

   B. _____ refers to the olfactory bulb, tract, and striae; pyriform area; intermediate olfactory area; hippocampal formation; and fornix.

   C. _____ includes the thalamus, hypothalamus, pituitary gland (hypophysis), and optic tract.

   D. _____ refers to the midbrain.

   E. _____ includes the pons and cerebellum.

   F. _____ refers to the medulla.

13. On the figure below, identify the parts of the neuron indicated.

A. _____

B. _____

C. _____

D. _____

E. _____

F. _____

G. _____

H. _____

I. _____

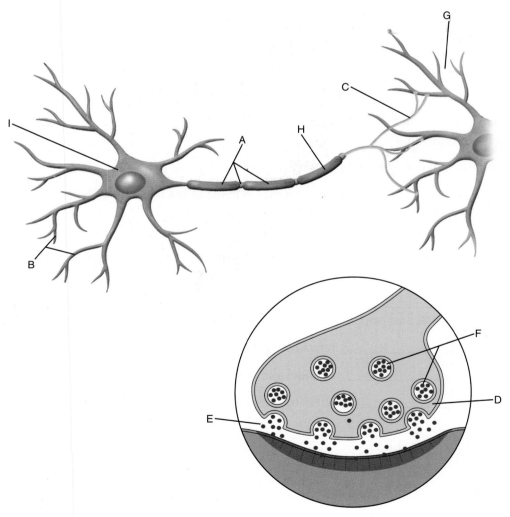

Source: From Seikel/Drumright/King. *Anatomy & Physiology for Speech, Language, and Hearing, 5th Ed.* ©Cengage, Inc. Reproduced by permission.

14. On the figure below, identify the parts of the cerebrum indicated.

A. _____ lobe

B. _____ lobe

C. _____ lobe

D. _____ lobe

E. _____ gyrus

F. _____ gyrus

G. _____ sulcus

H. _____ sulcus

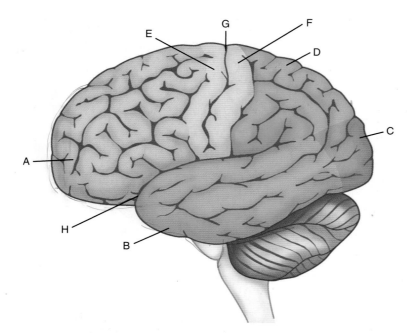

Source: From Seikel/Drumright/King. *Anatomy & Physiology for Speech, Language, and Hearing*, 5th Ed. ©Cengage, Inc. Reproduced by permission.

15. On the figure below, identify the parts of the surface of the cerebrum.

A. _____ gyrus

B. _____

C. _____ gyrus

D. _____ area

E. _____ area

F. _____ area

G. _____ gyrus

H. _____ gyrus

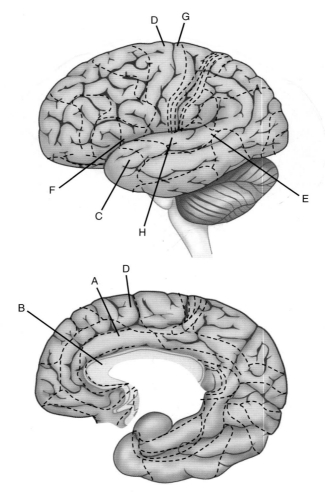

Source: From Seikel/Drumright/King. *Anatomy & Physiology for Speech, Language, and Hearing, 5th Ed.* ©Cengage, Inc. Reproduced by permission.

16. On the figure below, identify the components of the ventricle system indicated.

A. _____

B. _____

C. _____

D. _____

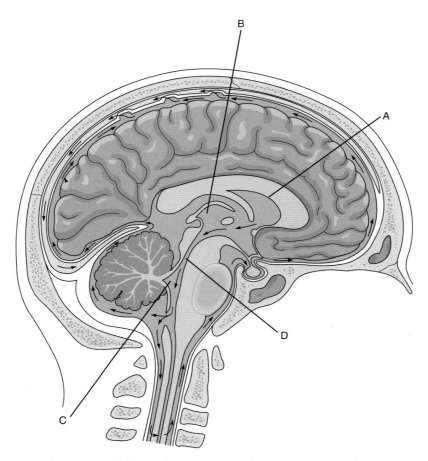

Source: From Seikel/Drumright/King. *Anatomy & Physiology for Speech, Language, and Hearing, 5th Ed.* ©Cengage, Inc. Reproduced by permission.

17. On the figure below, identify the arteries and the structure indicated.

A. _____ artery

B. _____ artery

C. _____ artery

D. _____ artery

E. _____ artery

F. _____ artery

G. _____ artery

H. _____ artery

I. _____

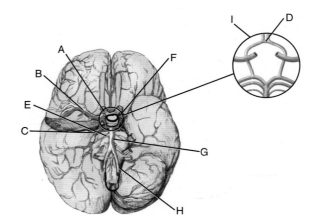

Source: From Seikel/Drumright/King. *Anatomy & Physiology for Speech, Language,
and Hearing, 5th Ed.* ©Cengage, Inc. Reproduced by permission.

18. Redundancy is nature's safety net. Identify as many redundant systems as you can within
the nervous system.

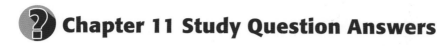

Chapter 11 Study Question Answers

1. The **CEREBRUM** governs voluntary actions.

2. The **CEREBELLUM** is responsible for coordinating movement.

3. **PROPRIOCEPTION** is the sense of muscle and joint position.

4. **GANGLIA** are groups of cell bodies in the PNS with functional unity.

5. **KINESTHETIC** sense is the sense of the body in motion.

6. Special senses include **OLFACTION, VISION, GUSTATION**, and **AUDITION**.

7. The **CENTRAL NERVOUS** system includes the cerebrum, cerebellum, subcortical structures, brain stem, and spinal cord.

8. The **PERIPHERAL NERVOUS SYSTEM** consists of the 12 pairs of cranial nerves and 31 pairs of spinal nerves, as well as the sensory receptors.

9. The **AUTONOMIC NERVOUS SYSTEM** governs involuntary activities of involuntary muscles.

10. The **SOMATIC NERVOUS SYSTEM** governs voluntary activities.

11. Information directed toward the brain is termed **AFFERENT** whereas information directed from the brain is termed **EFFERENT**.

12. Developmental divisions are identified as follows:

    A. **TELENCEPHALON** refers to the "extended" or "telescoped" brain, and includes the cerebral hemispheres, the white matter immediately beneath it, the basal ganglia, and the olfactory tract.

    B. **RHINENCEPHALON** refers to the olfactory bulb, tract, and striae; pyriform area; intermediate olfactory area; hippocampal formation; and fornix.

    C. **DIENCEPHALON** includes the thalamus, hypothalamus, pituitary gland (hypophysis), and optic tract.

    D. **MESENCEPHALON** refers to the midbrain.

    E. **METENCEPHALON** includes the pons and cerebellum.

    F. **MYELENCEPHALON** refers to the medulla.

13. The parts of the neuron indicated are as follows:

    A. **AXON**

    B. **DENDRITE**

    C. **TELODENDRIA**

    D. **TERMINAL END BOUTON**

    E. **SYNAPTIC CLEFT**

    F. **SYNAPTIC VESICLES**

    G. **POSTSYNAPTIC NEURON**

    H. **MYELIN SHEATH**

    I. **SOMA**

14. The parts of the cerebrum indicated are as follows:

    A. **FRONTAL** lobe

    B. **TEMPORAL** lobe

    C. **OCCIPITAL** lobe

    D. **PARIETAL** lobe

    E. **PRECENTRAL** gyrus

    F. **POSTCENTRAL** gyrus

    G. **CENTRAL** sulcus

    H. **LATERAL** sulcus

15. The parts of the surface of the cerebrum are as follows:

    A. **CINGULATE** gyrus

    B. **CORPUS CALLOSUM**

    C. **SUPERIOR TEMPORAL** gyrus

    D. **SUPPLEMENTARY MOTOR** area

    E. **WERNICKE'S** area

    F. **BROCA'S** area

    G. **PRECENTRAL** gyrus

    H. **HESCHL'S** gyrus

16. The components of the ventricle system indicated are as follows:

    A. **LATERAL VENTRICLE**

    B. **THIRD VENTRICLE**

    C. **FOURTH VENTRICLE**

    D. **CEREBRAL AQUEDUCT**

17. The arteries and the structure indicated are as follows:

    A. **ANTERIOR CEREBRAL** artery

    B. **MIDDLE CEREBRAL** artery

    C. **POSTERIOR CEREBRAL** artery

D. **ANTERIOR COMMUNICATING** artery

E. **SUPERIOR CEREBELLAR** artery

F. **INTERNAL CAROTID** artery

G. **BASILAR** artery

H. **VERTEBRAL** artery

I. **CIRCLE OF WILLIS**

18. Redundancy takes many forms within the nervous system. One of the most obvious is the presence of two cerebral hemispheres, although they are not functionally equal, as we will see in Chapter 12. The fact that the corticospinal tract divides into anterior and lateral corticospinal tracts indicates some safety in spreading the "risk" around. Likewise, the circle of Willis within the cerebrovascular system is an important safety valve. What about the fact there are identical nuclei within each half of the brain stem? How about the fact that the upper face is bilaterally innervated? Can you think of any other redundancies?

Bibliography

Akshoomoff, N. A., & Courchesne, E. (1992). A new role for the cerebellum in cognitive operations. *Behavioral Neuroscience, 106*(5), 731–738.

Albin, R. L. (1995). The pathophysiology of chorea/ballism and parkinsonism. *Parkinsonism and Related Disorders, 1*(1), 3–11.

Allen, N. J., & Eroglu, C. (2017). Cell biology of astrocyte-synapse interactions. *Neuron, 96*(3), 697–708.

Amaral, D., & Lavenex, P. (2007). Hippocampal anatomy. In P. Andersen, R. Morris, D. Amaral, T. Bliss, & J. O'Keefe (Eds.), *The hippocampus book* (pp. 37–114). New York, NY: Oxford University Press.

Andersen, P., Morris, R., Amaral, D., Bliss, T., & O'Keefe, J. (2007). The hippocampal formation. In P. Andersen, R. Morris, D. Amaral, T. Bliss, & J. O'Keefe (Eds.), *The hippocampus book* (pp. 3–6). New York, NY: Oxford University Press.

Azevado, F. A. C., Carvalho, L. R. B., Gringberg, L. T., Farfel, J. M., Ferretti, R. E. L., Leite, R. . . . Herculano-Houzel, S. (2009). Equal numbers of neuronal and non-neuronal cells make the human brain an isometrically scaled-up primate. *Journal of Comparative Neurology, 513*, 532–541.

Bach, P., Peelen, M. V., & Tipper, S. P. (2010). On the role of object information in action observation: An fMRI study. *Cerebral Cortex, 20*(12), 2798–2809.

Bowman, J. P. (1971). *The muscle spindle and neural control of the tongue.* Springfield, IL: Charles C. Thomas.

Brodmann, K., & Garey, L. J. (2007). *Brodmann's: Localisation in the cerebral cortex.* New York, NY: Springer.

Church, J. A., Coalson, R. S., Lugar, H. M., Petersen, S. E., & Schlaggar, B. L. (2008). A developmental fMRI study of reading and repetition reveals changes in phonological and visual mechanisms over age. *Cerebral Cortex, 18*, 2054–2065.

Craig, A. D. (2002). How do you feel? Interoception: The sense of the physiological condition of the body. *Nature Reviews Neuroscience, 3*, 655–666.

Dalgleish, T. (2004). The emotional brain. *Nature Reviews Neuroscience, 5*, 582–589.

de Vries, H. E., Kuiper, J., de Boer, A. G., Van Berkel, T. J. C., & Breimer, D. D., (1997). The blood–brain barrier in neuroinflammatory disease. *Pharmacological Reviews, 49*(2), 143–156.

Di Cesare, G., Marchi, M., Errante, A., Fasano, F., & Rizzolatti, G. (2017). Mirroring the social aspects of speech and actions: The role of the insula. *Cerebral Cortex, 28*(4), 1348–1357.

Dronkers, N. F. (1996). A new brain region for coordinating speech articulation. *Nature, 384*(6605), 159–161.

Ehrsson, H. H., Spence, C., & Passingham, R. E. (2004). That's my hand! Activity in premotor cortex reflects feeling of ownership of a limb. *Science, 305*(5685), 875–877.

Farrer, C., Frey, S. H., Van Horn, J. D., Tunik, E., Turk, D., Inati, S., & Grafton, S. T. (2007). The angular gyrus computes action awareness representations. *Cerebral Cortex, 18,* 254–261.

Ffytch, D. H. (2005). Perisylvian language networks of the human brain. *Annals of Neurology, 57,* 8–16.

Fields, D. (2004, April). The other half of the brain. *Scientific American,* 53–61.

Fields, R. D. (2007). Sex and the secret nerve. *Scientific American Mind, 18,* 20–27.

Fischer, H., Andersson, J. L., Furmark, T., & Fredrikson, M. (1998). Brain correlates of an unexpected panic attack: A human positron emission tomographic study. *Neuroscience letters, 251*(2), 137–140.

Fuller, G. N., & Burger, P. C. (1990). Nervus terminalis (cranial nerve zero) in the adult human. *Clinical Neuropathology, 9*(6), 279–283.

Gilman, S., & Winans, S. S. (2002). *Manter and Gatz's essentials of clinical neuroanatomy and neurophysiology* (10th ed.). Philadelphia, PA: F. A. Davis.

Horn, J. P., & Swanson, L. W. (2012). The autonomic motor system and the hypothalamus. In E. R. Kandel, J. H. Schwartz, T. M. Jessell, S. A. Siegelbaum & A. J. Hudspeth, (Eds.), *Principles of neural science* (5th ed., pp. 1056–1078). New York, NY: McGraw-Hill.

Jespersen, S. N., & Ostergaard, L. (2012). The roles of cerebral blood flow, capillary transit time heterogeneity, and oxygen tension in brain oxygenation and metabolism. *Journal of Blood Flow and Metabolism, 32*(2), 264–277.

Kaiser, D. A. (2010). Cortical cartography. *Biofeedback, 38*(1), 9–12.

Kandel, E. R. (2012). From nerve cells to cognition: The internal representation of space and action. In K. R. Kandel, J. H. Schwartz, T. M. Jessell, S. A. Siegelbaum, & A. J. Hudspeth (Eds.), *Principles of neural science* (5th ed., pp. 370–392). New York, NY: McGraw-Hill.

Kanwisher, N., McDermott, J., & Chun, M. M. (1997). The fusiform face area: A module in human extrastriate cortex specialized for face perception. *Journal of Neuroscience, 17*(11), 4302–4311.

Karlsen, A. S., & Pakkenberg, B. (2011). Total numbers of neurons and glial cells in cortex and basal ganglia of aged brains with Down syndrome—a sterological study. *Cerebral Cortex, 21*(11), 2519–2524.

Kobayashi, M. (2006). Functional organization of the human gustatory cortex. *Oral Bioscience, 48*(4), 244–260.

Kringelbach, M. L., & Rolls, E. T. (2004). The functional neuroanatomy of the human orbitofrontal cortex: Evidence from neuroimaging and neuropsychology. *Progress in Neurobiology, 72,* 341–372.

Lutz, A., Greischar, L. L., Perlman, D. M., & Davidson, R. J. (2009). BOLD signal in insula is differentially related to cardiac function during compassion meditation in experts vs. novices. *NeuroImage, 47,* 1038–1046.

Mackay, L. E., Chapman, P. E., & Morgan, A. S. (1997). *Maximizing brain injury* recovery. Gaithersburg, MD: Aspen.

Mariën, P., Baillieux, H., De Smet, H. J., Engelborghs, S., Wilssens, I., Paquier, P., & De Deyn, P. P. (2009). Cognitive, linguistic and affective disturbances following a right superior cerebellar artery infarction: A case study. *Cortex 45*(4), 527–536.

Møller, A. R. (2003). *Sensory systems: Anatomy and physiology.* New York, NY: Academic Press.

Naqvi, N. H., Rudrauf, D., Damasio, H., & Bechara, A. (2007). Damage to the insula disrupts addiction to cigarette smoking. *Science, 315*(5811), 531–534.

Noback, C. R., Strominger, N. L., Demarest, R. J., & Ruggiero, D. A. (2005). *The nervous system: Structure and function* (6th ed.). Totowa, NJ: Humana Press.

O'Brown, N. M., Pfau, S. J., & Gu, C. (2018). Bridging barriers: A comparative look at the blood–brain barrier across organisms. *Genes and Development, 32*(7–8), 466–478.

Pakkenberg, B., & Gunderson, H. J. G. (2011). Total number of neurons and glial cells in human brain nuclei estimated by the dissector and tractionator. *Journal of Microscopy, 10*(1), 1–20.

Papantchev, V., Hristov, S., Todorova, D., Naydenov, E., Paloff, A., Nikolov, D., Tschirkov, A., & Ovtscharoff, W. (2007). Some variations of the circle of Willis, important cerebral protection in aortic surgery—A study in Eastern Europeans. *European Journal of Cardiothoracic Surgery, 31*(6), 982–989.

Penfield, W., & Roberts, L. (1959). *Speech and brain mechanisms.* Princeton, NJ: Princeton University Press.

Pickles, J. O. (2012). *An introduction to physiology of hearing* (4th ed.). Bingley, UK: Emerald Group.

Sajja, V. S., Hlavac, N., & VandeVord, P. J. (2016). Role of glia in memory deficits following traumatic brain injury: Biomarkers of glia dysfunction. *Frontiers in Integrative Neuroscience, 10,* 7.

Schaltenbrand, G., & Woolsey, C. N. (1964). *Cerebral localization and organization.* Madison, WI: University of Wisconsin Press.

Seikel, J. A., Drumright, D. G., & King, D. W. (2015). *Anatomy & physiology for speech, language, and hearing.* Clifton Park, NJ: Cengage Learning.

Seikel, J. A., Konstantopoulos, K., & Drumright, D. G. (2020). *Neuroanatomy and neurophysiology for speech and hearing sciences*. San Diego, CA: Plural Publishing.

Stolov, W. C., & Clowers, M. R. (1981). *Handbook of severe disability: A text for rehabilitation counselors, other vocational practitioners, and allied health professionals*. U.S. Government Printing.

Strominger, N. L., Demarest, R. J., & Laemle, L. B. (2012). *Noback's human nervous system, seventh edition: Structure and function*. New York, NY: Springer.

Sugiura, L., Ojima, S., Matsuba-Kurita, H., Dan, I., Tsuzuki, D., Katura, T., & Hagiwara, H. (2011). Sound to language: Different cortical processing of the first and second language in elementary school children as revealed by a large scale study using fNIRS. *Cerebral Cortex, 21*(10), 2374–2393.

Suzuki, A., Stern, S. A., Bozdagi, O., Huntley, G. W., Walker, R. H., & Alberini, C. M. (2011). Astrocyte-neuron lactate transport is required for long-term memory formation. *Cell, 4*(5), 810–823.

Tremblay, M. E., Cookson, M. R., & Civiero, L. (2019). Glial phagocytic clearance in Parkinson's disease. *Molecular Neurodegeneration, 14*(1), 16.

Tsao, D. Y., Freiwald, W. A., Tootell, R. B. H., & Livingstone, M. S. (2006). A cortical region consisting entirely of face-selective cells. *Science, 311*, 670–674.

Uddin, L. Q., Nomi, J. S., Hebert-Seropian, B., Ghaziri, J., & Boucher, O. (2017). Structure and function of the human insula. *Journal of Clinical Neurophysiology, 34*(4), 300–306.

Whitlock, K. E. (2004). Development of the nervus terminalis: Origin and migration. *Microscopic Research Techniques, 65*(1–2), 2–12.

Winans, S. S., Gilman, S., Manter, J. T., & Gatz, A. J. (2002). *Manter and Gatz's essentials of clinical neuroanatomy and neurophysiology* (10th ed.). Philadelphia, PA: F. A. Davis.

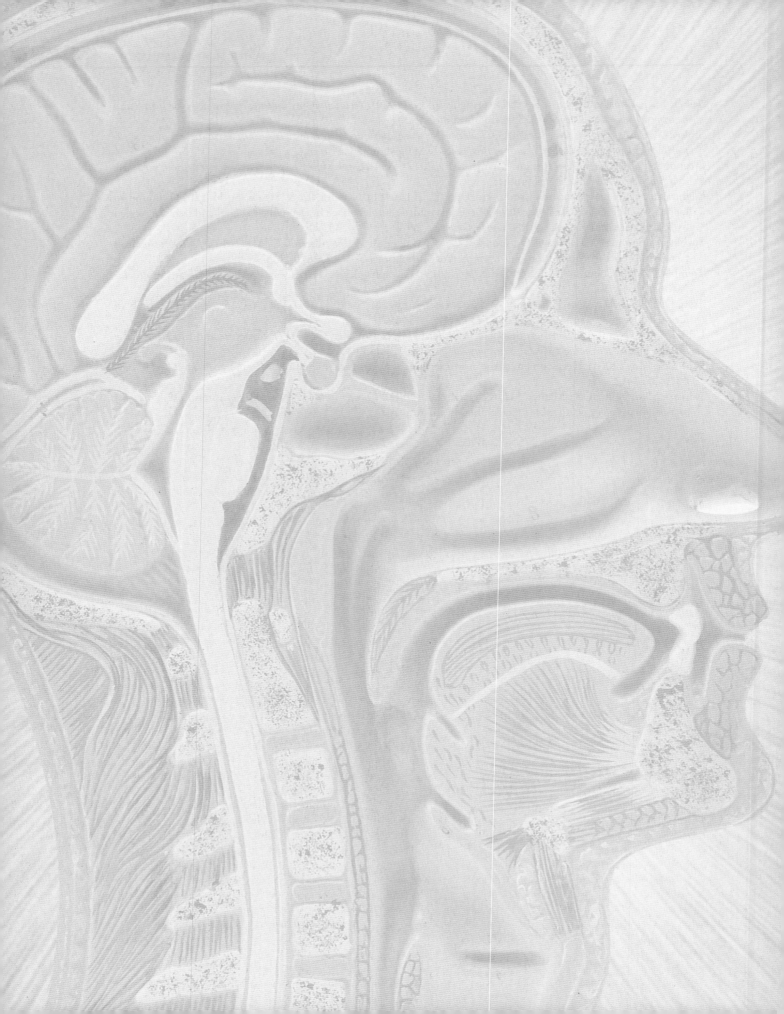

Neurophysiology

Although extraordinary advances over the past 30 years have vastly expanded our understanding of the workings of the brain, we still have a great deal to learn. We will set out in this chapter to provide at least some of the pieces of the puzzle. Knowledge of how the nervous system functions is the key to successful treatment by audiologists and speech-language pathologists. All speech-language therapy works within the limits of the client's nervous system, because behavior, motivation, learning, and especially speech and language functions depend on the ability to process information and respond to it. We hope that this introduction to nervous system physiology will tempt you to spend your life examining it.

We approach our discussion of nervous system function from the bottom up, looking first at the simplest responses of the system (communication between neurons) and working our way up to the all-important functions of the cerebral cortex (Table 12–1). The **single-neuron response** and the **spinal reflex arc** associated with the spinal cord represent the basic level of information processing, and the brain stem structures provide control of balance and **multi-segment** and high-level **brain stem reflexes**. Communication among structures of the nervous system is by means of tracts composed of neurons. The diencephalon supports attention to stimulation and basic (but highly organized) responses to danger. The cerebellum provides exquisite **integration of sensory information** and **motor planning**, and participates in cognitive processing and learning (Akshoomoff & Courchesne, 1992), but the cerebrum is the site of **consciousness**, **planning**, **ideation**, and **cognition**. When you are caught off guard by a loud noise, your lower (primary) neural processes will register the noise, cause you to orient to it, cause you to flinch, and even possibly cause you to move away from it. Only your cerebrum evaluates the input to determine the nature and meaning of the noise. Your eyes can receive light reflected off the Mona Lisa; your brain stem's visual pathways can process information concerning shapes, forms, textures, and colors—but it takes your cerebrum to wonder why she is smiling.

Instrumentation in Neurophysiology

The physiology of the nervous system is extraordinarily complex. The structures we are attempting to measure are exquisitely tiny, and the number

Table 12–1

Structures of Nervous System and General Functions	
Structure	**General Function**
Neurons	Single-neuron communication among tissues, organs, and other structures
Spinal reflex arc	Subconscious response to environmental stimuli
Multi-segment spinal reflexes	Complex subconscious response to environmental stimuli
Tracts	Transmission of information to cerebrum or periphery
Brain stem	Mediation of high-level reflexes and maintenance of life function; activation of cranial nerves
Diencephalon	Mediation of sensory information arriving at cerebrum and provision of basic autonomic responses for body maintenance
Cerebellum	Integration of somatic and special sensory information with motor planning and command for coordinated movement
Cerebrum	Processing of conscious sensory information, planning and executing voluntary motor act, analyzing stimuli, performing cognitive functions, decoding and encoding linguistic information

of structures we want to examine boggle the mind. A wide array of instruments and techniques have been developed to help us peer into this marvelous system.

Many methods attempt to view the structure and function of the brain in a macroscopic way. These methods have resolution down to the millimeter level (i.e., the level that we would have with the naked eye, were we to have the opportunity to view the tissue itself). We are all familiar with the beautiful display of the brain presented through the lens of magnetic resonance imaging (MRI). This method uses very strong magnets to align nuclei of the atoms of your body, and the results can be analyzed to produce two- or three-dimensional images that far exceed those available through x-ray radiographic techniques. MRI is particularly useful for soft tissue, such as that found in the brain, and contrast agents can help physicians identify different structures (such as tumors, or characteristics of the blood supply). A positive benefit of MRI is that it does not use radiation, and therefore has significantly reduced risk for the patient. A modification of the MRI is functional MRI (fMRI), which measures blood flow to tissue. The notion of fMRI is that blood flowing to tissue reflects increased metabolic activity, which implies function of the tissue. Thus, if someone is hearing words and the left-hemisphere Wernicke's area is active ("lights up"), researchers imply that Wernicke's area is important for listening to words. If the same subject is given warble tones to listen to and the right superior temporal gyrus is active, the researcher may conclude that these two types of stimuli are processed differentially by the brain. fMRI summates information over a 2- to 3-second period, so that temporal resolution is limited. (fMRIs are also very, very noisy, which reduces their functionality for intricate psycho-acoustical studies.) Specific pathways of the brain can be visualized using diffusion tensor imaging, providing striking evidence of tracts within the brain (e.g., Mueller et al., 2013). MRI and fMRI provide resolution down to about 1 mm, which is remarkable. (Realize, also, that the cortex is between 1 and 5 mm thick, has a volume of 11,300 cubic millimeters, and holds 17,000,000,000 neurons. That 1 mm resolution will include activity between 1.5 million and 7.5 million neurons.)

Another macroscopic view is provided by computer-aided tomography (CT or CAT). CT scans use low-dose irradiation to create three-dimensional images of the tissue under study. The patient may swallow a contrast medium that enhances aspects of the tissue, such as the vascular supply. CT scans are quite useful for imaging problems with the cerebrovascular supply and can show evidence of hemorrhage or ischemia (blockage) that has caused a cerebrovascular accident. Density of tissue will cause differences in the image, so tumors can be more readily seen through CT scans than MRI. Variants of the CT scan include single-photon emission computed tomography (SPECT) and positron emission tomography (PET). PET is similar to fMRI, in that it reveals blood flow, although requiring use of ionizing radiation. PET allows researchers to label neurotransmitters and observe active sites, which is a significant advantage over fMRI.

Magnetoenceophalography (MEG) measures the magnetic fields generated by the brain and provides excellent temporal resolution (but poor spatial resolution). The most common implementation of MEG is through superconducting quantum interference devices (SQUIDs).

There are many microscopic methods available to researchers, some of which we discussed in Chapter 10. Time-honored electroencephalography (EEG) remains a clinical and research staple. EEG measures the brain-wave activity over the scalp, revealing frequencies of activity at a significant distance from the generator source. Auditory brain stem responses (ABR) are an example of evoked EEG activity, wherein audiologists measure the brain's EEG relative to an auditory stimulus, specifically brain stem activity. Event-related potentials (ERP) record cortical activity using a large array of electrodes. Unlike ABR, ERP allows researchers and clinicians to more accurately define the neural generator for responses to stimuli (Johnson, 2009). Using these methods, for instance, a researcher can produce verbal or visual stimuli that differ in some strategic way (e.g., verb versus noun) and identify the primary sites of activation and changes that occur over time relative to the stimuli. Single-cell measurement has been a staple of neuro-physiological research for decades, and recent advances in microvisualization methods have allowed researchers to view the activity of small volumes of

nodes of Ranvier but generally are absent in the myelinated regions. The myelin insulates the fiber so that even if there were channels, they would serve no function, because ions cannot pass through them. The nodes of Ranvier are precisely spaced, based on the diameter of the axon, to promote maximum conduction time.

Thus, the membrane becomes depolarized at one node, and the effect of that depolarization is felt at the next node where the membrane depolarizes as well. The propagating action potential is passed from node to node, and this jumping is referred to as **saltatory conduction**. Clearly, in long fibers, many precious milliseconds can be saved by skipping from node to node.

When the impulse reaches the terminal point on an axon, a highly specialized process begins. The synaptic vesicles within the terminal end boutons release a neurotransmitter substance that permits communication between two neurons. A **neurotransmitter** is a substance that causes either the excitation or inhibition of another neuron or the excitation of a muscle fiber. When the AP reaches the terminal point, the vesicles are stimulated to migrate to the membrane wall, where they dump their neurotransmitter through the membrane into the synaptic cleft (Figure 12–3).

The neurotransmitter travels across the synapse very quickly (100 microseconds) and is emptied into the cleft to activate receptor proteins on the **postsynaptic neuron**. The presence of neurotransmitters in the cleft triggers ion channels to open. Neurotransmitters fit into specific ion channels,

Neurotransmitters

There are four major classes of neurotransmitters: amino acids, acetylcholine, monoamines and neuropeptides (Table 12–2).

Amino acids can be either excitatory or inhibitory, and include **glutamate (GLU)** and **aspartate (ASP)** as excitatory neurotransmitters and **gamma-amino butyric acid** (GABA) and **glycine** as inhibitory neurotransmitters. Glutamate is the most prevalent excitatory neurotransmitter in the CNS, but excessive glutamate is a neurotoxin. Many sedatives act on GABA receptors. **Acetylcholine** (ACH) is used by neurons to activate muscles. ACH is also found in the striatum, and is critical to memory function: it declines as Alzheimer's disease progresses. It is a critical neurotransmitter of the reticular activating system of the brain stem/thalamus, mediating consciousness, arousal, sleep and wakefulness.

Monoamines include catecholamines and serotonin. **Dopamine** (DA) is responsible for inhibition in the hypothalamus, brain stem, and basal ganglia. Alterations in DA are seen in Parkinson's disease, schizophrenia, and attention deficit hyperactivity disorder (ADHD).

Norepinephrine (NE) (aka noradrenaline) is classified as a hormone and a neurotransmitter. As a "stress hormone," NE is released under acute physical and/or psychological stress, causing increased heart rate and fear-based vigilance. NE is critical to sensory focus and attentional shift, and is involved in reward and attention. **Serotonin** is important for regulation of mood, depression, and appetite, as well as memory, sleep, and learning. Selective serotonin reuptake inhibitors (SSRIs) alleviate depression by keeping serotonin in the nervous system longer.

Neuropeptides include both hormones and neurotransmitters. They include opioids (sedatives), oxytocin, and insulin. Neuropeptides are actively involved in sensory perception, emotion, pain, and stress responses.

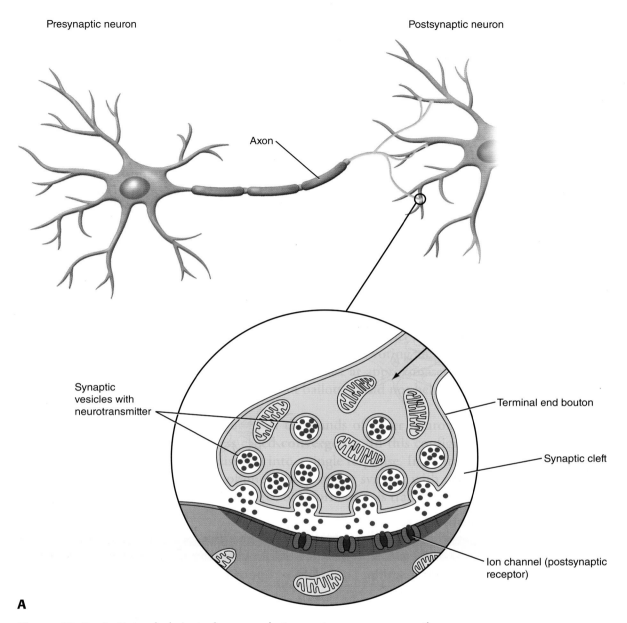

Presynaptic neuron

Postsynaptic neuron

Axon

Synaptic vesicles with neurotransmitter

Terminal end bouton

Synaptic cleft

Ion channel (postsynaptic receptor)

A

Figure 12–3. A. Expanded view of synapse between two neurons. *continues*

and if a given neurotransmitter does not match a receptor channel protein, the postsynaptic neuron does not fire. That is, the neurotransmitter is a key and the receptor is a lock: If the key does not fit, the gate will not open.

The neurotransmitter may have either an excitatory or an inhibitory effect on the neuron. **Excitatory effects** increase the probability that a neuron will depolarize, whereas **inhibition** decreases that probability. An excitatory stimulation generates an **excitatory postsynaptic potential (EPSP)**, whereas inhibitory stimulus produces an **inhibitory postsynaptic potential (IPSP)**. Excitation causes depolarization, whereas inhibition causes **hyperpolarization**, greatly elevating the threshold of firing. Generally, inhibitory synapses are found on the soma. Synapses on the dendrites

- The **absolute refractory period** after excitation is an interval during which the neuron cannot be excited to fire, whereas it may fire during the **relative refractory period**, given adequate stimulation.

- Myelinated fibers conduct the wave of depolarization more rapidly than demyelinated fibers, primarily because of **saltatory conduction**.

Muscle Function

A similar process occurs at the **neuromuscular junction**, the point where a nerve and muscle communicate. In this case, the product of the communication is a muscle twitch rather than an AP. The basic unit of skeletal muscle control is the **motor unit**, consisting of the motor neuron, its axon, and the muscle fibers it innervates.

Figure 12–4 shows a neuromuscular junction, which looks very much like a synapse. In this case, however, there is a **terminal endplate** on the axon, with a synaptic cleft as before. The neurotransmitter **acetylcholine** is released into the active zone, and a **miniature end plate potential (MEPP)** is generated. If there are sufficient numbers of MEPPs, a muscle action potential is generated. This is directly analogous to that of a synapse, in that it takes many activated regions to excite a muscle fiber. In addition, we will see that we must activate many muscle fibers to actually move a muscle and do work.

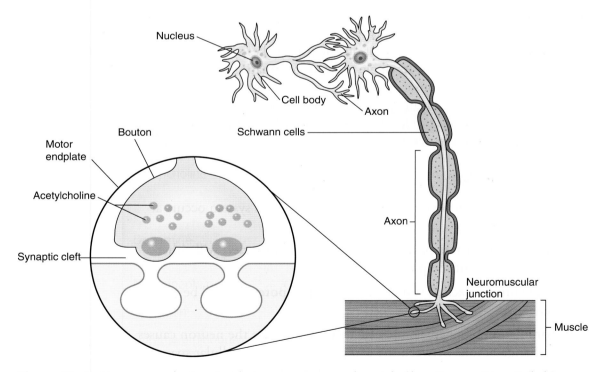

Figure 12–4. Neuromuscular junction between neuron and muscle fiber. *Source:* From Seikel/Drumright/King. *Anatomy & Physiology for Speech, Language, and Hearing, 5th Ed.* ©Cengage, Inc. Reproduced by permission.

You know that movement requires muscular effort, and that muscles can only contract, shortening the distance between two points. This is a good opportunity to examine that function at a microscopic level.

If you were to look at a cotton rope, you would see that the rope is actually made up of smaller ropes, wrapped in a spiral. If you were to look closer, you could see that those smaller spiral ropes are made up of individual strings, and your microscope would show you that those strings were made of cotton fibers that had been spun into thread. There are successively smaller elements from which the rope is made, and they all have a similar orientation and structure. The same is true for the muscle.

As you can see from Figure 12–5, the skeletal (striated) muscle is a long ropelike structure made up of strands of muscle fiber, each running the length of the muscle and having many nuclei. Each muscle fiber is made up of long **myofibrils**, and myofibrils are composed of either **thin** or **thick myofilaments**.

Thin myofilaments are composed of a pair of **actin** protein strands coiled around each other to form a spiral or helix. Double strands of tropomyosin that are laced with molecules of troponin wrap around this helix. Thick myofilaments are composed of myosin molecules arranged in a staggered formation. These two components (actin and myosin) are key players in movement: The actin and myosin filaments slide past one another during muscle contraction, with **bridging arms** reaching from the myosin to the actin. The tropomyosin and troponin facilitate the bridging arms, as you will see.

When the myofilaments group together to form muscle myofibrils, a characteristic striated appearance is seen. This is the product of alternating dark and light myofilaments. Each of these combined units is known as a **sarcomere**. The sarcomere is the building block of striated muscle. An area known as the **Z line** marks the margin of the sarcomere, and the thin filaments are bound at this point. The thick filaments are centered within the sarcomere, much like overlapping bricks in a wall. The **A band** is the region of overlap between thin and thick fibers at rest, and the **H zone** in the center of the sarcomere is a region with only thick filaments. The two myofilaments slide across each other as the muscle shortens, bringing the centers of the thin and thick filaments closer together. Here is how that happens.

When the muscle is at rest, the regulatory proteins of tropomyosin on the thin filaments block the binding sites, prohibiting the formation of cross-bridges. The regulatory proteins are guards that prohibit the myosin and actin from interacting. For a cross-bridge to form, the tropomyosin must be moved out of the way to free up the binding sites, and that function is performed by calcium. When calcium is present in the environment, it changes the configuration of the proteins, revealing the binding site on the thin filaments and facilitating the development of cross-bridges. Calcium has the "password" that causes the tropomyosin "guards" to move away from the binding sites and to permit cross-bridges to form. What causes the calcium to enter the environment, though?

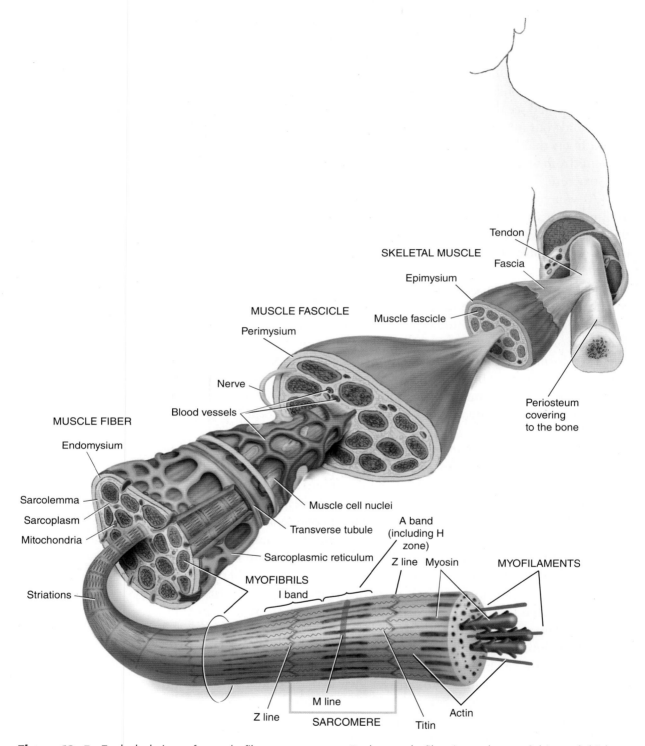

Figure 12–5. Exploded view of muscle fiber components. Each muscle fiber is made up of thin and thick filaments. *Source:* From Seikel/Drumright/King. *Anatomy & Physiology for Speech, Language, and Hearing, 5th Ed.* ©Cengage, Inc. Reproduced by permission.

Calcium is found within the sarcoplasmic reticulum of the muscle cytoplasm. (Sarcoplasmic reticulum is a form of the cellular endoplasmic reticulum.) An AP generated at the neuromuscular junction is conveyed deep into the muscle cell by a series of transverse tubules that are in contact with the sarcoplasmic reticulum. The AP depolarizes the membrane of the sarcoplasmic reticulum, permitting calcium ions to be released. Tropomyosin and troponin are critical to the formation of bridges that causes the muscle fibril to shorten in length. When the tropomyosin and troponin are activated by calcium, they change shape, which reveals the binding site for myosin. This, in turn, allows myosin to form a bridge with the thin filaments. Adenosine triphosphate (ATP) provides the energy to the bridging arm (that is the same energy that you run out of when you become fatigued from overwork), which reaches across to a binding site on the thin filaments, pulls, and releases even as other arms are pulling and releasing. When the AP terminates, calcium is taken back up into the sarcoplasmic reticulum, the binding site is once again hidden, and contraction ceases. That is, an AP at the neuromuscular junction causes the release of calcium into the environment of actin and myosin. Calcium causes the binding sites to be revealed so that cross-bridges can be formed between the two molecules—at that point, muscle contraction begins.

It seems like a lot of work to contract a muscle, and it is. Work requires energy, and ATP supplies it. The actual contraction is much like pulling yourself up a mountainside using a rope. You grab the rope (cross-bridge) and pull, hand-over-hand, drawing yourself upward. Your arms are like the myosin arms, the rope is like the thin filament of actin, and you are the thick filament. This is the **sliding filament model** of muscle contraction.

In this process, the center of the sarcomere (the H zone) disappears as the sarcomere shortens. There are about 350 heads on each thick filament that can bridge across to the thin filaments, and each bridge can perform its hand-over-hand act five times per second. If you remember that it takes many myofilaments to make up one muscle fiber, and that a muscle bundle is made up of many muscle fibers, you will begin to realize the magnitude of activity involved in moving your little finger.

Muscle Control

This information still does not tell us how a muscle does its job. When the AP is generated and the sarcoplasmic reticulum releases calcium, there is an all-or-none response, and the muscle twitches. From your study, you already know that muscles come in all sizes, from the massive to the minute. In addition, muscles must perform vastly different functions, ranging from gross, slow movement to quick, precise action. How do we manage this?

The answer lies largely in the allocation of resources. For fine movement, only a limited number of muscle fibers need be recruited, because you are not trying to move as much mass. In contrast, heavy lifting requires the recruitment of many muscle fibers. This makes sense if you consider the effort involved in moving objects. It takes only one person to move a chair, but it might take four or five individuals to lift a piano.

Neuromotor innervation accounts for much of the allocation of resources: Each muscle fiber is innervated by one motor neuron, but each motor neuron may innervate a large number of muscle fibers. The more motor neurons that are activated, the greater the number of fibers that will contract. The use of many motor nerves to activate a muscle is called **multiple motor unit summation**.

Another mechanism of control comes from a functional difference between how various muscles act. There are two basic types of muscle fibers: slow twitch fibers and fast twitch fibers. As their name implies, **slow twitch fibers** take a longer time to move, whereas fast twitch fibers are capable of much more rapid movement. Slow twitch muscle fibers remain contracted five times longer than do fast twitch fibers, perhaps because calcium remains in the cytoplasm for longer periods. Slow twitch fibers are typically found in muscles that must contract for long periods of time, such as those used to support your body against gravity. Fast twitch muscles, in contrast, are used to meet rapid contraction requirements. Now remember our discussion of the tongue anatomy and physiology. Recall that the tongue tip moves much more rapidly than the massive dorsum, but it is not *only* the mass of the musculature that determines the speed of response. The rapidly moving tongue tip is supplied with *fast twitch fibers*, but the slow-moving deep tongue muscles have *slow twitch fibers*.

There is another significant difference between slow and fast twitch fibers. One neuron may innervate thousands of slow twitch fibers, but neurons serving fast twitch fibers may innervate only 10 or 20 muscle fibers. With this difference in innervation ratio, you can get extremely fine control: If you need to tense the vocal folds quickly for pitch change, you want to be able to control precisely the fraction of a millimeter required to keep your voice from going sharp while singing. This control comes from being able to activate progressively more motor units in fine steps. In contrast, maintaining an erect posture requires less precision and more stamina.

✓ To summarize:

- Activation of a muscle fiber causes the release of calcium into the environment of **thick myofilaments**, revealing the binding sites on the **thin filaments** that permit **cross-bridging** from the thick filaments.

- The action of the bridging causes the myofilaments to slide past one another, thereby shortening the muscle.

- **Slow twitch** muscle fibers remain contracted longer than **fast twitch** fibers, with the former being involved in the maintenance of posture and the latter in fine and rapid motor functions.

Muscle Spindle Function

We touched on the activities of the muscle spindle in Chapter 11 but let us discuss its function more thoroughly. If you examine Figure 12–6, you can

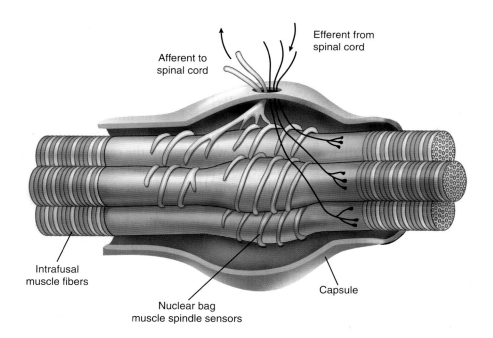

Afferent to
spinal cord

Efferent from
spinal cord

Intrafusal
muscle fibers

Nuclear bag
muscle spindle sensors

Capsule

Figure 12–6. Schematic representation of a muscle spindle. *Source:* From Seikel/ Drumright/King. *Anatomy & Physiology for Speech, Language, and Hearing, 5th Ed.* ©Cengage, Inc. Reproduced by permission.

see the major players in posture and motor control in general. It is sobering to realize that the lowest level of motor response (the stretch reflex) is intimately related to the highest levels of motor response requiring extraordinary skill and dexterity, such as the fine motor control of the fingers. Discussion of the muscle spindle will provide the background necessary to talk about higher-level motor control.

The role of the muscle spindle is to provide feedback to the neuromotor system about muscle length and thus information about motion and position (Bowman, 1971). Before we explain that function, let us examine the structure of this important sensory element.

There are two basic types of striated muscle fibers with which we must be concerned. **Extrafusal muscle** fibers make up the bulk of the muscles discussed over the past several chapters. Deep within the structure of the muscle is another set of muscle fibers, referred to as **intrafusal muscle fibers**. These fibers have a parallel course to the extrafusal fibers and would not really be obvious on gross examination of a muscle. Close examination would reveal short intrafusal fibers that attach to the muscle and are capable of sensing changes in the length of the muscle. At or near the **equatorial region** of the intrafusal muscle fibers are the stretch sensors themselves, with the combination of muscle and sensor known as the **muscle spindle**, so named because of its spindle shape.

The intrafusal fibers may be classified as being either thin or thick. Thick muscle fibers are typically outfitted with a capsule that contains nuclear bag fibers, and thin muscle fibers house nuclear chain fibers. **Nuclear bag fibers** are groups of stretch receptors collected in a cluster at the equatorial region of the intrafusal muscle fiber. **Nuclear chain fibers** are configured as a "chain" or row of stretch sensors (not shown in figure) in the equatorial region. These two configurations serve different functions, as we will see. The placement

The term nuclear bag fiber *refers to the portion of the muscle spindle that is formed by a cluster of stretch sensors situated on the equatorial region of the muscle fiber.*

Table 12–3

A Sample of Reflexes Mediated by the Spinal Cord and the Brain Stem	
Spinal Reflexes	
Palmar grasp reflex	Placing object on ventral surface of fingers causes fingers to flex (up to 3–4 months).
Sucking reflex	Stroking lips laterally causes sucking action (ends at 6 months to 1 year).
Knee-jerk tendon	Rapid stretching of patellar tendon by tapping on knee at tendon causes extension of leg (present after 6 months).
Flexor withdrawal	In supine position, head in mid position; leg flexes when sole of foot is stimulated (ends at 2 months).
Extensor thrust	In supine position with head in mid position, one leg extended and one leg flexed; leg remains flexed when sole is stimulated (ends at 2 months).
Crossed extension	In supine position with head in mid position, one leg extended and one leg flexed; when extended leg is flexed, the opposite leg will extend (before 2 months) or remain flexed (after 2 months).
Crossed extension	In supine position with head in mid position and legs extended; stimulation of medial leg surface causes adduction (ends at 2 months).
Brain Stem Reflexes	
Asymmetrical tonic neck reflex (ATNR)	In supine position with arms and legs extended and head in mid position; if head is turned, arm on face side extends, arm on opposite side flexes (ends 4–6 months).
Symmetrical tonic neck reflex	In quadrupeds, on tester's knee; ventroflex (toward belly), no change in arm/leg tone (before 6 months) or arms flex or increase tone and legs extend or increase tone (after 6 months).
Tonic labyrinthine supine reflex	In supine position with arms and legs extended; passive flexing of arms and legs does not increase tone (before 6 months) or does increase tone (after 6 months).
Tonic labyrinthine prone reflex	In prone position with head in mid position; no increase in flexor tone (before 4 months) or cannot dorsiflex head, retract shoulders, or extend arms and legs (after 4 months).
Associated	In supine position, have individual squeeze object; increases tone in opposite arm and hand (before 6 months) or produces no change in opposite-side tone (after 6 months).
Positive supporting reactions	In standing position, bounce individual on soles of feet; no increase in leg tone (up to 8 months) or increase in extensor tone (after 8 months).
Neck righting reflex	In supine position with head in mid position and arms and legs extended; rotate head, and body will rotate (before 6 months) or not rotate (after 6 months).
Body righting; acting on the body	In supine position with head in mid position, arms and legs extended; rotate head to one side, and body rotates as a whole (before 6 months), or head turns, then shoulders, and finally pelvis (after 6 months).
Labyrinthine righting; acting on the head	Blindfolded and suspended in prone; head does not rise (before 2 months) or rises with face vertical and mouth horizontal (after 1 month).

Table 12–3

continued	
Optical righting	Held in space in prone, head does not rise (before 2 months) or rises to face vertical and mouth horizontal (after 2 months).
Moro reflex	In semi-reclined position, drop head backward; arms extend, arms rotate, fingers extend and abduct (under 4 months).
Landau reflex	Held in space supported at thorax in prone; raise head and spine, and legs extend and remain in flexed position (present from 3 to 12 months).
Positive extensor thrust (parachute reaction)	In prone position with arms extended overhead, suspended in space by pelvis; move suddenly downward; arms extend, fingers abduct and extend to protect head (after 6 months).
Rooting reflex and sucking reflex	Stroke the side of the mouth at the corner of the lips laterally; the infant will orient toward the fingers with a sucking motion of the lips (before 6 months).
Jaw reflex	Pull down on the mandible briskly or draw down on the masseter with deep pressure; the mandible will snap to close (before 6 months).

Note that several variations have been eliminated for brevity, as have specific stimulus conditions.
Source: For a thorough review of reflexes, elicitation procedures, and normal and pathological responses, see Bly (1994) and Fiorentino (1973).

What if you move your legs purposefully? How do the muscle spindles oppose *that* movement? When a new posture is reached, the intrafusal muscle contracts to adjust the tension on the spindle, accommodating the new posture. Likewise, the muscle spindle afferent information is delivered to the cerebral cortex and cerebellum. When voluntary movement is initiated, both alpha and gamma systems are activated. There is speculation that the gamma system receives information from the cortex concerning the desired or *target* muscle length, and thus the gamma system provides feedback to the cortex when this length has been achieved. Thus, the gamma system may be a regulatory mechanism for voluntary movement: Damage to this system has devastating effects.

Golgi Tendon Organs

Another type of sensor, which is less well understood, is the Golgi tendon organ (GTO), a sensor located at the tendon and sensitive to the degree of tension on the muscle. If the muscle is passively stretched, it takes a great deal to excite a GTO. However, if a muscle is contracted, the GTO is quite sensitive to the tension placed on it.

The GTO probably works in close conjunction with the muscle spindle. The muscle spindle is active any time a muscle is lengthened, while the GTO is sensitive to the *tension* placed on the muscle. If a muscle is tensed isometrically, the lengthening is minimal but the GTO reacts to the tension placed on it by contraction. Likewise, if a muscle is passively stretched, the muscle spindle responds but the tendon organ does not.

Synaptic Pruning

A normal and natural process, called *synaptic pruning*, involves elimination of synapses that are no longer needed. This pruning, which results in a massive loss of synapses, axons, and neurons, occurs at three significant points in a person's life: prenatally, during childhood, and at puberty. All these prunings occur as a direct result of experience. You may have heard the statement "use it or lose it." This is the starkest manifestation of it, because literally if you do not use a synapse, you will lose it. This is not bad, mind you, because if you never pruned back on connections in your brain, your thought processes would be overwhelmed by the noise of those residual connections. As it is, the process of learning (experiencing stimuli) causes synapses to increase in strength, and the process of deprivation (not experiencing stimuli) causes synapses to die off. This is an elegant process that supports memory and learning, and keeps our brain from becoming overwhelmed.

Neuroscience has long held that the blood–brain barrier, arising from the protective function of astrocytes, kept the immune system from operating within the brain. Research by Chun and Schatz (1999) has shown that not only are there identity markers for neural tissues (major histocompat-ibility complex [MHC] markers) within the brain, but it now appears that these MHC markers team up with a molecule (C1q) secreted by neurons to prune synapses that are not needed. Astrocytes secrete thrombospondin to support development of synapses. The C1q marks the synapses as "junk," and macrophages collect and dispose of them.

This synaptic pruning poses some interesting and intriguing questions about neurogenic disorders. It is possible that aberrant C1q function is at the root of demyelinating diseases such as multiple sclerosis. Indeed, individuals who have early signs of Alzheimer's dementia have already lost over half of their synapses, and the C1q molecule is present in overwhelming numbers. Similarly, it is hypothesized that children with autism may have excessive numbers of synapses, as demonstrated by increased cerebral volume. One research group (Belmonte et al., 2004) posited that maternal infection during prenatal development may trigger an immune dysfunction in the brain of the fetus that may later result in inadequate synaptic pruning. One of the long-held observations about autism is the extraordinary response of the individual to sensory overload, and this would be supported by the pruning hypothesis.

This localization of function has some very complex manifestations in the nervous system. As an example, the fusiform gyrus is just lateral to the parahippocampal gyrus. It is also known as the fusiform face area and appears to be specialized in recognizing faces of individuals (Tsao, Freiwald, Tootell, & Livingstone, 2006). Indeed, there is mounting evidence that *single neurons* within this area are dedicated to specific faces of people. That is, there are neurons that recognize, for instance, your grandmother (indeed, they have been called "grandmother neurons"). These neurons recognize the canonical version of your grandmother, however, and not just a single picture of her. For instance, if you were to see a picture of your grandmother that you had never seen before, the same neuron would fire in response to it. (Let's be careful here, however: That single neuron has received input from a large number of other neurons, so its development of that canonical version of your grandmother arises from many inputs.) Evidence of the "grandmother neuron" emerged from physiological, single neuron studies of individuals undergoing craniotomy (open skull surgery) for epileptic seizures. In this treatment (electrocorticography), individuals are fitted with a grid of electrodes that are placed on the surface of the brain and that record electrical discharge. Patients must be hospitalized as they wait for a seizure to be recorded. Because many epileptic seizures focus on the temporal lobe, researchers recognized that this population would be ideal for studying the face-sensitive neurons. These face-sensitive neurons are the localizationist's dream because they represent the type of specificity that defines that model of neural processing.

We will take a regional approach to review of the function of the cerebral cortex. Although, clearly, regions of the cerebral cortex, such as the motor strip, are highly specialized for specific functions, other regions of the cortex are less well defined. To further confound things is the fact that the developing brain is **plastic**, meaning that it undergoes change as a result of experience or stimulation. At one time the scientific community was convinced that the brain you were born with never changed, but rather simply declined as a result of sickness and aging. Early work by Marianne Diamond and colleagues (e.g., Diamond, Johnson, Protti, Ott & Kajisa, 1985) showed that neurons continued to develop not only during the postnatal as a result of environmental stimulation, but that there was even neuron development throughout life. The notion of neural plasticity was revolutionary (even heretical to some researchers) and quickly became a bedrock concept for learning and brain change. We know that the brains of infants who receive trauma are more likely to overcome damage to function than those of adults receiving the same trauma. This and other evidence has led to theories of **equipotentiality**, which state that the brain functions as a whole. One could strike a balance with the notion of **regional equipotentiality**. According to this theory, there seems to be a functional unity by regions, but the degree of functional loss to an individual receiving trauma is also related to the total volume of damaged tissue. Our discussion will focus on the functional regions and association pathways of the brain, and on the interconnections among regions. The current view of neural function is a system-wide view, where regions of the brain are activated or entrained to complete a task or function. Thus, for instance, the task of concentration may include the temporoparietal junction, the dorsolateral prefrontal cortex, and the orbitofrontal cortex, but the preparation to act on information derived through attention involves entraining the premotor cortex, supplemental motor area, and other areas.

Lead Exposure

We have known for many years that lead exposure is bad for children. Excessive exposure to lead causes permanent brain damage, resulting in mental retardation, learning disability, attention deficit, and memory problems. Recently, however, researchers have found an even more insidious route for lead effects. Basha et al. (2005) found that when infant monkeys were given milk with low levels of lead, at 23 years of age they developed the plaques associated with Alzheimer's disease. If the monkeys had the genetic markers for Alzheimer's susceptibility, they were twice as likely to develop the plaques.

The cortex appears to be organized around regions of **primary activity of a cortical region**, such as the primary receptive area for somatic sense, primary motor area, primary auditory cortex, and primary region of visual reception (Figure 12–8). Adjacent to these are **higher-order areas of processing**. That is, there are secondary, tertiary, and even quaternary areas of higher-order processing adjacent to the primary receptive areas for sensation. There are also higher-order areas of processing for motor function, as we will see. Beyond the higher-order areas of processing are **association areas** in which the highest form of human thought occurs. That is, we receive information from our senses at primary reception areas and we extract the information received and put it together with other information associated with the modality at higher-order areas of processing. This information is passed to association areas for the highest level of cognitive processing.

The **primary reception area for vision (VI)** is located within the calcarine fissure of the occipital lobe (area 17). At that location, precise maps of information received at the retinae are projected. The secondary visual processing region is considered area 18 of the occipital lobe, with even **higher-level processing regions for vision** found in the temporal lobe (areas 20 and 21) and the occipital lobe (area 19 and the region anterior to it). Area 7 of the parietal lobe performs higher-level processing of visual

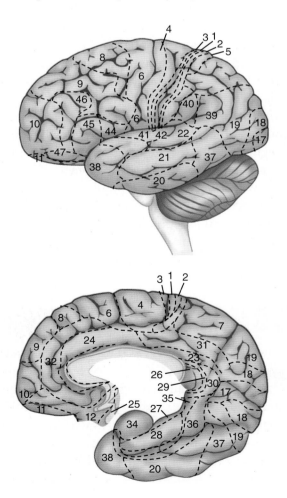

Figure 12–8. Brodmann's area map of lateral and medial cerebrum. *Source:* From Seikel/Drumright/King. *Anatomy & Physiology for Speech, Language, and Hearing, 5th Ed.* ©Cengage, Inc. Reproduced by permission.

Parkinson's Disease

Parkinson's disease is a neuromuscular disease that results in tremors, muscular rigidity, difficulty initiating movement, and dementia. The physical cause of the disease is known to be the loss of cells in the substantia nigra, the "black substance" within the cerebral peduncles of the midbrain. While researchers are comfortable with the cause of the disease, the cause of the damage to the substantia nigra is elusive. It has long been felt that some sort of environmental etiology was at work, but evidence is emerging to show that Parkinson's is caused through pesticides. In a five-country study of Parkinson's patients, Betarbet et al. (2000) found that the use of pesticides was strongly related to a later development of Parkinson's disease.

There is good news regarding Parkinson's disease, however, in that the injection of glial line neurotrophic factor (GDNF) into the brain tissue of Parkinson's patients resulted in significant and long-term gains in motor function. All patients injected showed remarkable benefits in motor and cognitive functions. Unfortunately, the company that owns the patent for GDNF removed the drug from clinical trials because of fears concerning safety. Prior treatments using neural tissue transplants have also been quite successful but remain experimental because of ethical dilemmas concerning the source of the tissue (aborted fetuses).

Deep brain stimulation has been beneficial in the treatment of Parkinson's disease, reducing tremor and increasing motor function for speech, ambulation, and swallowing.

lations. Dyspraxia occurs in the absence of the muscular weakness typical of an individual with motor strip damage, but the ability to contract the musculature voluntarily is impaired. One may also experience **oral apraxia**, which is a deficit in the ability to perform nonspeech oral gestures, such as imitatively puffing up the cheeks or blowing out a candle. A word of caution is due, however: Lesions are rarely so focal; it is much more often the case that frontal lobe damage that causes dyspraxia will be of a magnitude to also include regions of the motor strip. That is, dyspraxia and dysarthria very often co-occur.

If an individual has damage to the posterior parietal cortex, the result will be difficulty focusing on the target of an action. This individual will have difficulty locating objects in space and may even ignore or neglect the side of the body served by the damaged parietal lobe tissue, because the person cannot use that information. In addition, the *supramarginal gyrus* is involved in spatiomotor tasks in nonhumans (identifying whether physical orientation of an object is functionally correct) (Bach, Peelen, & Tipper, 2010), but appears intimately involved in phonological processing developmentally in humans (Sugiura et al., 2011).

Afferent Inputs

The motor strip is populated by giant Betz cells, and this area receives input from the thalamus, sensory cortex, and premotor area. Regions involved in fine motor control (such as those activating facial regions or the fingers) are very richly represented. There is heavy sensory input to this motor region, underscoring the notion that the control of movement is strongly influenced by information about the ongoing state and position of the musculature.

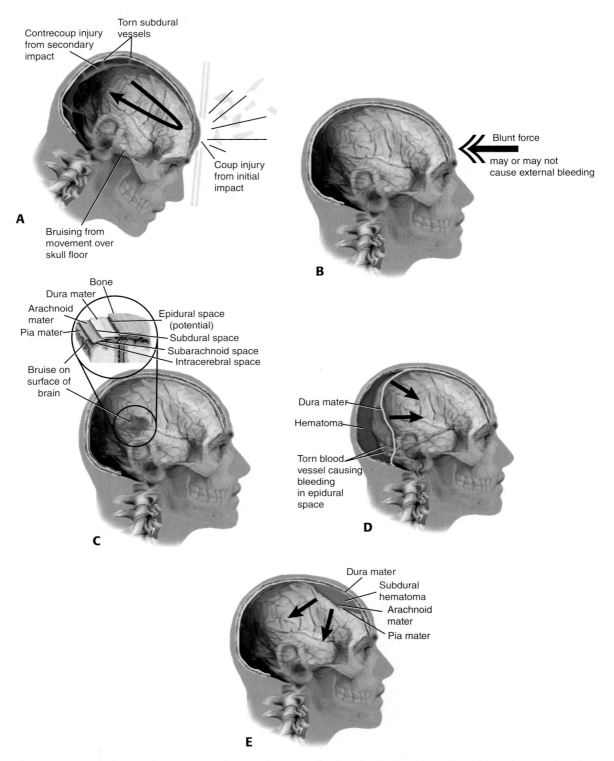

Figure 12–10. Effects of trauma on the cerebrum and related structures. **A.** Closed head injury (CHI) producing a direct effect (coup) on frontal region and a rebound effect (contracoup) in the occipital region. **B.** Blunt force trauma to the frontal region causing neural damage, but which may not manifest as external damage. **C.** Cerebral contusion (bruising of the brain). **D.** Subdural hematoma arising from broken blood vessels deep to the dura mater. **E.** Epidural hematoma, arising from broken blood vessels superficial to the dura mater. *Source:* From Seikel/Drumright/King. *Anatomy & Physiology for Speech, Language, and Hearing, 5th Ed.* ©Cengage, Inc. Reproduced by permission.

A Story with a Happy Ending

Not all stories of cerebrovascular accident end with dysfunction or disability. This is a story of cerebrovascular accident with a happy ending. While at a public event in a rural area one Saturday, a dear friend developed a debilitating headache. When her headache did not improve after an hour of nursing it in the cab of her truck, her husband began the long drive home. Her husband wisely decided to stop by the local hospital to check whether everything was in order, and the emergency physician suggested magnetic resonance imaging (MRI) to help determine the source of the pain. As the MRI was activated, she became unconscious.

As we later learned, she had a history of aneurysms in her family and had been examined frequently and repeatedly to ensure that there were no surprises in her future. Despite these precautions, an aneurysm had developed at the base of her brain and hemorrhaged as the MRI was activated. Life-flight took her to a metropolitan center that specialized in the management of hemorrhage, and friends and family watched anxiously as she slowly became aware of her surroundings. To everyone's great joy and relief, her recovery was remarkably complete, and she was able to return to her life and work unencumbered. The quick action of the emergency room medical team and the stroke unit at the receiving hospital gave her the chance to be called the "miracle woman" by all who know her.

fluent **aphasia**. Similarly, we have come to recognize that damage to Broca's area (areas 44 and 45) severely disrupts the oral manifestation of language (speech). Through cortical mapping and precise lesion studies, researchers have described these conditions and the sites of lesions more precisely, providing us with some insight into how the cerebral cortex functions.

As you know, Heschl's gyrus of the temporal lobe has the primary responsibility of auditory reception. The region adjacent to it in the superior temporal gyrus is a higher-order processing region, and the hippocampus is involved with memory. Portions of the inferior and middle temporal gyri are regions of higher-level integration of visual information. Wernicke's area is posterior to this, technically comprised of the posterior superior gyrus of the temporal lobe, but we know that language function involves a markedly larger area, generally including the temporal-occipital-parietal association areas.

Damage to Heschl's gyrus may result in cortical deafness, the inability to hear information that has passed through the lower auditory nervous system (Narayanan, Majeed, Subramaniam, Narayanan, & Navaf, 2017). Lesions of the higher-order processing region adjacent to AI will produce a deficit in processing complex auditory information, and if the lesion involves the inferior temporal lobe (area 28), the individual may experience a memory deficit associated with visual information. You may wish to review the information in Chapter 10 on the auditory pathway and higher cortical functioning related to auditory stimuli.

With the notion of the auditory and visual input function of the temporal lobe in mind, let us examine lesions involving Wernicke's area. **Wernicke's aphasia** is referred to as a *fluent aphasia*, because individuals with this condition have relatively normal flow of speech. Their expressive

& Roane, 2005; Raz & Buhle, 2006). The executive attentional network involves activation of the right dorsolateral prefrontal cortex (DLPFC: BA 9, 46) and the right temporo-parietal juncture (TPJ). Damage to the TPJ is nearly always present with misidentification syndromes, which all include some form of failure to identify an element of one's personal existence. In hemispheric neglect (also known as left neglect), the individual fails to attend to the left half of the visual field and the left side of the body. The individual is capable of seeing that portion of the visual field and can become aware of the left side of the body when attention is drawn to it, but that awareness is lost almost immediately. Asomatognosia involves lack of awareness that a person owns half of the body or a limb, often the left arm. This confusion can be improved through calling it to the attention of the patient. When people have somatoparaphrenia, they believe that a part of their body belongs to someone else, and there are often delusions and confabulations about who the body part belongs to. The person with this condition usually can't be convinced that his or her perception is inaccurate. A person with Capgras syndrome believes that a relative, friend, or spouse has been replaced by an imposter. When patients have anosognosia, they have lack of awareness of a disease state. These individuals may have hemispatial neglect or paralysis, but deny that there is a problem. This condition poses a real problem for therapy, as you can imagine. Because the attentional network is localized to the right hemisphere, it is possible that the reduced activation of the right hemisphere is at least partially responsible for many of the deficits seen in networks and processes not otherwise involved in the lesion (Seikel, 2018). For a thorough review of misidentification syndromes, see Feinberg and Roane (2005).

✅ To summarize:

- The **hemispheres** of the brain display clear functional differences.
- The **left hemisphere** in most individuals is dominant for language and speech, processes brief-duration stimuli, and performs detailed analysis.
- The **right hemisphere**, in contrast, appears to process information in a more holistic fashion, preferring spatial and tonal information.
- **Face recognition** appears to be a right-hemisphere function.
- Lesion studies have shown that damage to **Wernicke's area** in the dominant hemisphere usually results in a receptive language deficit with relatively intact speech fluency, whereas damage to **Broca's area** results in the loss of speech fluency manifested as Broca's aphasia.
- Damage to the **arcuate fasciculus** connecting these two regions will result in **conduction aphasia**, and damage to all of these regions will produce **global deficit**.
- **Verbal dyspraxia** may result from damage to Broca's area, but has also been seen with lesions to the supplementary motor area, frontal operculum, and insula.

- **Nondominant hemisphere lesions** often result in a deficit in the **pragmatics**, especially related to monitoring the facial responses of communication partners, information carried in the intonation of speech, and communicative nuance.
- **Frontal lobe lesions** may result in deficits in judgment and in response inhibition, whereas damage to the **hippocampus** will affect short-term memory, especially as it relates to auditory information.

Motor Control for Speech

The production of speech is an extraordinarily complex process. We tend to view area 4 as the prime mover, but it would be more accurate to view it as the location where the very complex planning, programming, and preparation reach fruition. Movement is initiated at the motor strip, but only after it has been conceived, and after the steps involved for muscle activity have been prepared. To further confound things, control of speech musculature must be precisely coordinated, a process involving afferent input from the muscles. You will want to refer to our discussion of the DIVA model in Chapter 7.

Input to the motor strip arises from the premotor regions that are involved in the preparation of the motor act. The premotor gyrus and supplemental motor area receive input concerning the state of the musculature from the postcentral gyrus, and it appears that the knowledge of articulator position in space is established there. In addition, Broca's area (areas 44 and 45) communicates with the TOP by means of the arcuate fasciculus and is intimately involved in articulatory planning. The supramarginal gyrus of the parietal lobe appears to be involved in phonological processing. The prefrontal association area receives input from diffuse sensory integration regions of the cerebrum, and this information is used to make decisions concerning execution of the motor act (such as inhibiting a response). Prefrontal and premotor regions project to the precentral gyrus, as does Broca's area, so that both immediate planning and cognitive strategies associated with speech influence the output.

The primary motor cortex (MI) receives information concerning the state of muscles, tendons, and tissue through several means. The sensory cortex (SI) receives this information in a well-organized fashion. Area 3 receives muscle afferent information from Group Ia fibers terminating in the thalamus and from mechanoreceptors of the skin that are apparently very important for the speech muscles of the face. Area 1 receives mechanoreceptor input as well, and area 2 receives joint sense. This information is all directed to the MI, either directly or via other SI areas, apparently to modulate the motor command based on current status.

This sensory information obviously is not the only information processed by the MI. The premotor region (lateral area 6) is involved in organization of the motor act for skilled, voluntary movement, and its output is directly routed to the MI in both hemispheres. It receives somatic and visual information and apparently integrates this into its motor plan. The SMA

18. Damage to _____ area in the dominant hemisphere usually results in a receptive language deficit with relatively intact speech fluency.

19. Damage to _____ area in the dominant hemisphere often results in loss of speech fluency manifested as Broca's aphasia.

20. Damage to the _____ fasciculus will result in conduction aphasia.

21. A client of yours had a stroke and reveals some muscular weakness on the left side of her body. Her speech is precisely articulated, but the intonation is flat. She complains that, despite her lack of physical problems, she has noticed that her friends don't call anymore. Where is the site of lesion, and where should therapy be directed?

Chapter 12 Study Question Answers

1. **ACTION POTENTIAL** is a change in electrical potential that occurs when a cell membrane is stimulated adequately to permit ion exchange between the intra- and extracellular spaces.

2. The **ABSOLUTE REFRACTORY PERIOD** is the time during which the cell membrane cannot be stimulated to depolarize.

3. The **RELATIVE REFRACTORY PERIOD** is a period during which the membrane may be stimulated to excitation again, but only with greater than typical stimulation.

4. The **NODES OF RANVIER** of the axon myelin promote saltatory conduction.

5. The substance known as **NEUROTRANSMITTER** is discharged into the synaptic cleft, stimulating the postsynaptic neuron.

6. Activation of a muscle fiber causes the release of calcium into the environment of **THICK** myofilaments.

7. **SLOW** twitch muscle fibers remain contracted longer than **FAST** twitch fibers.

8. **MUSCLE SPINDLES** provide feedback to the neuromotor system about muscle length, tension, motion, and position.

9. Higher cognitive processing occurs generally in **ASSOCIATION** areas.

10. The **TEMPORO-OCCIPITAL-PARIETAL ASSOCIATION** area is involved in language function.

11. **FLACCID** dysarthria results from damage to LMNs, whereas UMN lesions result in **SPASTIC** dysarthria.

12. **HYPERKINETIC** dysarthria is the result of damage to the inhibitory processes of the extrapyramidal system.

13. **ATAXIC DYSARTHRIA** arises from cerebellar damage.

14. The **PREFRONTAL** area of the cerebrum appears to be involved in higher function related to motor output (such as inhibition of motor function and the ability to change motor responses), whereas the **TEMPORAL-OCCIPITAL-PARIETAL** association area is involved in language function.

15. The **LIMBIC ASSOCIATION** area integrates information related to affect, motivation, and emotion.

16. The **LEFT** hemisphere in most individuals is dominant for language and speech, processes brief-duration stimuli, and performs detailed analysis.

17. The **RIGHT** hemisphere appears to process information in a more holistic fashion, preferring spatial and tonal information.

18. Damage to **WERNICKE'S** area in the dominant hemisphere usually results in a receptive language deficit with relatively intact speech fluency.

19. Damage to **BROCA'S** area in the dominant hemisphere often results in loss of speech fluency manifested as Broca's aphasia.

20. Damage to the **ARCUATE** fasciculus will result in conduction aphasia.

21. This individual suffered frontal lobe damage of the right hemisphere. Speech was unaffected because the left hemisphere dominates speech and many language functions. Nonetheless, she has a reduction in the ability to examine the context of communication (right hemisphere) and may be insensitive to cues that her friends are giving her that would otherwise cause her to change some communication strategy. An important goal of therapy would be to increase her awareness of the pragmatic cues and to develop strategies to increase her sensitivity to context.

Bibliography

Akshoomoff, N. A., & Courchesne, E. (1992). A new role for the cerebellum in cognitive operations. *Behavioral Neuroscience, 106*(5), 731–738.

Andermann, M. L., Kerlin, A. M., Roumis, D. K., Glickfeld, L. L., & Reid, R. C. (2012). Functional specialization of mouse visual cortical areas. *Neuron, 72*(6), 1025–1039.

Androulakis, X. M., Krebs, K. A., Jenkins, C., Maleki, N., Finkel, A. G., Rorden, C., & Newman, R. (2018). Central executive and default mode network intranet work functional connectivity patterns in chronic migraine. *Journal of Neurological Disorders, 6*(5), 393.

Bach, P., Peelen, M. V., & Tipper, S. P. (2010). On the role of object information in action observation: An fMRI study. *Cerebral Cortex, 20*(12), 2798–2809.

Basha, M. R., Wei, W., Bakheet, S. A., Benitez, N., Siddiqi, H. K., Ge, Y. W., . . . Zawia, N. H. (2005). The fetal basis of amyloidogenesis: Exposure to lead and latent overexpression of amyloid precursor protein and β-amyloid in the aging brain. *Journal of Neuroscience, 25*(4), 823–829.

Belmonte, M. K., Allen, G., Beckel-Mitchener, A., Boulanger, L. M., Carper, R. A., & Webb, S. J. (2004). Autism and abnormal development of brain connectivity. *Journal of Neuroscience, 24*(42), 9228–9231.

Betarbet, R., Sherer, T. B., MacKenzie, G., Garcia-Osuna, G., Panov, A. V., & Greenamyre, J. T. (2000). Systemic pesticide exposure reproduces features of Parkinson's disease. *Nature Neuroscience, 3*, 1301–1306.

Blakemore, C., & Cooper, G. F. (1970). Development of brain depends on the visual environment. *Nature, 228*, 477–478.

Bly, L. (1994). *Motor skills acquisition in the first year.* Tucson, AZ: Therapy Skill Builders.

Bowman, J. P. (1971). *The muscle spindle and neural control of the tongue.* Springfield, IL: Charles C. Thomas.

Chun, J., & Schatz, D. G. (1999). Developmental neurobiology: Alternative ends for a familiar story? *Current Biology, 9*(7), R251–R253.

Corkin, S. (2002). What's new with the amnesic patient H.M.? *Nature Reviews Neuroscience, 3*(2), 153–160.

Cotman, C. W., & McGaugh, J. L. (1980). *Behavioral neuroscience.* New York, NY: Academic Press.

Diamond, M. C., Johnson, R. E., Protti, A. M., Ott, C., & Kajisa, L. (1985). Plasticity in the 904-day-old male rat cerebral cortex. *Experimental Neurology, 87*(2), 309–317.

Duffy, J. R. (2005). *Motor speech disorders* (2nd ed.). St. Louis, MO: Mosby.

Dworkin, J. P. (1991). *Motor speech disorders.* St. Louis, MO: Mosby.

Feinberg, T. E., & Roane, D. M. (2005). Delusional misidentification. *Psychiatric Clinics, 28*(3), 665–683.

Finn, E. S., Shen, X., Scheinost, D., Rosenberg, M. D., Huang, J., Chun, M. M., . . . Constable, R. T. (2015). Functional connectome fingerprinting: Identifying individuals using patterns of brain connectivity. *Nature Neuroscience, 18*(11), 1664–1671.

Fiorentino, M. R. (1973). *Reflex testing methods for evaluating CNS development.* Springfield, IL; Charles Thomas.

Gonzalez-Castillo, J., Hoy, C. W., Handwerker, D. A., Robinson, M. E., Buchanan, L. C., Saad, Z. S., & Bandettini, P. A. (2015). Tracking ongoing cognition in individuals using brief, whole-brain functional connectivity patterns. *Proceedings of the National Academy of Sciences, 112*(28), 8762–8767.

Hickok, G. (2012). Computational neuroanatomy of speech production. *Nature Reviews Neuroscience, 13*(2), 135–145.

Hilts, P. J. (1996). *Memory's ghost: The nature of memory and the strange tale of Mr. M.* Simon and Schuster.

Hubel, D. H. (1979). The visual cortex of normal and deprived monkeys. *Scientific American, 67,* 532–543.

Johnson, J. (2009). Late auditory event-related potentials: Children with cochlear implants. *Developmental Neuropsychology, 34*(6), 701–720.

Kandel, E. R., Schwartz, J. H., & Jessell, T. M. (2000). *Principles of neural science* (4th ed.). New York, NY: McGraw-Hill.

Keene, D. L., Whiting, S., & Ventureyra, E. C. (2000). Electrocorticography. *Epileptic Disorders, 2*(1), 57–63.

Kupferman, I. (1991). Localization of higher cognitive and affective functions: The association cortices. In E. R. Kandel, J. H. Schwartz, & T. M. Jessell (Eds.), *Principles of neural science* (3rd ed., pp. 823–838). Norwalk, CT: Appleton & Lange.

Lazar, S. W., Kerr, C. E., Wasserman, R. H., Gray, J. R., Greve, D. N., Treadway, M. T., . . . Fischl, B. (2005). Meditation experience is associated with increased cortical thickness. *Neuroreport, 16*(17), 1893–1897.

Lutz, A., Greischar, L. L., Rawlings, N. B., Ricard, M., & Davidson, R. J. (2004). Long term meditators self-induce high amplitude gamma synchrony during practice. *Proceedings of the National Academy of Sciences, 101*(46), 16369–16373.

Mackay, L. E., Chapman, P. E., & Morgan, A. S. (1997). *Maximizing brain injury recovery.* Gaithersburg, MD: Aspen.

Martinez, L. M., Wang, Q., Reid, R. C., Pillai, C., Alonso, J. M., Sommer, F. T., & Hirsch, J. A. (2005). Receptive field structure varies with layer in primary visual cortex. *Nature Neuroscience, 8*(3), 372–379.

McKay, L. C., Janczewski, W. A., & Feldman, J. L. (2005). Sleep-disordered breathing after targeted ablation of preBotzinger complex neurons. *Nature Neuroscience, 8,* 1142–1144.

Miller, K J., denNijs, M., Shenoy, P., Miller, J. W., Rao, R. P. N., & Ojemann, J. G. (2007). Real-time functional brain mapping using electrocorticography. *NeuroImage, 37,* 504–507.

Mueller, S., Kesser, D., Samson, A. C., Kirsch, V., Blautzik, J., Grothe, E., . . . Meindl, T. (2013). Convergent findings of altered functional and structure brain connectivity in individuals with high functioning autism: A multimodal MRI study. *PLoS One, 8*(6), e67329.

Myers, P. (1999). *Right hemisphere damage.* San Diego, CA: Singular Publishing Group.

Naqvi, N. H., Rudrauf, D., Damasio, H., & Bechara, A. (2007). Damage to the insula disrupts addiction to cigarette smoking. *Science, 315*(5811), 531–534.

Narayanan, S., Majeed, K. A., Subramaniam, G., Narayanan, A., & Navaf, K. M. (2017). A case of cortical deafness due to bilateral Heschl gyrus infarct. *Case Reports in Medicine,* 6816748.

Penfield, W., & Roberts, L. (1959). *Speech and brain-mechanisms.* Princeton, NJ: Princeton University Press.

Raz, A., & Buhle, J. (2006). Typologies of attentional networks. *Nature Reviews Neuroscience, 7*(5), 367–379.

Schuell, H., Jenkins, J., & Jiménes-Pabon, E. (1964). *Aphasia in adults: Diagnosis, prognosis, and therapy.* New York, NY: Hoeber.

Seikel, J. A. (2018). An attentional view of right hemisphere dysfunction. *Clinical Archives of Communication Disorders, 3*(1), 76–88.

Stam, C. J., Van Straaten, E. C. W., Van Dellen, E., Tewarie, P., Gong, G., Hillebrand, A., . . . Van Mieghem, P. (2016). The relation between structural and functional connectivity patterns in complex brain networks. *International Journal of Psychophysiology, 103,* 149–160.

Sugiura, L., Ojima, S., Matsuba-Kurita, H., Dan, I., Tsuzuki, D., Katura, T., & Hagiwara, H. (2011). Sound to language: Different cortical processing of the first and second language in elementary school children as revealed by a large scale study using fNIRS. *Cerebral Cortex, 21*(10), 2374–2393.

Tsao, D. Y., Freiwald, W. A., Tootell, R. B. H., & Livingstone, M. S. (2006). A cortical region consisting entirely of face-selective cells. *Science, 311,* 670–674.

Von Bohlen und Halbach, O., & Dermietzel, R. (2006). *Neurotransmitters and neuromodulators.* Weinheim, Germany: Wiley-VCH.

Whittle, S., Yap, M. B., Yücel, M., Fornito, A., Simmons, J. G., Barrett, A., . . . Alan, N. B. (2008). Prefrontal and amygdala volumes are related to adolescents' affective behaviors during parent-adolescent interactions. *Proceedings of the National Academy of Sciences, USA, 105*(9), 3652–3657.

Anatomical Terms

Anatomical position:	Upright, palms forward, eyes directly ahead, feet together
Anterior:	Toward the front of the body or subpart
Asthenia:	Weakness
Bifurcation:	A fork; split into two parts
Caudal:	Toward the tail or coccyx
Central:	Relative to the center of a structure
Cranial:	Toward the head
Deep:	Away from the surface
Distal:	Further from the trunk or thorax; further from the attached end
Dorsal:	Pertaining to the back of the body or the posterior surface
Extension:	Straightening or moving out of the flexed position
External:	Toward the exterior of a body
Flexion:	The act of bending
Frontal plane:	Divides the body into anterior and posterior halves
Horizontal plane:	Divides the body or body part into upper and lower halves
Inferior:	The lower point; nearer the feet
Insertion:	Distal attachment of a muscle; typically the most mobile point of attachment
Internal:	Enclosed or on the interior
Lateral:	Away from the midline of the body or subpart
Medial/mesial:	Toward the midline of the body or subpart
Origin:	Proximal attachment of a muscle; typically the least mobile point of attachment
Palmar:	Pertaining to the palm of the hand
Peripheral:	Relative to the periphery or away from the center
Plantar:	Pertaining to the sole of the foot
Posterior:	Toward the back of the body or subpart
Prone:	Body in horizontal position with face down
Proximal:	Closer to the trunk or thorax; nearer to the attached end
Radial:	Pertaining to the radius bone
Sagittal plane:	Divides the body or body part into right and left halves
Superficial:	Near the surface

Superior: The upper point; nearer the head

Supine: Body in horizontal position with face up

Ventral: Pertaining to the belly or anterior surface

Useful Combining Forms

-a-	Without; lack of	**-culum**	Diminutive form of a noun
ab-	Away from	**-culus**	Diminutive form of a noun
ad-	Toward	**-cyte**	Cell
-algia	Pain	**de-**	Away from
amphi-	On both sides	**dextro-**	Right
an-	Without; lack of	**-dynia**	Pain
ana-	Up	**dys-**	Bad; with difficulty
angio-	Blood vessels	**e-**	Out from
ante-	Before	**ec-**	Out of
antero-	Before	**ecto-**	On the outer side; toward the surface
apo-	Away from	**-ectomy**	Excision
arthr-	A joint	**-emia**	Blood
bi-	Two	**endo-**	Toward the interior; within
blast-	Germ	**ento-**	Toward the interior; within
brachy-	Short	**ep-**	Upon or above something else
brady-	Slow	**epi-**	Upon or above something else
capit-	Head, or toward the head end	**etio-**	Cause or origin
-carpal	Wrist	**ex-**	Out of, toward the surface
-cele	Tumor	**extero-**	Aimed outward or nearer to the surface
cephalo-	Head, or toward the head end	**extra-**	Outside
circum	Around	**-gen**	Producing
-cle	Implies something very small	**-genic**	Producing
com-	With or together with	**hemi-**	Half
con-	With or together with	**hyper-**	Above; increased, or too much of something
contra-	Opposite	**hypo-**	Below; decreased, or too little of something
cor-	Heart		
corp-	Body	**idio-**	Peculiar
crur-	Cross; leglike part	**-ilos**	Diminutive form of a noun
crus-	Cross; leglike part	**infra-**	Below
cryo-	Cold	**inter-**	Between
-cule	Implies something very small		

intero-	Aimed inward or farther from the surface
intra-	Within
intro-	Into
ipsi-	Same
iso-	Equal
-itis	Inflammation or irritation
-ium	Diminutive form of a noun
latero-	Side
lepto-	Thick
leuco-	White
levo-	Left
macro-	Large
medio-	Middle
megalo-	Large
meso-	Middle
meta-	After; mounted or built upon
micro-	Small
mono-	Single
morph-	Form
my-	Pertaining to muscle
myelo-	Pertaining to spinal cord
myo-	Pertaining to muscle
naso-	Nose
neo-	New
neuro-	Nerve
oculo-	Eye
-oma	Morbid condition of a part, often a tumor
oro-	Mouth
ortho-	Straight
-osis	Condition
osseo-	A hardened or bony part, but not strictly
osteo-	Bone
pachy-	Thick
palato-	Palate
para	Beside; partial
patho-	Abnormal in some way
-pathy	Disease
ped-	Child; foot
-penia	Poverty
per-	Through; passing through; before
peri-	Around
-phage	Eating
-phagia	Eating
-pher-	Bearing or carrying
-plasia	Growth
-plastic	Capable of being molded
-plasty	Molding, forming
-poiesis	Making
poly-	Many
post-	After; behind
postero-	Behind
pre-	Before; in front of
pro-	Before; in front of
proto-	Primitive; simple form
quadra-	Four
quadri-	Four
-raphy	Suturing or stitching
re-	Back or again; curved back
retro-	Backward, toward the rear
-rrhea	A flowing
scirrho-	Hard
sclero-	Hard
-sclerosis	Hardening
scolio-	Curved
semi-	Half
sinistro-	Left
soma-	Pertaining to the body
somato-	Pertaining to the body
steno-	Narrow
strepto-	Swift
sub-	Under
sup-	Under; moderately

super-	Above; excessively	**-tomy**	Cutting
supra-	Above, upon	**trans-**	Beyond or on the other side
sym-	With or together	**tri-**	Three
syn-	With or together	**-trophic**	Related to nourishment
tachy-	Swift; fast	**-trophy**	Growth, usually by expanding
-tarsal	Ankle	**-tropy**	Implies seeking or heading for something
telo-	Far from, toward the extreme		
tetra-	Four	**uni-**	One

Muscles of Respiration

Thoracic Muscles of Inspiration

Primary Inspiratory Muscle

Muscle:	**Diaphragm** (sternal head, costal head, and vertebral head)
Origin:	Sternal head: Xiphoid process of the sternum; costal head: the inferior margin of the rib cage (ribs 7 through 12); vertebral head: the corpus of L1, and the transverse processes of L1 through L5
Course:	Up and medially
Insertion:	Central tendon of diaphragm
Innervation:	Phrenic nerve arising from cervical plexus of spinal nerves C3, C4, C5
Function:	Depresses central tendon of diaphragm, enlarges vertical dimension of thorax, distends abdomen

Accessory Thoracic Muscles of Inspiration

Muscle:	**External intercostal**
Origin:	Inferior surface of ribs 1 through 11
Course:	Down and obliquely in
Insertion:	Upper surface of rib immediately below
Innervation:	Intercostal nerves: thoracic intercostal nerves arising from T1 through T6 and thoracoabdominal intercostal nerves from T7 through T11
Function:	Elevates rib

Muscle:	**Internal intercostal, interchondral portion**
Origin:	Upper margin of ribs 2 through 12
Course:	Up and in
Insertion:	Lower surface of the rib above
Innervation:	Intercostal nerves: thoracic intercostal nerves arising from T1 through T6 and thoracoabdominal intercostal nerves from T7 through T11
Function:	Elevates ribs 2 through 12

Note that the internal intercostal muscles are considered muscles of expiration, with the exception of those muscles of the interchondral portion of the rib cage, which pull the rib cage up and are therefore considered accessory muscles of inspiration.

Muscle: **Rhomboideus minor**
Origin: Spinous processes of C7 and T1
Course: Down and laterally in
Insertion: Medial border of scapula
Innervation: Spinal C4, C5 from the dorsal scapular nerve of upper root of brachial plexus
Function: Stabilizes shoulder girdle

Muscle: **Trapezius**
Origin: Spinous processes of C2 to T12
Course: Fans laterally
Insertion: Acromion of scapula and superior surface of clavicle
Innervation: XI accessory, spinal branch arising from spinal cord in the regions of C3 and C4
Function: Elongates neck, controls head

Thoracic Muscles of Expiration

Muscle: **Internal intercostal, interosseous portion**
Origin: Superior margin of ribs 2 through 12
Course: Up and in
Insertion: Inferior surface of rib above
Innervation: Intercostal nerves: thoracic intercostal nerves arising from T2 through T6 and thoracoabdominal intercostal nerves from T7 through T11
Function: Depresses ribs 1 through 11

Note that the interosseous portion of the internal intercostal is a muscle of expiration, although the interchondral portion of the internal intercostal muscle is considered to be a muscle of inspiration.

Muscle: **Innermost intercostal**
Origin: Superior margin of ribs 1 through 11; sparse or absent in superior thorax
Course: Up and in
Insertion: Inferior surface of rib above
Innervation: Intercostal nerves: thoracic intercostal nerves arising from T2 through T6 and thoracoabdominal intercostal nerves from T7 through T11
Function: Depresses ribs 1 through 11

Muscle: **Transversus thoracis**
Origin: Inner thoracic lateral margin of the sternum
Course: Laterally
Insertion: Inner chondral surface of ribs 2 through 6
Innervation: Thoracic intercostal nerves and thoracoabdominal intercostal nerves and subcostal nerves derived from T2 through T6 spinal nerves
Function: Depresses rib cage

Posterior Thoracic Muscles

Muscle: **Subcostal**
Origin: Inner posterior thorax; sparse in the upper thorax; from inner surface of rib near angle
Course: Down and lateral
Insertion: Inner surface of second or third rib below
Innervation: Intercostal nerves of thorax, arising from the ventral rami of the spinal nerves
Function: Depresses thorax

Muscle: **Serratus posterior inferior**
Origin: Spinous processes of T11, T12, L1 through L3
Course: Up and lateral
Insertion: Lower margin of ribs 7 through 12
Innervation: Intercostal nerves from T9 through T11 and subcostal nerve from T12
Function: Contraction tends to pull rib cage down, supporting expiratory effort

Abdominal Muscles of Expiration

Anterolateral Abdominal Muscles

Muscle: **Transversus abdominis**
Origin: Posterior abdominal wall at the vertebral column via the thoracolumbar fascia of the abdominal aponeurosis
Course: Lateral
Insertion: Transversus abdominis aponeurosis and inner surface of ribs 6 through 12, interdigitating at that point with the fibers of the diaphragm; inferior-most attachment at the pubis
Innervation: Thoracic and lumbar nerves from the lower spinal intercostal nerves (derived from T7 to T12) and first lumbar nerve, iliohypogastric and ilioinguinal branches
Function: Compresses abdomen

Muscle: **Internal oblique abdominis**
Origin: Inguinal ligament and iliac crest
Course: Fans medially
Insertion: Cartilaginous portion of lower ribs and the portion of the abdominal aponeurosis lateral to the rectus abdominis
Innervation: Thoracic and lumbar nerves from the lower spinal intercostal nerves (derived from T7 to T12) and first lumbar nerve, iliohypogastric and ilioinguinal branches
Function: Rotates trunk, flexes trunk, compresses abdomen

Muscle: **External oblique abdominis**

Origin: Osseous portion of the lower seven ribs

Course: Fans downward

Insertion: Iliac crest, inguinal ligament, and abdominal aponeurosis lateral to rectus abdominis

Innervation: Thoracoabdominal nerve arising from T7 through T11 and subcostal nerve from T12

Function: Bilateral contraction flexes vertebral column and compresses abdomen; unilateral contraction results in trunk rotation

Muscle: **Rectus abdominis**

Origin: Originates as four or five segments at pubis inferiorly

Course: Up to segment border

Insertion: Xiphoid process of sternum and the cartilage of ribs 5 through 7, lower ribs

Innervation: T5 through T11 intercostal nerves (thoracoabdominal) subcostal nerve from T12 (T5 supplies upper segment, T8 supplies the second, T9 supplies remainder)

Function: Flexion of vertebral column

Posterior Abdominal Muscles

Muscle: **Quadratus lumborum**

Origin: Iliac crest

Course: Fans up and in

Insertion: Transverse processes of the lumbar vertebrae and inferior border of rib 12

Innervation: Thoracic nerve T12 and L1 through L4 lumbar nerves

Function: Bilateral contraction fixes the abdominal wall in support of abdominal compression

Muscles of Upper Limb

Muscle: **Latissimus dorsi**

Origin: Lumbar, sacral, and lower thoracic vertebrae

Course: Fans up

Insertion: Humerus

Innervation: Brachial plexus, posterior branch; fibers from the regions C6 through C8 form the long subscapular nerve

Function: For respiration, stabilizes posterior abdominal wall for expiration

Muscles of Phonation

Intrinsic Laryngeal Muscles

Muscle: **Aryepiglotticus muscle**
Origin: Continuation of the oblique arytenoid muscle from the arytenoid apex
Course: Back and up as muscular component of aryepiglottic fold
Insertion: Lateral epiglottis
Innervation: X vagus, recurrent laryngeal nerve
Function: Constricts laryngeal opening

Muscle: **Lateral cricoarytenoid**
Origin: Superior-lateral surface of the cricoid cartilage
Course: Up and back
Insertion: Muscular process of the arytenoid
Innervation: X vagus, recurrent laryngeal nerve
Function: Adducts vocal folds, increases medial compression

Muscle: **Transverse arytenoid**
Origin: Lateral margin of the posterior arytenoid
Course: Laterally on posterior surface of arytenoid
Insertion: Lateral margin of posterior surface, opposite arytenoid
Innervation: X vagus, recurrent laryngeal nerve
Function: Adducts vocal folds

Muscle: **Oblique arytenoid**
Origin: Posterior base of the muscular processes
Course: Obliquely up on posterior surface of arytenoid
Insertion: Apex of the opposite arytenoid
Innervation: X vagus, recurrent laryngeal nerve
Function: Pulls the apex medially, adducts the vocal folds

Muscle: **Posterior cricoarytenoid**
Origin: Posterior cricoid lamina
Course: Superiorly
Insertion: Posterior aspect of the muscular process of arytenoid cartilage
Innervation: X vagus, recurrent laryngeal nerve
Function: Abducts vocal folds

Cranial Nerves

Classes of Cranial Nerves

GSA General somatic afferent: Related to pain, temperature, mechanical stimulation of somatic structures (skin, muscles, joints)

GSE General somatic efferent: Innervates skeletal (striated) muscles

GVA General visceral afferent: From receptors in visceral structures (e.g., digestive tract)

GVE General visceral efferent: Autonomic efferent fibers

SSA Special somatic afferent: Special senses—sight, hearing, equilibrium

SVA Special visceral afferent: Special senses of smell, taste

SVE Special visceral efferent: Innervation of muscle of branchial arch origin: larynx, pharynx, face

Cranial Nerves and Sources

I. Olfactory

SVA: Sense of smell
Source: Mitral cells of olfactory bulb

II. Optic

SSA: Vision
Source: Rod and cone receptor cells synapse with bipolar interneurons that synapse with the multipolar ganglionic neuron;

III. Oculomotor

GSE: All extrinsic ocular muscles except superior oblique and lateral rectus
Source: Oculomotor nucleus

GVE: Light and accommodation reflexes
Source: Edinger-Westphal nucleus

IV. Trochlear

GSE: Superior oblique muscle of eye (turns eye down when eye is adducted)
Source: Trochlear nuclei

V. Trigeminal

GSA: Exteroceptive afferent for pain, thermal, and tactile stimuli from face, forehead, mucous membrane of mouth and nose, teeth cranial dura; proprioceptive (deep pressure, kinesthesis) from teeth, gums, temporomandibular joint, stretch receptors of mastication

Source: Principal sensory nucleus of trigeminal nerve (touch discrimination) and spinal nucleus of trigeminal nerve (pain and temperature), mesenthalic nucleus of trigeminal nerve (proprioception)

GSA, ophthalmic branch: Sensory only; from cornea, iris, upper eyelid, external nose, conjunctiva, anterior scalp back to lamdoidal suture

Source: Principal sensory nucleus of trigeminal nerve (touch discrimination) and spinal nucleus of trigeminal nerve (pain and temperature), mesenthalic nucleus of trigeminal nerve (proprioception)

GSA, maxillary branch: Sensory only; from lower eyelid, alar portion of nose, palate, upper jaw, cheek, part of temple, upper lip

Source: Principal sensory nucleus of trigeminal nerve (touch discrimination) and spinal nucleus of trigeminal nerve (pain and temperature), mesenthalic nucleus of trigeminal nerve (proprioception)

GSA, mandibular branch: Sensory and motor; skin of mandible and lower teeth, mucosa, cheeks, temporomandibular joint, anterior two thirds of tongue, lower lip, part of pinna, part of temple, lower labial gingivae

Source: Principal sensory nucleus of trigeminal nerve (touch discrimination) and spinal nucleus of trigeminal nerve (pain and temperature), mesenthalic nucleus of trigeminal nerve (proprioception)

SVE: To muscles of mastication (internal and external pterygoid, temporalis, masseter), tensor tympani, tensor veli palatine

Source: Principal sensory nucleus of trigeminal nerve (touch discrimination) and spinal nucleus of trigeminal nerve (pain and temperature), mesenthalic nucleus of trigeminal nerve (proprioception)

SVE: To muscles of mastication, tensor tympani, tensor veli palatini

Source: Motor nucleus of trigeminal

VI. Abducens

GSE: Lateral rectus muscle for ocular abduction

Source: Abducens nucleus

VII. Facial

SVE: To facial muscles of expression: platysma, buccinator, muscles of pinna, facial muscles around eye and forehead

Source: Motor nucleus of VII

SVA: Taste, anterior two-thirds of tongue

Source: Solitary nucleus

GSA: Cutaneous sense of EAM and skin of ear

Source: Trigeminal nuclei

GVE: Lacrimal gland (tears); sublingual and submandibular salivary glands; mucous membrane of mouth and nose

Source: Superior salivatory and lacrimal nuclei

VIII. Vestibulocochlear

SSA, cochlear (auditory) portion: Sensors are hair cells; cell bodies are in spiral ganglion; axons are of VIII nerve, in auditory portion; input divides so that all frequencies are represented in anteroventral cochlear nucleus (AVCN), posteroventral cochlear nucleus (PVCN), and dorsal cochlear nucleus (DCN); transfer of auditory sensation to central nervous system

Source: Spiral ganglion terminating in cochlear nucleus

SVA, vestibular portion: From semicircular canals, utricle, saccule; project to vestibular nuclei of medulla and subsequently to all levels of brain stem, spinal cord, cerebellum, thalamus, and cerebral cortex; maintenance of extensor tone, antigravity responses, balance, sense of position in space; coordinated eye/head movement through projection to III oculomotor, IV trochlear, VI abducens cranial nerves

Source: Vestibular ganglion terminating in superior, lateral, medial and inferior vestibular nuclei of medulla and pons

IX. Glossopharyngeal

GVA: Somatic (tactile, thermal, pain sense) from posterior one-third of tongue and pharynx (mediating gag reflex), tonsils, mastoid cells

Source: Solitary nucleus

SVA: Taste, posterior one-third of tongue

Source: Inferior salivatory nucleus

GSA: Somatic sense of middle ear, auditory tube, fauces, nasopharynx, uvula

Source: Trigeminal nuclei

SVE: Innervation of stylopharyngeus, superior pharyngeal constrictor

Source: Inferior salivatory nucleus

GVE: Parotid gland

Source: Inferior salivatory nucleus

X. Vagus

GSA: Cutaneous sense from EAM

Source: Trigeminal nuclei

GVA: Sensory from pharynx, larynx, trachea, esophagus, viscera of thorax, abdomen

Source: Solitary nucleus

SVA: Taste buds near epiglottis and valleculae

Source: Solitary nucleus

GVE: To parasympathetic ganglia, thorax, abdomen

Source: Dorsal motor nucleus of X

SVE: Striated muscles of larynx and pharynx

Source: Nucleus ambiguus

XI. Accessory

SVE, cranial portion: Joins with X vagus to form recurrent laryngeal nerve to innervate intrinsic muscles of larynx

Source: Nucleus ambiguus of medulla

SVE, spinal portion: Innervates sternocleidomastoid and trapezius

Source: Cranial portion: nucleus ambiguus of medulla; Spinal portion: anterior horn of C1 through C5 spinal nerves; unite and ascend; enter skull via foramen magnum; exit with vagus at jugular foramen

Source: Anterior horn of C2 through C5 spinal segments.

XII. Hypoglossal

GSE: Muscles of tongue

Source: Nucleus of hypoglossal nerve

Glossary

3rd ventricle See **third ventricle**

4th ventricle See **fourth ventricle**

VI abducens nerve a.k.a. abducent nerve; nerve mediating abduction of eyeball

VI abducent nerve a.k.a. abducens nerve; nerve mediating abduction of eyeball

IX glossopharyngeal nerve Cranial nerve associated with sensation of tongue and pharynx; a critical nerve for swallowing function

X vagus nerve Cranial nerve involved with vocal fold action, as well as numerous autonomic functions

XI accessory nerve Cranial nerve working in conjunction with IX glossopharyngeal and X vagus to innervate muscles of pharynx and velum

XII hypoglossal nerve Cranial nerve serving muscles of the tongue

-a- Without; lack of

ab- Away from

A band Region of overlap between thin and thick filaments of muscle

abdomen /'æbdəmən/ Region of the body between the thorax and pelvis

abdominal aponeurosis The aponeurotic complex of the anterior abdominal wall that forms points of origination for abdominal musculature

abdominal fixation Process of impounding air within the lungs through inhalation and forceful vocal fold adduction that results in increased intra-abdominal pressure

abdominal viscera /æb'damənl'vɪsɚ-ə/ Organs of the abdominal region

abduction /æb'dʌkʃən/ To draw a structure away from midline

abductor paralysis Paralysis of the muscles of abduction, specifically posterior cricoarytenoid muscles

absolute refractory period Phase of depolarization during which a neuron cannot be stimulated to discharge

accessory cuneate nucleus of medulla Nucleus mediating kinesthetic sense, muscle stretch, and proprioceptive sense from the lower body

acetylcholine /ə'sitlkolin/ Neurotransmitter involved in communication among several classes of neurons and between nerve and muscle

acoustic branch a.k.a. auditory nerve; auditory branch of the vestibulocochlear nerve

acoustic reflex a.k.a. stapedial reflex; contraction of stapedius muscle in response to auditory stimulation

acoustic stria Brain stem auditory pathways arising from the cochlear nucleus

actin One of two muscle proteins

action potential Electrical potential arising from depolarization of a cell membrane

active expiration Expiration arising from muscular activity

ad- Toward

adduct /æ'dʌkt/ to draw two structures closer together or to move toward midline

adduction Process of drawing two structures closer together or moving a structure toward midline

adductor paralysis Paralysis of the muscles of adduction of the vocal folds

adenoids /'ædnɔɪdz/ Lymphoid tissue within the nasopharynx

adequate stimulus Stimulation of sufficient intensity or frequency to cause a response

functional view View of a structure or system with reference to its function in the body

fundamental frequency The lowest frequency of vibration of the vocal folds or of a harmonic series

funiculus /fə'nɪkjuləs/ Small, cordlike structure

fusimotor efferent fibers a.k.a. gamma motor neurons; fibers innervating intrafusal muscle

gag reflex Reflex elicited by tactile stimulation of the faucial pillars, posterior pharyngeal wall, or posterior tongue near the lingual tonsils, with the result being elevation of the velum, protrusion of the tongue, and closure of the larynx

gamma motor neurons a.k.a. fusimotor efferent fibers; fibers innervating intrafusal muscle

ganglia Group of cell bodies having functional unity and lying outside of the central nervous system

ganglion /'gæŋgliən/ Mass of nerve cell bodies lying outside of the central nervous system

gastronomy Surgical placement of a tube into the stomach to provide nutrition.

gastroesophageal reflux Condition in which gastrointestinal contents are re-introduced into the esophagus and pharynx.

-gen Producing

general somatic afferent Sensory nerves that communicate sensory information, such as pain, temperature, mechanical stimulation of skin, length and tension of muscle, and movement and position of joints, from skin, muscles, and joints

general visceral afferent Nerves that transmit sensory information from receptors in visceral structures, such as the digestive tract

-genic Producing

geniculotemporal radiation a.k.a. auditory radiation; fibers from medial geniculate body of the thalamus that terminate at Heschl's gyrus of the temporal lobe

genioglossus muscle Muscle making up the bulk of the tongue, arising from inner mandibular surface at symphysis and coursing to tip and dorsum

geniohyoid muscle Muscle originating at mental spines of mandible and projecting to corpus hyoid

genu /'dʒɛnu/ Knee

genu of internal capsule Point of union between posterior and anterior limbs of internal capsule, containing corticobulbar tract

gingiva /'dʒɪndʒɪvə/ Gum tissue

glia Support tissue of the brain

glial cells Neural tissue with a wide variety of functions in the nervous system, including recycling of neurotransmitter, waste removal, and encapsulation of damaged areas of tissue; also involved in long-term memory function

global aphasia Severe aphasia that includes significant deficits in both expression and comprehension

Globose nuclei Afferent nucleus of the cerebellum

globose nucleus of cerebellum Central nucleus projecting to the red nucleus

globus pallidus Most superficial nucleus of basal ganglia, involved in regulation of muscle tone

glomerulus In the olfactory bulb, the collection of axons converging on a single olfactory neuron

glosso-epiglottic fold Epithelial covering of the lateral and medial glossoepiglottic ligaments, which produces the prominent valleculae between the tongue and epiglottis

glossopalatine muscle a.k.a. palatoglossus muscle; muscle coursing from the sides of posterior tongue to velum

glottal Referring to the glottis

glottal fry Phonatory mode characterized by low fundamental frequency and syncopated beat

glottis /'glatəs/ The space between the true vocal folds

Golgi cells of cerebellum Cells projecting dendrites into the molecular layer and axons into the granular layer of the cerebellum; soma receive input from both climbing fibers and Purkinje cells; axons synapse with granule cell dendrites

Golgi tendon organs (GTOs) Tension sensors within tendons

gooseflesh, goose bumps Autonomic skin response resulting in erection of skin papillae

gracilis tubercle a.k.a. clava of medulla; bulge in posterior medulla caused by nucleus gracilis

granular layer of cerebellum Deepest cell layer of cerebellum

gray matter Cell bodies and dendrites of neurons

greater cornu a.k.a. greater horn; the larger of the two cornu or horns of the hyoid bone, projecting posteriorly

greater horn a.k.a. greater cornu; the larger of the two cornu or horns of the hyoid bone, projecting posteriorly

greater wing of sphenoid bone Processes of sphenoid bone arising from the posterior corpus sphenoid, making up part of the eye socket

gross anatomy Study of the body and its parts as visible without the aid of a microscope

group Ia primary afferent fibers Means by which nuclear bag fibers transmit information to spinal cord

gustation /ɡəsteɪʃən/ Sense of taste

gyri Plural of gyrus; significant prominence or outfolding of tissue

gyrus Outfolding of tissue in cerebral cortex

habenular nuclei of epithalamus Nuclei of epithalamus that receive input from the septum, hypothalamus, brain stem, raphe nuclei, and ventral tegmental area via the habenulopeduncular tract and stria medullaris

habitual pitch The perceptual correlate of vocal fundamental frequency habitually used by an individual

hamulus /'hæmjuləs/ Hook

hard glottal attack Glottal attack that uses excessive muscular force, potentially damaging phonatory anatomy

hard palate The bony portion of the roof of the mouth, made up of the palatal processes of the maxillae and the horizontal plates of the palatine bones

head Proximal portion of a bone

head of caudate nucleus Anterior-most portion of caudate nucleus

hearing The process of receiving and transducing acoustic information as sensation

helicotrema /'hɛlɪkotrimə/ Hooklike region of the cochlea, forming the minute union of the scala vestibuli and scala tympani

hemi- Half

hemiballism /hɛmi'balɪzm/ Hyperkinetic condition involving involuntary and uncontrollable flailing of extremities of the right or left half of the body

hemispheric specialization The concept that one cerebral hemisphere is more highly specialized for a particular function than that seen in the opposite hemisphere

hertz, Hz Cycles per second

Heschl's gyrus Primary reception area of the temporal lobe, BA 41

Hg Mercury

hiatus /'haɪeɪtəs/ Opening

higher-order processing areas for vision (VII) of cerebral cortex The regions involved in higher-order feature extraction for vision, including BA 20 and 21 of the temporal lobe, BA 19 of the occipital lobe, and BA 7 of the parietal lobe

higher-order processing areas of the cerebral cortex Areas of the cortex that receive primary activity information and process it further, such as extraction of features

high-level reflexes Those reflexes mediated at the level of the brain stem

high spontaneous rate Auditory nerve fibers demonstrating a high rate of spontaneous discharge and low threshold of stimulation

hippocampus Structure of limbic lobe involved in memory

histogram Display of data arrayed with reference to its frequency of occurrence

histology Study of tissue through microscopy

homunculus /ho'mʌnkjuləs/ Literally, "little man"; referring to the spatiotopic array of fiber distribu-

intensity Magnitude of sound, expressed as the relationship between two pressures

inter- Between

interaural intensity difference The difference between signal intensity arriving at left and right ears of a listener

interaural phase difference The difference in arrival time of an auditory signal arriving at left and right

interchondral /ɪntə'kandr əl / The region between the cartilaginous portions of the anterior rib cage

intercostal Between the ribs

interhemispheric fissure a.k.a. cerebral longitudinal fissure or superior longitudinal fissure; the fissure that completely separates left and right cerebral hemispheres

intermaxillary suture a.k.a. median palatine suture; suture joining palatal processes of the maxilla

intermediate acoustic stria Auditory pathway arising from cochlear nucleus and terminating in superior olivary complex

intermediate layer of tympanic membrane a.k.a. fibrous layer of tympanic membrane; middle layer of tympanic membrane consisting of radiating fibers and circular fibers

intermediate tendon In digastricus muscle, the tendon that forms the attachment for the posterior and anterior digastricus to the hyoid bone

internal Within the body

internal auditory meatus Canal through which auditory nerve passes into cranial vault

internal capsule Region of cerebral projection fibers immediately superior to the cerebral peduncles of the midbrain, at the level of the basal ganglia and thalamus

internal carotid arteries Major vascular supply to the cerebral cortex, giving rise to the anterior and middle cerebral arteries

internal carotid artery of cerebrovascular supply Artery arising from common carotid artery, serving cerebrovascular system

internal pterygoid muscle a.k.a. medial pterygoid muscle; muscle arising from medial pterygoid plate

and fossa of the sphenoid and inserting into the inner surface of the ramus of the mandible

interneurons Neurons that provide communication between two neurons in a chain

intero- Aimed inward or farther from the surface

interoceptor /ɪntəo'sɛptə/ Sensory receptor activated by stimuli from within the body (contrast with exteroceptor)

interpeduncular fossa Indentation between the cerebral peduncles from which III oculomotor nerve exits

interspike interval Neural response histogram providing detail of the timing between individual neural discharges

interstitial /ɪntə'stɪʃəl/ Space between cells or organs

interthalamic adhesion Connection between left and right thalamus

intertragic incisure /ɪntə'treɪdʒɪk ɪn'saɪzə/ Region between tragus and antitragus

interventricular foramen of Monro Passageway connecting the lateral and third ventricles

intervertebral foramen Foramen through which spinal nerve exits and/or enters spinal cord

intonation The melody of speech, provided by variation of fundamental frequency during speech

intra- Within

intracellular Within the cell

intracellular resting potential Electrical potential within hair cells, being −70 mV relative to the endolymph

intracellular space Space within individual cells

intrafusal muscle fibers /ɪntrə'fuzl̩/ Muscle to which the muscle spindle is attached

intraoral /ɪntrə'orl̩/ Within the mouth

intraosseous eruption Eruption of tooth through bone

intraparietal sulcus Significant superior-lateral sulcus of parietal lobe, involved in body perception relative to guided movement of hand, making up part of the "where" visual stream

intrapleural pressure /ɪntrə'plə-əl/ Pressure measured within the pleural linings of the lungs

intrinsic laryngeal ligaments Ligaments within the larynx that bind the cartilages of the larynx together

intrinsic laryngeal muscles Muscles whose attachments are to other structures within the larynx, including lateral cricoarytenoid, posterior cricoarytenoid, transverse arytenoid, oblique arytenoid, cricothyroid, thyroarytenoid (thyrovocalis and thyrmomuscularis), thyroepiglottic, aryepiglottic, and superior thyroarytenoid muscles

intrinsic muscles of the tongue Muscles of the tongue that have both origin and insertion within the tongue

intro- Into

ion A particle carrying positive or negative charge

ion transport Movement of ions across a membrane

ipsi- Same

ipsilateral Same side

ipsilateral stimulation That pattern of stimulation wherein stimulation of a structure in the auditory nervous system arises from stimulus being received in the ear on the same side of the body as the structure

ipsilaterally Nerve fibers coursing and terminating on the same site as origin of the fiber

ischemia Cessation of blood flow

iIsland of Reil a.k.a. insular cortex; region located deep to the cerebral operculum

iso- Equal

isometric Muscle action that does not result in movement

isthmus /'ɪsməs/ A narrow passageway between cavities

-itis Inflammation or irritation

-ium Diminutive form of a noun

jejunostomy: The placement of a feeding tube into the small intestine

joint Articulation

jugum of sphenoid bone Anterior aspect of body of sphenoid

kinesthesia /kɪnɛsˈθiʒə/ Including sense of range, direction, and weight

kinesthetic sense Sense of movement

kinocilium /kɑɪnoˈsɪliəm/ Unitary cilium found on each hair cell of vestibular mechanism

labial surface of tooth The superficial surface of upper and lower teeth coming in contact with the lips

labioverted /ˈleɪbiovɚtd/ Tilted toward the lip

labyrinth Maze

labyrinthine hair receptors Mechanoreceptors within the vestibular mechanism that sense body movement

lacrimal gland Tear gland

lamdoidal suture of parietal bones Suture uniting the parietal and occipital bones

lamina /ˈlæmənə/ A flat membrane or layer

laminae Layers

laryngeal depressors Muscles that lower the larynx

laryngeal elevators Muscles that raise the larynx

laryngeal saccule Pouch of anterior laryngeal ventricle that contains mucus-producing and secreting epithelia

laryngeal stridor Harsh sound produced during respiration as a result of turbulence at the level of the vocal folds or within the respiratory passageway

laryngeal ventricle See **ventricle of larynx**

laryngectomee Person undergoing laryngectomy surgery

laryngectromy Partial or total removal of the larynx

laryngitis Inflammation of vocal folds

laryngologist /lɛrɪnˈgalodʒɪst/ Specialist in the study of vocal pathology

laryngopharynx a.k.a. hypopharynx; space bounded anteriorly by epiglottis and inferiorly by esophagus

laryngoscope /lɛˈrɪngoskop/ Instrument of visualization of the larynx and associated structures

larynx Structure housing the vocal folds and other phonation-related structures

lateral Toward the side

lateral apertures a.k.a. foramina of Luschka; left and right openings, lateral to median aperture, connecting the fourth ventricle and the cerebrospinal space outside of the cerebellum

lateral corticospinal tract Lateral differentiation of the corticospinal tract arising from the decussation of the corticospinal tract at the pyramids in the medulla

lateral cricoarytenoid muscle Muscle coursing from the muscular process of the arytenoid to superior surface of the cricoid cartilage, serving as the primary adductor of the vocal folds

lateral funiculus Lateral column of spinal cord

lateral geniculate body (LGB) Nucleus of thalamus involved in visual function

lateral glossoepiglottic ligament Lateral ligament binding the tongue to the epiglottis, forming the lateral aspects of the valleculae

lateral incisors Incisors lateral to central incisors

lateral ligament of malleus Ligament binding malleus to temporal bone, arising from the lateral process of the malleus

lateral process of malleus Process of malleus on lateral surface, providing attachment for the lateral malleolar ligament

lateral pterygoid muscle a.k.a. external pterygoid muscle; muscle arising from the lateral pterygoid plate of sphenoid bone and coursing back to insert into the pterygoid fossa of mandible

lateral pterygoid plate of sphenoid bone Laterally placed posterior prominence of sphenoid bone

lateral semicircular canal a.k.a. horizontal semicircular canal; sensory component of vestibular mechanism that senses movement roughly in the transverse plane of the body

lateral spinothalamic tract Tract conveying pain and thermal sense within the spinal cord

lateral sulcus a.k.a. Sylvian fissure; fissure dividing temporal lobe from frontal and anterior parietal lobes

lateral superior olive Nuclear aggregate of superior olivary complex involved in processing interaural intensity differences

lateral thyrohyoid ligament Ligament that runs from the superior cornu of the thyroid to the posterior tip of the greater cornu of the hyoid bone

lateral ventricles Paired spaces within the cerebral cortex

latero- Side

leg 1. The lower anatomical extremity, particularly the region between the knee and ankle. 2. A device used for raising grain from ground level to the top of a bin, consisting of a continuous flexible belt with a series of metal buckets or scoops

lemniscal pathway Pathway cord from medial lemniscus to thalamus

lentiform nucleus a.k.a. lentiform nucleus; combination of globus pallidus and putamen

lepto- Thick

lesion /ˈliʒən/ A region of damaged tissue or a wound

lesser cornu a.k.a. lesser horn; the smaller of the two cornu or horns of the hyoid bone, projecting superiorly from the corpus or the hyoid

lesser horn a.k.a. lesser cornu; the smaller of the two cornu or horns of the hyoid bone, projecting superiorly from the corpus or the hyoid

lesser wing of sphenoid of sphenoid bone Processes arising from corpus and clinoid processes of sphenoid bone, partially covering the optic canal

leuco- White

levator anguli oris muscle Muscle arising from canine fossa of maxilla and coursing to insert into upper and lower lips

levator labii superioris alaeque nasi muscle Muscle coursing vertically along lateral margin of nose, arising from frontal process of maxilla

levator labii superioris muscle Muscle originating from infraorbital margin of maxilla, coursing down and in to the upper lip

levator veli palati a.k.a. levator veli paltine or levator veli palatini; palatal elevator, making up bulk of velum

levator veli palatine a.k.a. levator veli palatini levator veli palate or palatal elevator, making up bulk of velum

levator veli palatini a.k.a. levator veli palate or levator veli paltine; palatal elevator, making up bulk of velum

lever advantage The benefit derived through reduction of the length of the long process of stapes relative to the manubrium malli

levo- Left

ligaments Fibrous connective tissue connecting bones or cartilage

limb apraxia The inability to perform volitional gestures using the limbs

limbic association cortex The cortical association areas that include Brodmann areas 23, 24, 38, 28, and 11, the parahippocampal gyrus and temporal pole, cingulate gyri of the parietal and frontal lobes, and orbital surfaces of the inferior frontal lobe; system involved with motivation, emotion, and memory, making it an ideal association area

limbic system The central nervous system structures responsible for mediation of motivation and arousal, including the hippocampus, amygdala, dentate gyrus, cingulate gyrus, and fornix

lingual Referring to the tongue

lingual frenulum a.k.a. lingual frenum; bands of connective tissue joining inferior tongue with mandible

lingual nerve of V trigeminal nerve Portion of V trigeminal that mediates somatic sensation of anterior two-thirds of tongue and floor of mouth

lingual papillae Prominences on posterior surface of tongue

lingual surface of tooth Surface of tooth adjacent to tongue

lingual tonsils Lymphoid tissue on palatine surface of tongue

linguaverted /ˈlɪŋgwəvɚtd/ Tilted toward the tongue

lingula Vestigial middle lobe of the left lung

literal paraphasias Phoneme substitutions found in aphasia (note that "literal" is an old medical reference to "letters," preceding our concepts of phonemes being the units of speech)

lobar bronchi Bronchial passageways connecting the main stem bronchi with individual lobes of the lungs

Lobe Major portion of a structure (e.g., frontal lobe of brain, superior lobe of lung)

localization The process of identification of a sound source presented in free field

localizationist a.k.a. materialists; theoreticians who view the brain as having very specific regions with clearly identified roles

long association fibers Association fibers of cerebral cortex that connect lobes of the same hemisphere

long process of incus Process of incus that runs approximately parallel to the manubrium malli

loudness The psychological correlate of sound intensity

lower extremity Portion of the body made up of the thigh, leg, ankle, and foot

lower motor neuron The final common neurological pathway leading to the muscle, including the anterior horn cell of the spinal cord, nerve roots, and nerves

low spontaneous rate Auditory nerve fibers with low rate of spontaneous discharge and relatively high threshold of stimulation

lumbar puncture Insertion of aspiration needle into subarachnoid region of spinal cord, usually below L4

lumbar vertebra Vertebra of the lumbar spinal column

lymphoid tissue /ˈlɪmfɔɪd/ Tissue comprising lymphatic organs, including tonsils and adenoids

macro- Large

macula /ˈmækjələ/ Sensory organ of saccule and utricle

macula cribrosa media Perforations in spherical recess of vestibule through which vestibular nerve passes to the saccule of the membranous labyrinth

mainstem bronchi First division of the bronchial tree

malleolar facet Point of union between malleus and incus

malleus /ˈmæliəs/ Initial bone of the ossicular chain

mandible Lower jaw, including dental arch

mandibular foramen Opening on posterior inner surface of the mandible through which V trigeminal enters mandible to serve teeth and gums

mandibular fossa of temporal bone Fossa of temporal bone with which condyle of mandible articulates

mandibular nerve of the V trigeminal Lowest branch of the V trigeminal nerve

mandibular notch Notch between condylar and coronoid process of mandible

manometer Device for measuring air pressure differences

manubrium /məˈnubriəm/ Process of malleus forming the major attachment to the tympanic membrane

manubrosternal angle The point of articulation of manubrium sterni and corpus sterni

mass The characteristic of matter that gives it inertia

masseter muscle Most superficial of muscles of mastication, running from the zygomatic arch to the ramus of the mandible

mastication Chewing

mastoid air cells Cells comprising much of the mastoid process and extending to the floor of the middle ear cavity

mastoid portion of temporal bone Posterior portion of temporal bone

mastoid process of temporal bone Bony process posterior to external auditory meatus

Materialists a.k.a. localizationist; theoreticians who view the brain as having very specific regions with clearly identified roles

maxilla Upper jaw

maxillary nerve of the V trigeminal Intermediate branch of the V trigeminal nerve

maxillary process of zygomatic bone Process of zygomatic bone that articulates with maxilla

maxillary sinus Largest of the sinuses of the maxilla

maximum phonation time The duration an individual can sustain a phonation

meatal atresia Developmental absence of external auditory meatus

meatus /miˈeɪtəs/ Passageway

meatus acousticus externus Outer ear canal; external auditory meatus

mechanoreceptors Sensory receptors sensitive to mechanical stimulation such as pressure on the skin

medial a.k.a. mesial; toward the midline of the body or subpart

medial compression The degree of force that may be applied by the vocal folds at their point of contact

medial geniculate body (MGB) Nucleus of thalamus involved in auditory function

medial lemniscus of pons Somatic sense pathway within pons

medial longitudinal fasciculus (MLF) Group of fiber tracts within spinal cord that includes the rubrospinal tract

medial pterygoid muscle a.k.a. internal pterygoid muscle; muscle arising from medial pterygoid plate and fossa of the sphenoid and inserting into the inner surface of the ramus of the mandible

medial pterygoid plate of sphenoid bone Medially placed posterior prominence of sphenoid bone

medial superior olive Nuclear aggregate of superior olivary complex involved in processing interaural time (phase) differences

medial surface of tooth a.k.a. mesial; surface directed toward midpoint between central incisors, along dental arch

medial vestibular nucleus of medulla Nucleus associated with vestibular function

median Middle

median aperture a.k.a. foramen of Magendie; midline opening connecting the fourth ventricle and the cerebrospinal space outside of the cerebellum

median fibrous septum of tongue Dividing wall between right and left halves of tongue that serves as the point of origin for the transverse muscle of the tongue

median glossoepiglottic ligament Middle ligament binding the tongue to the epiglottis, structurally dividing the left and right valleculae

median palatine suture a.k.a. intermaxillary suture; suture joining palatal processes of the maxilla

median pharyngeal raphe Midline connective tissue that forms union of left and right pharyngeal musculature

median raphe of hard palate Division point between left and right halves of hard palate

median raphe of medulla Point of decussation of fibers from the principal inferior olivary nucleus

median sulcus of tongue Midline sulcus dividing tongue into left and right halves

median thyrohyoid ligament Ligament coursing from the anterior corpus hyoid to the upper border of the anterior thyroid

mediastinal /mɪdɪˈəstaɪn̩l/ Referring to the middle space; in respiration, referring to the organs separating the lungs

mediastinal pleurae Parietal pleural lining covering the mediastinum

medio-, medius Middle

medulla a.k.a. medulla oblongata; the inferior-most segment of the brain stem

medulla oblongata a.k.a. medulla; the inferior-most segment of the brain stem

medullary reticulospinal tract Tract arising from the medulla and descending through the lateral lemniscus of the spinal cord, supporting postural control of lower limb muscles

megalo- Large

melogenesis imperfeca Congenital condition in which enamel of tooth is thin or missing

membranous glottis /mɛmˈbrənəs ˈglatəs/ The anterior three-fifths of the vocal fold margin; the soft tissue of the vocal folds (note that the term *glottis* is loosely used here, because glottis is actually the space between the vocal folds)

membranous labyrinth /mɛmˈbrənəs ˈlæbɪrɪnθ/ Membranous sac housed within bony labyrinth of inner ear, holding the receptor organs of hearing and vestibular sense

meningeal infection /məˈnɪndʒiəl/ Infection of the meningeal linings of the brain and spinal cord

meningeal linings a.k.a. meninges; connective tissue linings of the brain, including dura mater, arachnoid mater, and pia mater

meninges /məˈnɪndʒiz/ a.k.a. meningeal linings; connective tissue linings of the brain, including dura mater, arachnoid mater, and pia mater

mental symphysis a.k.a. symphysis menti; the juncture of the fused paired bones of the mandible

mentalis muscle Muscle arising from region of incisive fossa of the mandible, coursing down to insert into the skin of the chin below

mesencephalon /mɛsɛnˈsɛfəlan/ The midbrain

mesial /ˈmiziəl/ a.k.a. medial; toward the midline of the body or subpart

mesial surface of tooth a.k.a. medial; surface directed toward midpoint between central incisors, along dental arch

mesioverted /misioˈvɚtd/ Tilted toward the midline

meso- Middle

meta- After; mounted or built upon

metencephalon /mɛtɛnˈsɛfəlan/ Embryonic portion of brain from which cerebellum and pons originate

micro- Small

microdontia Abnormally small tooth size

microglia Glial cells responsible for phagocytosis, or scavenging of necrotic tissue in the nervous system

micron One thousandth of a millimeter; one millionth of a meter

micropotential a.k.a. miniature postsynaptic potential (MPSP); depolarization of a small portion of a neuron membrane

microscopic anatomy Study of structure of the body by means of microscopy

microtia Small auricle

middle cerebellar peduncle a.k.a. brachia pontis; middle pathway for information to and from cerebellum

middle cerebral arteries Major arteries arising from internal carotid artery; responsible for serving

neuraxis /nə-ˈæksɪs/ The axis of the nervous system, representing the embryonic brain axis

neuro- Nerve

neurogenic Of neurological origin

neurology Neurology study of the diseases of the nervous system

neuromotor dysfunction Neurological condition in motor ability arising from lesion within the nervous system or at the myoneural junction

neuromuscular junction The point of contact between a muscle fiber and the nerve innervating it

neurons Nerve cell tissue whose function is to transmit information from one neuron to another, from neurons to muscles, or from sensory receptors to other neural structures

neurotransmitters Substance that is released into synaptic cleft upon excitation of a neuron

neutroclusion /ˈnutrokluʒən/ Normal molar relationship between upper and lower dental arches

Nissen fundoplication Surgery placing a tissue valve in the lower esophageal sphincter to eliminate regurgitation of stomach contents

nodes of Ranvier /ˈnodz ʌv ˈranvieɪ/ Regions of myelinated fibers in which there is no myelin

nodulus of cerebellum Central region of the anterior cerebellum, making up part of the flocculonodular lobe

non-pyramidal cells Small neurons involved in sensory function or intercommunication between brain regions

nuclear bag fibers Stretch receptors clustered at the equatorial region of the intrafusal muscle fiber

nuclear chain fibers Row of stretch sensors at the equatorial region of the intrafusal muscle fiber; surrounded by bags that may have either primary Ia or group II secondary afferent fibers

nucleus /ˈnukliəs/ An aggregate of neuron cell bodies within the central nervous system

nucleus ambiguus Nucleus giving rise to the IX glossopharyngeal, X vagus, and XI accessory nerves

nucleus cuneatus Nucleus of fasciculus cuneatus

nucleus interpositus of cerebellum Combination of emboliform and globose nuclei of cerebellum

nucleus pulposus: Gel-like center of the vertebral disc capsule

nucleus solitarius of medulla Nucleus of the X vagus nerve

oblique Diagonal

oblique arytenoid muscle a.k.a. oblique interarytenoid muscle; muscle coursing from the posterior apex of one arytenoid to the posterior base of the other arytenoid, serving as adductor of the vocal folds

oblique interarytenoid muscle a.k.a. oblique arytenoid muscles; muscle coursing from the posterior apex of one arytenoid to the posterior base of the other arytenoid, serving as adductor of the vocal folds

oblique line of thyroid Point of attachment on the thyroid cartilage of the thyrohyoid and sternothyroid muscles

occipital horn of lateral ventricles a.k.a. posterior horn of lateral ventricles; portion of lateral ventricles extending into the occipital lobe

occipitomastoid suture of temporal bone Suture joining mastoid region with occipital bone

occlusal surface /əˈkluzl̩/ The surface of teeth within opposing dental arches that make contact

occlusion Process of bringing upper and lower teeth into contact

oculo- Eye

olfaction The sense of smell

olfactory bulb Nuclei of the olfactory nerve

olfactory sulcus Sulcus on inferior surface of the frontal lobe along which optic tract passes

oligodendrocytes Glial cells that are instrumental in production of myelin in the central nervous system

olive of medulla Bulge between the ventrolateral and dorsolateral sulci, caused by the inferior olivary nuclear complex, which consists of nuclei serving to localize sound in space

olivocerebellar fibers Fibers that arise from the inferior olivary and medial accessory olivary nucleus of the medulla and project to the contralateral cerebellum, terminating as climbing fibers

olivocochlear bundle /alɪvoˈkoklɪɚ/ Collective term for crossed and uncrossed olivocochlear bundles, the efferent auditory nerve fibers involved in processing auditory signal in noise

-oma Morbid condition of a part, often a tumor

omohyoid muscle Laryngeal depressor with two bellies: the inferior belly arising from the scapula and inserting into an intermediate tendon; the superior belly arising from the intermediate tendon and inserting into the hyoid; together, the two bellies that depress the hyoid

onset response Neural response in which there is an initial burst of activity related to the onset of a stimulus, followed by silence

opening stage of phonation In the cycle of phonation, the stage in which the vibrating vocal folds are opening up

ophthalmic nerve of the V trigeminal Superior branch of the V trigeminal nerve

optic canal of sphenoid bone Canal within sphenoid through which optic nerve passes

optic chiasm Decussation point for optic nerve

Optic radiation Portion of the visual pathway projecting from lateral geniculate body of thalamus

optic tracts Extension of the optic nerve coursing around the crus cerebri following the decussation at the optic chiasm

optimal pitch The perceptual characteristic representing the ideal or most efficient frequency of vibration of the vocal folds or powers

oral apraxia Difficulty using the facial and lingual muscles for nonspeech acts in absence of muscular weakness or paralysis

oral cavity The region extending from the orifice of the mouth in the anterior, and bounded laterally by the dental arches and posteriorly by the fauces

oral diadochokinesis /ˈdaɪədokokɪ ˈnisɪs/ A task involving repetition of movements requiring alternating contraction of antagonist muscles associated with speech (lips, mandible, tongue)

oral-peripheral examination a.k.a. oral mechanism examination; procedure for examining structure and function of the oral mechanism with particular interest in functionality related to speech

Oral mechanism examination a.k.a. oral-peripheral examination; procedure for examining structure and function of the oral mechanism with particular interest in functionality related to speech

oral surface of tongue a.k.a. palatine surface of tongue; superior surface of the portion of the tongue within the oral cavity

orbicularis oris inferior muscle Muscle underlying lower lip of oral cavity

orbicularis oris muscle Muscle underlying lips of oral cavity

orbicularis oris superior muscle Muscle underlying upper lip of oral cavity

orbital margin of zygomatic bone Portion of zygomatic bone that contributes to the eye socket

orbital plates of ethmoid bone The ethmoid component of the eye socket

orbital portion of frontal bone Process of the frontal bone that makes up a portion of the eye socket

orbital process of palatine bone Process making up the lower portion of the eye socket

orbital region a.k.a. pars orbitale; region of inferior frontal lobe overlying the eyes

orbital surface On inferior surface of the frontal lobe, region overlying the eyes

organ of Corti Sensory organ of hearing within inner ear

organelles Specialized structures of a cell (e.g., mitochondria)

organs Aggregates of tissues with functional unity

orienting reflex Reflex elicited by touching the side of a newborn's cheek, with the result being that the infant's tongue moves in the direction of the stimulus

orifice Mouth or opening

origin Proximal attachment of a muscle; point of attachment of a muscle with relatively little movement

oro- Mouth

orofacial myofunctional therapy a.k.a. oromyo-functional therapy; therapy directed toward remediating problems of muscular imbalance

second bicuspid In adult arch, tooth distal to first bicuspid, with two cusps

second molar Tooth distal to first molar in adult arch

segmental Divided into segments

segmental spinal arc reflex Reflex system arising at the spinal cord level; involved in reflexive contraction of skeletal muscle as result of passive stretching

selective enhancement Relative benefit of auditory signal arising from resonance of the auditory mechanism

sellar /ˈsɛlɚ/ Saddlelike

sella turcica of sphenoid bone a.k.a. pituitary fossa of sphenoid bone, hypophyseal fossa; inferior space of sphenoid in which pituitary gland resides

semi- Half

semicircular canals Canals of the vestibular system, responsible for sensation of movement of the head in space

sensation Awareness of body conditions

septal cartilage Anterior cartilaginous component of the nasal septum

septum /ˈsɛptəm/ A divider

serous Pale, yellow body fluid

shaft of rib The long, relatively straight component of a rib, between the neck and the angle of the rib

shearing action The bending action of the hair cells arising from the relative movement of the basilar membrane and tectorial membrane during auditory stimulation

shedding teeth a.k.a. deciduous teeth or milk teeth; teeth within the deciduous arch that are shed during development

short association fibers Association fibers of cerebral cortex that connect gyri of the same hemisphere

short process of incus Posteriorly projecting process of incus

shoulder girdle Another term for pectoral girdle

single neuron response Measurement of response of a single neuron

sinistro- Left

sinus A cavity or passageway

skeletal muscle Striated or voluntary muscle

sliding filament model of muscle contraction Process in which cross-bridges connect actin and myosin of parallel myofilaments, pulling the fibers closer together

slowly adapting sensors Those sensors that continue responding once stimulated, such as pain sensors

slow twitch fibers Fibers that are slow acting and remain contracted longer than fast twitch fibers; typically found in postural muscles

smooth muscle Sheet-like muscle with spindle-shaped cells; makes up the muscular tissue of the digestive tract and blood vessels

sodium inactivation Closure of sodium channels in cell wall, prohibiting transport of sodium

sodium–potassium pump Biological mechanism by which sodium and potassium are actively moved through a cell wall

soft palate a.k.a. velum; the musculotendinous structure separating the oropharynx and nasopharynx

solitary tract nucleus Nucleus of brain stem; the inner portion including axons from the VII facial, IX glossopharyngeal, X vagus cranial nerves

soma A cell body

somatic muscle Skeletal muscle; striated muscle

somatic nervous system The voluntary component of the nervous system

somatic sense Body sense

somato- Pertaining to the body

somatosomatic synapse Synapse of the soma of one neuron with the soma of another

somesthetic /somǝsˈθæɛtɪk/ Pertaining to awareness of body sensation

sound Audible disturbance in a medium

sound wave The acoustical manifestation of physical disturbance in a medium

source-filter theory The theory of vowel production that states that a voicing source is generated by the vocal folds and routed through the vocal tract where it is shaped into the sounds of speech

spastic dysarthria Dysarthria arising from upper motor neuron lesion, resulting in spasticity, hypertonicity, hyperreflexia reflexes, and muscular weakness

spatial orientation Knowledge of body position in space

spatial summation Phenomenon of many near-simultaneous synaptic activations, representing many points of contact arrayed over the surface of the neuron

spatiotopic /speɪʃioˈtɑpɪk/ The physical array of many of the regions of the cerebral cortex that defines the specific region of the body represented (e.g., the pre- and postcentral gyri)

specialization Given task or function (e.g., language) restricted to a specific hemisphere

special senses Olfaction, audition, gustation, and vision

special somatic afferent Cranial nerves that serve the special body senses, such as vision and hearing

special visceral efferent Cranial nerves that innervate striated muscle of branchial arch origin, including the larynx, pharynx, soft palate, face, and muscles of mastication

spectral analysis Analysis of an acoustical signal to determine the relative contribution of individual frequency components

speculum /ˈspɛkjuləm/ Instrument used to examine orifices and canals

sphenoid sinuses Air-filled sinuses in sphenoid bone

spherical recess of vestibule Recess in inner ear vestibule that contains perforations through which vestibular nerve passes to the saccule of the membranous labyrinth

spheroid /ˈsfɪrɔɪd/ Shaped like a sphere

spike rate Rate of discharge of a neuron

spinal column The vertebral column

spinal cord The nerve tracts and cell bodies within the spinal column

spinal cord segment A segment of the spinal cord corresponding to a vertebral region

spinal meningeal linings Meningeal linings of the spinal cord

spinal nerves Nerves arising from the spinal cord

spinal tract nucleus of V trigeminal Sensory nucleus of V trigeminal served by input from IX glossopharyngeal nerve

spinocerebellum a.k.a. paleocerebellum; portion of cerebellum made up of anterior lobe of cerebellum and posterior lobe related to arm and leg

spinous process Posterior-most process of vertebra

spiral ligament Region of scala media to which stria vascularis is attached

spiral limbus Region of scala media from which the tectorial membrane arises

spiritualists a.k.a. equipotentialists; theoreticians who view brain function as being distributed broadly, with very little or no localization of function

spirometer /spaɪrˈamətɚ/ Device used to measure respiratory volume

splenium of corpus callosum The posterior portion of the corpus callosum through which information for the temporal and occipital lobes passes

spongy bone Bone that contains the marrow that produces red and white blood cells as well as the blood plasma matrix

squamosal suture of parietal bones Suture uniting parietal and temporal bones

squamous portion of temporal bone Fan-shaped portion of temporal bone

s-segment Lateral superior olive of superior olivary complex

Stahl's ear Pointy, elfin-shaped ears

stapedius /stəˈpidiəs/ Muscle of middle ear that acts on the stapes

stapes /ˈsteɪpiz/ The final bone of the ossicular chain

stapedial reflex a.k.a. acoustic reflex; contraction of stapedius muscle in response

stellate cells of cerebellum Cells in cerebellum that communicate with Purkinje cells

steno- Narrow

stereocilia /stɛrio'sɪliə/ Minute cilia protruding from the surface of hair cells

stereognosis /'stɛriagnosəs/ Ability to recognize objects through tactile sensation

sternal notch a.k.a. suprasternal notch; the notch on the superior aspect of the manubrium sterni

sternohyoid muscle Hyoid depressor coursing from the sternum to the hyoid bone

sternothyroid muscle Muscle arising from the sternum and inserting into the thyroid cartilage and depressing the thyroid cartilage and larynx

stiffness The strength of the forces within a given material that restore it to its original shape on being distended

stoma Mouth of an opening; in larygectomee, stoma is short for tracheostoma

strepto- Swift

stress In speech, the product of relative increase in fundamental frequency, vocal intensity, and duration

striated Striped

striatum Combination of putamen and caudate nucleus of basal ganglia

stria vascularis /'striə væskju'lɛrɪs/ Vascularized tissue arising from the spiral ligament of the scala media

strohbass Glottal fry; pulse register

styloglossus muscle Muscle arising from styloid process of temporal bone and inserting into inferior sides of tongue

stylohyoid ligament Ligament attaching styloid muscle with hyoid bone

stylohyoid muscle Muscle coursing from styloid process of mandible to hyoid bone

styloid process of temporal bone Process protruding beneath the external auditory meatus and medial to the mastoid process

stylopharyngeus Muscle arising from styloid process of temporal bone and inserting into pharyngeal constrictors and thyroid cartilage

sub- Under

subcortical nuclei Nuclei of thalamus with no direct communication with the cerebral cortex

subdural hematoma Release of blood through hemorrhage beneath the dura mater

subglottal /sʌb'glatl̩/ Beneath the glottis

subglottal pressure air pressure generated by the respiratory system beneath the level of the vocal folds

sublingual fold Fold on lower surface of tongue that marks salivary glands

sublingual gland Salivary gland beneath tongue

submandibular gland Salivary gland posterior to sublingual gland

substantia nigra Dopamine-producing cells within cerebral peduncles; critical for function of the basal ganglia

subthalamic nucleus Nucleus on inner surface of internal capsule that receives input from globus pallidus and motor cortex; involved in control of striated muscle

successional tooth Tooth in adult dental arch that replaces a homologous deciduous tooth

sulci Plural of sulcus; significant in-folding of tissue

sulcus /'sʌlkəs/ A groove

summating potential A sustained, direct current (DC) shift in the endocochlear potential that occurs when the organ of Corti is stimulated by sound

sup- Under; moderately

super- Above; excessively

superadded tooth Tooth in adult dental arch not represented in deciduous arch

superficial Near the surface

superficial sensation Sensation of the surface tissue of the body

superior The upper point; nearer the head

superior cerebellar artery of cerebrovascular supply Artery arising from basilar artery, serving cerebellum

superior cerebellar peduncle a.k.a. brachia conjunctiva; superior pathway for information to and from cerebellum

superior lobe of cerebellum a.k.a anterior lobe; anterior-most lobe of cerebellum

superior colliculus Midbrain relay for visual stimuli

superior cornu of thyroid Superior-most processes of the thyroid cartilage, providing the point of articulation between the greater cornu of the hyoid bone and thyroid cartilages

superior frontal gyrus Gyrus bordering the longitudinal fissure in superior aspect of frontal lobe

superior laryngeal nerve (SLN) of X vagus Branch of X vagus innervating cricothyroid muscle for laryngeal pitch change

superior ligament of incus Ligament binding incus to temporal bone, arising from the superior surface of the incus and coursing to the epitympanic recess

superior ligament of malleus Ligament binding malleus to temporal bone, arising from the head of the malleus

superior longitudinal fissure a.k.a. cerebral longitudinal fissure; interhemispheric fissure; the fissure that completely separates left and right cerebral hemispheres

superior longitudinal muscle of tongue Superior-most muscle on surface of tongue, coursing from median fibrous sulcus to lateral surface

superior medullary velum Pontine surface providing superior border of fourth ventricle

superior nasal conchae Superiorly placed process of ethmoid bone, found in nasal cavity

superior olivary complex in pons Important auditory nuclear complex within the pons, responsible for localization of sound in space

superior orbital fissure of sphenoid bone Canal of the sphenoid bone through which the IV trochlear nerve passes

superior parietal lobule Superior-most gyrus of the parietal lobe

superior petrosal ganglion Ganglion of IX glossopharyngeal nerve

superior pharyngeal constrictor muscle Muscle coursing from pterygomandibular raphe to median pharyngeal raphe

superior temporal gyrus Superior-most gyrus of the temporal lobe

superior temporal sulcus Sulcus separating superior and middle temporal gyri

superior thyroarytenoid muscle Auxiliary intrinsic musculature of larynx that is inconsistently present, arising from the inner angle of the thyroid cartilage and coursing to the muscular process of the arytenoid, and being an extension of the thyroarytenoid (thyromuscularis)

supernumerary teeth Teeth in addition to the normal number

supination /supɪˈneɪʃən/ Placement in the supine position

supine /ˈsupaɪn/ Body in horizontal position with face up

supplementary motor area (SMA) Upper and medial portions of Brodmann area 6, involved in aspects of motor planning

supplementary motor area of cerebral cortex (SMA) The superior and medial portions of Brodmann area 6, which is involved in complex motor acts, including rehearsal and initiation of motor function

supra- Above, upon

suprahyoid muscles Muscles attached to the hyoid bone and a structure superior to the hyoid bone

supramarginal gyrus Portion of inferior parietal lobule

suprasternal notch a.k.a. sternal notch; the notch on the superior aspect of the manubrium sterni

supraverted /suprəˈvɚtɪd/ Turning up

surface anatomy Study of the body and its surface markings, as related to underlying structures

surfactant /sɚˈfæktənt/ A chemical agent that reduces surface tension

suture /ˈsutʃɚ/ The demarcation of union between two structures through immobile articulation

sylvian fissure a.k.a. lateral sulcus; fissure dividing temporal lobe from frontal and anterior parietal lobes

sym- With or together

sympathetic nervous system a.k.a. thoracolumbar system; the portion of the autonomic nervous system that responds to stimulation through energy expenditure

sympathetic trunk ganglia Collection of cell bodies coursing parallel to the vertebral column

symphysis /sɪmfɪsɪs/ A type of union of two structures that were separated in early development, resulting in an immobile articulation

symphysis menti a.k.a. mental symphysis; the juncture of the fused paired bones of the mandible

syn- With or together

synapse /'sɪnæps/ The junction between two communicating neurons

synaptic cleft the region between two communicating neurons into which neurotransmitter is released

synaptic vesicles /sɪ'næptɪk 'vɛsəklz/ The saccules within the end bouton of an axon, containing neurotransmitter substance

synergist /'sɪnɚdʒɪst/ A muscle working in conjunction with another muscle to facilitate movement

synostosis Articulation of adjacent bones by means of ossification of a suture

synovial fluid /sɪnoviəl/ The fluid within a synovial joint

system A functionally defined group of organs

systemic anatomy The description of individual parts of the body without reference to disease conditions

tachy- Swift; fast

tactile Referring to the sense of touch

tactile sense The specific sense of touch, mediated by sensors within the epithelial lining

tail of caudate nucleus Posterior-most portion of caudate nucleus

-tarsal Ankle

tectorial membrane /tɛk'toriəl/ The membranous structure overlying the hair cells of the cochlea

tectospinal tract Tract arising in superior colliculus of midbrain that terminates in the cervical spinal cord, mediating visual orientation by head turning

tectum Portion of posterior midbrain behind the cerebral aqueduct

tegmentum of pons Posterior portion of pons

tegmen tympani of temporal bone Thin plate of bone above tympanic antrum

teleceptors /'tɛlɛsɛptɚz/ Sensory receptors responsive to stimuli originating outside the body

telencephalon /tɛlɛn'sɛfəlan/ Embryonic structure from which cerebral hemispheres and rhinencephalon develop

telo- Far from, toward the extreme

telodendria /tɛloden'driə/ The terminal arborization of an axon

temporal fossa of temporal bone Indentation of external temporal bone to which temporalis muscle attaches

temporalis muscle Muscle deep to masseter arising from temporal fossa and inserting into the coronoid process of mandible

temporal-occipital-parietal (TOP) association cortex The cortical association area that includes portions of the temporal, parietal, and occipital lobes (Brodmann areas 39 and 40; and portions of 19, 21, 22, and 37), and that is involved in integration of auditory, visual, and somatosensory information into language function

temporal operculum Portion of temporal lobe overlying insula

temporal process of zygomatic bone Process of zygomatic bone that articulates with the temporal bone

temporal summation Phenomenon in which small number of regions depolarize virtually simultaneously

temporofacial division of VII facial nerve Branch of VII facial giving rise to temporal and zygomatic branches

tendinous intersections Tendinous slips forming the separation between individual muscles of the rectus abdominis muscle group.

tendon /'tɛndən/ Connective tissue attaching muscle to bone or cartilage

tensile strength The quality of a material that provides resistance to destructive pulling forces

tensor tympani /'tɛnsɚ 'tɪmpənɪ/ Middle ear muscle acting on the malleus

tensor veli palatine a.k.a. tensor veli palatini tensor veli paltati tensor veli palatini; or dilator of auditory tube coursing from scaffoid fossa and medial and lateral pterygoid plates of sphenoid bone to lateral auditory tube

tensor veli palatini a.k.a. tensor veli palati or tensor veli palatine; dilator of auditory tube coursing from scaffoid fossa and medial and lateral pterygoid plates of sphenoid bone to lateral auditory tube

Tensor veli palati a.k.a. tensor veli palatini tensor veli palatine; dilator of auditory tube coursing from scaffoid fossa and medial and lateral pterygoid plates of sphenoid bone to lateral auditory tube

tentorium cerebelli Dura mater structure separating the cerebral cortex from the cerebellum

teratogen /tɛ'rætodʒən/ An agent that causes abnormal embryonic development

terminal device a.k.a. end effector; in motor function, the articulator responsible for completion of the motor act

terminal end bouton Terminal portion of axon, notably housing synaptic vesicles

terminal endplate Terminal component of an axon that is exciting a muscle fiber

terminal respiratory bronchioles The last bronchioles in the respiratory tree, connecting the respiratory tree to the alveoli

terminal sulcus Sulcus on posterior tongue separating the oral surface of the tongue from the palatine surface

termination of phonation Completion of the period during which vocal folds are vibrating for a given segment

tetra- Four

thalamus Major sensory relay; dominant component of diencephalon

thermoreceptors Sensors responsive to temperature

thick myofilaments Myosin component making up myofibril, made of the protein myosin, and which forms the scaffold for muscle fiber contraction

thin myofilaments Component making up myofibril, made up of the protein actin, forming the binding site for thick myofilaments

third ventricle Cerebral ventricle residing between the paired thalami

thoracic vertebra Vertebra of the thoracic spinal column

thoracolumbar system a.k.a. sympathetic nervous system; the portion of the autonomic nervous system that responds to stimulation through energy expenditure

thorax The part of the body between the diaphragm and the seventh cervical vertebra

thrombosis Obstruction caused by thrombus

thrombus Foreign body, such as a blood clot or bubble of air, that obstructs a blood vessel

thyroarytenoid muscle Muscle coursing from the thyroid cartilage, just below the thyroid notch, to the vocal process of the arytenoid cartilage; muscle that is further divided into thyrovocalis and thyromuscularis muscles by speech and hearing scientists

thyroepiglottic ligament Ligament coursing from the inner surface of the thyroid cartilage to the epiglottis

thyroepiglottic muscle Auxiliary intrinsic musculature of larynx, coursing from posterior attachment of the thyrovocalis muscles to the lateral epiglottic cartilage

thyrohyoid membrane The membranous laryngeal spanning the space between the greater cornu of the hyoid bone and the lateral thyroid

thyrohyoid muscle Muscle arising from the thyroid cartilage and inserting into the hyoid bone; elevates the thyroid cartilage or depresses the hyoid bone

thyroid angle Point of articulation of the paired thyroid laminae

thyroid cartilage The major cartilage of the larynx

thyroid notch Superior-most point of thyroid angle

thyromuscularis muscle Lateral-most muscle of the thyroarytenoid muscle; responsible for relaxation of the vocal folds

thyropharyngeus Muscle component of cricopharyngeal muscle arising from oblique line of thyroid lamina and coursing to median pharyngeal raphe of the posterior pharyngeal wall

thyrovocalis muscle Medial-most muscle of the thyroarytenoid muscle; responsible for tension of the vocal folds

tidal volume The volume inspired and expired during normal, quiet respiration

tip of tongue a.k.a. apex; anterior-most portion of tongue

tissue recoil The property of tissue that causes it to return to its original form after distention and release

-tomy Cutting

tongue Primary articulatory structure of speech, made up primarily of genioglossus muscle but also including numerous other extrinsic and intrinsic muscles

tongue thrust Anterior protrusion of tongue during swallow

tongue tie a.k.a. ankyloglossia; condition in which lingual frenulum is short, restraining movement of tongue

tonic Pertaining to muscular contraction

tonicity Partial contraction of musculature to maintain muscle tone

tonic lengthening of muscle spindle Condition in which muscle spindle length is held constant after change

tonotopic arrangement /tonə'tapɪk/ The arrangement of auditory nerve fibers such that fibers innervating the apex process low-frequency information, while fibers in the basal region process high-frequency information

tonotopicity Characteristic of cochlea wherein sensitivity to the frequency spectrum is arrayed with higher frequencies near base of cochlea and lower frequencies near apex

torque Rotary twisting

torsiversion /torsə'vɚʒən/ Rotating a tooth about its long axis

torso The trunk of the body

torus tubarius Ridge of tissue encircling the orifice of the auditory tube

total lung capacity Sum of tidal volume, inspiratory reserve volume, expiratory reserve volume, and residual volume

tracheostoma Opening placed surgically in the trachea

tracheostomy Process of surgically placing an opening in trachea

tracts A bundle of nerve fibers in the central nervous system

tragus /'treɪgəs/ Flap-like landmark of auricle approximating the concha

trajectories Predicted or actual movement paths for an articulator

trans- Beyond or on the other side

transduce To change from one form of energy to another

transducer Mechanism for converting energy from one form to another

transport stage Stage of deglutition in which bolus is moved from oral to pharyngeal space

transverse At right angles to the long axis

transverse dimension of thorax expansion The anteroposterior and lateral dimensional expansion of the thorax generated by contraction of the accessory muscles of inspiration

transverse interarytenoid muscle a.k.a. transverse arytenoid muscle; muscle coursing from lateral posterior aspect of one arytenoid to the lateral posterior aspect of the other arytenoid; serving as adductor of the vocal folds

transverse muscle of tongue Muscles originating at median fibrous septum of tongue and coursing laterally to insert into the side of the tongue

transverse process Lateral process of vertebra

trapezoid body of pons Pons level relay within the auditory pathway

traveling wave The wave-like action of the basilar membrane arising from stimulation of the perilymph of the vestibule

tremor Minute, involuntary repetitive movements

tri- Three

triangular fossa /ˈtraɪæŋgjulɚ fasə/ Region between the crura anthelicis

triangularis a.k.a. depressor anguli oris muscle; muscle originating along lateral margins of mandible on the oblique line and inserting into corner of upper lip and orbicularis oris superior

trifurcate /ˈtraɪfɚˌkeɪt/ To divide into three parts

tritiate cartilage a.k.a. triticeal cartilage; variably present cartilage between the superior horn of the thyroid cartilage and the greater horn of the hyoid bone

triticeal cartilage a.k.a. tritiate cartilage; variably present cartilage between the superior horn of the thyroid cartilage and the greater horn of the hyoid bone

trochlear process a.k.a. cochleariform process; bony outcropping around which courses the tendon of tensor tympani

trochleariform process /trakliˈarəform ˈprasɛs/ Bony outcropping of middle ear from which the tendon for the tensor tympani arises

trunk of corpus callosum a.k.a. body; the major, central portion of the corpus callosum

-trophic Related to nourishment

-trophy Growth, usually by expanding

-tropy Implies seeking or heading for something

true rib a.k.a. vertebrosternal ribs; consisting of those ribs making direct attachment with the sternum (ribs 1 through 7)

trunk The body excluding head and limbs

tubercle /ˈtubɚkl/ A small rounded prominence on bone

tunnel of Corti Region of the organ of Corti produced by articulation of the rods of Corti

turbulence Disturbance within fluid or gas caused by irregularity in its passage

tympanic antrum of temporal bone Portion of petrous portion of temporal bone that communicates with the mastoid portion

tympanic membrane The membranous separation between the outer and middle ear, responsible for initiating the mechanical impedance-matching process of the middle ear

tympanic portion of temporal bone Portion of temporal bone including the anterior and inferior walls of the external auditory meatus

tympanic sulcus Groove in external auditory meatus portion of temporal bone into which fits the fibrocartilaginous of the tympanic membrane

type Ia sensory fibers Primary afferent fibers from the muscle spindle

type Ib sensory fibers Primary afferent fibers from Golgi tendon organs

type III sensory fibers Sensory fibers conducting pain, pressure touch, and coolness sensation

umbo /ˈʌmbo/ The most distal point of attachment of the inner tympanic membrane to the malleus

uncrossed olivocochlear bundle (UCOB) Efferent fibers arising from superior olive of brain stem that remain ipsilateral, serving efferent function of cochlea through action on the inner hair cells

uncus Gyrus of the inferior cortex, within which the amygdala resides

uni- One

unilateral One side affected

unilateral upper motor neuron (UUMN) dysarthria Dysarthria with signs of spastic dysarthria presented unilaterally and typically with less severity than bilateral spastic dysarthria

unipolar neuron a.k.a. monopolar neuron; neuron with a single, bifurcating process arising from the soma

upper extremity The arm, the forearm, wrist, and hand

upper motor neurons Any motor neuron in a neuron chain that does not terminate on a muscle

urinary system The system of the body involved in elimination of waste through urination

utricle /ˈjutrɪkl/ Regions of vestibule housing the otolithic organs of the vestibular system

uvula Midline structure of velum or soft palate, consisting of the musculus uvulae

vagal trigone of medulla Bulge in posterior medulla caused by nucleus of X vagus

vagus nerve X cranial nerve

from stimulation of a large number of hair cells simultaneously, eliciting nearly simultaneous individual action potentials in the VIII nerve

wisdom tooth Third molar, in adult arch

Wormian bones of parietal bones Irregular bones created by bifurcations of the lambdoidal suture

xerostomia a.k.a. dry mouth; reduced sensation of salivary output

yellow cartilage Cartilaginous connective tissue that has reduced collagen and increased numbers of elastic fibers. See **elastic cartilage**

yellow elastic tissue Tissue that is found in locations where connective tissue must return to its original shape after being distended

Z line Margin of sarcomere

zygomatic arch Arch consisting of the temporal process of zygomatic bone and zygomatic process of temporal bone, and to which masseter attaches and through which temporalis passes

zygomatic major muscle Muscle arising lateral to zygomatic minor on zygomatic bone that courses obliquely down to insert into the corner of the orbibularis oris

zygomatic minor muscle Muscle coursing down from facial surface of zygomatic bone, inserting into upper lip

zygomatic process of frontal bone Process of frontal bone that articulates with the zygomatic bone

zygomatic process of maxilla The maxillary process abutting the zygomatic bone